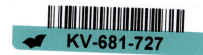

1994
YEAR BOOK OF
SPORTS MEDICINE®

Statement of Purpose

The YEAR BOOK Service

The YEAR BOOK series was devised in 1901 by practicing health professionals who observed that the literature of medicine and related disciplines had become so voluminous that no one individual could read and place in perspective every potential advance in a major specialty. In the final decade of the 20th century, this recognition is more acutely true than it was in 1901.

More than merely a series of books, YEAR BOOK volumes are the tangible results of a unique service designed to accomplish the following:

• to *survey* a wide range of journals of proven value

• to *select* from those journals papers representing significant advances and statements of important clinical principles

• to provide *abstracts* of those articles that are readable, convenient summaries of their key points

• to provide *commentary* about those articles to place them in perspective

These publications grow out of a unique process that calls on the talents of outstanding authorities in clinical and fundamental disciplines, trained literature specialists, and professional writers, all supported by the resources of Mosby, the world's preeminent publisher for the health professions.

The Literature Base

Mosby subscribes to nearly 1,000 journals published worldwide, covering the full range of the health professions. On an annual basis, the publisher examines usage patterns and polls its expert authorities to add new journals to the literature base and to delete journals that are no longer useful as potential YEAR BOOK sources.

The Literature Survey

The publisher's team of literature specialists, all of whom are trained and experienced health professionals, examines every original, peer-reviewed article in each journal issue. More than 250,000 articles per year are scanned systematically, including title, text, illustrations, tables, and references. Each scan is compared, article by article, to the search strategies that the publisher has developed in consultation with the 270 outside experts who form the pool of YEAR BOOK editors. A given article may be reviewed by any number of editors, from one to a dozen or more, regardless of the discipline for which the paper was originally published. In turn, each editor who receives the article reviews it to determine whether or not the article should be included in the YEAR BOOK. This decision is based on the article's inherent quality, its probable usefulness to readers of that YEAR BOOK, and the editor's goal to represent a balanced picture of a given field in each volume of the YEAR BOOK. In addition, the editor indicates when to include figures and tables from the article to help the YEAR BOOK reader better understand the information.

Of the quarter million articles scanned each year, only 5% are selected for detailed analysis within the YEAR BOOK series, thereby assuring readers of the high value of every selection.

The Abstract

The publisher's abstracting staff is headed by a physician-writer and includes individuals with training in the life sciences, medicine, and other areas, plus extensive experience in writing for the health professions and related industries. Each selected article is assigned to a specific writer on this abstracting staff. The abstracter, guided in many cases by notations supplied by the expert editor, writes a structured, condensed summary designed so that the reader can rapidly acquire the essential information contained in the article.

The Commentary

The YEAR BOOK editorial boards, sometimes assisted by guest commentators, write comments that place each article in perspective for the reader. This provides the reader with the equivalent of a personal consultation with a leading international authority—an opportunity to better understand the value of the article and to benefit from the authority's thought processes in assessing the article.

Additional Editorial Features

The editorial boards of each YEAR BOOK organize the abstracts and comments to provide a logical and satisfying sequence of information. To enhance the organization, editors also provide introductions to sections or individual chapters, comments linking a number of abstracts, citations to additional literature, and other features.

The published YEAR BOOK contains enhanced bibliographic citations for each selected article, including extended listings of multiple authors and identification of author affiliations. Each YEAR BOOK contains a Table of Contents specific to that year's volume. From year to year, the Table of Contents for a given YEAR BOOK will vary depending on developments within the field.

Every YEAR BOOK contains a list of the journals from which papers have been selected. This list represents a subset of the nearly 1,000 journals surveyed by the publisher and occasionally reflects a particularly pertinent article from a journal that is not surveyed on a routine basis.

Finally, each volume contains a comprehensive subject index and an index to authors of each selected paper.

The 1994 Year Book Series

Year Book of Allergy and Clinical Immunology: Drs. Rosenwasser, Borish, Gelfand, Leung, Nelson, and Szefler

Year Book of Anesthesiology and Pain Management: Drs. Tinker, Abram, Kirby, Ostheimer, Roizen, and Stoelting

Year Book of Cardiology®: Drs. Schlant, Collins, Engle, Gersh, Kaplan, and Waldo

Year Book of Chiropractic: Dr. Lawrence

Year Book of Critical Care Medicine®: Drs. Rogers and Parrillo

Year Book of Dentistry®: Drs. Meskin, Currier, Kennedy, Leinfelder, Berry, and Roser

Year Book of Dermatologic Surgery: Drs. Swanson, Glogau, and Salasche

Year Book of Dermatology®: Drs. Sober and Fitzpatrick

Year Book of Diagnostic Radiology®: Drs. Federle, Clark, Gross, Madewell, Maynard, Sackett, and Young

Year Book of Digestive Diseases®: Drs. Greenberger and Moody

Year Book of Drug Therapy®: Drs. Lasagna and Weintraub

Year Book of Emergency Medicine®: Drs. Wagner, Burdick, Davidson, McNamara, and Roberts

Year Book of Endocrinology®: Drs. Bagdade, Braverman, Poehlman, Kannan, Landsberg, Molitch, Morley, Odell, Rogol, Ryan and Nathan

Year Book of Family Practice®: Drs. Berg, Bowman, Davidson, Dietrich, and Scherger

Year Book of Geriatrics and Gerontology®: Drs. Beck, Reuben, Burton, Small, Whitehouse, and Goldstein

Year Book of Hand Surgery®: Drs. Amadio and Hentz

Year Book of Hematology®: Drs. Spivak, Bell, Ness, Quesenberry, and Wiernik

Year Book of Infectious Diseases®: Drs. Keusch, Wolff, Barza, Bennish, Gelfand, Klempner, and Snydman

Year Book of Infertility and Reproductive Endocrinology: Drs. Mishell, Lobo, and Sokol

Year Book of Medicine®: Drs. Bone, Cline, Epstein, Greenberger, Malawista, Mandell, O'Rourke, and Utiger

Year Book of Neonatal and Perinatal Medicine®: Drs. Klaus and Fanaroff

Year Book of Nephrology®: Drs. Coe, Favus, Henderson, Kashgarian, Luke, Myers, and Curtis

Year Book of Neurology and Neurosurgery®: Drs. Bradley and Crowell

Year Book of Neuroradiology: Drs. Osborn, Eskridge, Grossman, and Harnsberger

Year Book of Nuclear Medicine®: Drs. Hoffer, Gore, Gottschalk, Rattner, Zaret, and Zubal

Year Book of Obstetrics and Gynecology®: Drs. Mishell, Kirschbaum, and Morrow

Year Book of Occupational and Environmental Medicine: Drs. Emmett, Frank, Gochfeld, and Hessl

Year Book of Oncology®: Drs. Simone, Longo, Ozols, Steele, Glatstein, and Bosl

Year Book of Ophthalmology®: Drs. Laibson, Adams, Augsburger, Benson, Cohen, Eagle, Flanagan, Nelson, Rapuano, Reinecke, Sergott, and Wilson

Year Book of Orthopedics®: Drs. Sledge, Poss, Cofield, Frymoyer, Griffin, Hansen, Johnson, Simmons, and Springfield

Year Book of Otolaryngology–Head and Neck Surgery®: Drs. Paparella and Holt

Year Book of Pain: Drs. Gebhart, Haddox, Jacox, Payne, Rudy, and Shapiro

Year Book of Pathology and Clinical Pathology®: Drs. Gardner, Bennett, Cousar, Garvin, and Worsham

Year Book of Pediatrics®: Dr. Stockman

Year Book of Plastic, Reconstructive, and Aesthetic Surgery: Drs. Miller, Cohen, McKinney, Robson, Ruberg, and Whitaker

Year Book of Podiatric Medicine and Surgery®: Dr. Kominsky

Year Book of Psychiatry and Applied Mental Health®: Drs. Talbott, Frances, Breier, Meltzer, Perry, Schowalter, and Yudofsky

Year Book of Pulmonary Disease®: Drs. Bone and Petty

Year Book of Rheumatology: Drs. Sergent, LeRoy, Meenan, Panush, and Reichlin

Year Book of Sports Medicine®: Drs. Shephard, Drinkwater, Eichner, Torg, Col. Anderson, and Mr. George

Year Book of Surgery®: Drs. Copeland, Deitch, Eberlein, Howard, Luce, Ritchie, Seeger, Souba, and Sugarbaker

Year Book of Thoracic and Cardiovascular Surgery: Drs. Ginsberg, Lofland, and Wechsler

Year Book of Transplantation: Drs. Sollinger, Eckhoff, Hullett, Knechtle, Longo, Mentzer, and Pirsch

Year Book of Ultrasound: Drs. Merritt, Babcock, Carroll, Goldstein, and Mittelstaedt

Year Book of Urology®: Drs. Gillenwater and Howards

Year Book of Vascular Surgery®: Dr. Porter

1994

The Year Book of
SPORTS MEDICINE®

Editor-in-Chief
Roy J. Shephard, M.D., Ph.D., D.P.E.
School of Physical and Health Education and Professor of Applied Physiology,
Department of Preventive Medicine and Biostatistics, University of Toronto

Editors
Col. James L. Anderson, PE.D.
Director of Physical Education, United States Military Academy, West Point
Barbara L. Drinkwater, Ph.D.
Research Physiologist, Department of Medicine, Pacific Medical Center, Seattle
Edward R. Eichner, M.D.
Professor of Medicine, University of Oklahoma Health Sciences Center,
Oklahoma City
Francis J. George, A.T.C., P.T.
Head Athletic Trainer, Brown University, Providence
Joseph S. Torg, M.D.
Professor of Orthopedic Surgery, and Director, Sports Medicine Center,
University of Pennsylvania, Philadelphia

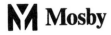 Mosby

St. Louis Baltimore Boston Chicago London Madrid Philadelphia Sydney Toronto

Vice President and Publisher, Continuity Publishing: Kenneth H. Killion
Director, Editorial Development: Gretchen C. Murphy
Acquisitions Editor: Linda Steiner
Illustrations and Permissions Coordinator: Maureen A. Livengood
Director of Editorial Services: Edith M. Podrazik, R.N.
Senior Information Specialist: Terri Santo, R.N.
Information Specialist: Nancy Dunne, R.N.
Senior Medical Writer: David A. Cramer, M.D.
Senior Project Manager: Max F. Perez
Project Supervisor: Tamara L. Smith
Senior Production Editor: Wendi Schnaufer
Production Coordinator: Sandra Rogers
Editing Coordinator: Rebecca Nordbrock
Proofroom Supervisor: Barbara M. Kelly
Vice President, Professional Sales and Marketing: George M. Parker
Marketing and Circulation Manager: Barry J. Bowlus
Marketing Coordinator: Lynn Stevenson

1994 EDITION
Copyright © December 1994 by Mosby–Year Book, Inc.

Printed in the United States of America
Composition by International Computaprint Corporation
Printing/binding by Maple-Vail

Mosby–Year Book, Inc.
11830 Westline Industrial Drive
St. Louis, MO 63146

Editorial Office:
Mosby–Year Book, Inc.
200 North LaSalle St.
Chicago, IL 60601
International Standard Serial Number: 0162-0908
International Standard Book Number: 0-8151-7704-6

Table of Contents

Mosby Document Express

Copies of the full text of the original source documents of articles abstracted or referenced in this publication are available by calling Mosby Document Express, toll-free, at **1 (800) 55-MOSBY.**

With Mosby Document Express, you have convenient, 24-hour-a-day access to literally every article on which this publication is based. In fact, through Mosby Document Express, virtually any medical or scientific article can be located and delivered by FAX, overnight delivery service, international airmail, electronic transmission of bitmapped images (via Internet), or regular mail. The average cost of a complete, delivered copy of an article, including up to $4 in copyright clearance charges and first-class mail delivery, is $12.

For inquiries and pricing information, please call the toll-free number shown above. To expedite your order for material appearing in this publication, please be prepared with the code shown next to the bibliographic citation for each abstract.

Journals Represented

Mosby subscribes to and surveys nearly 1,000 U.S. and foreign medical and allied health journals. From these journals, the Editors select the articles to be abstracted. Journals represented in this YEAR BOOK are listed below.

Acta Endocrinologica
Acta Paediatrica
Age and Ageing
American Family Physician
American Heart Journal
American Journal of Cardiology
American Journal of Epidemiology
American Journal of Knee Surgery
American Journal of Perinatology
American Journal of Public Health
American Journal of Roentgenology
American Journal of Sports Medicine
American Review of Respiratory Disease
Anesthesiology
Annals of Emergency Medicine
Annals of Internal Medicine
Archives of Andrology
Archives of Physical Medicine and Rehabilitation
Arthroscopy
Bone and Mineral
British Heart Journal
British Journal of Cancer
British Journal of Sports Medicine
British Medical Journal
Canadian Association of Radiologists Journal
Canadian Journal of Applied Physiology
Canadian Medical Association Journal
Cancer
Chest
Circulation
Clinical Biomechanics
Clinical Chemistry
Clinical Investigator
Clinical Orthopaedics and Related Research
Clinical Pediatrics
Digestive Diseases and Sciences
Ergonomics
European Heart Journal
European Journal of Applied Physiology and Occupational Physiology
European Journal of Clinical Pharmacology
Fertility and Sterility
Foot and Ankle
Gynecologic and Obstetric Investigation
ICA International Review of Chiropractic
Injury
International Journal of Epidemiology
International Journal of Obesity
International Journal of Sports Medicine
Isokinetics and Exercise Science
JOGNN: Journal of Obstetric, Gynecologic, and Neonatal Nursing

Journal of Applied Physiology: Respiratory, Environmental and Exercise
  Physiology
Journal of Arthroplasty
Journal of Athletic Training
Journal of Biomechanics
Journal of Bone and Joint Surgery (American Volume)
Journal of Bone and Joint Surgery (British Volume)
Journal of Cardiopulmonary Rehabilitation
Journal of Clinical Endocrinology and Metabolism
Journal of Clinical Epidemiology
Journal of Emergency Medicine
Journal of Family Practice
Journal of Gerontology
Journal of Hand Surgery (American)
Journal of Hand Surgery (British)
Journal of Heart and Lung Transplantation
Journal of Musculoskeletal Pain
Journal of Neurology, Neurosurgery and Psychiatry
Journal of Occupational Medicine
Journal of Orthopaedic Research
Journal of Orthopaedic and Sports Physical Therapy
Journal of Rheumatology
Journal of Shoulder and Elbow Surgery
Journal of Sports Medicine and Physical Fitness
Journal of Sports Sciences
Journal of Sports Traumatology and Related Research
Journal of Trauma
Journal of Urology
Journal of Vascular Surgery
Journal of the American Board of Family Practice
Journal of the American College of Cardiology
Journal of the American Medical Association
Journal of the American Podiatric Medical Association
Medecine du Sport
Medicine and Science in Sports and Exercise
Metabolism
Nephron
New England Journal of Medicine
New York State Journal of Medicine
Orthopaedic Review
Orthopedics
Pediatric Nursing
Physical Therapy
Physician and Sportsmedicine
Radiology
Regional Anesthesia
Scandinavian Journal of Work, Environment and Health
Spine
Sports Medicine
Western Journal of Medicine

STANDARD ABBREVIATIONS

The following terms are abbreviated in this edition: acquired immunodeficiency syndrome (AIDS), central nervous system (CNS), cerebrospinal fluid (CSF), computed tomography (CT), electrocardiography (ECG), human immunodeficiency virus (HIV), and magnetic resonance (MR) imaging (MRI).

Erratum

To our readers,

In the 1993 YEAR BOOK OF SPORTS MEDICINE, editor John Sutton, M.D., based a comment on incorrect data regarding the length of the study he was reviewing. Both the publisher and Dr. Sutton apologize for this error.

The reader is referred to Abstract 7–1, "Growth Hormone, IGF-I, and Testosterone Responses to Resistive Exercise," by R.R. Kraemer, J.L. Kilgore, G.R. Kraemer, and V.D. Castracane, on pages 399–401 of the 1993 YEAR BOOK OF SPORTS MEDICINE. Dr. Sutton has revised his comment to read as follows:

▶ Most studies of the endocrine response during exercise have concerned the effects of endurance exercise, and it is only recently that attention has turned to resistance exercise. In this study, the observations of changes in growth hormone (GH) are particularly interesting, and the authors have also quantified insulin-like growth factor I (IGF-I), which is synthesized in the liver, responds to GH, and is the mediator through which GH exerts many of its effects. As can be seen from Figures 1 and 2, there was a significant increase in GH during exercise and the immediate postexercise period; however, there was no change in IGF-I. As shown in the figures, measurements that extended +95 minutes, 5 hours 35 minutes, 22.20 hours, and 23.30 hours postexercise noted no changes in GH or IGF-I.

The importance of this study is the length of time during which the authors measured IGF-I after exercise. It is a pity that samples in periods of 6, 8, 10, 12, 14, 16, 18, and 20 hours were omitted, as this would have made the study more complete and left no doubt about IGF-I responsiveness. Nevertheless, 2 previous studies of IGF-I after resistance exercise followed IGF-I for a far shorter time (1, 2). Timing is of fundamental importance because there is normally a delay of several hours between infusions of GH and increases in IGF-I plasma. In fact, previously only 1 study—using a bioassay for IGF-I (somatomedin)—has followed the changes in blood for sufficient time to document any changes (3, 4). That study used dynamic exercise, and although increases in GH were noted, there was no increase in somatomedin.

Testosterone is another important anabolic hormone, but there were no significant changes in testosterone in this study. In considering the likely effects of endogenous anabolic agents for the increase in muscle bulk associated with resistance exercise, mean hormonal concentrations may be far more significant than any short-term perturbations that arise after an individual training session.—J.R. Sutton, M.D.

References

1. Kraemer WJ, et al: *Int J Sports Med* 12:228, 1991.
2. Kraemer WJ, et al: *J Appl Physiol* 69:1442, 1990.
3. Stuart M, et al: *Proc Endocrinol Soc Aust* 15:21, 1971.
4. Sutton JR, et al: Hormonal adaptation to physical activity, in Bouchard C, et al (eds): *Exercise, Fitness and Health.* Champaign, Illinois, Human Kinetics, 1989, pp 217–259.

Introduction

This year's edition of the YEAR BOOK OF SPORTS MEDICINE contains a fascinating selection of research that has been screened and evaluated by the editorial team. The epidemiology of injuries and the application of the resulting information to preventive measures continue to grow in importance, although some studies of the prevalence and incidence of injuries still need to be more specific about the severity of the lesions that have been incurred. An enormous toll of injuries still could be prevented by simple measures such as insisting that children wear helmets when bicycling. New studies included this year involve the incidence of problems in such growing sports as bungee-cord jumping, mountain biking, and roller blading. Brain damage in boxers continues to be the subject of controversy. Interest is also growing concerning the risk of late arthritic change in athletes, with soccer players apparently showing particular vulnerability in this regard.

The evaluation of surgical treatment is becoming increasingly sophisticated, and some authors now apply multivariate analyses to their data. Several papers on shoulder dislocation highlight the problem of achieving a satisfactory repair; many studies report high recurrence rates. One of the most frequent citations in the area of injury rehabilitation this year is the technique of closed-chain exercise, in which afferent neural structures are allowed to contribute to motor learning and re-education of the injured part. If the goal is to increase strength, such procedures must be used in conjunction with resistance exercise.

Physicians who are involved in the assessment of muscle strength continue to debate the relationship between cross-sectional area and the developed torque. New techniques such as MRI are making significant contributions to this debate. There is also growing awareness of the instrumental problems that may arise, e.g., from a lack of alignment of measuring equipment with the joint axis, from a change of damping coefficients, or from an alteration of temperature conditions when recording a surface electromyogram. Mathematical models are now being applied not only to the prediction of muscle forces, but also to demonstrate the impact of fatigue on such forces.

Those involved in cardiac rehabilitation have given much thought to patient compliance with exercise programs, and it is interesting to see that similar concern is now developing in terms of patient compliance with strength training programs. Shoes designed to develop strength have been examined and have been found wanting in terms of their impact on ankle strength and flexibility. A number of commonly used methods of strengthening the abdominal muscles have been declared dangerous. Water damage to casts continues to plague the orthopedic surgeon, and an interesting solution to this difficulty is suggested in the form of a Gore-Tex waterproof cast liner.

In the area of cardiorespiratory fitness, increasing interest is being seen regarding the replacement of formal exercise programs by lifestyle exercise programs. These programs incorporate vigorous physical activity into everyday living. Tactics are also being discussed for influencing hard-to-reach populations, such as ethnic minorities. Evidence continues to accumulate on the economic benefits of an active lifestyle; this volume contains a report from a Japanese company substantiating this view. There have been suggestions that too much training can cause problems of postural hypotension; however, a paper discussed in this edition shows that problems are seen only at very high intensities of training.

Gender verification continues to be a source of controversy for female competitors and their coaches, with the International Olympics Committee continuing to require such tests despite growing evidence that they lack validity. A paper by Hipkin questions whether conditions causing virilism should be grounds for disqualification from women's competitions. The role of fatness in determining the age of menarche continues to be a subject of debate. Cortisol may also be implicated in this process as well as contributing to the associated osteoporosis.

Women continue to sustain more injuries than men in army training, although it remains likely that the problem is a lack of fitness rather than sex per se. Colonel Anderson laments that still too few studies report data on female subjects. Many women now exercise during pregnancy, and it is disturbing that only 16% of one sample of patients had learned of American College of Obstetricians and Gynecologists guidelines for exercise from their physicians. An increasing number of papers describe practical regimens for the testing of elderly patients, along with programs for improving muscular and cardiorespiratory function, augmenting flexibility, correcting osteoporosis, and increasing the quality of daily living. Whether it is possible to build up a bank of bone by exercising as a young adult continues to be debated. However, claims that the aging of aerobic power and cardiac function can be halted by very vigorous exercise are coming under increasing scrutiny.

Divers are cautioned against the risks of air embolism, which can develop in quite shallow water. There are also reports of prolonged disturbances of lung function with deeper dives, which are possibly a manifestation of oxygen toxicity. Hyponatremia, provoked by excessive rehydration, continues to be a problem in ultramarathon runners, whereas ice hockey players can be exposed to significant concentrations of nitrogen dioxide, sometimes above recommended limits, from the exhaust fumes of ice-smoothing machinery.

On the metabolic front, debate continues as to whether the optimal body weight increases with age. A paper on gastroesophageal reflux points to an occasional diagnostic problem in older, coronary-prone exercisers. Loperamide is suggested as a useful treatment of the "runner's trots," and further papers show the value of regular exercise in individuals with diabetes. If one can believe questionnaire responses, steroid use has reached epidemic proportions in North America. Higher level athletes are adopting more sophisticated approaches (e.g., the abuse of human growth hormone) to avoid detection, and the battle continues in an attempt to find means of detecting and discouraging such abuse.

The favorable influence of exercise in hypertension is now well established, but an intriguing article suggests that low-intensity exercise is most beneficial in the morning, whereas more vigorous exercise is helpful later in the day. Among the articles on coronary patients, there is an interesting contribution on making education materials readable for those with limited education. Many articles attempt to increase the precision of diagnosis and prognosis, with specific emphasis on the impact of recent meals and personality on test outcome. Factors triggering sudden death during exercise, including a high risk between 9 A.M. and noon, are particularly fascinating. Two papers speak to issues in the rehabilitation of patients who have undergone heart and lung transplants, and one large-scale study from Britain makes a convincing argument for the value of regular exercise in stroke prevention.

Failure to observe elementary rules of hygiene continues to cause the spread of enteric disease among team members. However, evidence also continues to accumulate on the value of exercise in the prevention and treatment of a variety of medical conditions, including multiple sclerosis, certain forms of cancer, HIV infection, and fibromyalgia.

Roy J. Shephard, M.D., Ph.D.

Exercise Programs in Chronic Chest Disease

ROY J. SHEPHARD, M.D., PH.D., D.P.E.

School of Physical and Health Education, Department of Preventive Medicine and Biostatistics, Faculty of Medicine, University of Toronto

Introduction

Chronic obstructive lung disease (COLD) is now the fifth most common cause of death in North America, and it is also responsible for a great deal of disability. Unlike other forms of chronic disease, its prevalence is rising as the average age of the population increases (1). Nevertheless, exercise programs for the patient with chronic chest disease are much less widespread and less well developed than programs for those who have sustained a myocardial infarct. In this editorial, we will examine the contribution of chronic chest disease to the total burden of illness in elderly patients, and we will consider the impact of such disease on both specific respiratory parameters and overall functional ability. We will look at implications for the definition of "normal health" in the elderly patient, will consider the need to distinguish different types of chest disease, and will assess the contribution of cigarette smoke and other air contaminants to the overall burden of morbidity. Finally, specific recommendations will be offered for an exercise-centered rehabilitation program adapted to the needs of patients with COLD.

Aging: Normal or Pathologic?

The distinction between normal and pathologic aging is difficult in older patients. Indeed, some geriatricians have defined aging as an "increased probability of death" (2). If deaths per 1,000 members of the population are plotted against age, there is an exponential increase that begins in early middle age. Such deaths reflect not only a reduced resistance to death from a fixed incidence of illness, but also an increase in the prevalence of morbidity, caused by a combination of reduced resistance to acute infections, a slowing of recovery from such infections, and the accumulation of chronic disorders such as COLD. Thus, aging could almost equally well be characterized as "an increased probability of morbidity."

Cardiovascular disease is the most common cause of death in the latter half of life. However, as the age of the patient increases, cancers (including cancer of the lung) also become increasingly important, as do other disorders of the respiratory system. Timiras (3) looked at the primary causes of death in a general hospital and in a specialized geriatric unit. In the former, 12% to 13% of deaths were attributed to respiratory disease, and 24% to 29% to cancer. In the latter type of institution, all patients were older than 80 years of age, and problems of the respiratory system accounted for 24% to 25% of deaths, whereas cancer was identified as the primary cause of death in only 7% to 10% of patients.

The increase of respiratory problems with aging would hardly be surprising, given no more than the cumulative impact of repeated bouts of acute respiratory infection, cigarette smoking, and exposure to contaminants of the urban and the occupational environment. However, such noxious influences are further compounded by an age-related deterioration of immune function, with a resulting reduction in resistance to both bacterial and viral infections.

Functional Impact of Chronic Disease

Brown and Shephard (4) noted that about one half of female department store employees aged 40–70 years were affected by some type of chronic disorder. In about one quarter of those evaluated, the problem was considered to have had an adverse effect on cardiorespiratory function and the performance of endurance exercise. Reported diagnoses included chronic bronchitis and healed tuberculosis, along with hypertension, rheumatic carditis, anemia, thyroidectomy, and retropulsion of a cervical intervertebral disk.

In the group aged 40–49 years, the women with chronic disease had a maximal oxygen intake 90.1% of that found in their healthy peers, and in the group aged 50–59 years, the average for the subjects with disease had dropped to 86.5% of that for healthy workers. It remains unclear whether the decrement of oxygen transport was entirely caused by an inherent, disease-related limitation of cardiorespiratory function; more probably, those affected by disease had also become less active, thus allowing their physical condition to deteriorate relative to healthy fellow-workers. The younger members of the diseased group may have noticed little impact on their ability to undertake the ordinary activities of daily living, but a 13% to 14% loss of function would impose an increasing functional limitation as their age advanced.

All of the group studied by Brown and Shephard (4) were able to cope with full-time jobs in a department store, and the prevalence of both chronic disease and disability would probably have been higher if the entire population of those aged 40–70 years had been canvased. The Canadian Health Promotion Survey (5) found that only 23.5% of men and 16.8% of women older than 65 years of age rated their health as "excellent." Moreover, 30.5% of men and 37.1% of women over 65 years of age noted a disease-related limitation of their current physical activity.

The frequency of activity limitation varies from one country to another, depending on the success of national policies for prevention, treatment, and rehabilitation of those with chronic disease. However, a reduction in the quality of life as a result of physical disabilities is not unique to Canada. The United States National Health Interview Survey of 1983 (6) also found that ill-health restricted physical activity in 40% of those older than 65 years of age.

SPECIFIC EFFECTS ON RESPIRATORY FUNCTION

A history of COLD apparently has a major impact on the rate of aging of lung function. Anderson et al. (7) used multiple regression equations to develop norms relating vital capacity to height and age. The respective prediction formulas for vital capacity in healthy men and for those with a history of respiratory disease were as follows:

vital capacity—normal $= -4.21 + 5.63$ (H,m) $- 0.0174$ (A,yr)
vital capacity—disease $= -3.47 + 5.63$ (H,m) $- 0.0483$ (A,yr)

The implication is that by the age of 65 years, the vital capacity for a man of 1.7-m stature would be 4.23 L at body temperature and ambient pressure, and saturated with water vapor (BTPS) if he were healthy, but only 2.96 L if he had a history of chest disease (a 30% greater decrement of pulmonary function in the individual with chest disease). In effect, COLD has increased the rate of aging of vital capacity by a factor of 3, from 17.4 to 48.3 mL/year. Parallel formulas for females show that with a stature of 1.55 m, the vital capacity would be 2.65 L for a healthy 65-year-old, but only 1.85 L for a woman of the same age who had a history of chest disease. Again, chronic chest disease has caused a 30% greater decrement of pulmonary function during the span of normal working life.

How far does the reduction of pulmonary function restrict functional capacity? In a young adult, unpleasant breathlessness does not normally develop until the tidal volume amounts to some 50% of the vital capacity; tidal volumes of this order are seen during voluntary hyperventilation, but they are unlikely during normal daily exercise. However, as age advances, the margin between the ventilatory demands of exercise and the threshold of dyspnea narrows. Thus, breathlessness becomes the main factor limiting daily physical activity in many senior citizens. Even assuming that pathologic changes in the lungs do not augment a patient's sensitivity to dyspnea, the loss of vital capacity in COLD is likely to halt exercise at a 30% lower work rate than in a healthy patient of the same age.

The individuals examined by Anderson and associates (7) were of average physical fitness and included a proportion of cigarette smokers. Probably because of the correlation between COLD and smoking, their data showed little independent functional impact of cigarette smoking once allowances had been made for the adverse effect of COLD. The much slower loss of lung function seen in their disease-free group seems typical of normal aging. Comparable figures have been observed in other healthy populations, including fit nonsmokers (8, 9) and those following an active lifestyle in areas with little exposure to either urban or occupational pollutants (10).

IMPLICATIONS FOR REFERENCE STANDARDS

Normative scores for the aging of respiratory function differ markedly, depending on the care that has been taken to exclude diseased patients from the sample tested. If everyone with COLD is eliminated, there is the further dilemma that the supposed normative sample is then very atypical of the elderly population living in large urban areas. This raises a difficult philosophical question: Should functional norms be based on a rarely attained potential of health (with the risk that current efforts at disease prevention will be discredited), or should the standard be set at a more readily attainable value that is compatible with current public health resources?

Many investigators have erred in the direction of setting unattainable health standards. Typically, study recruits have been health-conscious, lifelong nonsmokers. Moreover, they have come from upper socioeconomic groups, thus avoiding a lifetime of exposure to domestic and occupational air pollution and escaping many other sources of chronic ill-health that are encountered by the average and the socially-disadvantaged citizen. Currently, life-expectancy measurements (and by implication chronic disease, including COLD) show a substantial socioeconomic gradient in most developed countries (11, 12). Deciding what is normal in an elderly individual thus becomes very arbitrary. One operational dividing line between normal and pathologic aging is the ability to maintain full-time employment (4), although this criterion can no longer be used once the age of mandatory retirement has been passed. Another option is to base norms on those rating their health as good, very good, or excellent; this approach still excludes 23.6% of men and 28.8% of women older than age 65 years (5). A third possibility is to exclude those who have reported functional limitations about the home. Finally, separate analyses could be made for the healthy elite and the total population (13).

Overall Effects of Chronic Chest Disease

The aging respiratory system becomes progressively more vulnerable to bacterial and viral infections because of a decrease in the speed of tracheal mucociliary transport (14) and an impaired immunologic response to microorganisms such as pneumococcus (15). Factors that translate an acute infection into the complex syndrome of COLD are poorly understood, but they may reflect, in part, an age-related deterioration in immune function.

The functional consequences of COLD include an exaggeration of the normal age-related decrease of vital capacity (caused by a combination of fibrotic disease of the lung tissues, ankylosis of sternocostal joints, progressive shortening and distortion of the thoracic vertebral column, and expiratory closure of the airways); an excessive slowing of peak expiratory flow rates (caused by an inflammatory narrowing of the air passages, bronchial hyper-reactivity, and expiratory collapse of the airways); chronic bronchitis (hypertrophy and chronic inflammation of the bronchial lining, with hyperactivity of the mucus-producing glands and an accumulation of phlegm); and emphysema (with a breakdown of the fine interalveolar septae, hyperinflation of the chest, a loss of alveolar surface area, destruction of pulmonary capillaries, and an increase of pulmonary vascular resistance). Attempts are often made to distinguish these problems pathologically, but in many patients they co-exist (16).

The end results of the disease process are a poor dynamic ventilatory capacity, a poor distribution of inspired gas, an impaired alveolar gas exchange, an excessive respiratory work rate, early fatigue of the chest muscles, and an unpleasant exercise-induced dyspnea that leads to a vicious cycle of habitual inactivity, a weakening of both the thoracic and other skeletal muscles, and progressively increasing breathlessness whenever exercise is attempted. The syndrome of COLD is thus an important and commonly overlooked reason for a pathologic response to exercise in the older patient (17, 18).

Specific Disease Conditions

CHRONIC BRONCHITIS

A diagnosis of chronic bronchitis reflects a case of COLD in which infection, inflammation, and mucus production are dominant features. The typical patient has a chronic or recurrent productive cough on most days for a minimum of 3 months per year, with frequent superimposed episodes of infection and chronic fibrotic reactions in the lung parenchyma. Cigarette smoking, repeated exposure to air pollution or industrial dusts, and a cold, damp climate all seem to be precipitating factors. The problem is exacerbated if the individual has inherited an abnormal alpha-antitrypsin phenotype. Antitrypsins normally counter the destruction of lung tissue when proteolytic enzymes are released from inflammatory cells. Vulnerability to proteolytic enzymes is greatest in individuals with the Pi Z antitrypsin variant (19). However, homozygotes are sufficiently rare that they cannot account for all cases of COLD; the impact of heterozygosity and of other genetic variants also merits attention.

There is substantial evidence for a household transmission of poor pulmonary function scores (20), but it is unclear whether this reflects undetected genetic influences or is merely a result of environmental factors such as exposure to cigarette smoke from an early age.

The cross-sectional analysis done by Anderson et al. (7) suggested a substantial effect of COLD on the aging of respiratory function. In contrast, Fletcher et al. (21) found no relationship between such indices of chronic bronchitis as chest colds in the previous 6 months, sputum purulence, hemophilus influenza antibodies, or mucus hypersecretion and the rate of loss of lung function during the course of a short-term prospective study.

EMPHYSEMA

In emphysema, the dominant processes are an abnormal enlargement of the terminal air-spaces, destruction of the small pulmonary blood vessels, and a resultant impairment of alveolar gas exchange. There is also an exaggeration of the normal, age-related deterioration in the elastic properties of the lung parenchyma, so that the chest becomes hyperinflated and the bronchi become unusually vulnerable to collapse during a vigorous expiration. Other manifestations of the disorder include extensive intrapulmonary trapping of gas and the rupture of alveoli, the latter perhaps arising from repeated bouts of coughing.

Because aging induces changes in the structure of elastic tissue, the condition may be in part an expression of normal senescence. By the age of 60 years, about one half of the population shows some evidence of emphysema at postmortem examination. However, the proportion of individuals who have respiratory symptoms is much smaller. Risk factors include chronic bronchitis and its various determinants.

CHRONIC OBSTRUCTIVE LUNG DISEASE

Because there is difficulty in distinguishing the two conditions from each other, chronic bronchitis and emphysema are commonly described jointly as COLD. The onset of the disorder is insidious, in marked contrast to the critical event of a myocardial infarction.

At first, the patient is conscious of no more than a little breathlessness while hurrying, and he or she may be inclined to dismiss this as no more than a normal expression of aging. In the early stages, compensation for the poor distribution of gas and the restriction of alveolar exchange is possible at the expense of an increase of ventilation (particularly tidal volume) (22) and some breathlessness (the group known as "fighters" or "pink puffers") (23). Nevertheless, much of the available maximal oxygen intake becomes consumed by the vigorous efforts of the respiratory muscles. As the condition advances, vigorous expiration ever more readily induces collapse of the airways, and the potential for compensatory hyperventilation is progressively lost. In such individuals, any attempt at physical activity leads to a dramatic decrease in arterial oxygen tension (the group known as "nonfighters" or "blue bloaters"). Light exercise then provokes a distressing dyspnea (24), pulmonary pressures increase, and the resultant ischemia can lead to myocardial failure or cardiac arrest.

The principles of exercise testing in COLD are much as in other medical conditions. Arterial blood gases, the alveolar-arterial oxygen partial pressure gradient, and the dead space/tidal volume ratio during a progressive cycle ergometer evaluation give a good indication of the efficiency of gas exchange. Heart rates tend to be high during submaximal exercise, but the stroke volume is less than anticipated. The poor cardiac performance reflects reduced preloading of the heart (because of prolonged inactivity, with a reduction of blood volume); a poor myocardial contractility (as a result of myocardial ischemia); and increased afterloading (secondary to weakened skeletal muscles). The rating of perceived exertion is increased at any given heart rate because of severe breathlessness and patient beliefs about the severity of the disorder (25). The peak heart rate is lower than in a healthy individual of comparable age, in part because of myocardial ischemia, and in part because exercise is halted by breathlessness before the heart is fully taxed. Therefore, attempts to predict physical condition from the heart rate observed during submaximal tests have little value. Alternative tactics in clinical assessment are to report a "symptom-limited" maximal test result, to predict maximal oxygen intake from maximal voluntary ventilation and the ventilatory equivalent for oxygen (26) or from lung function, age and breathlessness (27), or to report the work rate observed at a fixed and relatively low heart rate (for instance the PWC130).

In patients who are unable to operate a cycle ergometer, an arm-crank ergometer may provide a useful alternative test (28). In clinical practice, useful information can also be obtained by measuring the distance walked in 6 minutes, or by carrying out a shuttle-walking test (29).

HYPERACTIVE AIRWAYS

Exercise bronchospasm is sometimes envisaged as a problem seen in young athletes that is provoked by the inspiration of cold dry air during physical activity (30). However, COLD is also associated with "twitchy airways," perhaps because repeated bacterial infections modify T-cell function. Precipitants of bronchospasm include exposure to dusty, polluted, and allergen-filled air. Hyper-responsiveness does not seem to exacerbate the aging of pulmonary function in otherwise healthy adults (31), but it may do so in the patient with COLD (21). Barter and Campbell (32) and Britt et al. (33) found that the 5-year decline of lung function was closely matched to methacholine sensitivity. Confounding factors in such studies are the low initial level of function in the hyper-reactors and the close association between bronchospasm and a history of cigarette smoking.

Cigarette Smoking

Cigarette smoking is perhaps the most important cause of a pathologic aging of respiratory function. It has been said to account for 80% of the interindividual variability in respiratory function scores, and it accounts for 46% to 70% of the population-attributable risk of chronic bronchitis (34). Auerbach et al. (35) showed a clear dose/response relationship between the number of cigarettes smoked and the degree of emphysema. This has obvious lessons for prevention. There is plainly much interindividual variability in the adverse functional consequences of smoking. This is caused in part by issue of dose—the number and type of cigarettes smoked per day, the number and depth of puffs taken per cigarette, and the length of the butt when the cigarette is extinguished.

Longitudinal studies are complicated by changes in the number and type of cigarettes consumed as a study proceeds. Thus, Fletcher et al. (21) noted the loss of forced expiratory volume in 1 second during an 8-year period was greater for men who initially were smoking more than 15 cigarettes per day than for those who were smoking 5–15 cigarettes. However, those initially reporting a consumption of more than 25 cigarettes per day did not show a further exacerbation of functional loss, perhaps because the onset of symptoms had encouraged the most vulnerable of the heavy smokers to stop smoking or to reduce their cigarette consumption before the study began. Higenbottam et al. (36) found no difference of functional loss between those smoking high- and low-tar cigarettes, and they hypothesized that much of the harmful impact of cigarette smoke on lung aging was attributable to components of the gas phase such as ozone and nitrogen oxides.

The main biological reason for the interindividual variation in loss of lung function is the congenitally determined absence of alpha-1 antitrypsin. In some smokers, lung volumes decrease only a little faster than in nonsmokers, but in others, a dramatic loss leads to the early onset of disability and death (37). The overall goal of prevention must be to make smoking a socially unacceptable behavior, but in the short term, it would also be helpful to identify those patients in whom smoking has a particularly adverse impact on function. Some authors have suggested that changes occur first in the peripheral airways (38), but it is unclear whether such changes are pathologic or are merely a reversible spasm or edematous change that disappears on ceasing smoking (39, 40).

In any event, tests of small-airway function are not easy to undertake, and for the present, early detection of vulnerable individuals is probably best based on simple measurements of 1-second forced expiratory volumes. Long-term follow-up studies are needed to determine what proportion of individuals with currently subnormal function progresses to having overt COLD. Speizer and Tager (37) have emphasized that smoking during adolescence may set the stage for poor respiratory function in later adult life, because those who smoke as teenagers fail to show the anticipated continuing increase of lung volumes through to 24 years of age.

There is substantial interindividual variation in the response to smoking cessation. The mechanical benefits may be quite rapid. Rode and Shephard (41) observed a normalization of the work of breathing within 24 hours of smoking cessation in young adults. However, a slower normalization of function would be anticipated in older patients who already have pathologic changes in the airways. The rate of aging of lung function subsequent to cessation of smoking depends in part on the cumulative cigarette exposure to the date of quitting. One patient may regain an almost normal pattern of aging, but a second patient who has smoked for a longer period may show a continuing accelerated deterioration of function that leads inexorably to disability and death.

Data from one longitudinal study (42) found that the rate of loss of forced expiratory volume in 1 second during a 5-year period was 28 mL less per year in those who quit than in those who continued smoking. This difference was independent of the date of quitting, suggesting that the beneficial impact on the aging of function was achieved quite rapidly. Likewise, in the Framingham study, the average rate of loss of vital capacity during a 10-year period was identical for female nonsmokers and for women who stopped smoking during the study decade; in the men who quit, the rate of loss was only slightly higher than in nonsmokers (43). Nevertheless, in both of these studies, the ex-smokers were left with the functional loss that they had accumulated during their years of smoking.

The possible influence of environmental tobacco smoke on the aging of lung function has aroused considerable controversy (44). One problem is that the method of classifying people as nonsmokers is usually based on a self-report, and the chance of erroneously classifying a smoker as a nonsmoker is higher if the spouse or other member of the household is a regular smoker. The current conclusion seems to be that, whereas passive smoking increases the prevalence of respiratory disease in young children, any effect on the lung function of adults is small and is unlikely to have a major functional impact.

Exercise-Centered Rehabilitation for COLD

PRINCIPLES OF THERAPY

Lung tissue that has been destroyed by accelerated aging cannot be replaced, except by a lung transplant. There are few donors relative to the prevalence of chronic chest disease, and the cost of such operations is currently at least $30,000, with a 2-year survival rate of only 60% to 70% (45).

Thus, the main aims of therapy must be primary prevention (avoidance of smoking and exposure to air pollutants); secondary prevention (avoidance of smoking, air pollutants, and episodes of infection after pulmonary damage has been incurred); and improvement of function through a comprehensive program of local and general conditioning in a manner that enhances the quality of the patient's remaining years of life.

NONSPECIFIC MEASURES

Annual influenza vaccination is now recommended for the patient with chronic respiratory disease, although polyvalent pneumococcal vaccines are of less proven efficacy (46). Careful monitoring for and treatment of acute infections by broad-spectrum antibiotics, plus postural drainage as required, will avoid or minimize exacerbation of the underlying condition. Attempts to reduce ventilation by the suppression of thyroid function (47) may relieve resting dyspnea, but they seem unlikely to improve exercise performance. Codeine and morphine derivatives reduce the perception of dyspnea, thereby increasing exercise tolerance (48, 49). One uncontrolled study claimed that vagotomy improved exercise performance in 2 of 5 patients, possibly by a reduction of cholinergic tone in the airways (50).

The likelihood of precipitating bronchospasm during training sessions can be reduced by an appropriate choice of exercise environment. In particular, rehabilitation class leaders should note that the ambient concentrations of ozone in large and polluted cities are lower in the early morning and evening than at midday. If bronchospasm still occurs, bronchodilator therapy should be tried. Because the patient is middle-aged or older, the sensitivity of the adrenoreceptors is diminished, and the ischemic myocardium is more vulnerable to arrhythmias. Inhaled anticholinergic agents such as ipratropium bromide may thus prove more useful than β-2 agonists (51). The β-2 agonists tend to cause pulmonary vasodilatation and may increase the mismatching of ventilation and perfusion, with a further decrease of arterial oxygen pressures (52). Theophylline is a useful adjuvant; it has a weak bronchodilator action (53), relieves respiratory muscle fatigue (54), and, at least in healthy individuals, stimulates mucociliary transport (55).

The use of corticosteroids is controversial. Only about 10% to 20% of patients with COLD seem to derive respiratory benefit from such treatment (56), and in our present context such gains could easily be offset by adverse effects on lean muscle mass. Mucolytics seem to be of little value (57), and ventilatory stimulants add to the already dangerously high loading of the right ventricle (58–60), worsening rather than improving effort tolerance (61). Attempts to change the ventilatory response to exercise by modifying the carbohydrate content of the diet (62) also have only a minimal effect on effort tolerance.

BREATHING EXERCISES

Appropriate breathing exercises can strengthen the chest muscles and increase their endurance in normal individuals (63), with a probable reduction in the perceived respiratory effort (64). In the patient with COLD, the endurance of the respiratory muscles and their resistance to fatigue are commonly (65–67) but not always (68, 69) improved by such programs. However, the average patient with COLD cannot undertake a sufficiently vigorous program of exercise to strengthen the respiratory muscles appreciably, whether using abdominal weights (65) or resisted inspiration (66).

A skilled physiotherapist can also teach mechanically more efficient patterns of ventilation that diminish the very high oxygen cost of breathing and/or increase ventilatory function (70). Tactics include increased use of the abdominal muscles to alter the shape of the thoracic cavity and store elastic energy for inspiration (71), a rapid inspiration followed by a slow expiration, and the pursing of the lips to minimize collapse of the airways during vigorous expirations. Patients rarely adopt the new breathing patterns spontaneously; nevertheless, they can be taught to use such measures to increase the mechanical efficiency of the chest muscles during bouts of vigorous effort (16, 72). A given level of ventilation is then achieved with a smaller local oxygen consumption, releasing a larger fraction of the available maximal oxygen intake for the use of the limb muscles.

ENERGY CONSERVATION

One important benefit of a successful training program is that the patient learns to walk with greater mechanical efficiency (16, 73, 74); for example, tentative, tottering steps are progressively replaced by much longer strides. The patient can be taught to carry out many daily activities in a better coordinated and mechanically more efficient manner, and the energy cost of tasks that involve displacement of the body can be further decreased by a loss of excess body weight. Plainly, the amount of daily activity that can be accomplished with an impaired oxygen transport system is directly proportional to the efficiency with which the patient converts chemical energy into the required external work.

OXYGEN THERAPY AND TRAINING

There have been suggestions that domiciliary oxygen therapy can extend the life span of the patient with COLD by 6–7 years (75). The ideal candidate seems to be the patient whose arterial oxygen pressure is less than 55 torr when breathing air (76), a patient in whom a large decrease of oxygen tension develops during exercise, with associated signs of myocardial ischemia such as anginal pain or deep ST segment depression. In such patients, the administration of oxygen during formal exercise sessions improves arterial oxygen pressures without necessarily relieving hypoxic pulmonary vasoconstriction (77).

Perhaps because of relief of airway spasm, a decrease of intratracheal pressure, and a resulting increase of effective right atrial filling pressure, the output of atrial natriuretic peptide during exercise is increased (78). The relief of bronchospasm may also reduce the oxygen cost of breathing (79). As a consequence of these various changes, the patient's confidence is increased to the point that the training threshold can be reached (80). If the oxygen is also provided for home use, the quality of life is enhanced (81), and an increase of habitual activity may further improve exercise tolerance (82).

Quite a low oxygen flow rate (1–2 L/min) is usually enough to bring the resting arterial oxygen pressure to 65–80 torr, but it is advisable to increase the flow rate during exercise to maintain a 30% inspired oxygen mixture. An oximeter can be used to determine the flow that is needed to maintain arterial oxygen saturation while exercising. The main basis of symptomatic relief is a relief of hypoxic drive to the respiratory control centers, with a resultant decrease of ventilation at any given rate of working (83).

GOALS OF GENERAL CONDITIONING PROGRAMS

Many patients with COLD initially have difficulty in walking faster than 2 km per hour, so that a program of supervised walking on the treadmill is unlikely to yield what would be regarded as a true conditioning response in either the cardiorespiratory system or the skeletal muscles (84, 85). Rather, the objectives of the general conditioning program are to decrease dyspnea, to increase the duration of exercise that can be tolerated at a single session, to enhance subjective well-being, and to reverse the vicious cycle of fear, inactivity, and progressive deconditioning.

Given that most patients with COLD are elderly, and many have been heavy smokers, the risk that exercise will precipitate a dangerous abnormality of cardiac rhythm is surprisingly low (86). Almost all authors have reported a marked symptomatic improvement when patients with COLD have participated in exercise-centered rehabilitation programs (17, 18, 87–91). However, the majority of studies have been small in scale and of short duration (3 months or less). With some exceptions (66, 89, 94), there have also been no controls. Thus, it has been difficult to determine how far any observed functional benefit was attributable to exercise per se, and how far it reflected ancillary features of the rehabilitation program such as breathing exercises, postural drainage, the better control of intercurrent respiratory infections, psychological encouragement, and an improvement of mood state.

Typically, there has been no objective evidence of improvements in respiratory function (94–97), although some studies have noted small increases of peak oxygen intake (66, 94, 98) or peak power output (90, 99) after training (possibly in part because the factor limiting peak effort shifts from dyspnea to central cardiac function). It is difficult to envisage how an exercise program could reverse the destruction of tissue in an emphysematous lung. It might enhance the local blood flow to the chest muscles (100, 101). In theory, it might also help the process of lung drainage and improve the ventilation of obstructed alveoli (92, 93). Thus, Cockcroft et al. (94) noted a decrease of both coughing and sputum volume in trained individuals. However, clearance of ^{99}Tc-labeled aerosol gives little support to the view that exercise facilitates mucus drainage (95).

Several authors have noted the contribution of lean tissue loss to the deterioration in physical condition in patients with COLD (87, 96, 102, 103). Lake et al. (88) further pointed out that any training response seemed specific to the muscles that had been trained. A strengthening of key skeletal muscles could reduce the afterloading of the left ventricle, giving the possibility of a larger peak stroke volume and some increase of maximal oxygen intake. More importantly, the improvement of peripheral blood flow with muscle strengthening might reduce acidosis and hyperventilation, so that the patient would become less conscious of dyspnea (99, 104). Thus, lean body mass is a determinant of overall functional capacity in COLD, independent of respiratory function (87).

Many patients with COLD are particularly dyspneic when using their arms (89, 105), in part because ventilation is greater for a given oxygen consumption during arm exercise (106), and in part because the shoulder muscles become fatigued by the exercise task (107), so that they can no longer contribute as effectively to ventilation (108, 109). An endurance training regimen for COLD should involve as large a muscle mass as possible (110), preferably including the arms as well as the legs (88, 89, 111, 112), and it should be supplemented by deliberate resisted exercises to increase muscle mass (113). Strengthening of the arm muscles will not only reduce perceived breathlessness (89), but, at least in younger and less disabled patients, it may also enhance ventilatory endurance (114). On the other hand, arm exercise alone is unlikely to allow a sufficient intensity of effort to improve cardiovascular function.

Above all, a successful training program restores the confidence and self-efficacy of the patient (25, 115); sensitivity to dyspnea will be decreased, and the vicious cycle of fear, diminishing physical activity, and loss of physical condition will be reversed. Nevertheless, the overall response to training remains discouraging in the typical patient who is severely disabled by COLD. There is no critical event to motivate a change of lifestyle, and in many individuals attempts at exercise are discouraged by an unpleasant dyspnea. Progress to the point that physical activity becomes intrinsically rewarding is slow and difficult. Compliance is poor, and there is a tendency for the patient to seek an escape by taking prolonged holidays away from the rehabilitation center or by indulging in alcoholism and drug abuse. Patients who show an increase of arterial oxygen saturation when exercising are the most likely to persist with and show a favorable response to training; adverse features of the initial examination include a low vital capacity and forced expiratory volume, an increased hemoglobin level, advanced age, pulmonary hypertension, and a history of respiratory failure.

If the exercise tolerance of the patient remains severely limited despite regular participation in an optimal rehabilitation program, mobility can apparently be improved by the prescription of a portable oxygen cylinder. However, it is unclear how much of the benefit of such oxygen therapy is physiologic and how much is psychological (116). The main problem is the small capacity of the cylinder (it is usually kept to a weight of less than 2 kg and yields a maximum of 100 liters of oxygen). Another possibility for extending the mobility of very breathless patients is to provide an ultra-lightweight tricycle (117).

Conclusion

Even elderly and severely disabled patients with COLD can profit substantially from an exercise-centered rehabilitation program (118), but the mechanisms of benefit remain somewhat obscure. The exercise prescription should not seek any massive improvement in cardiorespiratory function; rather, it should concentrate on reversing the vicious cycle of loss of self-confidence, physical inactivity, loss of lean tissue, and worsening dyspnea. When possible, the patient should also be taught to move and to breathe more efficiently, so that maximum use can be made of residual function. In many patients, an appropriate regimen will not only decrease dependency and enhance the quality of life (119, 120), but (despite a remarkably small impact on standard laboratory test scores) it will also have a helpful effect on the course of the disease process.

References

1. Higgins MW: Chronic airway disease in the United States: Trends and determinants. *Chest* 96:S328–S329, 1989.
2. Shock NW: Physical activity and the rate of aging. *Can Med Assoc J* 96:836–842, 1967.
3. Timiras PS: *Developmental Physiology and Aging.* New York: MacMillan, 1972.

4. Brown JR, Shephard RJ: Some measurements of fitness in older female employees of a Toronto department store. *Can Med Assoc J* 97:1208–1213, 1967.
5. Health & Welfare Canada: *Canada's Health Promotion Survey.* Ottawa: Health & Welfare Canada, 1988.
6. National Center for Health Statistics: *Current Estimates from the National Health Interview Survey: United States, 1983.* Vital and Health Statistics, 10:154. Washington, DC: US Dept of Health & Human Services, 1986.
7. Anderson TW, Brown JR, Hall JW, et al: The limitations of linear regressions for the prediction of vital capacity and forced expiratory volume. *Respiration* 25:140–158, 1968.
8. Morris JF, Koski A, Johnson LC: Spirometric standards for healthy non-smoking adults. *Am Rev Respir Dis* 103:57–67, 1971.
9. Niinimaa V, Shephard RJ: Training and oxygen conductance in the elderly. I. The respiratory system. *J Gerontol* 33:354–361, 1978.
10. Shephard RJ: *Human Physiological Work Capacity.* London: Cambridge University Press, 1978.
11. Siegerist H: *Civilisation and Disease.* Chicago: University of Chicago Press, 1962.
12. UK Dept of Health and Social Security. *Inequalities in Health. Report of a Working Group.* London: Dept. of Health & Social Security, 1980.
13. Andres R: Normal aging versus disease in the elderly. In: Andres R, Bierman EL, Hazzard WR, eds. *Principles of Geriatric Medicine.* New York: McGraw Hill, 1985, pp 38–41.
14. Wanner A: Clinical aspects of muco-ciliary transport. *Am Rev Respir Dis* 116:73–125, 1977.
15. Roghman KJ: Immune response of elderly patients to pneumococcus. *J Gerontol* 42:265–270, 1987.
16. Canadian Thoracic Society Workshop Group: Guidelines for the assessment and management of chronic obstructive pulmonary disease. *Can Med Assoc J* 147:420–428, 1992.
17. Shephard RJ: Training and the respiratory system—Therapy for asthma and other obstructive diseases. *Ann Clin Res* 14:S86–S96, 1982.
18. Van Herwaarden CLA: Exercise and training in chronic non-specific lung disease (CNLSD). *Int J Sports Med* 5:S54–S58, 1984.
19. Cohen BH: Chronic obstructive pulmonary disease: A challenge in genetic epidemiology. *Am J Epidemiol* 112:274–288, 1980.
20. Higgins M, Keller J: Familial occurrence of chronic respiratory disease and familial resemblance in ventilatory capacity. *J Chronic Dis* 28:239–251, 1975.
21. Fletcher C, Peto R, Tinker C, et al: *The Natural History of Chronic Bronchitis and Emphysema.* Oxford: Oxford University Press, 1976.
22. Fragoso CAV, Clark T, Kotch A: The tidal volume responses to incremental exercise in COPD. *Chest* 103:1438–1441, 1993.
23. Petty TL: Definition, identification, assessment and risk factors. In: Petty TL, ed. *Chronic Obstructive Pulmonary Disease.* New York: Dekker, 1978.
24. O'Donnell DE, Webb KA: Breathlessness in patients with severe chronic airflow limitation: Physiological correlations. *Chest* 102:824–831, 1992.
25. Morgan AD, Peck DF, Buchanan DR, et al: Effects of attitudes and beliefs on exercise tolerance in chronic bronchitis. *BMJ* 286:171–174, 1983.
26. Armstrong BW, Workman JM, Hurt HH, et al: Clinico-physiologic evaluation of physical working capacity in persons with pulmonary disease; rationale and application of a method based on estimating maximal oxygen consuming capacity from MBC and O_2V_e. *Am Rev Respir Dis* 93:223–233, 1967.
27. Mahler DA, Harver A: Prediction of peak oxygen consumption in obstructive airway disease. *Med Sci Sports Exerc* 20:574–578, 1988.
28. Martin TW, Zeballos RJ, Weisman IM: Use of arm crank exercise in the detection of abnormal pulmonary gas exchange in patients at low altitude. *Chest* 102:169–176, 1992.
29. Singh SJ, Morgan MDL, Scott S, et al: Development of a shuttle walking test of

disability in patients with chronic airways obstruction. *Thorax* 47:1019–1024, 1992.

30. Shephard RJ: Exercise-induced bronchospasm: A review. *Med Sci Sports* 9:1–10, 1977.
31. Burrows B, Lebowitz MD, Barbee RA: Respiratory disorders and allergy skin test reactions. *Ann Intern Med* 84:1134–1139, 1976.
32. Barter CE, Campbell AH: Relationship of constitutional factors and cigarette smoking to decrease in $FEV_{1.0}$. *Am Rev Respir Dis* 113:305–315, 1976.
33. Britt EJ, Cohen B, Menkes H, et al: Airway reactivity and functional deterioration in relatives of chronic obstructive pulmonary disease patients. *Chest* 77:S260, 1980.
34. Weiss ST: Chronic bronchitis, asthma and obstructive airways disease: Age, smoking, and other risk factors. In: Bossé R, Rose CL, eds. *Smoking and Aging.* Lexington, Mass: Lexington Books, 1984, pp 73–94.
35. Auerbach O, Hammond EC, Garfinkle L, et al: Relation of smoking and age to emphysema. Whole lung section study. *N Engl J Med* 286:853–857, 1972.
36. Higenbottam T, Shipley MJ, Clark TJH, et al: Lung function and symptoms of cigarette smokers related to tar yield and number of cigarettes smoked. *Lancet* 1:409–412, 1980.
37. Speizer FE, Tager IB: Epidemiology of chronic mucus hypersecretion and obstructive airways disease. *Epidemiol Rev* 1:124–142, 1979.
38. Macklem PT, Hogg JC, Thurlbeck WM: The flow resistance of central and peripheral airways in human lungs. In: Cumming G, Hunt LB, eds. *Form and Function in Human Lungs.* Baltimore, Md: Williams & Wilkins, 1968, pp 76–88.
39. McCarthy DS, Craig DB, Cherniack RM: The effect of modification of the smoking habit on lung function. *Am Rev Respir Dis* 114:103–113, 1976.
40. Buist AS, Ghezzo H, Anthonisen NR, et al: Relationship between the single breath N_2 test and age, sex and smoking habit in three North American cities. *Am Rev Respir Dis* 120:305–318, 1979.
41. Rode A, Shephard RJ: The influence of cigarette smoking on the work of breathing in near maximal exercise. *Med Sci Sports* 3:51–55, 1971.
42. Bossé R, Sparrow D, Rose CL, et al: Longitudinal effect of age and smoking cessation on pulmonary function. *Am Rev Respir Dis* 123:378–381, 1981.
43. Ashley F, Kannel WB, Sorlie PD, et al: Pulmonary function: Relation to aging, cigarette habit, and mortality. *Ann Intern Med* 82:739–745, 1975.
44. Shephard RJ: Respiratory irritation from environmental tobacco smoke. *Arch Environ Health* 47:123–130, 1992.
45. Patterson GA, Maurer JR, Williams TJ, et al: Comparison of outcomes of double and single lung transplantation for obstructive lung disease. *J Thorac Cardiovasc Surg* 101:623–632, 1991.
46. Williams HH: Continuing controversy: Pneumococcal vaccine and COPD. *Chest* 92:193–194, 1987.
47. Butland RJA, Pang JA, Geddes DM: Carbimazole and exercise tolerance in chronic airflow obstruction. *Thorax* 37:64–67, 1982.
48. Terry P, Tockman MS: Chronic airways obstruction. In: Andres R, Biermann EL, Hazzard WR, eds. *Principles of Geriatric Medicine.* New York: McGraw Hill, 1985, pp 571–578.
49. Light RW, Muro JR, Sato RI, et al: Effects of oral morphine on breathlessness and exercise tolerance in patients with chronic obstructive pulmonary disease. *Am Rev Respir Dis* 139:126–133, 1989.
50. Bradley GW, Hale T, Pimble J, et al: Effect of vagotomy on the breathing pattern and exercise ability in emphysematous patients. *Clin Sci* 62:311–319, 1982.
51. Ullah MI, Newman GB, Saunders KB: Influence of age on response to ipratropium bromide and salbutamol in asthma. *Thorax* 36:523–529, 1981.
52. Gross NJ, Bankwala Z: Effects of an anticholinergic bronchodilator on arterial blood gases of hypoxemic patients with chronic obstructive pulmonary disease:

Comparison with a beta adrenergic agent. *Am Rev Respir Dis* 136:1091–1094, 1987.

53. Bleecker ER, Johns M, Britt EJ: Greater bronchodilator effects of ipratropium compared to theophylline in chronic airflow obstruction. *Chest* 94:S3, 1988.
54. Murciano D, Aubier M, Lecocgiv Y, et al: Effects of theophylline on diaphragmatic strength and fatigue in patients with chronic obstructive pulmonary disease. *N Engl J Med* 311:349–352, 1984.
55. Wanner A: Effects of methylxanthines on airway mucociliary function. *Am J Med* 79:S16–S21, 1985.
56. Eliasson O, Hoffman J, Trueb FD, et al: Corticosteroids in COPD: A clinical trial and reassessment of the literature. *Chest* 89:484–490, 1986.
57. Guyatt GH, Townsend M, Kazim F, et al: A control trial of ambroxol in chronic bronchitis. *Chest* 92:618–620, 1987.
58. MacNee W, Connaughton J, Rhind JB, et al: A comparison of the effects of almitrine or oxygen breathing on pulmonary arterial pressures and right ventricular ejection fraction in hypoxic chronic bronchitis and emphysema. *Am Rev Respir Dis* 134:559–564, 1986.
59. Cheong TH, Magder S, Shapiro S, et al: Cardiac arrhythmias during exercise in severe chronic obstructive pulmonary disease. *Chest* 97:793–797, 1990.
60. Cox NJM, van Herwaarden CLA, Folgering H, et al: Exercise and training in patients with chronic obstructive lung disease. *Sports Med* 6:180–192, 1988.
61. Morrison DA, Adcock K, Collins CM, et al: Right ventricular dysfunction and the exercise limitation of chronic obstructive pulmonary disease. *J Am Coll Cardiol* 9:1219–1229, 1987.
62. Brown SE, Wiener S, Brown RA, et al: Exercise performance following a carbohydrate load in chronic airflow obstruction. *J Appl Physiol* 58:1340–1346, 1985.
63. Leith DE, Bradley M: Ventilatory muscle strength and endurance. *J Appl Physiol* 41:508–516, 1976.
64. Redline S, Gottfried SB, Altose MD: Effects of changes in inspiratory muscle strength on the sensation of respiratory force. *J Appl Physiol* 70:240–245, 1991.
65. Merrick J, Axen K: Inspiratory muscle function following abdominal weight exercises in healthy subjects. *Phys Ther* 61:651–656, 1981.
66. Pardy RL, Rivington RN, Despas PJ, et al: Inspiratory muscle training in patients with chronic airflow limitation. *Am Rev Respir Dis* 123:421–425, 1981.
67. Carter R, Coast JR: Respiratory muscle training in patients with chronic obstructive pulmonary disease. *J Cardiopulmon Rehabil* 13:117–125, 1993.
68. Belman MJ, Kendregan BA: Physical training fails to improve ventilatory muscle endurance in patients with chronic obstructive pulmonary disease. *Chest* 81:440–443, 1982.
69. Guyatt G, Keller J, Singer J, et al: Controlled trial of respiratory muscle training in chronic airflow limitation. *Thorax* 47:598–602, 1992.
70. Austin JHM, Ausubel P: Enhanced respiratory muscular function in normal adults after lessons in proprioceptive musculoskeletal education without exercises. *Chest* 102:486–490, 1992.
71. Dodd DS, Brancatisano T, Engel LA: Chest wall mechanics during exercise in patients with severe airflow obstruction. *Am Rev Respir Dis* 129:33–38, 1984.
72. Campbell EJM, Friend J: Action of breathing exercises in pulmonary emphysema. *Lancet* 1:325–329, 1955.
73. Pierce AK, Paez PN, Miller WF: Exercise training with the aid of a portable oxygen supply wtih emphysema. *Am Rev Respir Dis* 91:653–659, 1965.
74. Chester EH, Belman MJ, Bahler RC, et al: Multidisciplinary treatment of chronic pulmonary insufficiency. 3. The effect of physical training on cardiorespiratory performance in patients with chronic pulmonary disease. *Chest* 72:695–702, 1977.
75. Cooper CB, Waterhouse J, Howard P: Twelve year clinical study of patients with hypoxic cor pulmonale given long term domiciliary oxygen therapy. *Thorax* 42:105–110, 1987.
76. Anthonisen NR: Long-term oxygen therapy. *Ann Intern Med* 93:391–398, 1983.

77. Morrison DA, Stovall JR: Increased exercise capacity in hypoxemic patients after long-term oxygen therapy. *Chest* 102:542–550, 1992.

78. Mannix ET, Manfredi F, Palange P, et al: The effect of oxygen with exercise on atrial natriuretic peptide in chronic obstructive lung disease. *Chest* 101:341–344, 1992.

79. Mannix ET, et al: Oxygen may lower the oxygen cost of ventilation in chronic obstructive lung disease. *Chest* 101:910–915, 1992.

80. Olopade CO, Beck KC, Viggiano RW, et al: Exercise limitation and pulmonary rehabilitation in chronic obstructive pulmonary disease. *Mayo Clin Proc* 67:144–157, 1992.

81. Canadian Thoracic Society Workshop Group. Guidelines for the assessment and management of chronic obstructive pulmonary disease. *Can Med Assoc J* 147:420–428, 1992.

82. Bell CW, O'Donohue WJ, Dewan NA, et al: Effects of transtracheal oxygen therapy on exercise capacity. *J Cardiopulmon Rehabil* 8:449–452, 1988.

83. Stein DA, Bradley BL, Miller WC: Mechanisms of oxygen effects on exercise in patients with chronic obstructive pulmonary disease. *Chest* 81:6–10, 1982.

84. Belman MK, Kendregan BA: Exercise training fails to increase skeletal muscle enzymes in patients with chronic obstructive pulmonary disease. *Am Rev Respir Dis* 123:256–261, 1981.

85. Hughes RL, Davison R: Limitations of exercise reconditioning in COLD. *Chest* 83:241–249, 1983.

86. Cheong TH, Magder S, Shapiro S, et al: Cardiac arrhythmias during exercise in severe chronic obstructive pulmonary disease. *Chest* 97:793–797, 1990.

87. Schols AMWJ, Mostert R, Soeters PB, et al: Body composition and exercise performance in patients wtih chronic obstructive pulmonary disease. *Thorax* 46:695–699, 1991.

88. Lake FR, Henderson K, Briffa T, et al: Upper-limb and lower-limb exercise training in patients with chronic airflow obstruction. *Chest* 97:1077–1082, 1990.

89. Ellis B, Ries AL: Upper extremity exercise training in pulmonary rehabilitation. *J Cardiopulmon Rehabil* 11:227–231, 1991.

90. Swerts PMJ, Kretzers LMJ, Terpstra-Lindeman E, et al: Exercise training as a mediator of increased exercise performance in patients with chronic obstructive pulmonary disease. *J Cardiopulmon Rehabil* 12:188–193, 1992.

91. Carter R, Coast JR, Idell S: Exercise training in patients with chronic obstructive pulmonary disease. *Med Sci Sports Exerc* 24:281–291, 1992.

92. Oldenburg FA, Dolovich MB, Montgomery JM, et al: Effects of postural drainage, exercise and cough on mucus clearance in chronic bronchitis. *Am Rev Respir Dis* 120:739–758, 1979.

93. Wolff RK, Dolovich MB, Obminsky G, et al: Effects of exercise and eucapnic hyperventilation on bronchial clearance in man. *J Appl Physiol* 43:46–50, 1977.

94. Cockcroft AE, Saunders JJ, Berry G: Randomized controlled trial of rehabilitation in chronic respiratory disability. *Thorax* 36:200–203, 1981.

95. Olseni L, Midgren B, Wollmer P: Mucus clearance at rest and during exercise in patients with bronchial hypersecretion. *Scand J Rehabil Med* 24:61–64, 1992.

96. Mertens DJ, Kavanagh T, Shephard RJ: Exercise rehabilitation for chronic obstructive lung disease. *Respiration* 35:96–107, 1978.

97. Belman MJ: Exercise in chronic obstructive pulmonary disease. *Clin Chest Med* 7:585–597, 1986.

98. Punzal PA, Ries AL, Kaplan RM, et al: Maximum intensity exercise training in patients with chronic obstructive pulmonary disease. *Chest* 100:618–623, 1991.

99. Davey P, Meyer T, Coats A, et al: Ventilation in chronic heart failure: Effects of physical training. *Br Heart J* 68:473–477, 1992.

100. Mancini DM, Ferraro N, Nazzaro D, et al: Respiratory muscle deoxygenation during exercise in patients with heart failure demonstrated with near-infrared spectroscopy. *J Am Coll Cardiol* 18:492–498, 1991.

101. Thompson CH, Davies RJO, Kemp GJ, et al: Skeletal muscle metabolism during

exercise and recovery in patients with respiratory failure. *Thorax* 48:486–490, 1993.

102. Morrison WL, Gibson JNA, Scrimgeour C, et al: Muscle wasting in emphysema. *Clin Sci* 75:415–420, 1988.

103. Canny GC, Levison HR: Exercise response and rehabilitation in cystic fibrosis. *Sports Med* 4:143–152, 1987.

104. Casaburi R, Patessio A, Ioli F, et al: Reductions in exercise lactic acidosis and ventilation as a result of exercise training in patients with obstructive lung disease. *Am Rev Respir Dis* 143:9–16, 1991.

105. Ries AL, Ellis B, Hawkins RW: Upper extremity training in chronic obstructive pulmonary disease. *Chest* 93:688–692, 1988.

106. Rasmussen B, Klausen K, Clausen JP, et al: Pulmonary ventilation, blood gases and blood pH after training of the arms or the legs. *J Appl Physiol* 38:250–256, 1975.

107. Celli BR, Rassulo J, Make BJ: Dysynchronous breathing during arm but not leg exercise in patients with chronic airflow obstruction. *N Engl J Med* 314:1485–1490, 1986.

108. Criner GJ, Celli BR: Effect of unsupported arm exercise on ventilatory muscle recruitment in patients with severe chronic airflow obstruction. *Am Rev Respir Dis* 138:856–861, 1988.

109. Banzett RB, Topulos GP, Leith DE, et al: Bracing arms increases the capacity for sustained hyperpnea. *Am Rev Respir Dis* 138:106–109, 1988.

110. Weintraub N, Dolan G, Stratmann H: Hemodynamics and respiratory responses to maximal treadmill and arm ergometry exercise in men with chronic obstructive pulmonary disease. *J Cardiopulmon Rehabil* 13:25–30, 1993.

111. Tangri S, Woolf CR: The breathing pattern in chronic obstructive lung disease during performance of some common daily activities. *Chest* 63:126–127, 1973.

112. Couser JL, Martinez FJ, Celli BR: Pulmonary rehabilitation that includes arm exercise reduces metabolic and ventilatory requirements for simple arm elevation. *Chest* 103:137–141, 1993.

113. Simpson K, Killian K, McCartney N, et al: Randomised controlled trial of weightlifting exercise in patients with chronic airflow limitation. *Thorax* 47:70–75, 1992.

114. Keens TG, Krastins JRB, Wannamaker EM, et al: Ventilatory muscle endurance training in normal subjects and patients with cystic fibrosis. *Am Rev Respir Dis* 116:853–860, 1977.

115. Carter R, Coast RJ, Idell S: Exercise training in patients with chronic obstructive pulmonary disease. *Med Sci Sports Exerc* 24:281–291, 1992.

116. Howard P, Waterhouse JC: Breathlessness and oxygen therapy. *Clin Sci* 62:P28, 1981.

117. Woodcock AA, Johnson M, Geddes D: Cycling patterns in patients with chronic airflow limitation. *BMJ* 286:1184, 1983.

118. O'Donnell DE, Webb KA, McGuire MA: Older patients with COPD: Benefits of exercise training. *Geriatrics* 48:59–66, 1993.

119. Reardon J, Patel K, ZuWallack RL: Improvement in quality of life is unrelated to improvement in exercise endurance after outpatient pulmonary rehabilitation. *J Cardiopulmon Rehabil* 13:51–54, 1993.

120. Vale F, Reardon JZ, ZuWallack RL: The long-term benefits of outpatient pulmonary rehabilitation on exercise endurance and quality of life. *Chest* 103:42–45, 1993.

1 Prevention and Principles of Treatment

"All Physicians Are Not Created Equal." Understanding the Educational Background of the Sports Medicine Physician
Rich BSE (Arizona Sports Medicine Specialists, Phoenix)
J Athletic Train 28:177–179, 1993   139-94-1–1

Background.—The American Medical Society for Sports Medicine defines its specialty as "the application of principles and concepts of medicine to physical activity and those who participate in sports, games, and other physical activities." Sports medicine involves providing comprehensive medical and therapeutic care for individuals involved in fitness activities.

Discussion.—The field of sports medicine is not dominated by any particular specialty or specialty group. Rather, it is a group of connected specialties that include athletic training, physical therapy, exercise physiology, nutrition, sports psychology, coaching, and traditional medicine. Biomechanists, podiatrists, chiropractors, dentists, nurses, and administrators also may be connected with or contribute to a sports medicine practice. At present, any physician can declare himself or herself a sports medicine specialist, because practicing the medical aspects of sports medicine does not require special certification and primary care sports medicine is not a recognized specialty within the field of medicine. Sports medicine physicians should complete fellowship training or participate in appropriate continuing education courses, which are offered several times each year during annual and specialty meetings. Athletic trainers should familiarize themselves with the field of sports medicine and the educational background of sports medicine physicians as part of their responsibility in providing quality sports medicine care.

▶ The author has quoted Lamb's (1) statement, "Sports medicine has been referred to as an umbrella with different specialities representing the ribs of the umbrella and the athlete representing the stem." I have always believed that was a good description of this profession. It is the belief of many of the "ribs" of this umbrella that certification of physicians within this specialty of sports medicine is inevitable. Until that time, athletes and those of us who refer our athletes to physicians should know their qualifications and areas of expertise.—F.J. George, A.T.C., P.T.

Reference

1. Lamb DR: *Sports Med Bull* 19:8, 1984.

Emergency Equipment: What to Keep on the Sidelines
Rubin A (Southern California Permanente Med Group, Fontana)
Physician Sportsmed 21:47–54, 1993   139-94-1-2

Introduction.—The physician providing medical coverage at an athletic competition should have an emergency plan that covers personnel, procedures, and equipment. The equipment and planning will vary according to the type of sport, the level of competition, the availability of additional personnel with their own equipment, the time of year, the weather conditions, and the physician's responsibility for spectator and/or participant care. Communication capability with local Emergency Medical Services is essential. The availability of local services will often determine the type and extent of treatment given by the sideline physician.

Emergency Equipment Checklist.—The sideline physician's equipment should include pocket equipment for urgent care, carried on the individual or in a small fanny pack. Diagnostic equipment for evaluating less urgent problems includes a blood pressure cuff, an oto/ophthalmoscope, and an eye tray with topical anesthetic, fluorescein strips, and a blue light. The physician should be trained in advanced cardiac life support (ACLS). Appropriate life support equipment encompasses airway management, breathing apparatus, circulation maintenance, drugs for ACLS, and electrical monitoring devices. Equipment for neurologic, orthopedic, and wound care is needed. The physician must consider general team needs and specific individual needs for medications; for example, an athlete with asthma or diabetes will require a β-agonist inhaler or glucagon or a glucose replacement.

Conclusion.—The sideline physician's emergency plan must address appropriate personnel, procedures, and equipment. The standard emergency equipment should provide for simple diagnosis, life support, neurologic and orthopedic emergencies, wound care, and medication. The physician must also be aware of specific individual medication needs. A high level of emergency preparedness allows the physician to provide effective immediate care to an injured athlete or spectator.

▶ Be prepared. Plan ahead. There is nothing worse than being in an emergency situation and not having the necessary equipment available. Communication to activate the local Emergency Medical Services is a must. Practice and communicate with everyone you will be dealing with before an emergency arises, including administrators, parents, coaches, athletic trainers, and athletes. The more planning and practicing of emergency situations the physician does, the smoother the performance will be when the real situation arises.—F.J. George, A.T.C., P.T.

Surveillance of Serious Recreational Injuries: A Capture-Recapture Approach
Laporte RE, Kohl HW, Dearwater SR, Kriska AM, Anderson R, Aaron DJ, Olsen T, McCarty DJ (Univ of Pittsburgh, Pa)
Med Sci Sports Exerc 25:204–209, 1993   139-94-1–3

Background.—Serious injury from sports and recreation is a leading cause of morbidity and mortality in the United States. The need to develop national surveillance systems for sports injury was examined, and a method by which it can be accomplished was studied.

Method.—Existing surveillance systems for the prevention of communicable and noncommunicable diseases have proven to be highly effective in reducing the morbidity and mortality of common illnesses. However, in the case of surveillance of communicable disease, the voluntary reporting of events represents a passive surveillance system in which only 10% to 50% of events are ever recorded. As a sports injury model, this would not provide accurate data on incidence rates. The noncommunicable disease model relies on disease-specific population registries limited to geographic areas. It is successful in identifying 90% to 100% of the patients, but it is an expensive task. The problem in applying this system to sports injury surveillance is that there are too many injuries to record.

An alternative model is, therefore, required. The initial step is to evaluate the upper end of the injury severity spectrum—catastrophic injuries occurring not only in high school and college sports, but also as a result of voluntary unsupervised activity. Secondly, an effective method of surveillance must be drawn up using bodies that collect and record sports injuries. Several of these bodies already operate as independent sources; however, the collection of data is inaccurate and gives distorted information. One way to overcome such distortion would be the use of a system called capture-mark-recapture, a statistical technology that estimates the degree of undercount and controls for the variability of ascertainment. The goal of a sports injury surveillance system would be to use 2 or more reporting sources; e.g., members of the American College of Sports Medicine, certified athletic trainers, or other groups dealing with acute, serious injuries. A two-source model would provide the opportunity for pairwise comparisons across multiple lists.

Conclusion.—Until a means of accurately monitoring the incidence of sports injury is set up, the efficacy of sports injury prevention programs will not improve. Some suggestions of how this may be achieved were provided. However, at this stage, it is not the method that is important, but rather the recognition that an accurate surveillance system for serious sports injuries is required and that discussion needs to begin regarding how it can be accomplished.

Injuries in Recreational Adult Fitness Activities
Requa RK, DeAvilla LN, Garrick JG (Saint Francis Mem Hosp, San Francisco)
Am J Sports Med 21:461–467, 1993   139-94-1–4

Background.—The risk of musculoskeletal injury from recreational or fitness activities has not been systematically examined. Adult participants in recreational fitness activities were studied prospectively to assess their risk of injury.

Methods.—The study sample included 986 adults, (median age, 32 years) who were recruited from local fitness clubs and exercise studios. Study participants were followed for a 3-month period during which telephone interviewers called once per week to record all physical activity and any injury or complaint that had occurred during that week. Activities were coded as team sports, individual sports, aerobic dance, weights, or cardiovascular.

Results.—A total of 525 injuries and complaints, of which 475 were caused by sports participation, occurred during 60,629 hours of activity. The overall injury rate was 7.83 per 1,000 hours of sports activities. The overall rate for injuries that caused a change in participation was less than 2 per person per year. Participants in competitive team sports had the highest injury rate. Running had a higher risk of injury than many team sports. Those engaged in cardiovascular exercise had low to medium rates of injury, but injury rates varied by type of cardiovascular activity.

Subjects engaged in weight work also had low injury rates. The 5 most common types of injury were sprains, strains, inflammation, pain/aches, and contusions. The most commonly injured sites were the shoulder, low back, knee, leg, ankle, and the foot and toes. A history of a sports-related injury almost doubled the risk of reinjury. Those with a history of knee injury had an almost threefold higher rate of knee injury during the study.

Conclusion.—The risk of injury resulting from participation in most adult recreational fitness activities is relatively low.

▶ The major problem with this paper is that although the authors described types of injuries, injured sites, and injury rates, they failed to deal with the most important aspect: severity of injury.—J.S. Torg, M.D.

Sports and Osteoarthrosis of the Hip: An Epidemiologic Study
Vingård E, Alfredsson L, Goldie I, Hogstedt C (Karolinska Hosp, Stockholm;

Natl Inst of Occupational Health, Solna, Sweden)
Am J Sports Med 21:195–200, 1993   139-94-1-5

Study Design.—To determine whether long-term sports participation increases the risk of osteoarthrosis of the hip in men, a case-control study was performed on the sports activities of 233 men between the ages of 50 and 70 years who received a hip prosthesis because of severe idiopathic osteoarthrosis of the hip. The controls consisted of 302 men of the same age who were randomly selected from the general population. Interviews were conducted to determine sports participation, job history, and health status. The study subjects were interviewed regarding their exposure to each of 26 sports activities from the year of diagnosis, whereas the controls were evaluated from the year of the interview. The hours of exposure were then aggregated to 49 years of age.

Findings.—Men with high exposure to sports of all kinds combined (in hours) had a relative risk of having osteoarthrosis of the hip of 4.5, compared with men who had low exposure to sports. The activities that were most hazardous to the hip joint appeared to be track-and-field sports and racket sports. Men who had been exposed to high physical loads, both from sports and from their occupation, had a relative risk of 8.5, compared with those with low physical load in both activities. Potential confounding factors such as age, body mass index, and smoking were considered. Age was a confounding factor, but body mass index appeared to be an independent risk factor. Smoking was not associated with osteoarthrosis of the hip.

Conclusion.—Long-term exposure to participation in sports appears to be a risk factor among men for severe osteoarthrosis of the hip developing. The risk is further increased when combined with a heavy occupational load.

▶ The conclusions of this study were in keeping with those of Klünder et al. (1), who observed an increase in incidence of osteoarthrosis of the hip in retired soccer players compared with a comparable control group. Specifically, 53% of the soccer players had osteoarthritic changes on their radiographs, compared with 30% of the controls. The Vingård study also demonstrated that badminton, squash, and track-and-field events had the highest relative risk for osteoarthrosis later in life, whereas ice hockey was not associated with an increased risk of osteoarthrosis of the hip. A determination of the relative risk associated with American football, basketball, and baseball would be interesting.—J.S. Torg, M.D.

Reference

1.   Klünder KB, et al: *Acta Orthop Scand* 51:925, 1980.

Common Sports Hand Injuries: An Overview of Aetiology, Management and Prevention

McCue FC III, Meister K (Univ of Virginia, Charlottesville)
Sports Med 15:281–289, 1993   139-94-1-6

Introduction.—Injuries to the hand are common in sports, probably because the hand often absorbs the initial contact. As with other injuries, the key to a good outcome is prompt diagnosis, proper management, and an appropriate rehabilitation program.

Carpometacarpal Joint Dislocations.—These injuries generally result from hyperextension and/or hyperabduction forces across the volar aspect of the thumb metacarpal. Patients are seen with a diffusely swollen basilar joint area; pain and inability to pinch are present in patients with full dislocation. Evaluation should include standard anteroposterior and lateral roentgenograms. Closed reduction is followed by 6 weeks of immobilization; a transarticular Kirschner wire can be used when reduction is difficult to maintain.

Thumb Metacarpal Fractures, Joint Dislocations.—Metacarpal fractures of the thumb can be intra- or extra-articular. The most common pattern is Bennett's fracture dislocation. With proper protection, continued athletic participation can be allowed in many sports. Union usually occurs within 6 weeks and should be followed by a period of protective splinting. Closed reduction is usually sufficient for most dislocations, but those with ulnar or radial collateral injuries may require open repair and reconstruction.

Metacarpal Fractures, Fractures of the Phalanges.—The so-called boxer's fracture occurs through the shafts and the metacarpal neck. Multiple displaced metacarpal shaft fractures are an indication for open reduction. Anatomical reduction is required when the articular surface of the metacarpal head is involved. Most fractures of the phalanges can be treated by closed methods, with an attempt made to obtain as near an anatomical alignment as possible. Fractures that are too unstable or too comminuted should be managed by closed reduction and percutaneous Kirschner wire fixation or by open reduction and internal fixation.

Proximal Interphalangeal Joint (PIP) Injuries.—Nondisplaced intra-articular fractures of the PIP joint are treated with 3 weeks of immobilization followed by 4–6 weeks of protection. An attempt at closed reduction is advised for fracture dislocations of the PIP joint.

Volar Plate Injuries.—Hyperextension can cause acute injuries of the volar plate. These injuries should be treated with splinting for 2 weeks, with the PIP joint in 20–30 degrees of flexion. Surgical treatment is an option for deformities resistant to stretching and maintained beyond 40 degrees of flexion.

Distal Interphalangeal Joint Injuries and the Mallet Finger.—Dislocations of this joint should be reduced and splinted for at least 3 weeks. In mallet finger deformity, the extensor tendon can be attenuated or ruptured from the base of the distal phalanx, either with or without a piece of bone. Mallet fingers with fractures of more than 30% of the articular surface require open reduction and internal fixation.

▶ This is a comprehensive review article of sports hand injuries from the author who gave us the "coaches' finger" (1).—J.S. Torg, M.D.

Reference

1. McCue III FC, et al: *Am J Sports Med* 7:275, 1979.

Wrist and Hand Injuries in Platform Diving
le Viet DT, Lantieri LA, Loy SM (Paris)
J Hand Surg (Am) 18A:876–880, 1993   139-94-1–7

Introduction.—Olympic platform divers have developed 2 methods to permit a smooth entry into the water. In the first hand position, the fists are closed and the right thumb is in the left fist. The second, newer method uses an open hand position with the fingers and wrists extended, the forearms pronated, and the hands overlapped. Both hand positions have resulted in wrist injuries.

Methods.—Twenty-one divers who participated in the French diving championship in 1991 were interviewed. All were training and/or competing at the 10-m platform. The group had a mean age of 21 years and had been active in diving for a mean of 6 years. Three dove with the fists closed and 18 with the hands flat.

Results.—Eighteen divers complained of occasional or frequent wrist pain. In 9 patients, pain persisted outside of competition; 1 diver had to withdraw permanently from competitive diving. The open-hand technique was used by all but 1 of the 9 divers who had a sprain, fracture, or surgery and by all 9 divers who experienced pain even when not competing.

Discussion.—Both hand techniques used by the injured divers are designed to avoid splashes in the water. During training, these competitive divers complete as many as 240 dives per week. Those using the open-hand technique may experience pain on the dorsal side of the wrist as a result of repeated trauma of the wrist in hyperextension. In the closed-fist technique, the violence of the impact creates hyperextension and traction of the thumb that is held in the other fist. Kinetic analysis shows that the diver's hand is the principle element absorbing the energy when the body speed is suddenly braked at the moment of entering the water. The open-handed technique is more traumatic than the closed-fist method. A small 4 × 3 cm splint placed under strapping on the radial side of the wrist appears to be effective in preventing wrist injuries. Bandages held by a Velcro hook and loop fastener may also help to restrain the wrist when diving. Coaches need to be more aware of the risk of hand and wrist injuries and the means of preventing these problems.

▶ The cumulative effect of repetitive impact to the hands is put in perspective when one understands that the athlete can dive 20 times per hour up to 20 hours per week, resulting in 240 dives per week. Added to this, divers off the 10-m platform reach a speed of 51 km/hr when penetrating the water. This certainly results in significant repeated trauma to the wrist and/or hand.—J.S. Torg, M.D.

Pedal Cycling Fatalities in Northern Sweden
Öström M, Björnstig U, Näslund K, Eriksson A (Univ of Umeå, Sweden)
Int J Epidemiol 22:483–488, 1993   139-94-1-8

Introduction.—During recent years, about 12% of all traffic fatalities in Sweden have involved cyclists. Because the crash and injury mechanisms are often different in fatal vs. nonfatal bicycle accidents, the nature of the fatal crashes was examined.

Methods.—Data concerning all bicycle fatalities from 1975 to 1985 were collected for the 4 northern counties of Sweden, an area with a population of approximately 907,000 inhabitants. People who were pushing their bicycles at the time of the fatal accident were excluded. The Swedish government strongly recommends that a forensic pathologist perform a complete medicolegal autopsy in all cases of traffic fatalities. Thus, autopsy data were available in all but 4 of the 146 bicycle-related fatalities during the study.

Results.—Bicycle-related fatalities accounted for about 15% of all traffic fatalities in the region. Most (83%) crashes occurred during the summer months. During the months of June and August, nearly one third of those who died were children aged 16 years and younger. Most deaths resulted from injuries to the head; none of the bicyclists who died used a protective helmet. Nearly all (88%) of the fatal accidents involved a collision with a motor vehicle on a public road. The bicyclist was at a road junction in 49 of the crashes. In only 1 case was a mechanical fault discovered in the bicycle. Two thirds of the victims and 91% of the 115 motor vehicle drivers for whom information was available were male. Alcohol was considered to be a contributing factor in 9 bicyclists and in 5 motor vehicle drivers.

Conclusion.—The annual incidence of bicycle fatalities was 1.4 per 100,000 population. Children and the elderly were at greatest risk for fatal injuries, and male victims predominated in both of these age groups. Elderly individuals who survive the crash are at risk of delayed death from pulmonary complications. Trucks were heavily overrepresented in accidents involving motor vehicles. Measures likely to reduce bicycle fatalities are the use of protective helmets and the separation of bicyclists from motor vehicle traffic.

▶ Of the more than 1,000 bicycling deaths each year, three fourths are caused by head injuries. Half of those killed are school-age children. In a survey of caregivers of schoolchildren in Alabama, two thirds of responders thought that a head injury was likely if their child was in a mishap, but 91% of the kids had no helmet (1). In a 1991 telephone survey in Toronto, 81% of parents favored legislation mandating helmet use by child cyclists (2). In a study by the Johns Hopkins Injury Prevention Center evaluating bicyclists aged 15 years or older who died in accidents between 1987 and 1991, two thirds had been tested for alcohol use. Of those tested, nearly one fourth had blood alcohol concentrations of 100 mg/dL or higher—the legal limit for automobile drivers in most states. Helmet use would also reduce deaths associated with horseback riding (3).—E.R. Eichner M.D.

References

1. Jones CS, et al: *South Med J* 86:859, 1993.
2. Hu X, et al: *Can J Public Health* 84:163, 1993.
3. Hamilton MG, Tranmer BI: *J Trauma* 34:227, 1993.

Acute Injuries From Mountain Biking
Chow TK, Bracker MD, Patrick K (Loma Linda Univ, Calif; Univ of California, San Diego)
West J Med 159:145–148, 1993   139-94-1–9

Background.—With the change in focus of recreational bicycling, we can expect to see a subsequent change in injuries to cyclists. Previous studies of bicycling injuries have focused on children, urban settings, head injuries, and helmet use. The injuries sustained by mountain bikers who generally ride off-road were documented.

Method.—An anonymous questionnaire was mailed to the members of 2 California bicycling clubs (459 members in total) that encourage off-road recreational cycling. Four gift certificates from a bicycle shop were offered by lottery as an incentive to respond. The questionnaire asked about riders' experience, equipment use, bicycle maintenance habits, recent injuries and their treatment, and factors contributing to accidents. Riders reporting injuries were divided into 2 groups: those who sought medical attention (moderate and severe injuries) and those who did not (mild). The details of the accidents of each group were then compared to identify risk factors for serious injuries.

Results.—A total of 268 questionnaires were returned. Most riders were male, aged between 14 and 68 years. The mean number of years of experience mountain bicycling was 4.2 years. Most riders spent around 6.6 hours biking each week, most of which was off-road. Eighty-four percent of the respondents reported at least 1 injury. Fifty-one percent had sustained an injury in the past year. Almost 90% of the riders damaged extremities; 37% had injury to the trunk; head and neck trauma occurred in 12%. Most injuries were mild and could be self-treated. One quarter of the victims consulted a physician. A total of 4.4% were admitted to a hospital.

Most accidents occurred in June and July, generally during the middle of the day and in clear weather. Injuries occurred more commonly off-road and usually during a descent. Excessive speed and riding on unfamiliar terrain were the principal causes. Regarding upkeep of the bikes, more than half of the riders provided maintenance 6 times per year or more. Most wore helmets routinely (86%) and equipment failure only accounted for 7% of the accidents. Comparing patients with severe injuries to those with mild, no significant demographic details were found; however, the more seriously injured group cycled more off-road hours per week, yet were more likely to have had the accident on paved terrain.

Conclusion.—Eighty-four percent of the members of 2 cycling clubs reported mountain biking injuries. Most were minor injuries to extremities, but one quarter sought medical attention and nearly 5% were admitted to a hospital. There was a low occurrence of head injuries resulting from the high rate of helmet use. The major risk factor for cyclists appears to be motor vehicles on paved road; for mountain bikers, it appears to be excessive speed, particularly downhill on unfamiliar terrain.

▶ The results of this study, when compared with those of injuries occurring to regular bicyclists, suggest that all-terrain cyclists have more (but not necessarily more severe) injuries. Regarding the circumstances surrounding the accidents, injuries are more likely to occur off-road, and most happen while descending a grade and do not involve a collision.—J.S. Torg, M.D.

Hand Injuries on Artificial Ski Slope
Van Geertruyden JP, Goldschmidt DP (Hôpital Erasme, Brussels, Belgium)
J Hand Surg (Br) 18B:712–713, 1993   139-94-1–10

Background.—Few studies have been published on injuries incurred on artificial ski slopes, although there are ample data on snow skiing injuries. Nevertheless, reports of injuries under both conditions are traumatologically quite specific.

Methods.—Traumatologic data were collected on 50 consecutive patients treated for injuries incurred on an artificial ski slope during a 16-month period.

Results.—Of the 50 patients, 38 (76%) had hand or wrist injuries. There were 42 lesions—40 in the hand, 1 Colles' fracture, and 1 scaphoid fracture. Of the hand lesions, 31 were in the first ray; half of them were fractures and one third were sprains of the ulnar collateral ligament.

Discussion.—Hand and wrist lesions were much more common among those injured on artificial slopes than on snow. Hand injuries on snow were most frequently injuries of the ulnar collateral ligament of the first metacarpophalangeal joint. This is a rare injury on artificial slopes, where fractures, especially of the first ray, are most common. The hardness of the artificial ski slope may explain this increased hand trauma. In contrast, there are relatively few lower leg injuries on the artificial ski slope, perhaps because skis are not trapped in snow; therefore, torsion forces are not applied on the leg during falls.

▶ The artificial ski slope is a 100-m surface composed of 3-mm polyvinyl chloride bristles arranged in 2.5-mm wide strips and 7 × 7 mm squares. To maintain a gliding surface, the slope is continuously sprinkled with water. To the best of my knowledge, this is the second report of artificial ski slope injuries, the first having been published by Steedman (1). Although this study by Van Geertruyden and Goldschmidt is small and certainly not a well-controlled series, 76% of the injuries occurring on this slope were seen in one hospital emergency room.—J.S. Torg, M.D.

Reference

1. Steedman DJ: *Injury* 17:208, 1986.

Women's Gymnastics Injuries: A 5-Year Study
Sands WA, Shultz BB, Newman AP (Univ of Utah, Salt Lake City)
Am J Sports Med 21:271–276, 1993   139-94-1–11

Introduction.—Few epidemiologic studies of women's gymnastic injuries have considered the relationship between training methods and specific injuries. This information must be available, however, before injuries can be prevented. The distribution of injuries relative to time and training demands in a successful college-level women's gymnastic team was studied prospectively.

Subjects and Methods.—The study subjects were members of the NCAA Division I team at the University of Utah. Data were collected during the 5 competitive seasons from 1986 to 1991. Gymnasts provided information on injuries on Scantron computer dot sheets or on a computer terminal before each training session. They were asked to record the injured body part, the event or activity, and the date of injury.

Results.—Thirty-seven gymnasts participated in the study through the 5 seasons. Analysis of the total injuries/exposure ratios indicated that gymnasts trained with an injury approximately 71% of the time. A new injury could be expected about 9% of the time. The first-ranked cause of injury was the unknown/repetitive stress syndrome category; tumbling was ranked second and uneven bars third. The right side of the body was injured more than the left and the lower extremity more than the upper extremity. New injuries tended to increase during specific training periods and during competition preparation and performance, whereas total injuries increased until the middle of the season.

Conclusion.—The women's gymnastic team trained approximately 5 days per week, 4 hours per day, with 2 additional, separate workouts of weight training. The findings yielded a new injury ratio of 22.7 injuries per 1,000 hours and 176.9 new and continuing injuries per 1,000 hours. The high incidence of injury linked with competitions and full routines suggests that competition rules and the performance environment need to be evaluated. Coaches and team physicians should be extra vigilant during these periods.

Women's Intercollegiate Gymnastics: Injury Patterns and "Permanent" Medical Disability
Wadley GH, Albright JP (Univ of Iowa, Iowa City)
Am J Sports Med 21:314–320, 1993   139-94-1–12

Introduction.—Although injuries are quite common in the sport of gymnastics, few studies have investigated gradual-onset or overuse injuries and their residual effects on the athlete. These aspects of injury were examined in a prospective study of a women's college gymnastics team.

Subjects and Methods.—Twenty-six members of a Division I women's gymnastic team were followed from 1983 to 1987. Injuries sustained during this period were recorded by the team's athletic trainer and classified as having either acute or gradual onset. Data collected included the date and circumstances of the injury, tissue damage, previous injury history, and time lost from participation. Participants were sent a questionnaire 3 years after the study to determine the long-term effects of specific injuries.

Results.—There were 106 injuries recorded during the study. The average number of injuries per athlete per year was 2.1. New injuries accounted for 81% of reports; 19% were a recurrence of the same injury from the same or a previous season. Sixty injuries had a specific, acute onset, and 46 were considered to be of gradual onset. Only 16 injuries occurred during competition. The lower extremity was the most common site of injury (67%); strains and sprains accounted for 68% of all reports. Three of 6 gymnasts who injured ligaments of the knee had ruptures of the anterior cruciate ligament. The mean time loss from date of injury until return to full participation was 30.87 days. Twenty-two of 26 gymnasts were available for follow-up. Almost half (45%) of the respondents reported that their gymnastics-related injuries still bothered them 3 years after retiring from competition. Only 1 gymnast appeared to be free of residual symptoms or limitations. Acute- and gradual-onset injuries were equally likely to cause long-term effects. Pain and stiffness were common symptoms. None of the patients were limited in routine activities of daily living, however, and most (71%) still believed they were capable of high-intensity athletic activity.

Conclusion.—Women's gymnastics at the college level ranks with or above football and wrestling in injury risk. Such injuries, particularly those involving the back and ankle, are likely to have long-term effects.

▶ These 2 papers (Abstracts 139-94-1–11 and 139-94-1–12) provide interesting insights into the injury risk factors associated with women's gymnastics. The distribution of injuries as related to activities is similar to those found in the current literature. The high incidence of repetitive stress syndrome injuries as well as the relatively high incidence of injuries in the floor exercise are also in keeping with the findings of others.—J.S. Torg, M.D.

Ballet Injuries: An Analysis of Epidemiology and Financial Outcome
Garrick JG, Requa RK (Saint Francis Mem Hosp, San Francisco)
Am J Sports Med 21:586–590, 1993   139-94-1–13

Background.—Professional ballet dancers are at risk of sustaining career-ending injuries that may also have major financial consequences for the company that employs them. The epidemiology and financial outcome of ballet dancers' injuries were examined by analyzing insurance records.

Methods.—The workers' compensation insurance documents covering 3 dance seasons of a large professional ballet company were examined. An injury was defined as any condition that resulted in a financial outlay for medical expenses. Injuries not involving insurance payouts that were treated in-house were excluded from this analysis.

Results.—During the 3-year study, 104 dancers sustained 309 injuries, or 2.97 injuries per injured dancer. Twenty-four dancers—or 23% of the injured dancers—sustained 5 or more injuries each, accounting for 161 (51.9%) of all injuries. The total insurance payout was $398,396 or $1,289 per injury. Nine injuries (3%) resulting in medical costs exceeding $10,000 each were responsible for 37.8% of the total costs. The most frequently injured anatomical regions were the foot (23.9%), the lumbar spine (23%), and the ankle (13.3%).

Conclusion.—Future studies that identify risk factors for major injuries and lead to modifications to prevent such injuries may benefit not only the dancers, but also the companies that are financially responsible for them.

▶ The authors observe that among athletes of any sort, the reduction of injuries never attracts the interest that treatment of these injuries does. Perhaps the appreciation of the financial consequences of these injuries will stimulate new efforts aimed to enhance safety and reduce cost. I would suspect that the total insurance pay-out of $398,396 for one professional ballet company for a 3-year period should be an attention getter. However, with regard to insurance carriers and injury prevention, it has been my experience that the sole interest is to pay the bills and pass the costs on to the premium payers.—J.S. Torg, M.D.

Australian Snowboard Injury Data Base Study: A Four-Year Prospective Study

Bladin C, Giddings P, Robinson M (Victorian Ski Assoc. Victoria, Australia; Mt Hotham Med Centre, Victoria, Australia; Falls Creek Med Centre, Victoria, Australia)

Am J Sports Med 21:701–704, 1993   139-94-1-14

Background.—The popularity of snowboarding has increased dramatically despite ski resort owners' misgivings about injury rates, risks to others, and liability insurance. Estimates from Europe and North America suggest that as much as one third of the ski industry may soon be devoted to snowboarding. Snowboarding footwear includes soft- and hardshell boots with nonreleasable bindings. "Hybrid" boots have a hardshell base and a soft upper portion designed for ankle flexibility. Many beginners use ski boots on plate bindings that allow crossover between skiing and snowboarding. The incidence and pattern of snowboarding and ski injuries were investigated in a prospective study.

Method.—Information on snowboarding and skiing injuries was collected during 4 years at 3 ski resort medical centers in Australia. The recorded information included name, age, sex, level of experience, type of boots worn, and mode of injury (fall, collision). The site, type, and severity of injury; treatment; predicted workdays missed; days off the snow; and long-term disability were also recorded.

Results.—A total of 276 snowboarding injuries were reported, for a rate of 4.2 injuries per 1,000 visits. The injured snowboarders were 76% male and 24% female. The average age for both men and women was 21 years. Fifty-eight percent of the injuries occurred in novices. Fifty-seven percent of the injuries were in the lower extremities and 30% were in the upper extremities. The most common injuries were sprains (53%), followed by fractures (24%), and contusions (12%). Falls were the most common mode of injury. Snowboarders had 2.4 times as many fractures and fewer knee injuries than skiers, but they had more ankle injuries. Snowboarders' ankle injuries were more common with soft-shell boots, worn mostly by intermediate and advanced riders. Knee injuries and distal tibial fractures were more common with hard-shell boots, worn mostly by novices. The novices also had more upper extremity fractures.

Conclusion.—To prevent injury, beginners should take lessons and wear hybrid or soft-shell boots with stiff inner boots for ankle support.

Rental equipment must be properly fitted and adjusted because it can be a source of potential injury.

▶ Although it was not possible for the authors to determine injury rates, their findings are similar to those reported by Ganong et al. (1). Specifically, these two studies have documented snowboarding as an at-risk activity comparable to alpine skiing. They also emphasize the importance of adequate instruction and make recommendations for "foot-wear needed to balance the frequency and severity of different injuries." It is noted that Ganong et al. recommend rigid boots or inserts and release bindings, whereas Bladin et al. recommend soft-shell boots with stiff inner boots.—J.S. Torg, M.D.

Reference

1. Ganong RB, et al: *Physician Sportsmed* 20:114, 1992.

Injuries Resulting From Bungee-Cord Jumping
Hite PR, Greene KA, Levy DI, Jackimczyk K (Maricopa Med Ctr, Phoenix, Ariz; St Joseph's Hosp, Phoenix, Ariz)
Ann Emerg Med 22:1060–1063, 1993   139-94-1-15

Introduction.—Bungee jumping, which imitates a rite of passage in South American tribes, usually entails wearing a vest that is attached to the bungee cord and jumping off a platform 200–400 feet above the ground. After approaching the ground, the jumper rebounds and falls once or twice again before being lowered to the ground or retrieved by a balloon. In "reverse" jumping, the individual is held to the ground while the cord is stretched and then released in an upward trajectory.

Case 1.—Woman, 19, passed through the coiled cord when rebounding, and the cord became tightened about her neck on returning to descent, leading her to snap to an upright position and be suspended there. There was tenderness over C5, but cervical spine radiographs were normal, and the jumper did well (Fig 1–1).

Case 2.—Man, 28, while attempting a reverse jump, had his head snapped to the side when 1 side of the restraint failed. He noted immediate neck pain and an inability to move his legs, as well as reduced sensation from the sternum distally. A sensory level of C7-8 was noted, with no tendon reflexes in the lower limbs. A 3-mm anterior subluxation of C6 on C7 was found, with indications of a unilateral locket facet confirmed by CT examination. After reduction in traction, an MR study demonstrated cord contusion in the C6-7 region. The patient was placed in a halo vest but remained quadriplegic 5 months later.

Discussion.—These cases show the potentially severe injuries that can result from bungee jumping. Fatal hangings have been described. The

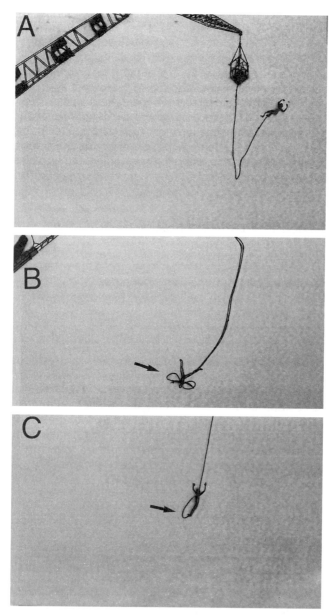

Fig 1–1.—Photographs taken from a VHS recording of patient 1's jump. Artist has emphasized cord and body position because of the reproduction quality. **A,** patient at beginning of the jump. **B,** at the peak of the first rebound, the loose cord has formed loops through which the patient has ascended (*arrow*). **C,** less than 2 seconds later, the patient is hung from a short segment of the cord, which has now wrapped tightly about her neck. The patient has interposed her hands between the cord and her neck (*arrow*). (Courtesy of Hite PR, Greene KA, Levy DI, et al: *Ann Emerg Med* 22:1060–1063, 1993.)

risks inherent in this activity may be greater than are recognized by the general population.

▶ This article represents the first report in the medical literature of injuries from bungee-cord jumping. I am aware of several other serious injuries reported in the lay press. I agree with the authors that "Formal epidemiologic studies of injuries resulting from this sport as well as regulation of bungee-jumping companies are suggested."—J.S. Torg, M.D.

Wheels-in-Line Roller Skating Injuries

Callé SC, Eaton RG (Columbia College of Physicians and Surgeons, New York)
J Trauma 35:946–951, 1993   139-94-1–16

Background.—There appears to be great potential for severe upper extremity trauma with wheels-in-line roller skating. No previous studies have described the at-risk population and identified the types of injuries incurred.

Methods.—The study surveyed 57 patients seen at the Roosevelt Hospital Hand Service, 65 metropolitan emergency room physicians, and 60 randomly selected members of the American Society of Hand Surgey regarding in-line skating injuries. Data collected included skating ability of the patient, use of protective gear, and circumstances and type of injury. The responses were added to national data on 444 cases collected by the Consumer Product Safety Commission.

Results.—Most injuries were to the upper extremity; lower extremity injuries were relatively rare. Fractures were the most common injuries. The wrist was the most common site for injury and for fracture. The Roosevelt survey identified the 3 most common types of wrist fracture: distal radius (45%), scaphoid (14%), and radial head (10%). Most of the distal radius fractures were severely comminuted and were incurred by men at an average age of 27 years. Women with upper extremity fractures had an average age of 34 years. Most patients were novice skaters and did not wear protective gear. Almost all of the patients experiencing upper extremity fractures did not wear wrist splints. Although fractures did occur with protective gear, the bone was not significantly displaced.

Conclusion.—In-line skating injuries can be severe. Novices should first master the techniques of skating and stopping in a controlled setting. All skaters should wear volar wrist splints and elbow pads. Because injury can occur even with splints, splint design should be evaluated.

▶ The new recreational activity, in-line roller skating, is increasing in popularity and, as indicated by this report, will produce its share of injuries. Of the injuries collected and documented by this study, 10 resulted in deaths. It appears that roller blading has the potential of becoming a significant health problem.—J.S. Torg, M.D.

High- Versus Low-Top Shoes for the Prevention of Ankle Sprains in Basketball Players: A Prospective Randomized Study

Barrett JR, Tanji JL, Drake C, Fuller D, Kawasaki RI, Fenton RM (Univ of Oklahoma, Oklahoma City)
Am J Sports Med 21:582–585, 1993   139-94-1–17

Introduction.—In theory, taping, ankle bracing, and high-top shoes can reduce the risk of ankle injuries in athletes by preventing extremes in range of motion. However, few studies have tested the truth of this theory. Whether wearing high-top shoes can prevent ankle sprains in basketball players was prospectively evaluated.

Methods.—The study sample comprised 622 college intramural basketball players, representing 44% of the total number of such athletes. After stratification for a history of previous ankle sprains, the subjects were randomized to receive a new pair of 1 of 3 types of basketball shoes: high-top, high-top with an inflatable air chamber, or low-top. The subjects were to wear the shoes only during basketball competition. They were followed during the 2-month intramural season for ankle sprains, which were documented by courtside athletic trainers.

Results.—Follow-up included 1,833 player-games and 39,302 minutes of player-time. There were 15 ankle sprains: 7 in standard high-top shoes, 4 in high-top shoes with an inflatable air chamber, and 4 in low-top shoes. Corresponding injury rates were 4.80, 2.69, and 4.06×10^{-4}, respectively, the differences being nonsignificant. The overall rate of injury was lower than expected. Variables from the history and physical examination did not predict the occurrence of ankle sprains.

Conclusion.—Shoe type—specifically high-top vs. low-top—does not appear to have any important effect on the rate of ankle sprains in basketball players. Future studies may assess the possible protective effects of high-top shoes with inflatable air chambers, of wearing new shoes, and of stretching and other methods to prevent ankle sprains.

▶ This study demonstrates the apparent complexity of what, on the surface, appears to be a relatively simple question, i.e., high- vs. low-top shoes as related to the prevention of ankle sprains in basketball. Garrick and Requa found high-top shoes to be more protective than low-top shoes. However, those study subjects had their ankles taped (1). Rovere et al. found low-top shoes to be more protective than high-top shoes when both were combined with lace-up ankle stabilizers (2). In this study by Barrett et al. an overall injury rate of 8.2 injuries per 1,000 player-games was seen, compared with that of 30.4 to 33.4 injuries per 1,000 player-games found in the study by Garrick and Requa. The proposed explanation for this discrepancy is that all of the players in Barrett's study played in "new basketball shoes."—J.S. Torg, M.D.

References

1. Garrick J, Requa R: *Med Sci Sports Exerc* 5:200, 1973.
2. Rovere G, et al: *Am J Sports Med* 16:228, 1988.

Medial Collateral Ligament Knee Sprains in College Football: Brace Wear Preferences and Injury Risk

Albright JP, Powell JW, Smith W, Martindale A, Crowley E, Monroe J, Miller R, Connolly J, Hill BA, Miller D, Helwig D, Marshall J (Indiana Univ, Bloomington; Univ of Illinois, Champaign-Urbana; Univ of Iowa, Iowa City; et al)
Am J Sports Med 22:2–11, 1994   139-94-1–18

Objective.—Despite extensive research, it remains unclear whether off-the-shelf knee braces are effective in preventing medial collateral ligament (MCL) strains in football players. Knowledge of the extrinsic—environmental or sport-related—factors is essential to the epidemiologic study of these injuries. This prospective, multicenter study of MCL sprains in college football players sought to account for all extrinsic factors relevant to these injuries.

Methods.—The study sample comprised 987 previously uninjured collegiate football players. All athletes were categorized according to how often they wore preventive knee braces. One hundred injuries occurred during the 3-year study, 47 of them in unbraced knees. The patterns of these injuries were analyzed to identify some extrinsic factors common to both braced and unbraced knees. Each athlete's attendance; brace wear choice; position group (line, linebacker, tight end); string group (player vs. nonplayer); and session (game vs. practice) were recorded. Tissue damage was confirmed for all reported MCL sprains.

Results.—Type of session, position group, and string group all had important effects on both the likelihood of brace wear and the risk of injury without a brace. Nonplayers in the line positions were most likely to wear a brace, whereas their unbraced MCL sprain rates were nowhere near those of line players. Offensive linemen most commonly wore a brace, followed by defensive linemen, linebackers, tight ends, and all categories of backs. Frequency of brace use did not change before, after, or during the study. Linebacker/tight ends, although they also had a high unbraced knee MCL injury rate, often preferred to remove their braces for games. Thus, braces usually were worn only when concern over the possibility of injury outweighed the desire for speed and agility.

Conclusion.—These findings emphasize the need to evaluate daily brace wear patterns in studies of MCL sprains in football players. Once this has been done, the database must be repartitioned to ensure that only similar groups are compared. Players must be analyzed separately from nonplayers.

Medial Collateral Ligament Knee Sprains in College Football: Effectiveness of Preventive Braces
Albright JP, Powell JW, Smith W, Martindale A, Crowley E, Monroe J, Miller R, Connolly J, Hill BA, Miller D, Helwig D, Marshall J (Indiana Univ, Bloomington; Univ of Illinois, Champaign-Urbana; Univ of Iowa, Iowa City; et al)
Am J Sports Med 22:12–18, 1994   139-94-1-19

Introduction.—Although it is far from certain whether protective knee bracing prevents medial collateral ligament (MCL) sprains in football players, braces continue to be used at the collegiate and professional level. The results of a 3-year study of the effectiveness of prophylactic knee braces in preventing MCL sprains among Division I college football players were evaluated.

Methods.—The analysis included 987 football players from the Big Ten conference, representing 155,772 knee exposures during a 3-year period. A brace was worn for about half of those exposures. Data on the players' position, string, type of session, and daily brace wear were recorded, and an incidence density ratio was created by use of the injury rates for braced vs. unbraced knees. The data were stratified at the same time they controlled for position, string, and type of session.

Findings.—Injury rates for braced and unbraced knees were significantly different in almost every position during practice, depending on whether the athlete was a player or nonplayer. After adjustment for position, string, and session, players wearing braces tended to have fewer knee injuries than those not wearing braces; however, the difference was not significant. In practices as well as games, starters and substitutes in the line positions, linebackers, and tight ends showed a significant trend toward a lower injury rate. The injury rate during games appeared to be higher for braced players in the skill positions, (e.g., backs and kickers).

Conclusion.—These findings suggest, but do not prove, that knee bracing protects college football players against MCL sprains. Any conclusive study of this issue will have to address the role of several associated risk factors. The risk of injury is highest for interior linemen during games and for nonplayers during practices. Linebackers and tight ends have nearly the same risk of injury as linemen, but they only wear braces half of the time.

▶ These 2 papers (Abstracts 139-94-1–18 and 139-94-1–19) report a sound, multicentered epidemiologic study dealing with a major current controversy. The position is taken that "Combining our findings with those of the West Point Study provides a strong suggestion that there is some minor influence of braces in the reduction of MCL injuries" (1). Unfortunately, the severity of the MCL injuries was not defined. Also, the relationship between brace use and anterior cruciate ligament injury was not discussed. The important factors of shoes and surfaces also were not factored into the equation. In view of this and considering the expense involved, it does not appear that these 2 papers either resolve the controversy or justify the use of prophylactic braces.—J.S. Torg, M.D.

Reference

1. Sitler M, et al: *Am J Sports Med* 18:310, 1990.

Injuries in Professional Rugby League: A Three-Year Prospective Study of the South Sydney Professional Rugby League Football Club
Gibbs N (South Sydney Orthopaedic and Sports Medicine Centre, Maroubra, Australia)
Am J Sports Med 21:696–700, 1993   139-94-1-20

Background.—Rugby league football is an extremely physical game played with no protective equipment. As a result, injuries from direct trauma are common, as are twisting injuries or muscle-tendon injuries from indirect trauma. In a 3-year prospective study, the incidence and nature of injuries sustained by rugby league players on 3 Australian teams were investigated.

Findings.—A total of 141 injuries that resulted in players missing subsequent games occurred during the 3 years. Minor injuries resulted in 1 missed game, moderate injuries in 2–4 missed games, and major injuries in 5 or more missed games. Of the 141 injuries, 37.6% were classified as minor, 34.8% as moderate, and 27.6% as major. The incidence of injury was 44.9 per 1,000 player-position game hours. This incidence is high compared with that of other sports. The number of knee injuries was more than twice that of the next most injured areas, groin, chest, shoulder, and spine. The most common specific injuries were to the medial collateral ligament of the knee and to the groin musculotendinous unit. Injuries to a lower extremity accounted for more than half of all the injuries.

Conclusion.—Compared with other sports, rugby has a high incidence of injury. The lack of protective clothing or helmets and the repetitive body contact contribute to the high injury rate.

▶ In addition to this study having been prospective, it is interesting to note that the author was present at all games and personally attended to and treated all injuries sustained. This being the case, it would appear that injury definition could have been based on both the anatomical part involved and the severity of injury.—J.S. Torg, M.D.

Total Knee Arthroplasty in Active Golfers

Mallon WJ, Callaghan JJ (Duke Univ, Durham, NC; Univ of Iowa, Iowa City)
J Arthroplasty 8:299–306, 1993   139-94-1-21

Background.—Many elderly patients undergo total knee arthroplasty (TKA) to alleviate arthritis, and many of these patients play golf for exercise. Because published data on activity and TKA loosening are not available, total joint arthroplasties in active golfers were assessed.

Methods.—Eighty-three golfers who had a single TKA with at least a 3-year follow-up and who played golf at least 3 times per week were surveyed. Postoperative anteroposterior and lateral radiographs were requested from the patients' surgeons and evaluated for evidence of TKA loosening.

Results.—Whereas 84.3% of patients reported no pain during play, 34.9% reported a mild ache after play. Radiographs for 54 golfers were obtained. Lucent lines were discernible in 53.7% of all prostheses, in 79.1% of cemented prostheses, and in 44.5% of uncemented prostheses. Radiographic loosening rates with hybrid TKA were significantly lower than those with cemented or uncemented prostheses. Nevertheless, pain during and after play did not differ signficantly among the 3 types of prostheses. Radiographic loosening did not differ significantly between left and right TKA; however, significantly more golfers with left TKA experienced more pain during and after play.

Discussion.—The higher incidence of left TKA pain during and after playing golf may relate to the increased torque on the left knee in right-handed golfers. Playing golf with a TKA on the target side need not be discouraged; however, these patients should be cautioned about possible pain during and after playing.

▶ This article is the authors' sequel to their report last year entitled, "Total Hip Arthroplasty in Active Golfers" (1). It also represents a significant contribution with regard to putting the activity status of the active golfer with a TKA into proper perspective.—J.S. Torg, M.D.

Reference

1. 1993 YEAR BOOK OF SPORTS MEDICINE, p 86.

The Effects of Ice and Compression Wraps on Intramuscular Temperatures at Various Depths

Merrick MA, Knight KL, Ingersoll CD, Potteiger JA (Northeast Physical Therapy Ctrs, Brookfield, Conn; Indiana State Univ, Terre Haute)
J Athletic Train 28:236–245, 1993   139-94-1-22

TABLE 1.—Average Temperatures at the Time of the Greatest Treatment Effect

Treatment	Skin Surface	Depth of Measurement Fat + 1 cm	Fat + 2 cm
Preapplication	32.50±1.15	36.28±0.74	36.59±0.71
Control	32.79±0.87	36.13±0.62	36.38±0.52
Compression only	34.38±0.66	36.25±0.51	36.47±0.47
Ice Only	7.24±1.19	26.58±3.66	28.21±2.34
Ice + Compression	4.94±0.68	23.54±3.33	26.46±3.04

Note: Values are °C ± 1 SD.
(Courtesy of Merrick MA, Knight KL, Ingersoll CD, et al: *J Athletic Train* 28:236–245, 1993.)

Background.—The principal use of cryotherapy (ice) in acute injury management is to lower the temperature of the injured tissue, thus reducing the metabolic rate and helping the tissue to survive the period of hypoxia after injury. Compression is often used with cryotherapy to increase external pressure on the tissue and prevent edema. Little is known about the effects of compression in conjunction with cryotherapy on intramuscular temperatures. Tissue cooling was examined at several depths during both cryotherapy and compression.

Method.—The effects of 4 treatment conditions were studied in 11 subjects: ice alone, compression alone, ice with compression, and control (no treatment). The subjects underwent all 4 conditions with a minimum of 1 day between treatments. Surface and intramuscular temperatures were recorded at 30-second intervals during 5 minutes of preapplication, 30-minute application, and a 20-minute postapplication. A repeated measure analysis of variance and Duncan post hoc tests were used to measure peak temperature differences between the treatment conditions and the depths of measurement.

Results.—Both ice and ice with compression were significantly colder than control or compression alone. Ice with compression was significantly colder than ice alone. The compression-only treatment led to a

TABLE 2.—Time at Which Greatest Treatment Effect Occurred

Treatment	Surface	Depth of Measurement Fat + 1 cm	Fat + 2 cm
Control	30.41±2.2	30.32±1.95	30.32±1.95
Compression only	29.32±1.49	30.73±6.40	31.41±6.38
Ice Only	29.73±1.34	35.95±3.75	39.23±5.09
Ice + Compression	30.82±1.25	32.86±1.93	35.32±4.72

Note: Time in minutes from the beginning of application phase ± 1 SD.
(Courtesy of Merrick MA, Knight KL, Ingersoll CD, et al: *J Athletic Train* 28:236–245, 1993.)

substantial increase in skin temperature, which returned to normal about 10 minutes after removal of the compression. (Tables 1 and 2).

Conclusion.—At all 3 depth measurements, ice with compression was significantly colder than ice alone. This can be explained by a number of factors. Compression causes the ice to be in closer contact with the skin. It also reduces blood flow and thus heat flow from other parts of the body. Third, the elastic wrap provides an insulating effect, and fourth, compression of tissue may increase its density, leading to greater conductive cooling. Not only was the ice and compression treatment colder than the others, it also reached its lowest temperature faster. The use of compression wraps to increase the rate of cooling would, therefore, be a valuable asset in the treatment of acute injuries.

▶ What is the best way to decrease tissue temperature when treating an acute injury? We have argued among ourselves for many years, deciding that "ice is best," "compression and ice are best," a "combination of ice and compression is best." The authors have given us proof that the combination of ice and compression is significantly better than any of the other methods. The authors state that not only is the combination colder but that the low temperature is reached faster. For acute injuries, don't be satisfied with just using an ice pack: use compression to provide colder tissue temperatures and to lower the temperature faster.—F.J. George, A.T.C., P.T.

A More Comfortable Cast?: A Trial of a Waterproof Liner
Selesnick H (Univ of Miami, Fla)
Physician Sportsmed 21:106–116, 1993   139-94-1-23

Purpose.—Although recent advances in orthopedics have decreased the need for cast immobilization, many patients still require casting to treat their injuries. Traditional fiberglass casts with stockinette and cast padding allow swimming and bathing, but the casts have to be dried afterward. The comfort, practicality, and possible cutaneous side effects of a waterproof cast liner that allows swimming, bathing, and hydrotherapy without special drying procedures were examined.

Methods.—The study population consisted of 140 patients (mean age, 30.7 years) who needed cast immobilization for nondisplaced fractures, stable fractures, and severe sprains. Sixty-nine patients had upper extremity injuries and 71 had lower extremity injuries. The Gore-Tex waterproof cast liners were applied directly to the skin. Patients and physicians completed satisfaction and cast performance surveys after cast removal.

Results.—All fractures healed without complications. At cast removal, the skin condition was rated good or exceptionally good in 95.7% of the patients and fair in the remaining 4.3%. One patient had mild skin blistering; 1 had a small, superficial skin ulcer; and 1 had a mild rash. None of the patients had skin infections. Mild erythema not requiring treatment was seen in 15 patients. Itching was minimal or not a problem for 80.6% of the patients. Odor was a problem for only 7.2% of the patients. Patients bathed an average of 7.3 times per week. Fifty-two patients swam an average of 3.4 times per week. Drying of the cast liner and fiberglass casting tape took less than 30 minutes for 33.3% of the patients, 31–60 minutes for 36.4%, and 1–2 hours for 26.5%. Patient and physician satisfaction ratings of the new cast liner were high.

Conclusion.—The use of Gore-Tex waterproof cast liners allows patients to maintain a more normal lifestyle compared with traditional cast types.

▶ We have been discouraging our athletes from getting their casts wet because of the drying and skin problems that can occur. It is the rare individual who will take the time to properly dry a cast so that skin problems can be avoided. The author states there are advantages and disadvantages to using the Gore-Tex waterproof cast liner. He states that "it is slightly more difficult to apply and it is more expensive than traditional stockinette and cast padding. . .[T]he additional cost to the physician was $12 to $20 for short-arm casts and $18 to $36 for short-leg casts. . .The material permits bathing, showering, sweating and swimming without any special drying procedures."

It appears that this material would be of great benefit to swimmers especially, but also to other athletes in training.—F.J. George, A.T.C., P.T.

2 Injuries of the Head, Neck, Spine, Nerves, and Abdomen

Does Amateur Boxing Lead to Chronic Brain Damage?: A Review of Some Recent Investigations
Haglund Y, Eriksson E (Karolinska Hosp, Stockholm)
Am J Sports Med 21:97–109, 1993   139-94-2-1

Background.—New rules and regulations for amateur boxing were introduced in Sweden during the 1970s to reduce the risks of amateur boxing. Despite the modified regulations, it was suggested that amateur boxing be forbidden. The Swedish Sports Foundation was subsequently commissioned to retrospectively investigate former Swedish amateur boxers whose careers started after the introduction of the new rules to see whether they had experienced chronic brain damage.

Method.—A total of 340 former amateur boxers were included in this study. All had applied for a boxing license between 1967 and 1977, and all had ended their career at least 1 year before the study began. Of the 340 participants, 25 boxers who had fought more than 30 matches (HM group) and 44 boxers who had fought less than 10 matches (LM group) were randomly selected. Two control groups, one consisting of 25 soccer players and the other 25 track-and-field athletes, were also selected. The soccer players chosen were considered to be typical headers by their managers. The boxers and controls underwent a complete neurologic examination except for ophthalmoscopy. A mini–mental-state examination was also carried out. Personality variables were measured and related to platelet monoamine oxidase activity. Computed tomography and MRI were used to evaluate cerebral morphological changes, along with clinical neurophysiologic examinations, comprising brain electric-activity mapping, and tests for sensory, motor, cognitive, and memory tasks. An overall assessment of intellectual impairment was made by a psychologist using a 3-point rating scale.

Results.—No significant differences were identified between the groups in any of the neurologic or physical examinations or in platelet monoamine oxidase activity. Boxers tended to have a lower degree of education and participated in less intellectual professions, but they were less impulsive and more socialized. There were no significant differences seen in CT and MRI studies of the different groups. However, a significantly higher incidence of slight or moderate electroencephalographic deviations was found among boxers. Neurophysiologic tests also revealed an inferior finger-tapping performance in boxers.

Conclusion.—No signs of serious brain damage were found among the former amateur boxers participating in this study. However, they did demonstrate some electroencephalographic and finger-tapping differences, which may indicate slight brain dysfunction. It is, therefore, extremely important that amateur boxing rules be followed, and perhaps they should be more strict.

▶ The authors have presented a comprehensive review of the historical, diagnostic, and clinical parameters of chronic brain damage resulting from boxing. It is pointed out that the severity of acute injury can vary from transient alterations of cognitive function to irreversible brain damage and death. Specifically, 645 fatalities have been identified worldwide from 1918 to 1983. The explanation of why more signs of chronic brain damage were not found in boxers is interesting. The authors hypothesize that "in amateur boxing there is a natural selection so that boxers who fight well and do not get hit so often can continue while those who are less successful give up and therefore, do not sustain chronic brain damage."—J.S. Torg, M.D.

Sports-Related Eye Trauma: Managing Common Injuries
Zagelbaum BM (North Shore Univ, Manhasset, NY)
Physician Sportsmed 21:25–40, 1993   139-94-2-2

Introduction.—Ocular injuries are a frequent occurrence in those engaging in sports activities; fortunately most of them are minor. Weekend athletes who are in suboptimal physical condition and schoolchildren who may be more enthusiastic than skillful are at the highest risk. The sports in which most ocular injuries occur are listed in the table.

Management.—Corneal abrasions, when confirmed by fluorescein dye, are treated with a topical broad-spectrum antibiotic and a pressure patch. Subconjunctival hemorrhage usually resolves spontaneously within 2 weeks and does not require treatment. A cycloplegic agent and topical steroid drops may be used to treat traumatic iritis. If an eyelid laceration is present, a complete ocular examination must be done to make sure that no other injury has occurred. Hyphema frequently is a marker of other eye damage. Discomfort is minimized by using a topical steroid or cycloplegic agent. In addition, an antifibrinolytic drug may be used to preserve the clot until the vessels heal. Foreign bodies may be removed by irrigation, with an applicator, or by using a foreign body spud or needle if the body is stuck on the cornea. A ruptured globe should always be considered when evaluating a patient with an injured eye. Any evidence of posterior segment injury—which usually results from severe blunt trauma—calls for prompt referral to an ophthalmologist.

Eye Injuries Sustained in Sports and Recreational Activities in the
United States in 1992

Activity	Number of Eye Injuries (percent of total)	
Basketball	8,304	(17.2)
Baseball	8,083	(16.8)
Swimming and pool sports	4,966	(10.3)
Racket and court sports*	4,161	(8.6)
Football	2,105	(4.4)
Ball sports (unspecified)	1,536	(3.2)
Soccer	1,469	(3.1)
Golf	1,320	(2.7)
Hockey (all types)	971	(2.0)
Volleyball	785	(1.6)
Subtotal	**33,700**	**(69.9)**
Other activities	14,490	(30.1)
Total	**48,190**	**(100.0)**

* Racket and court sports include racquetball, tennis, squash, paddleball, badminton, and handball.
(From Zagelbaum BM: *Physician Sportsmed* 21:25-40, 1993. Courtesy of the National Society to Prevent Blindness: 1992 Eye Injuries Associated With Sports and Recreational Products, Schaumburg, Illinois.)

Preventive Measures.—Protective eyewear, available for most sports, could prevent as many as 90% of all ocular injuries. A properly fitted and well-constructed device is essential. The best lens material is polycarbonate. Eyeglasses, contact lenses, and open eye guards do not protect the eyes. Protective eyewear is most often used in baseball, basketball, racket sports, ice hockey and, recently, football.

▶ Prevention is a major factor in the management of eye injuries. Most if not all eye injuries could be prevented if well-designed and properly fitted eye protection was worn in high-risk sports. The author states, "Open eye guards are of no value in racquetball and may increase injury by funneling a compressible ball into the orbit."

Many of our athletes wear contact lenses, and the author cautions, "Contact lens–related corneal abrasions should not be patched; if patched these patients may develop infectious keratititis. . ."—F.J. George, A.T.C., P.T.

A Discussion of the Issue of Football Helmet Removal in Suspected Cervical Spine Injuries

Segan RD, Cassidy C, Bentkowski J (Salisbury State Univ, Md)
J Athletic Train 28:294–305, 1993   139-94-2-3

The Problem.—Emergency medical technicians in some parts of the country routinely remove the football helmet during the initial care of athletes suspected of having an injured cervical spine. Sports medicine professionals, however, almost always discourage this practice when there is even the slightest possibility of the cervical spine being injured.

Pros and Cons.—Some believe that a helmet may interfere with the immobilization of the athlete, but a properly fitted helmet allows very little head motion. The possibility of missing a depressed skull fracture or cranial laceration is remote, because the resulting symptoms and signs may be discerned through the face mask and ear holes. It may be feared that the helmet will lead to hyperflexion of the cervical spine, but the shoulder pads offset the thickness of the helmet, resulting in neutral alignment of the cervical spine. Cervical hyperextension may result when the helmet is removed. Whereas removal of a motorcycle helmet may be necessary for proper airway management, the design of a football helmet permits resuscitative measures.

Recommendations.—There should be free communication between sports medicine staff members and local Emergency Medical Services systems and national associations. Those who provide emergency care should regularly practice the management of cervical spine injuries, including performance of cardiopulmonary resuscitation on a mannequin wearing football equipment. Further work is needed to determine how a face mask is most efficiently removed.

▶ This abstract should be read with the following article (Abstract 139-94-2-4). The controversy over helmet removal continues among sports medicine professionals and the Emergency Medical Services community as a whole. Is it necessary to remove a helmet before transporting an athlete with a cervical injury? My initial response is to leave the helmet in place if the athlete is breathing properly and then remove only the face mask, if necessary, to establish an airway. Please see my comments after the following abstracts.

There are radiologic studies now being done with normal individuals, on patients with quadriplegia caused by cervical injuries, and on cadavers to study the effects of helmet removal on cervical spine position. These studies are being done with and without shoulder pads. Studies like this should help us determine the best procedure to follow. A policy should be established at your institution and lines of communication between sports medicine personnel and emergency medicine technicians should be established.—F.J. George, A.T.C., P.T.

Management of the Critically Injured Football Player
Feld F (St. Margaret Mem Hosp, Pittsburgh, Pa)
J Athletic Train 28:206–212, 1993   139-94-2-4

Background.—Early recognition and treatment of life-threatening injuries in football players is crucial. A rapid and simple assessment method used by paramedics for trauma patients focuses on how and when equipment should be removed.

Assessment.—Assuming critical injuries to be cervical spine injury, respiratory distress, loss of consciousness, or sudden cardiac arrest, the following assessment can be accomplished in less than 30 seconds by trained personnel. First, airway patency should be determined and the cervical spine stabilized. It is vital to remove the mouthpiece at this point. If the airway is not patent, a jaw thrust maneuver must be carried out. Breathing should be checked: a rate of less than 10 or greater than 30 breaths per minute requires assisted ventilation. Pulse rate and quality should be measured, capillary refill and skin temperature assessed, and any bleeding controlled. The patient's consciousness can be measured by responses to verbal or painful stimuli. Pupil size and movement and strength of the extremities should be taken into account. Some clothing and equipment will have to be removed to examine the chest, although measures should be taken to prevent hypothermia in cold weather.

Management—Treatment involves airway management, oxygen administration, cervical spine immobilization, intravenous access, and cardiac monitoring with defibrillation and drug therapy in the case of cardiac arrest. Football equipment complicates some of these procedures. It is necessary to remove the face mask to assist respiration. To carry out cardiac monitoring, the jersey, shoulder pad strings, and straps must be cut. Defibrillation requires a completely exposed, dry chest. In the case of a player in cardiac arrest or with injuries that increase the chance of arrest, helmet and shoulder pads should be removed while keeping the cervical spine in an in-line neutral position. Players with cervical spine injuries without respiratory or cardiac involvement may be effectively immobilized with all equipment in place.

The following procedure should be used in removing equipment: The individual at the head holds the athlete's head in an in-line neutral position. A second individual removes the mouthpiece, and cuts jersey, shoulder pad strings, and chin strap. Jaw pads are also removed. The second individual slides one hand up the cervical spine, placing as much of the hand as possible under the occiput, and the other hand under the mandible, thus controlling stabilization. The individual at the head spreads the helmet at the ear holes and removes the helmet. Two additional individuals slide their hands between the scapula and posterior shoulder pad plate from each side and all 3 lift the thorax and head as a unit. The individual who was holding the helmet now removes the shoulder pads, and the patient is lowered to the ground.

Conclusion.—Although critical injuries are rare in football, it is vital that athletic trainers be prepared for them. This requires an effective and practiced emergency plan with a good working relationship with the local Emergency Medical Services agency, good assessment skill to allow for early recognition of critical injuries, and practice in the removal of all equipment.

▶ For more on this topic, please read Abstract 139-94-2-3. As I stated, there continues to be controversy over helmet and face mask removal. There are certain face masks that do not have to be removed before some types of airways can be used. There are tools that make face mask removal a safe and fairly easy procedure. As the author states, these emergency procedures must be practiced and reviewed on an annual basis. The proper emergency equipment must be available. Communication between sports medicine personnel and emergency medical technicians must be established as well as a protocol to follow. The author makes a very important point that face mask removal should not be our only concern. Practicing the removal of all football equipment is an important concern that should be addressed in a nonemergency practice session.—F.J. George, A.T.C., P.T.

Neck Injuries: Backboard, Bench, or Return to Play?
Anderson C (Hennepin County Med Ctr, Minneapolis)
Physician Sportsmed 21:23–34, 1993   139-94-2-5

Introduction.—Neck injuries that are obviously severe or clearly no more than minor strains can be dealt with according to established protocols. More difficult medical decisions are involved when an athlete sustains a neck injury of uncertain severity. Such situations were studied and an on-field process for assessing neck injuries was examined.

Frequency of Neck Injuries and Mechanisms During Sports.—Although neck injuries are common among athletes, most of these injuries are not catastrophic in nature. Football players, hockey players, and divers appear to be at greatest risk for serious neck injury. The most common mechanism in sports is axial loading. This occurs when a football player tackles headfirst and when a hockey player slides headfirst into the boards. Many types of movement, however, including flexion-rotation, hyperflexion, or extension, can result in significant neck injury.

On-Field Examination.—A player with a neck injury should not be removed from the field until the nature of the injury is determined. Airway, breathing, and circulation should be continually monitored. Serious injury is assumed if the patient has lost consciousness. The neck must be stabilized in such patients. It is important to remember that a significant neck injury may occur without pain, spasm, or tenderness. A backboard is used without neck manipulation in the case of neurologic symptoms. The cervical examination can start once motor and sensory deficits have been ruled out for any athlete not requiring a backboard (Fig 2–1).

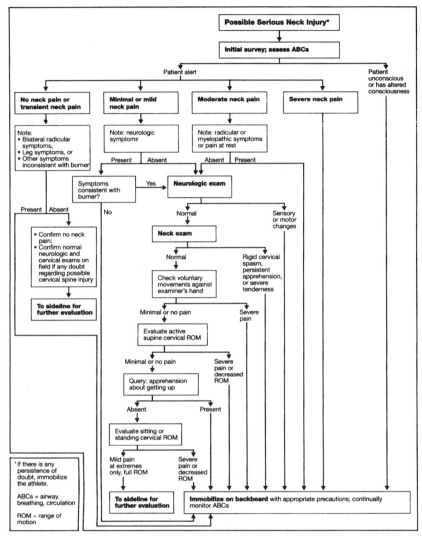

Fig 2–1.—On-field process of assessing neck injuries. (Courtesy of Anderson C: *Physician Sportsmed* 21:23–34, 1993.)

Return to Play and Follow-Up.—To return to play, an athlete must have a normal neurologic examination with emphasis on full, pain-free cervical range of motion and normal sensation, strength, and reflexes. The player is kept out of activity if any deficits are identified. Appropriate follow-up can vary widely, depending on the specific situation.

Prevention.—Rule changes and improvements in technique can help to prevent serious neck injuries in athletes. Strengthening before the season, use of protective equipment, and awareness of this risk of injury should all be encouraged. Finally, physicians, trainers, and coaches need to prepare for possible injuries by having appropriate personnel and equipment on-site.

▶ Abstracts 139-94-2-3 through 139-94-2-5 discuss emergency tech- niques that should be followed. Thankfully, the vast majority of cervical injuries are not serious or life-threatening, but they do pose a dilemma when making the decision to allow the athlete to return to participation. The author discusses guidelines to follow when making this decision. Also discussed are methods of preventing these injuries. The teaching of proper techniques is very, very important. Coaches should avoid teaching any technique that would jeopardize the head or cervical spine. *In football, an athlete must never be taught to use the helmet or face mask as the initial point of contact.*—F.J. George, A.T.C., P.T.

Spear Tackler's Spine: An Entity Precluding Participation in Tackle Football and Collision Activities That Expose the Cervical Spine to Axial Energy Inputs
Torg JS, Sennett B, Pavlov H, Leventhal MR, Glasgow SG (Univ of Pennsylvania, Philadelphia; Hosp for Special Surgery, New York; Campbell Clinic, Memphis, Tenn)
Am J Sports Med 21:640–649, 1993   139-94-2-6

Objective.—In previous work, criteria for the return to contact sports after cervical spine injuries were established after analysis of more than 1,500 tackle football injuries. Spear tackler's spine was established as a

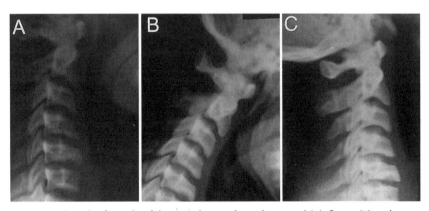

Fig 2–2.—Lateral radiographs of the cervical spine obtained in neutral (**A**), flexion (**B**), and extension (**C**) show reversal of the normal cervical lordosis, fixed from C2 to C6 in all positions. Extension is extremely limited. The C5-C6 interspace is narrowed, with deformity of the inferior endplate of C5, consistent with a Schmorl's node. The spinal canal is narrowed. (Courtesy of Torg JS, Sennett B, Pavlov H, et al: *Am J Sports Med* 21:640–649, 1993.)

distinct clinical entity and an absolute contraindication to return to tackle football and similar collision activities.

Background.—The cervical spine is repeatedly exposed to potentially injurious energy inputs during collision activities such as tackle football. Axial loading, implicated as the primary mechanism producing severe cervical spine injuries in this sport, occurs when the neck is slightly flexed and the normal cervical lordosis is straightened. At impact, the head is stopped, the trunk continues to move, and the cervical spine is crushed between the two. Spearing and the deliberate use of the top of the helmet as the initial point of contact have been banned in high school and college football, significantly decreasing the incidence of permanent cervical quadriplegia and cervical spine fractures. During the period from 1987 to 1990, however, 15 cases of spear tackler's spine were identified.

Methods.—Data obtained on the 15 patients included the mechanism of injury, sequential radiographic findings, initial neurologic complaints, management, and final neurologic status. All patients demonstrated the following findings: developmental narrowing of the cervical canal; persistent straightening or reversal of the normal cervical lordotic curve on erect lateral radiographs obtained in the neutral position (Fig 2–2); preexisting post-traumatic radiographic abnormalities of the cervical spine; and documentation of the use of spear tackling techniques.

Results.—Each of the football players initially was seen with complaints referable to the cervical spine, cord, or brachial plexus. Four patients subsequently sustained injuries resulting in permanent neurologic deficit. Eleven of the players had complete neurologic recovery but were precluded from further participation in contact activities. Seven had no specific treatment, 3 received cervical orthoses, and 1 underwent C3-4 anterior diskectomy and anterior fusion.

Conclusion.—Spear tackler's spine, as identified in this study, should preclude an individual from participation in collision activities such as tackle football, rugby, and ice hockey. These individuals are at risk of permanent neurologic injury from exposure of the cervical spine to axial energy inputs.

Upper Trunk Brachial Plexopathy: The Stinger Syndrome
Markey KL, Di Benedetto M, Curl WW (San Antonio, Tex; Univ of Virginia, Charlottesville; Wake Forest Univ, Winston-Salem, NC)
Am J Sports Med 21:650–655, 1993   139-94-2-7

Introduction.—Upper trunk brachial plexopathy, an injury referred to as a "stinger" or a "burner," is common among players of contact sports. A number of mechanisms and various treatments have been proposed for this injury. The cause of "stinger syndrome," or upper trunk brachial plexopathy, was determined.

Patients and Methods.—Between 1978 and 1982 at the United States Military Academy (USMA), most of these injuries were found among football players. In many cases the peripheral nerves as well as the brachial plexus were involved. Alterations of the protective shoulder pads or having the players wear high-riding pads decreased the incidence of the stinger syndrome. A 4-phase study of 261 tackle football players was undertaken to investigate the lesion. Fourteen players who appeared to have symptoms of brachial plexus injury and 18 additional football players underwent electromyography and nerve root stimulation studies. To test the hypothesis of the compressive nature of brachial plexus injuries, a total-contact neck-shoulder-chest orthosis was fashioned from thermoplastic material.

Results.—Relative to controls (USMA admission posture photographs), symptomatic players had a dropped or depressed shoulder. Atrophy of the supraspinous or deltoid muscle could be detected in some patients. Electromyographic analysis showed an increased amount of polyphasic waves. Evaluation of the musculocutaneous nerve supported the assumption that the lesion was at or near Erb's point, proximal to the site of actual supraclavicular fossa stimulation. Symptoms did not correlate with radiographic studies, grip strength, or neck size. Nerve conduction abnormalities, however, appeared to be related to symptoms of the syndrome. The orthosis was modified and has reduced the number of episodes of stingers.

Conclusion.—The stinger injury in football may be the only classic presentation of a compressive or percussive plexopathy or neuropathies of the upper extremity. The location of this lesion has been placed at Erb's point in the upper trunk of the brachial plexus, with frequent involvement of the accessory nerve at the superficial area in the neck. An orthosis may be effective in reducing the severity and recurrence of this injury.

► This is an excellent paper dealing with both the pathophysiology and prevention of neurapraxic injuries to the brachial plexus that occur in tackle football. The authors have correctly theorized that stingers or burners caused by mechanical insult to the brachial plexus result from compression rather than traction. In vitro studies in the bioengineering laboratories at the University of Pennsylvania have demonstrated that compressive deformation of a substance with a low modulus of rigidity actually results in elongation at the involved site. Our findings certainly substantiate the position of Markey et al. that "the pathophysiology of minor stretch versus percussion injury to a nerve may be indistinguishable except for the extent of the lesion." I also agree with the observation that a total-contact neck-shoulder-chest orthosis is effective in protecting against the stinger syndrome.—J.S. Torg, M.D.

Vertebral Ring Apophysis Injury in Athletes: Is the Etiology Different in the Thoracic and Lumbar Spine?

Swärd L, Hellström M, Jacobsson B, Karlsson L (East Hosp, Göteborg, Sweden; Univ of Göteborg, Sweden)
Am J Sports Med 21:841–845, 1993   139-94-2-8

Study Population.—The nature of apophyseal abnormalities in the thoracolumbar spine was studied in young male athletes (30 wrestlers, 26 gymnasts, 31 soccer players, and 30 tennis players), 26 female gymnasts, and 30 nonathletic men. The athletes were competitive at a high level. The men had a mean age of 20 years, and the women, 16 years.

Classification.—Apophyseal abnormalities were categorized as excavation of the apophyseal region (Fig 2–3), excavation with persisting apophysis, a persisting apophysis alone (Fig 2–4), or enlargement of the apophyseal region.

Findings.—Apophyseal abnormalities were seen only in athletes and were most prevalent in the wrestlers and female gymnasts. A persisting apophysis without excavation was always found at L2–L4. Most vertebrae with excavation were in the lower thoracic spine, particularly at T10. The caudal apophyses were most often involved in the lower thoracic spine, whereas in the lumbar spine, the cranial apophyses were affected. Two athletes, a tennis player and a female gymnast, had a displaced posterior caudal apophysis of L4.

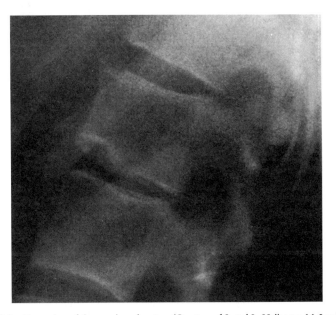

Fig 2–3.—Excavation of the apophyseal region. (Courtesy of Swärd L, Hellström M, Jacobsson B, et al: *Am J Sports Med* 21:841–845, 1993.)

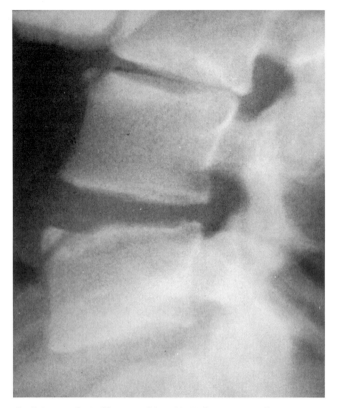

Fig 2–4.—Persisting apophysis. (Courtesy of Swärd L, Hellström M, Jacobsson B, et al: *Am J Sports Med* 21:841–845, 1993.)

Mechanisms.—Abnormalities of the anterior part of the vertebral ring apophysis appear to represent effects of trauma. In the lower thoracic and thoracolumbar regions, compression force probably is responsible, producing excavation with or without a persistent apophysis. In the lumbar spine, it is likely that traction force results in separation of the anterior part of the ring apophysis. This appears as a persisting apophysis or, after healing, as enlargement of the apophyseal region.

▶ This paper nicely defines the abnormalities involving the anterior aspect of the vertebral ring apophysis. It appears, however, that the biomechanical explanations for these abnormalities are at best conjectural.—J.S. Torg, M.D.

Percutaneous Discectomy in Athletes
Sakou T, Masuda A, Yone K, Nakagawa M (Kagoshima Univ, Japan)
Spine 18:2218–2221, 1993   139-94-2–9

Background.—Lumbar disk herniation is often the result of sports injury in young and middle-aged patients. When conservative therapy fails to relieve pain, surgery may be indicated. Percutaneous diskectomy is becoming the procedure of choice for this condition because it is simple and has few complications. However, the results of surgery have not been well studied when athletes who want to return to their sport are involved.

Materials and Methods.—Each probe had 2 sizes of dilators and a nucleotome tip containing an electric rotary shaver. These were used to remove 2–3 g of disk material from the center of the disk space in 543 patients, 13 of whom were athletes. The L4–L5 disk was repaired in 9 of these patient-athletes, the L5–S1 in 3, and both disk spaces were operated on in 1 patient. Patients were followed up for 2.3–3.9 years. The postoperative results were evaluated by Macnab's classification and the return of patients to their sport.

Results.—By Macnab's classification, the surgery produced excellent results in 4 patients, good results in 5, and poor results in 4. The 4 athletes with poor results ultimately underwent partial laminectomy. The 9 patients with acceptable results all returned to their sports; 4 of them returned to their former level of activity. The 10 patients who returned to sports activity began training 4 weeks after surgery, reaching stable levels of activity in 1–6 months. Roentgenographic studies showed that the disk space had narrowed after surgery in 18% of patients who underwent operation. Protrusion into the spinal canal was visibly reduced in 8 patients.

Discussion.—The technique of percutaneous diskectomy was validated. Its benefit lies largely in the minimal invasion of tissue, particularly of the neural tissue. This allows the procedure to be performed under local anesthesia and promotes the rapid return of athletes to sports activity.

Comparison of Operative Results of Lumbar Disc Herniation in Manual Laborers and Athletes

Matsunaga S, Sakou T, Taketomi E, Ijiri K (Kagoshima Univ, Japan)
Spine 18:2222–2226, 1993   139-94-2–10

Background.—In treating cases of lumbar disk herniation, either disk excision or 1 of several other treatment methods may be used. The results of a number of such procedures were evaluated. In addition, the limitations of the procedures in terms of the patient's ability to tolerate relatively high levels of mechanical stress were investigated.

Materials and Methods.—Eighty-two patients, 70 male and 12 female laborers, with herniated disks who complained of radicular pain and who engaged in activities that stressed the lower lumbar region had 1 of 3 procedures. These included 51 who had percutaneous diskectomy, 30 who had simple disk excision, and 29 who had disk excision followed by fusion of the involved spinal vertebrae. All the patients were followed up for at least 2 years after surgery; those who had the latter 2 treatments were followed up for at least 6 years.

Results.—When the simple disk excision group was compared with the spinal fusion group, the rates of return to manual labor were 53% and 89%, respectively. At 1 year, 75% of the simple disk excision group had returned to work; however, many laborers found it difficult to continue and eventually left work or changed their work because of fatigue in the lumbar region. Percutaneous diskectomy was associated with a shorter duration of illness before surgery and less narrowing of the intervertebral space after surgery; patients undergoing this procedure returned to work much faster than the others, but only at a rate of 58%.

Among 28 serious athletes also studied, 87% who had percutaneous diskectomy returned to their sport an average of 7.5 weeks after surgery, a better rate than for those undergoing simple excision (54%). Advancing age was associated with a poorer return-to-work rate after surgery; the best results for older patients were obtained with lumbar fusion.

Discussion.—Simple disk excision gives relatively poor results in patients whose work entails mechanical stress. This is probably because of physiologic dysfunction.

▶ These 2 papers (Abstracts 139-94-2–9 and 139-94-2–10) support the findings of Maroon et al. (1) that a percutaneous diskectomy is effective in the management of lumbar disk herniations in athletes. As pointed out, there are several advantages to this technique. It can be performed under local anesthesia, it has minimal violation of soft tissue, and the procedure is entirely outside the spinal canal without involvement of the dura mater or nerve root. It should be noted that the authors have developed a disk probe with an electric rotary shaver with an external diameter of 3 mm for this operation.—J.S. Torg, M.D.

Reference

1. Maroon JC, et al: *Physician Sportsmed* 16:61, 1988.

Systematic Evaluation of Brachial Plexus Injuries
Haynes S (Delaware SportsCare Physical Therapy, Inc, Newark)
J Athletic Train 28:263–267, 1993   139-94-2–11

Background.—Brachial plexus injuries are the most frequent nervous system injury found in football players, yet they are the least understood of cervical injuries. A systematic approach to evaluation of players is important for ensuring proper treatment.

Evaluation.—As with any injury, evaluation should start with ABCs (assessment of airway, breathing, and circulation). History-taking and observation then follow. This should include a description of the problem, including details about pain, mechanism of the injury regarding the position of head, neck, and arms, and assessment of neurologic symptoms. Palpation can be used to investigate tenderness, swelling, deformity, crepitation, warmth, pulses, muscle spasms, and the integrity of neurologic pathways.

The examination should start with the cervical spine to rule out spinal injury. The clavicle and shoulder should be palpated to rule out dislocation or fracture. The most common site of pain in brachial plexus injuries is tenderness in the upper trapezius. Finally, note any pain or motor loss in the normal ranges of movement, apply passive overpressure to the neck to assess the integrity of all structures, and carry out a compression test to check for nerve root irritation. The strength of all the major muscle groups should be tested before returning to play. Sensation can be checked by bilaterally rubbing the dermatomes to see whether one side feels different from the other.

Return-to-Play Criteria.—The athlete should have full, pain-free range of motion in the cervical spine. Full, pain-free neck strength and power to shoulders and arms should be obtained, and there should be normal sensation in all dermatomes. Finally, measures should be taken to prevent recurrence, such as checking helmet and pads, and beginning rehabilitation focused at strengthening the neck and shoulders.

▶ As the author states, we encounter a significant number of these injuries in football. Prevention is a major factor and all football players should be taught proper blocking and tackling techniques. They should never be instructed to use the face mask or helmet as the initial point of contact. In-season and out-of-season conditioning programs should emphasize neck and shoulder strengthening exercises. Before an athlete is allowed to return to participation after this injury he must exhibit complete, pain-free range of motion, normal strength, and no residual numbness or paresthesia.

We have tried just about every protective collar, pad, shoulder pad addition, and helmet strap that has come on the market. If the athlete does not recover completely from the initial injury, I have yet to find a protective device that will prevent the recurrence of this injury.—F.J. George, A.T.C., P.T.

Anterior Subcutaneous Transfer of the Ulnar Nerve in the Athlete
Rettig AC, Ebben JR (Methodist Sports Medicine Ctr, Indianapolis, Ind)
Am J Sports Med 21:836–840, 1993   139-94-2-12

Background.—Ulnar neuritis at the elbow, which responds poorly to conservative treatment, is a common diagnosis in athletes. The surgical alternatives currently used include simple decompression, subcutaneous anterior transfer, submuscular transfer, and medial epicondylectomy. Submuscular transfer has also been advocated for the treatment of this condition. The effectiveness of a subcutaneous subfascial transfer technique was evaluated in treating ulnar neuritis at the elbow.

Method.—A retrospective study was carried out on 20 active athletes who, having failed to respond to conservative treatment of ulnar neuritis, underwent subcutaneous ulnar nerve transfer. Preoperatively, all patients experienced paresthesia in the distribution of the ulnar nerve. Eight patients complained of a popping sensation in the medial epicondyle, and 5 described subjective weakness. Nineteen months after surgery, all patients completed a questionnaire to evaluate their elbow postoperatively with regard to pain, paresthesia, strength, mechanical symptoms, and overall function. A maximum of 20 points was given for each of the following categories: pain, numbness, and mechanical symptoms. A maximum of 10 points was given for strength, and 30 points for activity level. The patients were also asked to rate the elbow on a scale of 0 to 10, with 0 being worse than before surgery, 5 being no change, and 10 being excellent.

Results.—Nineteen of the 20 patients reported being symptom-free, or they had only minor infrequent pain or paresthesia that did not interfere with athletic activity 19 months after surgery. The average time for return to sports was 12.6 weeks. On a 20-point scale, with 20 representing a pain-free elbow, the patients rated their pain an average of 16. They rated numbness an average of 18 (where 0 represented persistent symptoms and 20 represented no symptoms). Mechanical symptoms were rated at a mean of 16, and average strength at 8. Finally, assessing overall activity, patients rated an average score of 26 on a 30-point scale. Ten patients scored 30, indicating no limitations. When patients were asked to rate their elbow overall on a scale of 0 to 10, the average score was 9. There were no complaints of deterioration or lack of improvement among the group.

Conclusion.—Good results can be obtained from both subcutaneous subfascial and submuscular ulnar nerve transfer in athletes. Subcutaneous subfascial ulnar nerve transfer is a reasonable alternative procedure that brings improved morbidity, rapid rehabilitation, and a high success rate in athletes with ulnar neuritis at the elbow.

▶ The authors' observations regarding the effectiveness of anterior subcutaneous transfer of the ulnar nerve in the athlete are credible. However, several shortcomings of the report bear pointing out. Preoperative nerve conduction studies were not obtained. This study was retrospective in nature without a control series. Most important, the pathology, if any, involving the nerve was not described.—J.S. Torg, M.D.

The Sports Hernia: A Cause of Chronic Groin Pain
Hackney RG (Princess Mary's Hosp, Royal Air Force Halton, Aylesbury,

Bucks, England)
Br J Sports Med 27:58–62, 1993   139-94-2-13

Introduction.—Chronic groin pain in athletes may be associated with a weakness of the posterior inguinal wall without a clinically recognizable hernia. Presentation is varied, and the condition does not respond well to conservative measures. Success has been achieved with surgical treatment of the sports hernia.

Patients and Methods.—The patients were 14 men and 1 woman who ranged in age from 18 to 38 years. The average duration of their symptoms before operation was 20 months. Conservative treatment, including rest, physiotherapy, and steroid injections, had failed to bring relief from pain. The decision to operate was initially based on patient history and findings of the physical examination. Recently, patients have also undergone a CT herniogram to attempt to discover the source of pain. The pain of a sports hernia is typically worse on one side, but it radiates laterally and across the midline, down the inside of the thigh into the adductor area, and, in men, into the scrotum and testicle. Adductor stretch is usually painful and the symphysis pubis is tender.

Results.—At operation, all patients had a weakening of the transversalis fascia with separation from the conjoined tendon. In 1 patient, the weakness amounted to a direct hernia. The internal ring was dilated and the inferior epigastric vessels were often clearly visible. Return to training begins gradually after surgery. Patients can start running at 4–5 weeks and daily training at 6 weeks. With a minimum follow-up of 18 months, these patients achieved a better than 80% return to full activity. The 2 patients who did not have an excellent result with surgery subsequently underwent adductor tenotomy and are optimistic about returning to full sports activity.

Conclusion.—Surgical repair to the posterior inguinal wall can relieve chronic groin pain in patients with sports hernia. This injury appears to be an overuse syndrome and has an extensive differential diagnosis. Many of these athletes had consulted a number of specialists and failed to respond to other treatments.

▶ Unquestionably, chronic groin pain is one of the major nemeses confronting both athlete and physician. As this article points out, "the syndrome of a weakness of the posterior inguinal wall without a clinically recognized hernia causing chronic groin pain has not been widely appreciated." It would appear that correct diagnosis is contingent on a high index of suspicion on the part of the examiner, with the diagnosis being substantiated by a CT herniogram. Several surgeons in the United States are reporting gratifying results using intraperoneal endoscopic surgical repair.—J.S. Torg, M.D.

The Alcock Syndrome: Temporary Penile Insensitivity Due to Compression of the Pudendal Nerve Within the Alcock Canal

Oberpenning F, Roth S, Leusmann DB, van Ahlen H, Hertle L (Univ of Münster, Germany)
J Urol 151:423–425, 1994   139-94-2-14

Background.—Perineal or genital insensitivity is usually associated with neurologic disorders caused by trauma or vascular, inflammatory, or tumor-producing diseases. This insensitivity is usually permanent. However, 2 patients were seen with temporary penile insensitivity probably induced by pudendal nerve compression within the Alcock canal caused by bicycling.

Patients.—Both patients were seen after long-term bicycle riding. Penile sensitivity was completely lacking; no penile functions were affected. Medical history was unremarkable. Extensive physical and genitourinary examinations revealed no abnormalities. Ultrasound and MRI of the penis, testes, perineum, and pelvis detected no evidence of trauma or pathologic condition. Radiodiagnostics of the pelvis and spine excluded malformation or skeletal nerve compression. Results of urinalyses and uroflowmetry were normal. Neurologic examination ruled out polyneuropathy and produced normal function. The 2 patients received no treatment but refrained from cycling and the symptoms resolved at 4 and 7 weeks.

Discussion.—Other perineal stress symptoms among cyclists have been reported. It is reasonable to suppose that the mechanical stress could affect the gliding capability in the Alcock canal, causing nerve friction. In addition, the repeated leg movements may distend the pudendal nerve where it surrounds the sacrospinal ligament. Nerve compression below the symphysis may also be involved. Because complete and spontaneous resolution was observed, no treatment is necessary, except temporary suspension of cycling. A change of seat could be beneficial.

▶ This article presents an interesting observation with a plausible anatomical explanation. Certainly, the transient nature of the phenomenon is reassuring.—J.S. Torg, M.D.

Deep Peroneal-Nerve Injury as a Result of Arthroscopic Meniscectomy: A Case Report and Review of the Literature

Rodeo SA, Sobel M, Weiland AJ (Hosp for Special Surgery, New York; Beth Israel North Hosp, New York)
J Bone Joint Surg (Am) 75-A:1221–1224, 1993   139-94-2-15

Introduction.—A number of large retrospective studies of arthroscopy-related complications have reported rates ranging from less than 1% to approximately 8%. Neurologic injury associated with arthroscopy appears to be quite rare, however, and most cases have involved temporary neurapraxia of the saphenous nerve. Peroneal nerve injury was seen in 1 patient after a routine arthroscopic meniscectomy.

Case Report.—Man, 28, sustained a twisting injury to his right knee. He underwent arthroscopy 4 months later because of persistent pain and swelling. Partial medial and lateral meniscectomies were performed; an incomplete tear of the anterior cruciate ligament was not repaired. The patient noted numbness of the dorsum of the foot and severe weakness of the toe and ankle extensors on the night after the operation. When motor loss persisted, the patient underwent electromyography and nerve-conduction studies. Both studies indicated absence of function of the right deep peroneal nerve.

One year after the injury the patient underwent exploration of the common peroneal nerve. The nerve was scarred, with a neuroma at the level of the joint line. Intact fibers of the nerve were preserved and a segment of sural nerve was harvested to provide 2 nerve grafts to bypass the resected area of the peroneal nerve. One year after the operation, the patient had regained sensation in the first web space in the distribution of the deep peroneal nerve and had partially recovered ankle dorsiflexion and toe extension.

Summary.—This is the first reported case of peroneal nerve injury after a routine arthroscopic meniscectomy. The injury appears to have been caused by the penetration of an instrument through a tear in the posterolateral aspect of the joint capsule that had been created during the arthroscopy. To avoid such complications, the surgeon must have a thorough knowledge of the relevant anatomy and exercise caution when using motorized instruments in the posterolateral aspect of the knee.

▶ Although peroneal nerve palsy has been reported after lateral meniscal repair, this report appears to be the first such injury occurring after a routine arthroscopic meniscectomy. The authors note that "Flexion of the knee to 90 degrees when instruments are passed into or out of the posterolateral aspect of the knee may decrease the risk of nerve injury by causing posterior displacement of the peroneal nerve . . .".—J.S. Torg, M.D.

Peripheral Nerve Injuries in Athletes: Treatment and Prevention
Lorei MP, Hershman EB (Lenox Hill Hosp, New York)
Sports Med 16:130–147, 1993   139-94-2-16

Background.—Although peripheral nerve lesions are rare, they may seriously delay or preclude an athlete from returning to sports.

Diagnosis.—An extensive physical examination is required for diagnosis of peripheral nerve lesions. It is necessary to study the walk for gait abnormalities and to carry out a complete motor, sensory, and reflex examination of the area of interest. Palpation can be helpful in defining joint and bone abnormalities and local tenderness. Diagnosis can be confirmed by electrophysiologic testing, including electromyography and nerve conduction studies.

Shoulder Injuries.—Spinal accessory nerve injury may be caused by a blow to the neck, resulting in trapezius paralysis with sparing of the sternocleidomastoid muscle. Scapular winging may result from paralysis of the serratus anterior caused by palsy of the long thoracic nerve. Suprascapular nerve lesions can produce symptoms similar to those seen in patients with rotator cuff tears, with pain and weakness in the cuff area. Axillary nerve injury commonly followed anterior shoulder dislocation.

Elbow Injuries.—Weight lifters may experience musculocutaneous nerve palsy in the elbow, bringing weakness in the elbow flexors and dysesthesias of the lateral forearm. Pronator syndrome is a median nerve lesion that occurs in the proximal forearm. Posterior interosseous nerve entrapment occurring at the arcade of Frohse is found in tennis players, producing symptoms of weakness in the wrist and metacarpophalangeal extensors. Baseball pitchers experience ulnar neuritis at the elbow.

Wrist Injuries.—Carpal tunnel syndrome is a common sports injury caused by median nerve compression in the carpal tunnel. Bicyclists also experience paralysis of the ulnar nerve at the wrist, resulting in grip weakness and numbness of the ulnar 1.5 digits.

Thigh Injuries.—Common thigh injuries include lateral femoral cutaneous nerve palsy, bringing numbness over the anterior thigh but no power deficit. High-energy sports sometimes result in femoral nerve injury occurring secondary to an iliopsoas hematoma. Sciatic nerve lesions may point to a concomitant dislocated hip.

Leg Injuries.—A direct blow or traction can cause peroneal nerve injury, bringing foot drop and numbness of the dorsum of the foot. Deep and superficial peroneal nerve palsies can be secondary to an exertional compartment syndrome. Tarsal tunnel syndrome, caused by dorsiflexion of the ankle, is a compressive lesion of the posterior tibial nerve found in runners and climbers. Dancers tend to experience Morton's interdigital neuroma, which responds well to a metatarsal pad.

Conclusion.—Although prophylactic measures have limited success in these injuries, the vast majority are temporary and respond well to conservative therapy, providing they are recognized and treated early.

▶ This article is a comprehensive review of the subject matter. Noteworthy is the observation of the authors that "Prophylactic measures are only modestly successful." They also point out that the vast majority of peripheral nerve injuries are transient and respond well to conservative therapy.—J.S. Torg, M.D.

Magnetic Resonance Imaging in the Diagnosis of Suprascapular Nerve Syndrome

Gerscovich EO, Greenspan A (Univ of California, Davis, Sacramento)
Can Assoc Radiol J 44:307–309, 1993   139-94-2-17

Objective.—Suprascapular nerve syndrome is a rare diagnosis. In patients with this condition, compromise of the nerve somewhere along its path causes nonspecific pain in the shoulder, neck, and/or anterior chest. Atrophy of the supraspinatus and/or infraspinatus muscle is a late sequela. Magnetic resonance imaging was used to diagnose suprascapular nerve syndrome at an early stage.

Case Report.—Man, 50, had severe pain over his left shoulder after lifting furniture 2 weeks before. He had no apparent muscle atrophy or limitation of motion and no tenderness over the area of the rotator cuff insertion and suprascapular notch. Magnetic resonance imaging was performed to assess possible rotator cuff injury. The only MRI abnormality was a discrete, lobulated mass superior and posterior to the glenoid fossa and immediately lateral to the scapular spine, corresponding to the position of the spinoglenoid notch. The mass, which measured $3 \times 3 \times 1.5$ cm, was diagnosed as a ganglion causing early suprascapular nerve syndrome. The patient's symptoms resolved with 3 weeks of conservative therapy, consisting of nonsteroidal anti-inflammatory drugs and limited activity of the extremity.

Conclusion.—Magnetic resonance imaging can differentiate subscapular entrapment neuropathy from the long list of other causes of shoulder pain. The fine soft tissue detail provided by MRI allows early diagnosis of suprascapular nerve syndrome, before the certain but late sign of muscle atrophy appears.

▶ As the authors indicate and other case reports have documented, the presence of a suprascapular ganglion may be unrelated to suprascapular nerve syndrome. Clinical evaluation is key in evaluating shoulder disorders, and MRI is only one of the means of determining the etiology of shoulder pain. Treatment must be related to the patient's symptoms and not based solely on the MRI findings.—J.S. Torg, M.D.

Abdominal Trauma: Occult Injury May Be Life Threatening

Colucciello SA, Plotka M (Carolinas Med Ctr, Charlotte, NC; Golden Glades Regional Med Ctr, Miami, Fla)
Physician Sportsmed 21:33–43, 1993   139-94-2-18

Introduction.—Sports-related trauma may account for as many as 10% of all abdominal injuries. A direct blow to the abdomen or flank during contact sports may injure the kidney, spleen, liver, pancreas, or small bowel. A fall or collision in either contact or noncontact activities also may injure the abdomen. These injuries frequently are occult, and repeated assessment may be required to recognize potentially life-threatening injuries.

Initial Evaluation.—As in any acute injury, the airway and circulation are assessed at the outset. An object that is impaled in the abdomen should not be removed on the field. At best, a single abdominal examination is only 65% accurate in cases of blunt abdominal trauma. Neither visual inspection nor auscultation are helpful in most cases of abdominal injury. A tender upper abdomen should suggest the possibility of liver or splenic injury. The patient should be told to return for treatment immediately if nausea or vomiting develops, anorexia ensues, or abdominal pain increases.

Off-the-Field Diagnosis.—Plain radiographs have limited value in evaluating abdominal trauma, and laboratory studies by themselves cannot establish or exclude injury. A declining hematocrit may indicate intra-abdominal bleeding. The serum amylase is not a sensitive or specific indicator of pancreatic trauma. Peritoneal lavage is a sensitive test for blood at this site, but it does not tell how much blood is present. Computed tomography is a useful means of estimating the extent of organ injury and the degree of intraperitoneal bleeding. It is indicated, however, only in hemodynamically stable patients.

▶ The authors describe 4 diagnostic pitfalls that we should consider when evaluating abdominal injuries: (1) failure to consider the possibility of intra-abdominal injury; (2) overreliance on a single initially benign abdominal exam; (3) overreliance on normal labs to rule out intra-abdominal injury; (4) attributing abdominal tenderness to abdominal wall injury. They go on to state, "Careful serial examinations (both on-field and off), vigilance even in the face of normal laboratory findings, and judicious use of diagnostic studies remain the best defense against missed injury."—F.J. George, A.T.C., P.T.

Inguinal Mass in a College Football Player: A Case Study
Rich BSE, Hough DO, Monroe JS, Nogle S (Michigan State Univ, East Lansing)
Med Sci Sports Exerc 25:318–320, 1993   139-94-2–19

Background.—Although surgical correction of inguinal hernia in a football player was required, the athlete was able to delay treatment until the end of the season.

Case Report.—Man, 22, a college football player, was seen 2 weeks before the start of the fall season with a slight bulge in his right groin. He experienced minimal discomfort at times other than during football practice, and the bulge disappeared when he was supine. A general surgeon confirmed the diagnosis of indirect inguinal hernia. There was no evidence of strangulation or compromise of bowel contents. The athlete, the starting punter on his team, was allowed to participate through the fall football season with the use of a truss. He was also asked to wear an athletic supporter at all times and advised not to placekick. The player was able to complete the season without any complications and underwent successful surgical repair at season's end.

Discussion.—Certain sports may predispose athletes to the development of hernias. Inguinal hernias make up 80% of all hernias and occur most commonly on the right side. The indirect type of inguinal hernia accounts for 50% to 75% of all hernias and is most frequently seen in younger men. Patients should be aware of the signs and symptoms of impending strangulation, a life-threatening complication. After conventional surgical repair, 8–12 weeks of healing are required before return to contact sports. Laparoscopic repair in properly selected cases may allow return to contact sports in 7–10 days.

Conclusion.—Physicians who care for athletes must be knowledgeable about inguinal hernias and their potential complications. Although some surgeons recommend repair as soon as possible after diagnosis, conservative management and delay of surgery are possible in some cases, depending on the size of the hernia, type of sport, and degree of symptoms.

▶ This case report illustrates that an athlete with groin pain and an inguinal bulge may mistake a hernia for a muscle strain. It also shows that one need not necessarily operate immediately on even a large indirect inguinal hernia in a starting punter. Hernias may occur more commonly in sports that markedly increase intra-abdominal pressure, such as weight lifting or shot putting, or in sports that involve vigorous twisting, such as in a tennis serve, soccer, or discus throwing. I have also seen acute bilateral inguinal hernias in patients who attempt to pull up from the water in waterskiing.—E.R. Eichner, M.D.

An Unusual Presentation of Liver Laceration in a 13-Yr-Old Football Player
Stricker PR, Hardin BH, Puffer JC (Univ of California, Los Angeles; Arkansas Children's Hosp, Little Rock)
Med Sci Sports Exerc 25:667–672, 1993   139-94-2–20

Background.—Abdominal injuries can occur in sports, particularly football. Serious abdominal injuries may occur in patients with only mild symptoms. In most reports, left-sided trauma results in splenic injury and right-sided trauma results in hepatic injury. A football player with an unusual mechanism of injury and presentation was studied.

Case Report.—Boy, 13 years, was injured playing football when an opponent's shoulder pad struck him in the left side of the abdomen while he was returning a punt. He had hyperventilation and severe abdominal pain and nearly fainted when helped to his feet. He was pale, with rapid pulse and breathing on examination. He was guarding the left side of his abdomen, with marked tenderness to palpation over his left lower ribs and left upper quadrant.

In the hospital, the patient had clear lung fields despite marked pain on deep inspiration. Pulse oximetry was 95% on room air; hemoglobin was 13 g/dL^{-1}; hematocrit was 38.8%; serum amylase was normal; and urinalysis was negative for blood. There were no rib fractures on chest or rib radiographs. Subcapsular laceration of the spleen was suspected, and abdominal CT was performed. The only abnormality on the contrast-enhanced scan was an abnormal area of low density in the right hepatic lobe, which was consistent with the diagnosis of liver contusion and laceration.

The patient was admitted and placed on intravenously administered fluids. His blood pressure and other vital signs remained stable, and his hematocrit was down to 37.7% after 12 hours. As the patient was still hemodynamically stable the next day, he was discharged with instructions to minimize activity for 3 weeks. His condition was good at 1-week follow-up. He was restricted from participation in contact sports for the rest of the season.

Discussion.—Serious abdominal injuries can occur as a result of sports participation. The physician must be aware of the potential for such injuries, because failing to suspect them may lead to a poor outcome. The severity of injury cannot always be determined from the initial physical examination. Any athlete who has serious abdominal injury needs rapid assessment and transport for definitive evaluation and treatment.

▶ The abdomen is unprotected and, thus, prone to injury during contact sports. Abdominal injuries, in fact, account for up to 10% of all sports injuries in some surveys. Severity of injury can be greater than suggested by initial symptoms or initial physical examination. Sports medicine physicians, then, must be alert to the potential of catastrophic injury from abdominal trauma. The CT scan is the best diagnostic test, as shown here. This case is unusual in that the blow was to the left side, the pain was on the left side, no symptoms were present on the right side, and the abdomen was soft on the right side but guarding was noted on the left. As the authors state, "this injury may represent an abdominal 'contra-coup' injury, with transmission of the force vector through the liver." See also Abstract 139-94-2–21 on renal laceration.—E.R. Eichner, M.D.

Renal Laceration: A Skateboarder's Symptoms Are Delayed
Stricker PR, Puffer JC (Univ of California, Los Angeles)
Physician Sportsmed 21:59–68, 1993   139-94-2–21

Purpose.—The abdominal viscera, particularly the kidneys, spleen, and liver, are commonly injured in sports. Athletes with quite serious injuries sometimes show only minor symptoms. A case of rib fracture and renal laceration in a skateboarder was examined.

Case Report.—Man, 19, fell while skateboarding downhill, hitting the curb with the right side of his body. The accident was followed immediately by pain on the right side of the chest, aggravated by deep breathing. At the time of examination, he was splinting the chest on the right side, where he had a 9 × 10 cm abrasion. Palpation in the area and compression of the rib produced pain. Chest radiography demonstrated a nondisplaced fracture at the posterolateral angle of the right ninth rib. He was sent home with acetaminophen with codeine and instructed to return if he had difficulty breathing or abdominal pain. Two days later, he returned with painless hematuria with mild right upper quadrant pain and costovertebral angle tenderness. Once the patient was hemodynamically stable, he underwent CT, which revealed a laceration of the right renal cortex with a perinephric hematoma and an edematous but intact collecting system. The patient refused hospitalization. When he returned 4 weeks later, his urinalysis was normal and blood pressure was 130/82 mm Hg.

Conclusion.—Rib fracture and renal laceration are uncommon complications of skateboarding accidents. In cases such as this, serious abdominal injuries can occur with only minor symptoms. Patients with any type of marked injury to the abdomen or thorax need careful observation and evaluation to detect any potentially catastrophic injury.

▶ This case of "skateboarder's kidney" emphasizes that injury to the abdominal viscera that appears to be minor can be serious. For evaluation, CT scan "is preferred over intravenous pyelogram because it is quicker, noninvasive, and more accurate in quantifying blood loss, gauging the extent of the lesion, and determining urinary extravasation," as well as evaluating other abdominal organs. The American Academy of Pediatrics recommends wearing helmets and pads, prohibiting skateboards on streets and highways, and restricting their use to those older than 5 years of age. See also Abstract 139-94-2–20 on liver laceration in a football player.—E.R. Eichner, M.D.

3 Injuries of the Shoulder, Arm, and Hand

Shoulder Arthroscopy With the Use of Local Anesthesia
Sperber A, Wredmark T (Huddinge Hosp, Sweden)
J Shoulder Elbow Surg 2:106–109, 1993   139-94-3-1

Introduction.—Shoulder arthroscopy using local anesthesia has not been performed as widely as arthroscopy of the knee, elbow, or ankle. In the extremely vascular shoulder joint, there is a risk that high uptake of induced medications and extra-articular fluid extravasation might lead to toxic serum levels of local anesthetic. The safety and efficacy of performing diagnostic shoulder arthroscopy with local anesthesia were evaluated.

Patients and Methods.—Two groups of patients were assessed. In group 1, 17 patients had general anesthesia during arthroscopy of the shoulder. They also received a continuous infusion of .2% lidocaine-chloride. Seventeen other patients (group 2) had arthroscopy performed with local anesthesia. They received a continuous infusion of .2% lidocaine-chloride in addition to 20 mL of 1% prilocaine-epinephrine injected into the soft tissues on the posterior aspect of the shoulder. The last 8 patients in group 2 received adjunctive diazepam. Those in the general anesthesia group had operative diagnoses of anterior instability (13), rotator cuff syndromes (2), and multidirectional instability (2). Patients in the local anesthesia group were suspected of having intra-articular problems; all had vague symptoms and normal radiographs.

Results.—Significant intra-articular causes were identified in both groups. Labral lesions were seen in 8 group 1 patients and Bankart lesions were seen in 5. Five group 2 patients had fraying of the labrum. Arthroscopy changed the preliminary diagnosis in 5 of the 14 group 2 patients in whom the procedure could be completed. Most group 1 patients had peak serum level values 15–30 minutes after initiation of the infusion; levels gradually decreased to approximately 0 after 4 hours. Arthroscopy could not be completed because of pain in 3 of the group 2 patients who did not receive diazepam.

Conclusion.—Shoulder arthroscopy using local anesthetic is very demanding for both patient and surgeon. Any sensation of pain leads to immediate muscle contraction and makes capsule penetration difficult. However, when carefully performed, using the beach-chair position and a mild sedative, shoulder arthroscopy without general anesthesia is possible. The absorption pattern of lidocaine is similar to that seen in the knee joint, and serum concentrations are well below toxic levels.

▶ I am in complete agreement with the authors that arthroscopy of the shoulder can be carried out with local anesthesia and intravenous sedation. Carrying this concept a step further, we routinely perform surgical arthroscopic procedures (e.g., resection of the acromioclavicular, subacromial decompression, rotator cuff débridement, and the resection of labral tears) using local anesthesia. It should be emphasized that these procedures should be done with the patient in the beach-chair position, and the choice of intravenous sedation is crucial. Specifically, minimal doses of fentanyl are preferred. Such CNS-disinhibiting drugs as midazolam are to be avoided because of their propensity to cause involuntary muscle spasm.—J.S. Torg, M.D.

The Results of Arthroscopic Debridement of Glenoid Labral Tears Based on Tear Location
Payne LZ, Jokl P (Yale Univ, New Haven, Conn)
Arthroscopy 9:560–565, 1993   139-94-3–2

Objective.—An attempt was made to relate the long-term results of primary arthroscopic labral débridement to the location of tears in patients whose shoulders were stable preoperatively.

Patients.—Fourteen patients with stable glenohumeral joints underwent arthroscopic débridement of a primary labral tear, all by the same physician. They included 11 men and 3 women with an average age of 30.7 years. Various conservative measures, including steroid injections, had been tried. The average duration of symptoms was 34 months, and the average follow-up after débridement was 2 years.

Management.—The labrum was divided into 5 sections to locate the major portion of each tear. All tears were débrided back to a smooth, stable rim of remaining labrum. Range-of-motion exercises began within 1 week of the procedure and progressed in several weeks to rotator cuff–strengthening exercises.

Results.—All patients had a longitudinal labral tear in the anterior or superior region. A partial rotator cuff tear was débrided in 5 patients, and 2 had bony/cartilaginous loose bodies removed. At final follow-up, 71% of the patients had an excellent or good outcome. Half of the patients deteriorated functionally between 6 months and final follow-up because of increased pain on overhead activities. Three patients with large anterosuperior tears had anatomical shoulder instability more than

6 months after labral débridement. There were no wound problems, infections, or neurovascular injuries.

Conclusion.—Arthroscopic débridement of primary tears of the glenoid labrum can be expected to give excellent or good functional results after 1 year or longer in about 70% of the patients. Patients should be followed closely, however, because they are at risk of delayed glenohumeral instability.

Arthroscopic Treatment of Glenoid Labral Tears
Cordasco FA, Steinmann S, Flatow EL, Bigliani LU (Columbia-Presbyterian Med Ctr, NY)
Am J Sports Med 21:425–431, 1993   139-94-3-3

Background.—Lesions of the anterior glenoid labrum are frequently associated with shoulder instability. With the increasing use of shoulder arthroscopy, many investigators have reported labral damage. The outcomes of arthroscopic débridement of labral tears in patients without overt preoperative instability were evaluated.

Patients and Methods.—The case records of 52 consecutive patients who had arthroscopic labral débridement were reviewed. The patients were 35 men and 17 women (mean age, 29 years). At surgery, 27 patients had superior labrum anterior and posterior lesions, and 20 had anteroinferior labral lesions. The remaining 5 patients had posterior labral lesions. None of the patients had a history of dislocation or clinically evident instability before surgery. The mean follow-up was 36 months.

Outcomes.—Seventy percent of the patients with superior labral lesions and 100% of those with anteroinferior and posterior lesions had instability on examination under anesthesia. One year after arthroscopy, 78% of the patients with superior lesions and 30% with anteroinferior lesions had excellent relief. At 2 years, these percentages declined to 63% and 25%, respectively. Only 45% of patients with superior labral lesions and 25% with anteroinferior lesions returned to their previous athletic performance level. Additional surgery was needed in 4 patients—2 for instability and 2 for impingement.

Conclusion.—Patients with glenoid labral tears often have occult instability. Although overall the outcomes were not encouraging, the procedure described may be indicated for short-term goals in competitive athletes or in those willing to accept some functional compromise.

▶ The observations and conclusions noted in these 2 papers (Abstracts 139-94-3-2 and 139-94-3-3) are remarkably similar to those we have reached in the past (1).—J.S. Torg, M.D.

Reference

1. Glasgow SG, et al: *Arthroscopy* 8:48, 1992.

Arthroscopic Treatment of Full-Thickness Rotator Cuff Tears: 2- to 7-Year Follow-Up Study

Ellman H, Kay SP, Wirth M (Univ of California, Los Angeles; Univ of Texas, San Antonio)
Arthroscopy 9:195–200, 1993   139-94-3–4

Purpose.—Arthroscopic subacromial decompression (ASD) is an effective treatment for shoulder impingement syndrome, but its efficacy for full-thickness rotator cuff tears has not been determined. Selected patients with shoulder impingement syndrome that had progressed to a full-thickness rotator cuff tear were treated with ASD to determine its usefulness.

Methods.—During a 6-year period, 40 patients with full-thickness rotator cuff tears underwent ASD and cuff débridement. Only older, relatively sedentary patients who did not want to undergo major surgery were included in the study. When grouped by rotator cuff tear size, as measured during arthroscopic inspection, 10 patients (average age, 63 years) had fixable cuff tears of less than 2 cm; 8 patients (average age, 66.7 years) had fixable but larger cuff tears of 2–4 cm; and 22 patients (average age, 73.9 years) had irreparable cuff tears greater than 4 cm in length. The 35-point UCLA shoulder rating scale was used to assess pain, function, range of motion, strength in forward flexion, and patient satisfaction.

Results.—The ASD and débridement improved pain and function scores in 90% of patients with small, fixable cuff tears as reflected by good or excellent scores on the UCLA shoulder rating scale. Furthermore, 90% of these patients were satisfied with the outcome. Only 50% of patients with larger rotator cuff tears had satisfactory UCLA outcome scores, and only 62.5% of these patients were satisfied with the outcome. Only 40.9% of patients with large, irreparable cuff tears received satisfactory UCLA ratings, but 86.4% of these patients were satisfied with the outcome.

Conclusion.—For treating small rotator cuff tears in a carefully selected subset of patients, ASD with cuff débridement can be useful. Open surgical repair remains the most effective approach, even for small cuff tears.

▶ The results of this study correlate well with those of Gartsman (1). Specifically, patients with tears less than 2 cm did well whereas those with larger massive tears greater than 4 cm did least well. The discrepancy in Ellman's study between poor UCLA rating scales and satisfactory subjective results in patients with large tears is explained by the fact that patients with massive tears cannot score well on the UCLA shoulder rating scale because of weakness and limitation of motion.—J.S. Torg, M.D.

Reference

1. Gartsman G: *J Bone Joint Surg (Am)* 72-A:169, 1990.

The Diagnosis and Treatment of Anterior Instability in the Throwing Athlete
Kvitne RS, Jobe FW (Kerlan-Jobe Orthopaedic Clinic, Los Angeles; Univ of Southern California, Los Angeles)
Clin Orthop 291:107–123, 1993   139-94-3–5

Pathogenesis.—Overhand or throwing sports place the shoulder at risk of injury from repeated high-energy forces. Progressive damage to the stabilizing structures of the shoulder begins when the frequency of stress exceeds the ability of tissues to repair themselves. Static restraints are attenuated during continued throwing, promoting anterior glenohumeral subluxation. In time, the dynamic stabilizers become fatigued and the humeral head then may subluxate anteriorly, contact the coracoacromial arch, and lead to subacromial impingement. In addition, the tendinous parts of the supraspinatus and infraspinatus muscles may impinge on the posterosuperior border of the glenoid rim.

Diagnosis.—To determine the cause of shoulder pain in the throwing athlete, it is necessary to precisely assess shoulder stability. With the patient lying supine, the arm is positioned in 90 degrees of abduction and 90 degrees of external rotation, and anteriorly directed force is applied gently to the posterior humeral head. In the same position, a posteriorly directed force may be applied to the anterior aspect of the proximal humerus to distinguish between primary impingement and primary instability with secondary impingement. Radiography may reveal a bony defect within the posterior part of the humeral head or a deficiency of the anterior-inferior glenoid rim in patients with acute traumatic glenohumeral dislocation or chronic recurrent instability.

Treatment.—Conservative measures suffice in most patients with chronic overuse injuries. Relative rest is urged initially, and the patient is given oral nonsteroidal anti-inflammatory medication and a program of physical therapy. In addition, the rotator cuff and scapular rotators are strengthened. If surgery is required by a young throwing athlete with shoulder pain, anterior capsulolabral reconstruction usually is an appropriate procedure for instability or occult subluxation.

Rehabilitation.—Exercises begin on the first postoperative day and continue for 6–12 months. Active internal rotation exercises are begun when the arm can be actively abducted to 90 degrees. Strengthening exercises continue for 2 months after surgery. In most cases, strength, power, and endurance are normal within 8–12 months, at which time maximal performance is possible.

▶ This paper is a beautifully illustrated review dealing with the diagnosis and management of anterior instability in the throwing athlete. The original article is strongly recommended for the interested reader.—J.S. Torg, M.D.

Long-Term Followup of the Modified Bristow Procedure
Banas MP, Dalldorf PG, Sebastianelli WJ, DeHaven KE (Univ of Rochester, NY)
Am J Sports Med 21:666–671, 1993   139-94-3–6

Background.—The modified Bristow procedure has been popular for the past 20 years. However, its use as a primary treatment for anterior glenohumeral instability is increasingly being discouraged. The long-term outcome of the modified Bristow procedure was evaluated in 78 patients.

Patients.—Between 1975 and 1987, the patients underwent 86 modified Bristow procedures for anterior shoulder instability. Complete follow-up data were available for 71 patients with 79 treated shoulders (92%). Eight patients had bilateral procedures. The patients ranged in age from 16 to 42 years at the time of operation. Follow-up ranged from 2 to 13.7 years. Indications were recurrent subluxation in 35 shoulders and recurrent dislocation in 44 shoulders. The average time between the initial injury and operation was 35 months.

Results.—Three patients had traumatic postoperative redislocations that required revision surgery. Eight other patients (10%) required secondary operations for screw removal because of persistent shoulder pain at an average of 27 months after primary operation. At the follow-up examination, none of the patients had sensory deficits in the operated extremity. Postoperative subjective shoulder function averaged 86% of the preinjury level. The results were rated as excellent or very good by 62 patients (88%), good by 6 (9%) patients, and poor by 2 (3%) patients. The Rowe scale for shoulder reconstruction recorded the results as good or excellent in 40 shoulders (85%), fair in 4 (9%), and poor in 3 (6%). All throwing athletes were able to return to throwing, although 54% of those with dominant shoulder involvement reported a decrease in throwing velocity.

Conclusion.—The modified Bristow procedure provides excellent long-term stability, satisfactory shoulder function, and minimal loss of internal and external rotation.

▶ The reported postsurgical redislocation rate of 4% with a postoperative follow-up of 8.6 years (range, 2–13.7 years) compares favorably with our initial report of the results of a modified Bristow procedure in 212 shoulders with a redislocation rate of 3.8% with a mean follow-up of 9 years (range, 2–11 years) (1). Subsequent evaluation of our group of patients revealed that with a follow-up of 12 years (range, 4.7–18 years), the number of postsurgical dislocations increased from 8 to 22 (10%). The conclusion that we draw from this is that the Bristow procedure does not appear to withstand the test of time. In addition to reported dislocations, Banas et al. report an additional 9 patients who experienced episodes of apparent subluxation, which means that they in fact had a 15% recurrent postoperative instability rate.—J.S. Torg, M.D.

Reference

1. Torg JS, et al: *J Bone Joint Surg (Am)* 69-A:904, 1987.

Arthroscopic Versus Open Bankart Procedures: A Comparison of Early Morbidity and Complications
Green MR, Christensen KP (Tripler Army Med Ctr, Hawaii)
Arthroscopy 9:371–374, 1993   139-94-3-7

Objective.—Arthroscopic Bankart repair to suture detached labra to the glenoid in patients wtih anterior shoulder instability is producing excellent results with few complications and minimal loss of motion. The morbidity associated with open vs. arthroscopic Bankart repair was compared retrospectively.

Methods.—Between 1988 and 1990, 38 patients with anterior shoulder instability underwent reattachment of the labrum to the glenoid. Twenty patients had arthroscopic Bankart repairs and 18 underwent open Bankart procedures. The factors measured and compared for this analysis included operative time, blood loss, narcotic use, hospital stay, days missed from work, and overall complications.

Results.—Arthroscopic Bankart repair was associated with a statistically significant reduction in all measured parameters. Three patients in the open surgery group had postoperative complications; there were none in the arthroscopic treatment group.

Conclusion.—The arthroscopic Bankart procedure is a safe alternative to open techniques in the treatment of anterior shoulder instability. The technique can be done on an outpatient basis, and it offers other important advantages when compared with the open Bankart procedure.

▶ The authors conclude that the arthroscopic Bankart procedure offers significant improvements in operative time, perioperative morbidity, and complications compared with the open technique. There are, however, two major problems with this study. First, it is basically a retrospective chart review. Second, the interval from surgery to follow-up is not stated. In that most procedures for anterior glenohumeral instability, either arthroscopic or open, failed to withstand the test of time, the results of this report must be viewed accordingly.—J.S. Torg, M.D.

Loss of External Rotation Following Anterior Capsulorrhaphy of the Shoulder

Lusardi DA, Wirth MA, Wurtz D, Rockwood CA Jr (United States Air Force Med Ctr, Lackland Air Force Base, San Antonio, Tex; Univ of Texas Health Science Ctr, San Antonio)
J Bone Joint Surg (Am) 75–A:1185–1192, 1993   139-94-3–8

Objective.—The rate of recurrent dislocation is the most commonly used criterion for failure of a surgical procedure for anterior instability of the shoulder. Other criteria have been identified as well, including excessively tight repair resulting in loss of motion. A retrospective study of 19 patients managed for loss of external rotation after reconstructive procedures for anterior glenohumeral instability was reported.

Patients.—The analysis included 20 shoulders in 19 patients who were treated surgically for severe loss of external rotation of the glenohumeral joint after anterior capsulorrhaphy for recurrent instability. Range of motion was restricted in all patients, and the shoulder was painful in 17. Posterior subluxation or dislocation of the humeral head was present in 7 cases, and mild-to-severe glenohumeral osteoarthrosis affected 16 shoulders.

Management consisted of anterior soft tissue release via a deltopectoral approach in all cases (Fig 3–1). A double thickness of the weakened capsule was created by advancing the lateral aspect of the capsule over the medial aspect. Any capsular defect was repaired with Dacron tape. Total arthroplasty was performed at the same time in 8 patients and

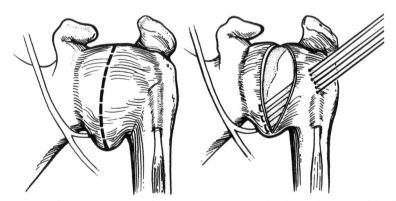

Fig 3–1.—Schematic drawings showing the operative technique for the anterior release. **Left,** after identification and protection of the axillary nerve, the capsule is divided vertically, midway between the glenoid and the humeral attachment, from top to bottom. **Right,** the medial aspect of the capsule is overlapped laterally and superiorly under the lateral aspect of the capsule. (Courtesy of Lusardi DA, Wirth MA, Wurtz D, et al: *J Bone Joint Surg (Am)* 75-A:1185–1192, 1993.)

hemiarthroplasty was done in 1 patient. Patients were followed up for an average of 4 years.

Outcomes.—Pain and range-of-motion scores improved in all 20 joints. No patient had more than mild pain, and all 10 shoulders with preoperative instability became stable. External rotation increased by an average of 45 degrees. There was no evidence of postoperative progressive osteoarthrosis in patients who had only mild or no degenerative changes at the time of presentation.

Conclusion.—Patients undergoing anterior reconstruction of the shoulder are at risk of limited external rotation. Operative release should be considered for patients with 0 degrees or less of external rotation at 6 months after anterior reconstruction. Patients without extensive osteoarthrosis can have soft tissue release alone to restore external rotation; those with more severe osteoarthrosis should also have shoulder arthroplasty.

▶ It should be noted that after the anterior release as described, no patient had symptoms consistent with recurrent anterior instability.—J.S. Torg, M.D.

Long-Term Results of Staple Capsulorrhaphy for Anterior Instability of the Shoulder
O'Driscoll SW, Evans DC (Mayo Clinic and Found, Rochester, Minn; Univ of Toronto)
J Bone Joint Surg (Am) 75–A:249–258, 1993   139-94-3–9

Objective.—Short-term results after open staple capsulorrhaphy of the shoulder have been encouraging, with a 90% to 97% success rate and few complications. The long-term results and complications of staple capsulorrhaphy of the shoulder were obtained.

Patients.—Between 1967 and 1986, 192 patients underwent 204 open staple capsulorrhaphies for recurrent anterior instability of the shoulder, including 88% with recurrent dislocations and 12% with recurrent subluxations. Stapling was combined with a Putti-Platt procedure in one third of the shoulders; a muscle-splitting approach was used in the others. The mean duration of follow-up was 10 years (range, 2–22 years).

Outcome.—Postoperative instability, either as dislocations or subluxations, occurred in 22% of patients, with recurrent episodes in more than half of these shoulders. One half of the failures occurred in the first 2 years, and the frequency of recurrence of instability increased logarithmically with the duration of follow-up, with a 30% failure rate by 20 years. Postoperative instability occurred significantly more often in shoulders that had stapling alone (29%), compared with those in which a modified Putti-Platt procedure had been added (8%). Loosening or migration of a staple or penetration of the articular cartilage by a staple occurred in 12% of shoulders, and the staple was removed in 9%. The rate of loosening or migration of barbed staples did not differ significantly from that of nonbarbed staples, but incorrect placement of staples was associated with a higher rate of recurrent instability. Pain, physical restrictions, and osteoarthrosis occurred more frequently in patients who had complications associated with a staple. Patients with a complication associated with a staple had greater reduction in average ranges of internal and external rotation than did patients without such complications.

Most patients (84% of the shoulders) believed that the operation had been worthwhile. However, half the shoulders were painful and 50% were different enough from normal to affect the patient's quality of life. In 6% of the shoulders, problems with the shoulder that had not been present before surgery caused patients to change occupations.

Conclusion.—Staple capsulorrhaphy for anterior instability of the shoulder is associated with unacceptably high rates of recurrent instability and serious or potentially serious complications associated with the staple. Hence, even when it is augmented by a Putti-Platt procedure, staple capsulorrhaphy is not recommended for anterior instability of the shoulder.

▶ This paper reiterates the well-recognized fact that open staple capsulorrhaphy of the glenohumeral joint for anterior stability has an unacceptable recurrence rate. In view of this, the question can be asked, if an open staple procedure does not withstand the test of time, why should the current arthroscopic stapling procedures perform differently?—J.S. Torg, M.D.

Arthroscopic Bankart Suture Repair
Grana WA, Buckley PD, Yates CK (Univ of Oklahoma, Oklahoma City; Marsh Brook Professional Ctr, Somersworth, NH)
Am J Sports Med 21:348–353, 1993   139-94-3-10

Background.—The Bankart lesion is a separation of the glenohumeral ligament–labrum complex from the anterior glenoid rim and scapular neck. Open repairs of this injury are accompanied by anterior shoulder scarring, which may be responsible for decreased laxity. Experience with an arthroscopic technique to repair the Bankart lesion was reported. An attempt was made to reproduce the results of open repair without its surgical morbidity and inherent loss of external rotation.

Patients and Methods.—Twenty-seven patients (average age, 21.7 years) underwent arthroscopic suture stabilization of anterior shoulder instability. None had previous surgery for the problem, radiographic evidence of significant loss of glenoid bone stock, or instability that was multidirectional or voluntary. Sixteen patients had dislocations and 11 had subluxation. Instability was acute in 4 patients and chronic in 23. Patients were followed for at least 12 months, and 70% were followed for more than 24 months. Reduction of the Bankart lesion was followed by a 3-week period of immobilization. Active range-of-motion and progressive resistive exercises were initiated at 3 and 6 weeks.

Results.—There were no complications related to the surgery. At arthroscopy, 13 patients had an associated Hill-Sachs lesion of the humeral head. A clinical evaluation rated outcome as excellent in 10 patients, good in 5, and poor in 12. Fourteen patients were able to return to their previous level of activity. No patient lost more than 15 degrees of external rotation. The repair failed in 12 patients at an average of 15 months after arthroscopy. In 9 cases, failure followed a significant trauma. Eight of these patients had not complied with the required 3 weeks of immobilization. Ten shoulders redislocated and 2 had recurrence of subluxation.

Conclusion.—The high failure rate of arthroscopic Bankart suture repair does not recommend the procedure, particularly in competitive athletes. A second surgery and rehabilitation after failed arthroscopy might mean the loss of additional sports participation. Success with the procedure was associated with the presence of a severe labral tear or bony Bankart lesions and compliance with immobilization.

▶ The authors attribute their 44% surgical failure rate to the inability of the procedure to address the plastic deformation that occurs in the glenohumeral ligament–labrum complex. I would agree with their statement that "until a technique is documented to correct this damage as precisely and reliably as an open reconstruction does, it cannot be recommended for general use."—J.S. Torg, M.D.

Suture Anchor Failure Strength: An In Vivo Study
Barber FA, Cawley P, Prudich JF (Plano Orthopedic and Sports Medicine Ctr, Tex; DonJoy Biomechanics Research Lab, Carlsbad, Calif; McKinney, Tex)
Arthroscopy 9:647–652, 1993   139-94-3–11

Objective.—Suture anchors increasingly are being used to secure tendons or ligaments to bone, and they are suitable for use in arthroscopic shoulder stabilization and rotator cuff repair. The characteristics of 4 anchors (Fig 3-2) were compared during and after implantation into the lateral femoral cortex of a castrated ram.

Methods.—Samples of Mitek G2, Zimmer Statak, Acufex TAG wedge, and the absorbable Arthrex expanding suture plug (ESP) were implanted under sterile conditions and harvested at varying intervals. Each bone-anchor-suture system was stressed to failure.

Observations.—The Mitek G2 (Fig 3-3) and Statak suture anchors failed by suture breakage throughout the 3-month study, at about 30 lb of resistance with no. 2 braided polyester suture. Problems were encountered during implantation of the TAG wedge, and the mode of failure varied with this suture anchor. A constant 30-lb level of failure was not

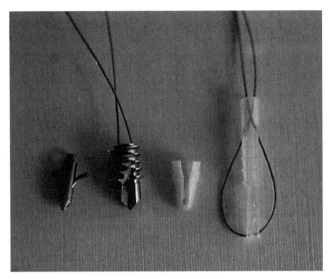

Fig 3–2.—The 4 suture anchors tested, left to right: the Mitek G2, Statak, TAG wedge, and Arthrex ESP. (Courtesy of Barber FA, Cawley P, Prudich JF: *Arthroscopy* 9:647–652, 1993.)

reached until 1 month after insertion. The ESP anchors also proved problematic both at the time of implantation and at failure testing. The ESP failed by anchor pull-out, suture breakage, and suture cut-out. A constant 30-lb failure level was achieved 6 weeks after insertion.

Conclusion.—The Mitek G2 and Zimmer Statak suture anchors proved easy to insert, and their level of failure was consistent over time.

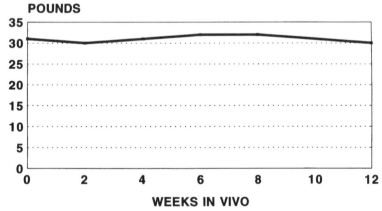

Fig 3–3.—The Mitek G2 suture anchor failed consistently by breaking the attached suture at a constant level throughout the 12-week period. (Courtesy of Barber FA, Cawley P, Prudich JF: *Arthroscopy* 9:647–652, 1993.)

Pull-Out Strength of Five Suture Anchors

Carpenter JE, Fish DN, Huston LJ, Goldstein SA (Univ of Michigan, Ann Arbor)

Arthroscopy 9:109–113, 1993   139-94-3-12

Purpose.—Suture anchors are used for attaching soft tissue to bone at sites where the use of screws or staples is impractical or not feasible. The biomechanical performance of 5 commercially available suture anchors was characterized and compared.

Study Design.—The anchor devices tested were the Acufex Rod TAG and Acufex Wedge TAG, the Mitek G1 and Mitek G2, and the Statak. The suture anchors were tested to failure on 12 fresh-frozen human cadaveric tibiae. The different anchors were randomly inserted in 16 positions around the proximal tibia at levels 1, 3, and 5 cm from the tibial joint surface. The load at failure and the mode of failure—anchor or suture—were recorded for each trial.

Results.—A total of 198 trials were completed, with 102 devices placed parallel and 96 placed perpendicular to the bone surface. Anchor insertion performed according to manufacturers' instructions was uncomplicated, except that 23% of the Acufex Rod TAG devices broke on insertion into thicker cortical bone. The anchors failed in 83 trials (42%) at an average force of 76.2 N, and the sutures failed in the remaining 115 trials (58%) at an average force of 124.2 N. Mitek G2 anchors had the lowest percentage of failures, whereas the Mitek G1 could be pulled out with significantly less force overall than any of the other anchors. Cortical bone thickness was weakly correlated with pull-out strength.

Conclusion.—Suture anchor devices fail over a wide range of forces. The direction of pull and the quality of bone at the insertion site appear to be major factors in overall anchor pull-out strength.

▶ These 2 studies, one using human cadaveric specimens (139-94-3-12) and the other an in vivo primate model (Abstract 139-94-3-11), present similar findings regarding the effectiveness of both the Mitek G2 and Statak suture anchors. This, of course, does not necessarily represent the performance of these devices in a clinical application.—J.S. Torg, M.D.

Pull-Out Strength of Suture Anchors for Rotator Cuff and Bankart Lesion Repairs

Hecker AT, Shea M, Hayhurst JO, Myers ER, Meeks LW, Hayes WC (Harvard Med School, Boston)

Am J Sports Med 21:874–879, 1993   139-94-3-13

Background.—Surgical reconstruction of anterior-inferior shoulder instability and rotator cuff injuries requires the secure fixation of soft tissues to bone. Current techniques entail the direct insertion of sutures

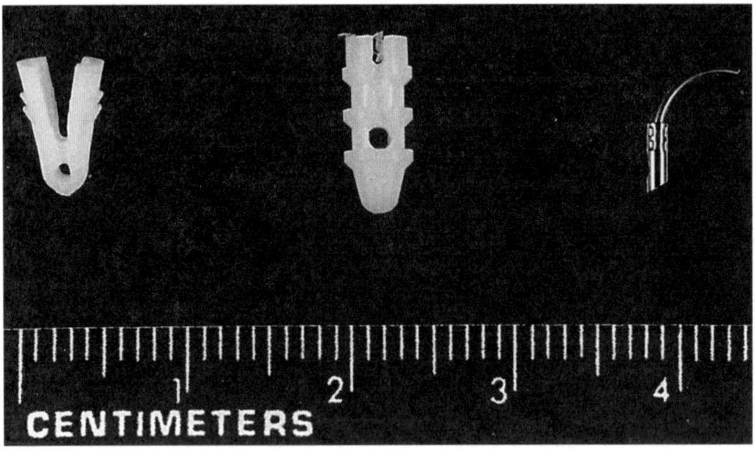

Fig 3–4.—The wedge, rod, and metallic suture anchors (*left to right*) used in the biomechanical tests. (Courtesy of Hecker AT, Shea M, Hayhurst JO, et al: *Am J Sports Med* 21:874–879, 1993.)

through transosseous tunnels, a complex approach that does not always provide adequately strong fixation.

Objective and Methods.—The immediate pull-out strength of 2 types of polyacetal suture anchors (wedge and rod forms) was compared with that of conventional suture-only attachment methods and a metallic suture anchor (Fig 3–4) in repair of Bankart lesions and rotator cuff tears in fresh-frozen human cadaveric shoulders. Bankart lesions were made by incision of the anterior capsule, and they were repaired by using sutures alone on 1 side and sutures with anchors on the other. Three fixation tunnels were created for the suture-only repair of either type of lesion. For the anchored suture repairs, 3 holes were drilled in the anterior glenoid ridge without violating the articular surface. The pull-out strength of the polyacetal and metallic anchors was tested in the tibial metaphyseal region 2 in cadaveric specimens.

Results.—With Bankart lesions and rotator cuff repairs, the fixation strength with sutures only or wedge or rod polyacetal suture anchors was comparable. Pull-out forces were similar for the 2 types of polyacetal anchor. The polyacetal anchors had higher pull-out forces than metallic anchors in the metaphyseal region of the tibia and in metaphyseal areas with thicker cortical walls.

Conclusion.—The wedge and rod types of polyacetal suture anchors provide adequate immediate fixation of soft tissue repairs in the human shoulder. This approach is less demanding than standard tunnel suturing methods and entails less surgical exposure.

▶ The authors' conclusion that "both polyacetal suture anchors provide adequate immediate fixation for soft tissue repairs in the human shoulder" is not supported by clinical data. That is, it cannot be inferred that results obtained in fresh-frozen cadaveric human shoulders can be applied to noncadaveric subjects.—J.S. Torg, M.D.

Efficacy and Pitfalls of the STATAK Soft-Tissue Attachment Device for the Bankart Repair

Tamai K, Sawazaki Y, Hara I (Dokkyo Univ, Tochigi, Japan; Hara Orthopedic Hosp, Tokyo)
J Shoulder Elbow Surg 2:216–220, 1993   139-94-3-14

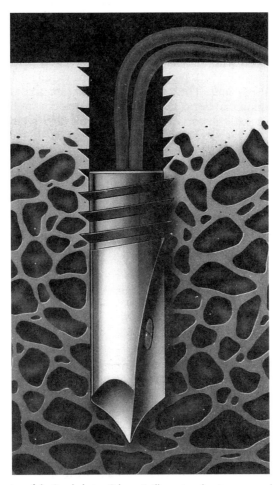

Fig 3–5.—Insertion of the Statak device. Schematic illustration showing correct placement of device within bone (reproduced from leaflet of Zimmer Division, Bristol-Meyers Squibb, Tokyo, Japan). (Courtesy of Tamai K, Sawazaki Y, Hara I: *J Shoulder Elbow Surg* 2:216–220, 1993.)

Background.—A transosseous suture technique (TOS) to attach capsular expansion to the bony glenoid rim commonly is used as part of a Bankart repair for recurrent anterior shoulder instability. The Statak soft tissue attachment device was developed as a substitute for the traditional TOS technique. The new Statak device was studied.

Patients.—The patient sample included 13 males and 2 females, aged 16–47 years, who underwent a Bankart repair with the Statak device (Fig 3–5) and 18 male and 4 female patients, aged 15–39 years, who had had a Bankart repair with the TOS technique before the Statak was introduced. All patients had unilateral post-traumatic recurrent anterior shoulder instability that had not responded to conservative treatment. The Rowe scoring system was used to evaluate the outcome 12–18 months after operation.

Results.—The mean operative time was 83 minutes for Statak-treated patients compared with 101 minutes for TOS-treated patients. The outcome after use of the TOS technique was rated excellent in 13 patients, good in 7, and fair in 2. The outcome with the Statak device was rated excellent in 8 patients, good in 4, fair in 2, and poor in 1. All 3 Statak-treated patients with an unsatisfactory outcome had recurrent subluxation that was attributed to incomplete insertion of the caudally placed device into the bone in 2 patients.

Conclusion.—Use of the Statak soft tissue attachment device significantly shortens the operative time of a Bankart repair. Careful determination of the drilling direction before using the device is essential.

▶ Although the authors state that surgeons who use the Statak device believed that it was technically less demanding, they further attribute the 3 postoperative subluxations that occurred in 15 patients to the fact that the device was "not inserted vertical to the bony surface." Subsequently, they proposed that the inserter head should make contact with the bony surface, thus preventing the metallic anchor from embedding below the cortical surface.—J.S. Torg, M.D.

Quadrilateral Space Syndrome: Findings at MR Imaging
Linker CS, Helms CA, Fritz RC (Univ of California, San Francisco)
Radiology 188:675–676, 1993   139-94-3-15

Background.—Quadrilateral space syndrome is a well-described cause of shoulder pain in which an isolated axillary nerve compressive neuropathy occurs in the quadrilateral space (Fig 3–6). One form of quadrilateral space syndrome occurs in young adults, with or without a history of trauma, as the result of axillary nerve compression by fibrous bands. Two such cases have been reported in baseball pitchers. The MRI findings of 3 patients with clinical signs of quadrilateral space syndrome were reported.

QUADRILATERAL SPACE

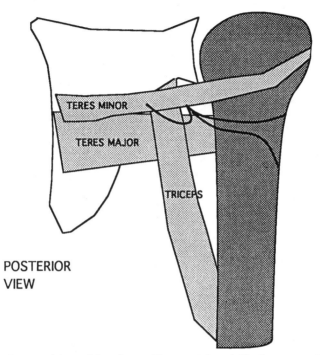

TERES MINOR

TERES MAJOR

TRICEPS

POSTERIOR
VIEW

Fig 3–6.—Diagram of the quadrilateral space. This space is bounded by the teres muscles, the long head of the triceps muscle, and the surgical neck of the humerus. The axillary nerve and the posterior humeral circumflex artery traverse this space. (Courtesy of Linker CS, Helms CA, Fritz RC: *Radiology* 188:675-676, 1993.)

Patients.—The patients were a female tennis player, a man who had fallen on his outstretched arm 6 months previously, and a male coal miner whose shoulder was struck by a heavy object; all patients were in their 40s. They complained of progressive shoulder pain that was exacerbated by abduction and/or external rotation. The MRI study revealed a normal rotator cuff but severe atrophy of the teres minor muscle in every patient (Fig 3-7). Axial images revealed an intact teres minor tendon. All patients showed mild clinical improvement with conservative therapy; none have gone on to surgery.

Conclusion.—In patients with symptoms of quadrilateral space syndrome, MRI can demonstrate selective atrophy of the teres minor muscle. Because teres minor muscle weakness is difficult to assess clinically,

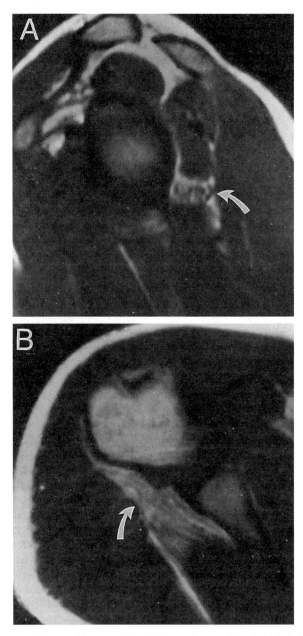

Fig 3–7.—A, oblique sagittal (repetition time, 700 ms; echo time, 20 ms [700/20]) (anterior is to the left); and **B,** axial (1,000/20) spin-echo MR images demonstrate high signal intensity within the teres minor muscle, consistent with fatty atrophy (*arrow*) in a female tennis player. (Courtesy of Linker CS, Helms CA, Fritz RC: *Radiology* 188:675–676, 1993.)

MRI may be a valuable diagnostic tool in this situation. The rotator cuff is normal and the teres minor tendon is intact in these patients.

▶ Magnetic resonance imaging has been shown in this, as well as in other reports, to accurately identify isolated muscle atrophy. Unfortunately, in this report only 3 cases were presented, there was no surgical confirmation, and no treatment was initiated. The authors' statement regarding the potential reversibility of this entity, once diagnosed, was not confirmed.—J.S. Torg, M.D.

Clinical Examination of the Shoulder Complex
Boublik M, Hawkins RJ (Steadman Hawkins Clinic, Vail, Colo; Univ of Colorado, Denver)
J Orthop Sports Phys Ther 18:379–385, 1993   139-94-3–16

Introduction.—Accurate diagnosis of the dysfunctional shoulder underlies effective treatment and rehabilitation. In most patients, a diagnosis can be made by a careful history and thorough physical examination, supplemented as needed by appropriate radiographic and laboratory studies.

General Assessment.—First, the attitude of the shoulder is noted, along with muscle symmetry and contours. Palpation is carried out in a regionalized manner. In examining shoulder motion, the scapulothoracic rhythm is inspected for winging or dyskinesia on forward elevation. Pushing against the wall or doing push-ups stresses the serratus muscle and demonstrates winging. If feasible, external rotation should be measured in the 90-degree abducted position. Internal rotation is estimated as the position reached by the outstretched thumb hitchhiking up the back. Muscle strength may be evaluated as the shoulder is put through ranges of motion.

Instability Testing.—Stability is evaluated by estimating the amount of passive translation between the humeral head and glenoid fossa, and by attempting to reproduce symptoms of subluxation by stressing the shoulder. The patient may first be examined while sitting, and the same tests are repeated in the supine position. The "load-and-shift" test is used to measure anterior and posterior translation of the humeral head. Inferior translation is estimated by grasping the elbow and applying inferior traction to the shoulder. If the crank test results in apprehension or pain, the fulcrum test is repeated with the patient supine. If symptoms are reproduced, a relocation test then is carried out, exerting posterior stress on the proximal humerus.

Other Tests.—Impingement of the supraspinatus tendon between the humeral head and the anteroinferior acromion may be demonstrated by forced passive elevation, or by active abduction in or just posterior to the coronal plane. Thorough vascular examination is necessary in cases of trauma, especially if the patient describes vague aching, heaviness, or fatigue radiating down the arm.

▶ The authors describe a good systematic method for evaluating shoulder problems. They stress the importance of history-taking, initial impression, regionalization, and scapulothoracic examination. The commentary is complete, with many pictures describing the evaluation procedures. The importance of a general physical examination to rule out disease processes that may cause shoulder pain is emphasized. An accurate diagnosis must be made before a well-defined, individualized rehabilitation program can be developed.—F.J. George, A.T.C., P.T.

Electromyographic Analysis and Its Role in the Athletic Shoulder
Glousman R (Kerlan-Jobe Orthopaedic Clinic, Inglewood, Calif)
Clin Orthop 288:27–34, 1993   139-94-3–17

Introduction.—Shoulder injuries to athletes frequently involve selective weakness of specific rotator cuff muscles, rather than generalized muscle impairment. Electromyographic (EMG) studies have questioned the applicability of single-plane motion analysis to sport-specific activities. Dynamic EMG evaluation of the mechanics of the shoulder has helped to formulate a base for the treatment and prophylaxis of athletic shoulder injuries.

Throwing.—Among the activities analyzed by dynamic EMG and high-speed film is the throwing motion. Professional throwing athletes, unlike amateurs, can selectively use the individual rotator cuff muscles. Thus, training may lead to efficient muscle use, improving endurance and avoiding overuse injury. In the throwing shoulder, the serratus anterior muscle, with the trapezius, controls the scapula, securing the glenoid as a stable platform for the humeral head. The activity of the serratus anterior is particularly important for upward rotation and scapular protraction during late cocking, allowing the scapula to keep pace with the humerus.

Instability in the Throwing Shoulder.—In pitchers with shoulder instability, serratus anterior activity is decreased throughout the pitching motion. This decreases the horizontal protraction of the scapula and allows the humerus to flex forward in the horizontal plane and rotate externally. This, along with early fatigue of the serratus anterior, places undue stress on the anterior restraints. If deficient scapular rotation decreases the space between the acromion and humeral head, functional impingement may develop and lead to rotator cuff tendinitis.

Discussion.—Studies of other sports—including swimming, tennis, and golf—have confirmed the importance of rotator cuff function. The emphasis and role of the individual muscles vary among sports. However, the action of the serratus anterior in stabilizing and protracting the scapula is a consistent finding. Comprehension and treatment of shoulder problems depend on a thorough understanding of the demands placed on the upper extremity by the patient's particular sport or activity.

▶ The author has done EMG studies with throwing athletes, swimmers, tennis players, and golfers and has made recommendations for training emphasis of the different muscles in each sport. He describes the importance of scapula stability to prevent rotator cuff impingement and the importance of adequate serratus anterior strength. He describes serratus anterior action as being consistent in scapula stabilization, regardless of the sport. We should heed Glousman's advice and include scapula stabilization exercises in all of our shoulder rehabilitation programs. In fact, scapula stabilization exercises should be initiated and performed satisfactorily before rotator cuff exercises are begun if the diagnosis is secondary shoulder impingement syndrome. Please read Abstract 139-94-3-18.—F.J. George, A.T.C., P.T.

Nonoperative Management of Secondary Shoulder Impingement Syndrome
Kamkar A, Irrgang JJ, Whitney SL (Laurel Rehabilitation and Sports Therapy, Uniontown, Pa; Univ of Pittsburgh, Pa)
J Orthop Sports Phys Ther 17:212–224, 1993   139-94-3-18

Purpose.—Shoulder instability and impingement syndrome are 2 common causes of shoulder pain in athletes. Impingement syndrome results from impingement of the rotator cuff tendons beneath the coracoacromial arch and is common in athletes who take part in repetitive overhead activities. Current knowledge on primary and secondary shoulder impingement syndromes and their nonoperative management was reviewed.

Classification.—Rotator cuff impingement has historically been attributed to repeated mechanical impingement. This type of impingement, known as primary impingement, may result from subacromial crowding, posterior capsular tightness, or excessive superior migration of the humeral head. In contrast, secondary impingement results from a relative decrease of the subacromial space caused by instability of the glenohumeral joint or scapulothoracic muscles. The distinction between primary and secondary impingement has important implications for treatment.

Secondary impingement caused by glenohumeral instability may result from weakness of the rotator cuff mechanism and biceps tendon, with subsequent overloading of the passive restraints of the glenohumeral joint during throwing. The active restraints attempt to stabilize the humeral head, abnormal translation of which leads to mechanical impingement, resulting in inflammation of the rotator cuff tendons. Impingement syndrome may overlap with glenohumeral instability. In patients with functional scapular instability, weakness of the scapulothoracic muscles leads to abnormal scapular positioning. If humeral elevation is

Suggested Exercises for the Scapulothoracic Muscles

Muscle	Suggested Exercises
Serratus anterior	Scapular plane abductions*, push up*, end range shoulder flexion in prone*, serratus anterior puncht
Upper trapezius	Shoulder shrug*, scapular plane abduction*
Middle trapezius	Rowing*, shoulder elevation and hyperextension in standing*, shoulder abduction and flexion in prone*, scapular retraction with horizontal abduction of the externally rotated shoulder in pronet
Lower trapezius	Scapular plane abduction and rowing*, shoulder depression and retraction in sitting*, elevation of the externally rotated arm which is positioned diagonally between flexion and abductiont
Levator scapulae	Shoulder elevation, abduction, flexion*, rowing*
Rhomboids	Rowing*, shoulder retraction, elevation and abduction* scapular retraction with horizontal abduction of the internally rotated shoulder in pronet
Latissimus dorsi	Press ups*, lat pull downt
Pectoralis major	Press ups*
Pectoralis minor	Press ups*

* Exercises based on electromyographic studies.
† Exercises based on anatomomechanical studies.
(Courtesy of Kamkar A, Irrgang JJ, Whitney SL: *J Orthop Sports Phys Ther* 17:212–224, 1993.)

not synchronized with scapular elevation and upward rotation, impingement of the rotator cuff may result. Weakness or fatigue of the serratus anterior muscle may lead to excessive winging or tipping of the scapula and, thus, to a relative decrease in the subacromial space.

Nonoperative Treatment.—Most regimens for shoulder rehabilitation emphasize strengthening of the rotator cuff muscles, along with restoring normal range of motion, endurance, and pain control. Restoration of scapulohumeral rhythm and strengthening of the rotator cuff and scapular rotators is central to treatment success. Increasing the strength of the scapular rotators ensures that the scapula will follow the humerus, conferring dynamic stability and synchrony of scapulohumeral rhythm (table).

Summary.—Secondary subacromial impingement can result from weakness of the scapulothoracic muscles via disruption of scapulohumeral rhythm, abnormal scapular positioning, and functional scapulothoracic instability. Nonoperative treatment for this problem aims to restore normal active and passive shoulder mobility, as well as scapulohumeral rhythm. Developing the strength and endurance of the shoulder muscles, including the scapulothoracic as well as the rotator cuff muscles, is a key part of successful treatment.

▶ The authors describe primary and secondary shoulder impingement syndromes and their rationale for specific rehabilitation programs. If the diagnosis of secondary shoulder impingement is made, then scapulothoracic muscle strengthening must be accomplished before significant rotator cuff strengthening is initiated. Shoulder posture is a very important factor in successful rehabilitation of this problem. We are constantly instructing our athletes with this problem to "Lift the shoulder up and roll it back." The authors have included a basic list of exercises for specific muscle strengthening.

A related study was abstracted in the 1993 YEAR BOOK OF SPORTS MEDICINE from the Kerlan Jobe Orthopaedic Clinic (1). My comments after that abstract were "there are exercises that can impinge on the rotator cuff muscles under the coracoacromial arch, especially abduction beyond 90 degrees, and often only to 70 or 80 degrees . . . . We advise no flexion or abduction beyond 90 degrees . . . until the symptoms have subsided."—F.J. George, A.T.C., P.T.

Reference

1. 1993 YEAR BOOK OF SPORTS MEDICINE, pp 40–41.

Current Concepts in the Rehabilitation of the Athletic Shoulder
Wilk KE, Arrigo C (HealthSouth Rehabilitation Corp, Birmingham, Ala; HealthSouth Sports Medicine and Rehabilitation Ctr, Birmingham, Ala)
J Orthop Sports Phys Ther 18:365–378, 1993   139-94-3-19

Introduction.—Current trends in rehabilitation are toward earlier protected motion and strengthening activities. Stabilizing exercises for the rotator cuff muscles are used to reestablish voluntary stability of the humeral head within the glenoid. Improved surgical and arthroscopic methods and better techniques of soft tissue fixation have made earlier and more aggressive rehabilitative procedures feasible. Functional stability is the key to pain-free shoulder function during sports activities.

Ways of Restoring Function.—The quality of glenohumeral motion relates directly to the state of the supraspinatus and infraspinatus muscles. The shoulder complex includes more than the shoulder joint itself; the scapulothoracic, acromioclavicular, and sternoclavicular joints should not be overlooked. The scapula provides proximal stability and allows good mobility of the distal segment. Scapulothoracic neuromuscular control exercises (Fig 3–8) are designed to challenge the scapular force couples. In addition to using dumbbells, plyometric exercises or stretch-shortening exercise drills are used to generate maximal muscular force. Closed-chain kinetic exercises, performed with the distal segment relatively fixed to an immovable object, are applicable to the upper extremity. Another approach is to perform external/internal rotator strengthening exercises in the scapular plane.

Key Rehabilitative Concepts.—Periodization refers to the year-round sequence and progression of sports and weight resistance training of athletes. The conditioning drills and sports training skills used at a given

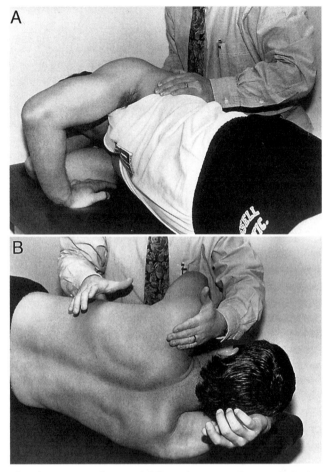

Fig 3–8.—Scapular neuromuscular control drills. **A,** the patient is lying involved side up, the shoulder is abducted to 90 degrees and internally rotated, and the hand is placed on the table. **B,** manual resistance is applied as the patient slowly protracts/retracts and elevates/depresses the scapula. (Courtesy of Wilk KE, Arrigo C: *J Orthop Sports Phys Ther* 18:365–378, 1993.)

time depend in part on the time of year. Quality skill training is emphasized during the competitive phase. Conditioning and strengthening exercises are emphasized in the preparation phase. The principle of individualization recognizes that each patient is unique, and that different sports activities require different rehabilitative techniques.

▶ The authors describe a number of shoulder and shoulder complex rehabilitation exercises. They recommend scapula and glenohumeral stabilization exercises through a group of exercises they refer to as "movement awareness drills." They have incorporated both closed-chain and plyometric exercises in their rehabilitation programs. They have also included the principles of periodization and individualization.

This is an excellent presentation of a shoulder rehabilitation program using the current concepts of scapulothoracic and scapulohumeral coordination. They use manual therapy and closed-chain and plyometric rehabilitation exercises in a well–thought-out program from initial injury to the final stages of rehabilitation.—F.J. George, A.T.C., P.T.

A Role for Hydrotherapy in Shoulder Rehabilitation
Speer KP, Cavanaugh JT, Warren RF, Day L, Wickiewicz TL (Hosp for Special Surgery, New York)
Am J Sports Med 21:850–853, 1993   139-94-3-20

Background.—Many patients undergoing shoulder rehabilitation seem to lose the ability to use the shoulder early in the course of rehabilitation. This inability is not simply the result of pain and anxiety but of a neurophysiologic difficulty in firing the muscles appropriately. Hydrotherapy has been found to be indispensable for patients with difficult shoulder rehabilitation who do not progress within established dry-land motion and strength protocols.

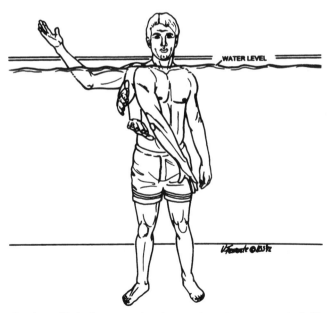

Fig 3–9.—An advanced hydrotherapy exercise using proprioceptive neuromuscular facilitation diagonal pattern no. 2. This exercise combines motions of external rotation, forward elevation, and abduction. Water baffles are a useful adjunct to increase resistance during this exercise. (Courtesy of Speer KP, Cavanaugh JT, Warren RF, et al: *Am J Sports Med* 21:850–853, 1993.)

Hydrotherapy Guidelines.—When a patient fails to progress according to expectations, hydrotherapy is added to the rehabilitation program. Under constant therapist supervision, the patient stands in a pool or other tank of water and performs shoulder exercises. The water level is at the base of the neck. Flotation devices are provided on request. Although the exercises are active, the effect of the water's buoyancy permits far gentler exercises than those done on dry land. The basic exercises include shoulder flexion and extension in the sagittal and scapular planes, with the arms kept completely submerged. Scapular protraction, retraction, elevation, and depression are also done. Proprioceptive neuromuscular facilitation upper-extremity patterns have also been introduced (Fig 3–9). Dry-land therapy is always continued along with hydrotherapy.

Conclusion.—The hydrostatic pressure on the arm during hydrotherapy may produce a glove effect on the involved arm. Combined with the water's buoyancy, this pressure may stimulate the proprioceptors of the skin and generate an effect like biofeedback to the patient. One problem with the use of hydrotherapy is that patients may feel secure too soon and push themselves too far through rehabilitation. Many patients have access to pools and continue hydrotherapy even after the physician has discontinued it. Patients need to be educated not to do too much too soon.

▶ We have all encountered the patient who has a great deal of difficulty with a shoulder rehabilitation program. The authors have made some good recommendations for easing through some of this difficulty with hydrotherapy exercises. We have access to a swimming pool and I plan to use some of their suggestions with my next difficult shoulder patient. The authors have cautioned us more than once to proceed gradually and not to overdo the program.—F.J. George, A.T.C., P.T.

Stretch-Shortening Drills for the Upper Extremities: Theory and Clinical Application
Wilk KE, Voight ML, Keirns MA, Gambetta V, Andrews JR, Dillman CJ
(HealthSouth Rehabilitation Corp, Birmingham, Ala; Univ of Miami, Coral Gables, Fla; Therex Corp, Denver; et al)
J Orthop Sports Phys Ther 17:225–239, 1993   139-94-3–21

Background.—Improving the muscle's ability to exert maximal force output in a minimal amount of time can enhance athletic performance. Plyometric exercise emphasizes quick powerful movements involving a prestretching of the muscle, thereby activating the stretch-shortening cycle. The stretch-shortening cycle occurs when elastic loading, through an eccentric muscular contraction, is followed by a burst of concentric muscular contraction. The concept was introduced in Russia in 1969 by

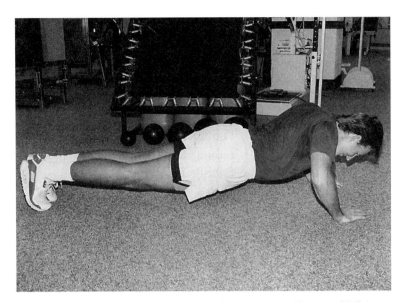

Fig 3–10.—Warm-up exercises; push-ups with 2 hands on the ground. (Courtesy of Wilk KE, Voight ML, Keirns MA, et al: *J Orthop Sports Phys Ther* 17:225–239, 1993.)

Verkhoshanski. Plyometric training increases the excitability of the neurologic receptors for improved reactivity of the neuromuscular system.

Plyometric Exercise.—The 3 phases of plyometric exercise are the setting or eccentric phase, the amortization phase, and the concentric response phase. The eccentric or setting phase begins when the athlete mentally prepares for the activity and lasts until the stretch stimulus is initiated. The amortization phase is the amount of time between the yielding eccentric contraction and initiation of a concentric force. In the concentric response phase, the athlete concentrates on the effect of the exercise and prepares for initiation of the second repetition.

Training Program.—A sample stretch-shortening program involves warm-up exercises, throwing movements, trunk extension/flexion exercises, and medicine ball wall exercises (Fig 3–10, table). Stretch-shortening exercise is used during the first and second preparation phases of training using Marveyev's model of periodization. Intense stretch-shortening exercise programs are contraindicated for the recreational athlete and athletes not involved in a weight training program.

Conclusion.—Intense stretch-shortening exercise is an advanced strengthening program to enhance the athletic performance of competitive athletes. An upper extremity stretch-shortening exercise program is especially useful in rehabilitating a competitive throwing athlete.

▶ Plyometrics or stretch-shortening exercises have been widely accepted in many lower extremity training programs. Recently we have begun to include

A Stretch-Shortening Exercise Program

I. <u>Warm-up Exercises</u>
    Med Ball Rotation
    Med Ball Side Bends
    Med Ball Wood Chops
    Tubing ER/IR
    Tubing Diagonal Patterns (D2)
    Tubing Biceps
    Push-Ups

II. <u>Throwing Movements</u>
    Med Ball Soccer Throw
    Med Ball Chest Pass
    Med Ball Step & Pass
    Med Ball Side Throw
    Tubing Plyos IR/ER
    Tubing Plyos Diagonals
    Tubing Plyos Biceps
    Plyo Push-Up (Boxes)
    Push-Up (Clappers)

III. <u>Trunk Ext/Flexion Movements</u>
    Med Ball Sit Ups
    Med Ball Back Extension

IV. <u>Medicine Ball Wall Exercises</u>
    Soccer Throw
    Chest Pass
    Side to Side Throw
    Backward Side to Side Throw
    Forward 2 hands Through Legs
    One Hand Baseball Throw

Abbreviations: IR, internal rotation; *ER*, external rotation.
(Courtesy of Wilk KE, Voight ML, Keirns MA, et al: *J Orthop Sports Phys Ther* 17:225–239, 1993.)

these principles and exercises in our upper extremity training programs. Throwing athletes and other athletes who use upper extremity strength, power, and coordination will benefit from these exercises. As with a lower extremity plyometric program, proper technique and supervision are very important to prevent injury with these exercises. The authors have included extensive photographs with accompanying descriptions of the exercises. Again a word of caution: Learn about plyometrics and their use before using them in a rehabilitation or training program.—F.J. George, A.T.C., P.T.

The Functional Anatomy of the Elbow Complex
Stroyan M, Wilk KE (Gary Nederveld & Associates, Port Huron, Mich; Health-South Rehabilitation Corp, Birmingham, Ala)
J Orthop Sports Phys Ther 17:279–288, 1993   139-94-3-22

Objective.—An understanding of the anatomy and biomechanics of the elbow complex is essential to the recognition and rehabilitation of elbow pathologies. A thorough description of the relative functional anatomy of the elbow complex was provided.

Arthrology of the Elbow Complex.—The elbow joint complex is composed of the humeroulnar, radioulnar, and superior and inferior radioulnar articulations. The 3 bones forming these articulations are the ulna, radius, and humerus. The humeroulnar joint can be described as a modified hinge joint. Its osseous structures include the distal humerus and the proximal ulna. The proximal ulna has a central bony projection known as the trochlear ridge. Another significant anatomical feature related to the humeroulnar articulation is the medial epicondyle, located proximal and medial to the trochlea. The humeroradial joint, often called a hinge/pivot joint, performs both flexion/extension and rotational movements. Rotation of the forearm is produced by the superior and inferior radioulnar joints. The head of the radius rotates during supination and pronation within a ring formed by the annular ligament and radial notch of the ulna.

Ligamentous Complexes and Muscles.—The elbow joint possesses medial and lateral ligamentous complexes. The ulnar collateral ligament on the medial side of the elbow consists of 3 parts: the anterior oblique, posterior oblique, and transverse portions. The lateral ligament complex consists of the radial collateral ligament, annular ligament, lateral ulnar collateral ligament, and the accessory lateral collateral ligament. The 23 muscles directly associated with the elbow joint can be classified into 4 main groups: the elbow flexors and extensors, the flexor-pronator group, and the extensor-supinator group. Muscles provide dynamic stabilization to the elbow and enable the hand to perform skilled, precise motions.

Neurologic Structures.—The 4 nerves that play significant roles in the elbow complex are the median, radial, musculocutaneous, and ulnar nerves. Recognition of problems involving compression requires a

knowledge of the origin and course of these nerves. Athletes who participate in throwing sports are susceptible to entrapment of the radial nerve
at the arcade of Frohse. Cutaneous innervation about the elbow is provided by a total of 5 sensory nerves.

▶ As with any joint in the body, the more the anatomy and biomechanics of
a joint are understood, the better will be our evaluation, differential diagnosis, treatment, and rehabilitation programs. Many of us consider the elbow to
be one of the most difficult joints to rehabilitate. This is a joint in which biomechanics play a very important role in injuries. For total rehabilitation and
to prevent further injury, the throwing or tennis stroke biomechanics must
change or the injury will certainly recur.—F.J. George, A.T.C., P.T.

Physical Examination of the Thrower's Elbow
Andrews JR, Wilk KE, Satterwhite YE, Tedder JL (Alabama Sports Medicine
& Orthopaedic Ctr, Birmingham; HealthSouth Rehabilitation Corp, Birming-
ham, Ala; American Sports Medicine Inst, Birmingham, Ala)
J Orthop Sports Phys Ther 17:296–304, 1993   139-94-3–23

Objective.—Various aspects of the physical examination of an athlete's
elbow—palpation of bony architecture and soft tissue, muscle testing,
isokinetic testing, neurologic testing, sensory examination, and some
special tests—were examined. Radiographic examination of the elbow
was also evaluated.

The Examination.—The physical examination should begin with a
complete and thorough history and proceed in a sequential fashion. Observation includes an evaluation of the skin and of the carrying angle of
the arm. The elbow is a stable hinge joint composed of 4 articulations:
the humeroulnar joint, the humeroradial joint, and the superior and inferior radioulnar joints. Knowledge of the bony architecture is required for
an accurate diagnosis of bony pathology.

The elbow can be divided into 4 parts for examination of the soft tissue: the medial, posterior, lateral, and anterior aspects. Passive movement of each range of motion should be checked for blockage and limitation. Side-to-side comparisons are important, and the "end feel" of
the movement should be assessed. Manual muscle tests are specific for
each of the muscles of the elbow. Isokinetic testing may be beneficial in
the athlete to measure muscular performance. The Tinel test, tests for
tennis elbow (lateral epicondylitis) and golfer's elbow (medial epicondylitis), the valgus extension overload test, and the test for ulnar collateral
ligament (UCL) stability are among the specialized tests discussed.

Radiographic Examination.—Anteroposterior and lateral plain radiographic views will determine joint integrity and identify fractures or loose
bodies. Internal and external oblique views are useful in detecting posterior olecranon osteophytes. A diagnostic CT arthrogram is valuable in

suspected cases of UCL tear. The CT scan may show partial undersurface tears not detected by a plain arthrogram. Magnetic resonance imaging is useful in diagnosing soft tissue inflammation, edema, and complete UCL tears.

Conclusion.—The examination sequence will yield a thorough evaluation of the athlete's elbow. Evaluation and rehabilitation of injuries are best accomplished by the combined efforts of the physician and therapist.

▶ Elbow injuries are common with throwing athletes, and the examiner must obtain a complete history, have extensive knowledge of the functional anatomy and biomechanics of the elbow (see Abstract 139-94-3-22), and have a well-organized physical examination to make a differential diagnosis. Only when that has been done can an appropriate treatment and rehabilitation regimen be instituted.—F.J. George, A.T.C., P.T.

Common Elbow Problems in the Athlete
Andrews JR, Whiteside JA (Univ of Virginia, Charlottesville)
J Orthop Sports Phys Ther 17:289–295, 1993   139-94-3-24

Introduction.—Athletic problems of the elbow include sprains, strains, contusions, fractures, dislocations, inflammations, and lacerations. Other miscellaneous pathologies are also seen, such as skeletal abnormalities, systemic diseases, soft tissue variations, and localized conditions. Some of the most common problems and the means by which they can be recognized were examined.

Pain in the Anterior, Lateral, Posterior, and Medial Compartments.—Anterior elbow pain and marked weakness in flexion can result from repetitious, overhead throwing motions. Pain in the anterior elbow is also linked to anterior capsular sprain, commonly caused by traumatic hyperextension of the elbow. Lateral elbow problems in the immature skeleton relate to compression forces, in conjunction with valgus medial stretching, on the capitellum of the humerus and adjacent radial head. In the golfer, lateral epicondylitis of the elbow is caused by over-practice/play and use of poor swing mechanics. The repetitive motions of throwing, vaulting, and swimming the backstroke, as well as the follow-through phase of pitching, can result in posterior compartment problems. Medial elbow pain, as in Little League, golfer's, and swimmer's elbow, can result from medial epicondylitis, ulnar collateral ligament sprain, flexor-pronator mass strain, and ulnar nerve neuritis.

Peripheral Nerve Problems.—The musculocutaneous, radial, median, and ulnar nerves are affected in some cases of elbow pain. Injuries can produce both motor and sensory deficits. Compression and entrapment of the lateral antebrachial cutaneous nerve are associated with repetitive overloading with extension or hyperextension of the elbow and pronation of the forearm. Conservative management and an active muscular rehabilitation are often the recommended treatment measures.

Dislocations, Fractures, and Vascular Problems.—Elbow dislocations are generally an injury of hyperextension and are common in football, gymnastics, and wrestling. The neurovascular status should be reexamined at the level of the elbow, wrist, and hand immediately after reduction of the dislocation. Posterior dislocations associated with radial head or coranoid fractures must be managed as a more serious complication. Intracondylar fractures are infrequently encountered in sports; more common are avulsion fractures, especially in the younger athlete engaging in contact sports. Vascular injuries usually occur as a result of repetitive trauma, anatomical compression, and occult vascular injury.

Conclusion.—Most elbow/forearm problems in the athlete result from repetitive overload stress combined with acute trauma. Prevention is an important facet to understanding elbow pathology. Some preventive measures are physical and psychological preparedness; year-round programs to develop strength, endurance, and flexibility; and rehabilitation of all previous injuries.

▶ The authors stress the role that off-season training programs play in the prevention of elbow injuries. Many elbow problems, with their biomechanical faults and evaluation techniques, are described.—F.J. George, A.T.C., P.T.

Rehabilitation of the Elbow in the Throwing Athlete

Wilk KE, Arrigo C, Andrews JR (HealthSouth Rehabilitation Corp, Birmingham, Ala; HealthSouth Sports Medicine & Rehabilitation Ctr, Birmingham, Ala; Alabama Sports Medicine & Orthopaedic Ctr, Birmingham)
J Orthop Sports Phys Ther 17:305–317, 1993   139-94-3–25

Thrower's Ten Program

1. Dumbbell exercises for the deltoid and supraspinatus musculature
2. Prone horizontal shoulder abduction
3. Prone shoulder extension
4. Internal rotation at 90° abduction of the shoulder with tubing
5. External rotation at 90° abduction of the shoulder with tubing
6. Elbow flexion/extension exercises (exercise tubing)
7. Serratus anterior strengthening—progressive pushups
8. Diagonal D_2 pattern for shoulder flexion and extension with exercise tubing
9. Press-ups
10. Dumbbell wrist extension/flexion and pronation/supination

(Courtesy of Wilk KE, Arrigo C, Andrews JR: *J Orthop Sports Phys Ther* 17:305–317, 1993.)

Background.—Although patients with elbow injuries commonly receive rehabilitation, the literature contains few descriptions of the process. The elbow joint is anatomically unique, posing a number of challenges to the rehabilitation professional. The process of rehabilitation for various elbow injuries and the rationales behind them were reviewed.

Immediate Motion.—Immediate motion is the first phase of elbow rehabilitation. It aims to reestablish pain-free range of motion, reduce pain and inflammation, and retard muscular atrophy. Early range-of-motion exercises nourish the articular cartilage and help in collagen tissue synthesis and organization. The humeroulnar and humeroradial joints are mobilized to counteract capsular restrictions. The primary goal of this phase is to obtain full elbow extension. Joint mobilization, along with other modalities, helps to relieve pain and inflammation. Submaximal isometric exercises help to retard muscular atrophy of the elbow and wrist.

Intermediate Exercise.—In the second phase, the goals are to advance elbow mobility, improve strength and endurance, and improve neuromuscular control. Full range of motion, minimal pain, and good elbow flexor and extensor strength are critical for progression to this stage. Stretching helps to maintain extension and flexion and promotes pronation and supination. Isotonic exercises are used to enhance strength and endurance. Neuromuscular control exercises are also added in this phase.

Advanced Strengthening.—The third phase consists of advanced strengthening activities, with the goal of preparing the athlete for unrestricted function. The foci of strengthening are total arm strength, power, endurance, and neuromuscular control, as well as preparation for a gradual return to throwing. The patient must have full, pain-free range of motion, no pain, and at least 70% strength before beginning advanced strengthening exercises, which focus specifically on the patient's activity or position. Advanced strengthening exercises emphasize the biceps muscle, an important stabilizer during the follow-through phase of throwing. Exercises to strengthen the triceps and the rotator cuff muscles are also included, as is the "Thrower's Ten" program for throwing athletes (table). Medicine ball training also begins in this phase.

Return to Activity.—This final phase ensures that the patient has adequate motion, strength, and functional capability before return to competition. It includes progressive functional drills and, for throwing athletes, an interval throwing program. The athlete must have full, pain-free range of motion and satisfactory isokinetic test results and physical examination.

Summary.—There are 4 phases of rehabilitation of the athlete with an elbow injury. Elbow extension must be emphasized early, and the elbow flexors, wrist flexors, and pronator muscles must be strengthened to deal with the stresses of the acceleration and follow-through phases of throwing. Strengthening of the rotator cuff muscles is another important component. Specific rehabilitation protocols for patients undergoing various operative procedures are presented.

▶ As you may have surmised from my previous comments on elbow joint injuries and rehabilitation, many of us believe this is one of the more difficult injuries to treat. The throwing athlete puts a tremendous amount of stress on the elbow joint, with a great deal of repetition. Many factors must be considered when treating these athletes to attain complete rehabilitation and prevent reinjury. Proper biomechanics must be stressed and followed. The author offers some excellent guidelines to follow before an athlete returns to participation.—F.J. George, A.T.C., P.T.

Tennis Elbow
Foley AE (Wright State Univ, Dayton, Ohio)
Am Fam Physician 48:281–288, 1993   139-94-3-26

Introduction.—The term "tennis elbow" has been used to describe pain at or near the origin of the extensor carpi radialis brevis, despite the fact that the pain actually is related to tennis playing in fewer than 5% of those affected. In younger patients, sports activities account for most cases of tennis elbow, but older patients more often have symptoms related to their work. The causes probably include traction, repeated microtrauma, and inflammation.

Diagnosis.—Tennis elbow is seen most often in 30- to 60-year-old white men and usually involves the dominant side. Symptoms generally have been present for 6–12 weeks before the patient seeks care. The diagnosis is made clinically. Typically, tenderness over the lateral epicon-

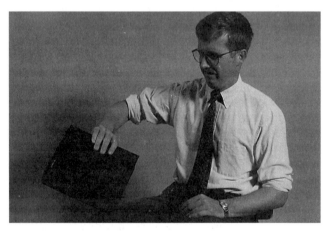

Fig 3–11.—Grasping a heavy book with the forearm pronated causes immediate pain in the elbow, followed quickly by elbow abduction, allowing the book to dip below the level of the elbow. (Courtesy of Foley AE: Am Fam Physician 48:281–288, 1993.)

dyle or slightly distally is found, which has the effect of reducing grip strength. The pain can be induced by resisting wrist extension. A heavy book may be used to confirm the diagnosis and to educate the patient; when the patient holds the book with the forearm pronated (Fig 3–11), immediate pain in the lateral epicondylar region results. The most common method of assessment is palpation at and distal to the affected epicondyle with resistance of wrist extension.

Treatment.—The patient is taught how to lift with the palm kept close to the body, thus protecting the elbow. A tennis-elbow band may be helpful; static and counterforce bands are available. In patients with marked symptoms, a cock-up splint may be placed at the wrist to provide 20 degrees of extension. Use of a nonsteroidal anti-inflammatory drug may also be helpful. Steroid injection may relieve disabling pain or symptoms that fail to respond to lesser measures. Application of ice afterwards may prevent a flare of pain.

Rehabilitation.—When the pain subsides, the patient should begin stretching exercises of the extensor forearm muscles, as well as strengthening exercises with a 1-lb weight. Formal rehabilitation may be indicated when epicondylitis is related to work or to sports activity. Surgery is reserved for patients with disabling and refractory symptoms.

▶ We have had good success using the following treatment and rehabilitation program for our athletes with lateral epicondylitis: (1) cold whirlpool—55 degrees; 20 minutes twice daily; (2) nonsteroidal anti-inflammatory medication; (3) tennis-elbow band—at least 2-in. wide—worn all waking hours; (4) stretching—wrist flexed with a varus force at the extended elbow joint; (5) soft tissue mobilization using a deep cross friction massage technique; and (6) strengthening exercises (wrist extension using light weights). Having read this article, we will include the author's suggestions on how to avoid further stress on the injury when lifting (see Fig 3–13).—F.J. George, A.T.C., P.T.

Lateral Extensor Release for Tennis Elbow: A Prospective Long-Term Follow-up Study
Verhaar J, Walenkamp G, Kester A, Van Mameren H, Van Der Linden T (Univ Hosp Maastricht, The Netherlands)
J Bone Joint Surg (Am) 75–A:1034–1043, 1993   139-94-3-27

Objective.—There are many effective operations available for the treatment of tennis elbow, including the lateral release of the common extensor origins, which is technically relatively simple. The long-term outcome after lateral extensor release for tennis elbow was examined in a prospective follow-up study.

Patients.—Fifty-seven of 63 patients with tennis elbow who underwent a lateral extensor release were followed up for a mean of 59 months. Indications for operation included severe pain that interfered with activities of daily living and occupation despite at least 6 months of conservative therapy.

Results.—The overall results were rated as excellent or good in 37% of patients at 6 weeks, in 69% at 1 year, and in 89% at 5 years. Satisfaction with the outcome was reported by 66% of patients at 1 year and by 91% of patients at 5 years. There were no recurrences. Analysis of the data did not identify any variables significantly related to either a good or a poor outcome.

Conclusion.—Lateral extensor release for tennis elbow is a relatively simple operation that should be the procedure of choice as well as being that with which all other operations are to be compared.

▶ The results and conclusions reached by the authors are in keeping with my own experience. To be noted, the procedure is performed with local anesthesia (1% lidocaine and epinephrine 1:10,000). Using this technique, it is possible to, so to speak "cut out the pain." That is, the completion of the release occurs when the patient is free of pain on the table.—J.S. Torg, M.D.

Undersurface Tear of the Ulnar Collateral Ligament in Baseball Players: A Newly Recognized Lesion
Timmerman LA, Andrews JR (American Sports Medicine Inst, Birmingham, Ala)
Am J Sports Med 22:33–36, 1994   139-94-3–28

Background.—Tearing injuries of the ulnar collateral ligament (UCL) of the elbow have been reported in throwing athletes. Seven patients had a newly recognized UCL injury—a lesion in which the undersurface of the anterior bundle is detached from the insertion site.

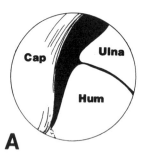 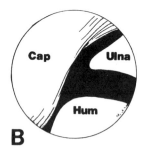

Fig 3–12.—Illustration of arthroscopic valgus instability test. **A,** arthroscopic view from anterolateral portal in a right elbow of the medial capsule (*Cap*), humerus (*Hum*), and ulna. There is no opening between the humerus and ulna. **B,** with valgus stress applied, the increase in space between the ulna and humerus is demonstrated. (Courtesy of Timmerman LA, Andrews JR: *Am J Sports Med* 22:33–36, 1994.)

Methods.—Evaluation of 25 baseball players with medial elbow pain included physical examination, stress radiography, CT arthrography, and MRI. Valgus instability was evaluated clinically, by examination with the use of anesthesia, and arthroscopically with the elbow flexed at 70 degrees. In 7 of the patients, the surgeon performed a longitudinal incision in line with the UCL fibers to visualize the capsular layers of the ligament's anterior bundle, revealing detachment and discolored degenerated tissue on the undersurface, although the superficial surface was intact. Cadaveric elbows were dissected to determine anatomical variation.

Results.—No abnormalities were detected in 6 of the 7 patients by radiography and MRI, in any patients by CT arthrography, and in 5 of the 7 by arthroscopy. Radiography revealed UCL calcification in 1 patient, and MRI showed some undersurface degeneration in 1 patient. Increased contrast leakage around the ulnar insertion of the UCL in 1 patient may have suggested the lesion. Arthroscopy allowed visualization of the lesion in only 2 patients. No difference in valgus instability was detected on examination with the patient wakeful or anesthetized. All 7 patients exhibited valgus instability with arthroscopic examination of the elbow flexed at 70 degrees (Fig 3-12). Cadaveric dissection excluded the possibility that the lesion was a normal anatomical variant.

Discussion.—Diagnosis of a UCL tear is difficult. Arthroscopic examination was most useful in evaluating valgus instability, but it did not allow adequate visualization of the anterior bundle. Although both CT arthrography and MRI can effectively detect full-thickness tears of the anterior bundle of the UCL, they were not sensitive to a partial tear. Even open surgical exploration may not reveal the lesion without the additional longitudinal incision.

▶ The authors state that the purpose of this study "is not to report on the results of treatment of this lesion, but instead to describe the nature of this abnormality involving the UCL." However, they do indicate that when valgus instability was found on clinical and arthroscopic examination with evidence of an incompetent anterior bundle of the UCL, "the decision was made to augment the ligament with autograft tendon." To be noted, neither follow-up nor results of the surgery are presented.—J.S. Torg, M.D.

Gamekeeper Thumb: Differentiation of Nondisplaced and Displaced Tears of the Ulnar Collateral Ligament With MR Imaging: Work in Progress
Spaeth HJ, Abrams RA, Bock GW, Trudell D, Hodler J, Botte MJ, Petersen M, Resnick D (Univ of New Mexico, Albuquerque; Univ of California, San Diego; Univ of Manitoba, Winnipeg, Canada; et al)
Radiology 188:553–556, 1993   139-94-3-29

Introduction.—Ulnar collateral ligament (UCL) injury of the first metacarpophalangeal joint—gamekeeper thumb—is a common injury. After

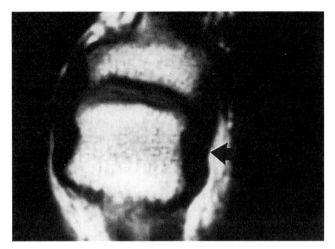

Fig 3–13.—T1-weighted MR image (500/20) of normal UCL (*arrow*). (Courtesy of Spaeth HJ, Abrams RA, Bock GW, et al: *Radiology* 188:553–556, 1993.)

rupture, the torn end of the UCL can become displaced superficially to the adductor pollicis aponeurosis, necessitating surgical repair. However, it is often difficult to detect displacement on plain radiographs. To determine whether MRI would be useful in the differentiation of displaced

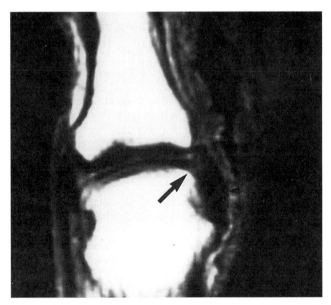

Fig 3–14.—T1-weighted MR image (500/20) shows nondisplaced tear (*arrow*) of the UCL. The adductor aponeurosis (*arrowhead*) covers the distal end of the UCL. (Courtesy of Spaeth HJ, Abrams RA, Bock GW, et al: *Radiology* 188:553–556, 1993.)

and nondisplaced UCL tears, both lesions were created in 29 nonembalmed, cadaveric specimens and examined with MRI.

Methods.—Of the 29 specimens, UCL tears were created in 16, 10 with displacement and 6 without. All specimens were examined in a blinded fashion by coronal MRI and anatomical slices.

Findings.—The normal UCL appeared as a low-signal-intensity band medial to the metacarpophalangeal joint (Fig 3-13). A nondisplaced tear appeared as a distally discontinuous UCL with intervening intermediate signal intensity and normal positioning (Fig 3-14). Displacement appeared as a folded or retracted UCL. The proximal margin of the adductor aponeurosis often appeared to abut the folded UCL, giving an appearance like a yo-yo on a string (Fig 3-15).

Results.—One control specimen was excluded because the UCL could not be identified. Magnetic resonance imaging identified displacement of UCL tears in all 10 cases. A displaced tear was also incorrectly identified in 1 control specimen. Therefore, MRI was 100% sensitive and 94% specific for the identification of displaced tears. Magnetic resonance imaging identified all nondisplaced tears. Three control specimens were incorrectly identified as nondisplaced tears. For all tears, sensitivity was 100% and specificity was 66%.

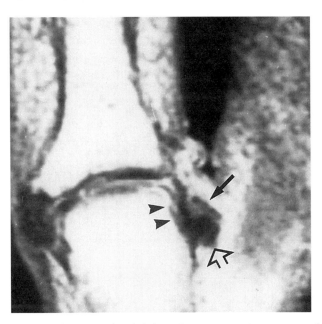

Fig 3–15.—T1-weighted MR image (500/20) shows the yo-yo on a string appearance of a displaced tear. The adductor pollicis aponeurosis (*arrowheads*) looks like a string holding a yo-yo, the balled-up, displaced UCL (*open arrow*). Note the thin region of low signal intensity (*filled arrow*), which represents an avulsed bone fragment. (Courtesy of Spaeth HJ, Abrams RA, Bock GW, et al: *Radiology* 188:553–556, 1993.)

Conclusion.—In this study, MRI was very sensitive in the diagnosis of the displacement of the ruptured UCL of the thumb. Therefore, MRI may be useful in the presurgical evaluation of patients with confusing clinical signs. A prospective study of a large series of patients is underway to delineate the benefits of MRI in the evaluation of this common injury.

▶ This work in progress demonstrates the exquisite soft tissue detail that is possible with MRI. Clinical information, however, is essential to achieve an examination of this quality and is mandatory if the proper study is to be obtained and appropriately performed.—J.S. Torg, M.D.

Skier's Thumb: The Significance of Bony Injuries

Hintermann B, Holzach PJ, Schütz M, Matter P (Hosp of Davos, Switzerland)
Am J Sports Med 21:800–804, 1993   139-94-3–30

Background.—The so-called skier's thumb is an acute injury of the ulnar collateral ligament (UCL) of the first metacarpophalangeal joint. It is generally agreed that a displaced fracture involving the attachment of the UCL is an indication for surgical repair.

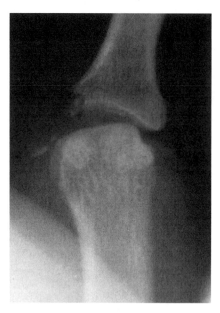 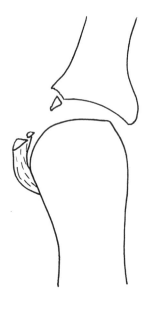

Fig 3–16.—Radiograph (**left**) and drawing (**right**) show skier's thumb injury with 2 osseous fragments, of which 1 corresponds to a bony avulsion of the UCL. The second fracture is an isolated bone fragment from the base of the proximal portion of the phalanx. (Courtesy of Hintermann B, Holzach PJ, Schütz M, et al: *Am J Sports Med* 21:800–804, 1993.)

Patients.—The anatomical findings were related to the outcome of acute skier's thumb injury in 63 consecutive patients who underwent surgery within 5 days of injury. Twenty-five patients had a fracture, whereas 38 had only ligamentous injury. The distal part of the UCL was ruptured in 34 of these patients, and the middle part of the ligament was ruptured in 4.

Findings.—Seven of the 25 patients with fracture had more than 1 fragment (Fig 3–16). Ten of the patients with a fracture had a purely ligamentous rupture of the UCL, with no connection between the fragment and the injured ligament. In these cases, the fragment originated from a fracture at the ulnar volar aspect of the base of the proximal phalanx. In 6 of the 10 patients, complete disruption of the UCL was recognized only with stress testing. In 17 cases, the fragment appeared on radiographs to be at the origin of the UCL. These were classified as a new type of injury, characterized by an isolated bony fragment combined with a ligamentous injury or bony avulsion of the UCL resulting in ulnar instability. Most injuries involving a distally ruptured UCL were treated by using the fishhook technique.

Implications.—Routine radiography does not allow reliable differentiation between an isolated fracture fragment of the phalangeal base and a bony avulsion of the UCL. Stress testing is necessary even when displacement is minimal. Fracture of the ulnar volar aspect of the proximal phalanx of the thumb may be associated with a completely disrupted UCL.

In Vitro Biomechanical Analysis of Suture Methods for Flexor Tendon Repair

Noguchi M, Seiler JG III, Gelberman RH, Sofranko RA, Woo SL-Y (Univ of Pittsburgh, Pa; Harvard Med School, Boston)
J Orthop Res 11:603–611, 1993   139-94-3–31

Background.—Rupture or gap formation after primary lacerated flexor digitorum profundus tendon repair may compromise the benefits of early mobilization. Several suture methods have been devised to allow early application of weight to the repair site. Biomechanical properties of 2 new suture methods were compared with those of 3 traditional methods in canine and human models.

Methods.—Flexor digitorum profundus tendons from 54 adult mongrel dogs and 54 adult human cadavers were lacerated and repaired using the Kessler, Tajima, or Tsuge 2-strand suture method, or the Savage or Lee 4-strand suture method (Fig 3–17). At time zero, gliding function and tensile properties of the repaired tendons were tested biomechanically.

Results.—For both canine and human specimens, the Savage and Tajima methods provided the highest value for gliding function and rotation. All suture methods provided comparable excursion. Suture failure

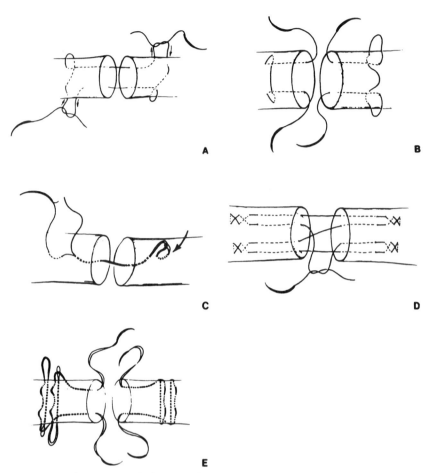

Fig 3–17.—The 5 suture methods compared in this study: the methods of Kessler (**A**), Tajima (**B**), Tsuge (**C**), Savage (modified 4-strand) (**D**), and Lee (**E**). (Courtesy of Noguchi M, Seiler JG III, Gelberman RH, et al: *J Orthop Res* 11:603–611, 1993.)

occurred with all methods, with the highest rates observed for the Savage and Lee methods. Canine linear stiffness per unit of load was highest with the Savage repair (16% of the control value), followed by the Kessler repair (14% of control). The Savage and Lee repairs provided the highest values for ultimate load and for energy absorbed per unit of length; both were more than 10% of control results. Among human specimens, only the Savage repair achieved more than 15% of the control value for linear stiffness per unit of length, although the Kessler and Tajima repairs were significantly superior to the Tsuge or Lee repairs. For energy absorbed per unit of length, the Savage and Lee methods provided 30% of the control value. Ultimate load was significantly higher with the Savage repair compared with the others.

Conclusion.—In vitro, the Savage repair is the suture of choice for tendon repair because it has the tensile characteristics needed to withstand early active mobilization and provides good gliding function. An in vivo comparison of these suture methods is needed to determine the effects of each suture method on healing.

▶ Of the 5 suture methods tested for the repair of a ruptured tendon, the authors found that the Savage modified 4-strand technique has the tensile characteristics to withstand early mobilization. This appears to be a fairly clear-cut study that should be helpful to surgeons. The authors did suggest that further study should be done to check on the effects of each suture method on healing.—Col. J.L. Anderson, PE.D.

4 Injuries of the Hip and Knee

Stress Fracture of the Femoral Neck in a Long Distance Runner: Biomechanical Aspects
Kupke MJ, Kahler DM, Lorenzoni MH, Edlich RF (Univ of Virginia, Charlottesville)
J Emerg Med 11:587–591, 1993   139-94-4-1

Background.—The increasing number of Americans participating in physical fitness programs has led to an increasing number of stress fractures being seen by emergency physicians. The diagnosis and treatment of a femoral neck stress fracture (Fig 4–1) in a long-distance runner were reviewed.

Case Report.—Woman, 27, a long-distance runner, reported a 7-day history of left thigh and groin pain exacerbated by running and walking. Local tenderness of the proximal thigh was noted, and extension, flexion, and lateral rotation of the hip produced considerable pain localized to that hip. No fracture or bony abnormalities were found on initial anteroposterior and lateral views of the left hip.

During the next 2 months her symptoms persisted, and she was referred to an orthopedic clinic. There, a ^{99m}Tc bone scan showed a density uptake in the left femoral neck. A radiographic study of the left hip confirmed a compression stress fracture of the femoral neck. Treatment consisted of weight-bearing restriction, musculoskeletal strength and flexibility maintenance, and aerobic con-

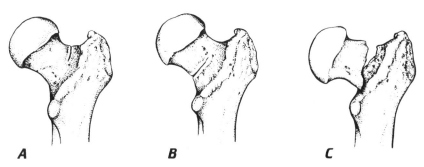

A   **B**   **C**

Fig 4–1.—Stress fracture of the femoral neck. **A,** tension side. **B,** compression side. **C,** displaced. (Courtesy of Kupke MJ, Kahler DM, Lorenzoni MH, et al: *J Emerg Med* 11:587–591, 1993.)

ditioning by aquatic therapy. Serial radiographs confirmed fracture healing. The patient's running shoes were examined and were found to have severe erosion of the lateral striking surface, which reduced shock absorption.

Conclusion.—Early diagnosis and conservative treatment enabled this athlete to resume running after the stress fracture had healed. The biomechanical cause of a compression-type stress fracture of the femoral neck may be associated with erosion of the running shoe sole, which reduces shock absorption and increases the potential for injury.

▶ Although unsupported by clinical data, the authors do present criteria for surgical vs. nonsurgical management of femoral neck stress fractures. Specifically, nonsurgical treatment is recommended for compression side fractures in that these injuries are unlikely to become displaced if treatment is initiated early. On the other hand, tension side stress fractures and complete nondisplaced fractures of the femoral neck are to be treated with internal fixation. Importantly, it is pointed out that displaced femoral neck fractures are associated with a high risk of avascular necrosis and nonunion. The attempt to attribute femoral neck stress fractures to eroded running shoes is not supported by either clinical or laboratory data.—J.S. Torg, M.D.

Relationship Between Changes in Length and Force in In Vitro Reconstructed Anterior Cruciate Ligament
Muneta T, Yamamoto H, Sakai H, Ishibashi T, Furuya K (Tokyo Med and Dental Univ)
Am J Sports Med 21:299–304, 1993   139-94-4–2

Introduction.—Successful reconstruction of the anterior cruciate ligament (ACL) rests on the correct choice of graft attachment sites on the tibia and femur. It is important to make sure that the graft will not be unduly loaded during joint flexion, but it has not been established that the change in length during isometric testing correlates with the stress on the graft when fixed between a given set of attachment sites.

Objective and Methods.—The effects of varying attachment sites on ACL grafts during unloaded flexion were examined in 8 cadaveric specimens. The grafts were attached to anteromedial and central sites on the tibia and to anterior, central, and over-the-top femoral sites (Fig 4–2). The changes in graft length were monitored at 15-degree increments from full extension to 150 degrees of passive flexion by using the degree of displacement of an inextensible 2-mm cord. After reconstruction of the ligament with a Kennedy Ligament Augmentation Device, graft forces were measured at the same flexion angles by using a buckle transducer (Fig 4–3).

Observations.—The femoral attachment site influenced both the change in graft length and force on the ACL graft more than did the tibial site. The change in length correlated closely with force measurements

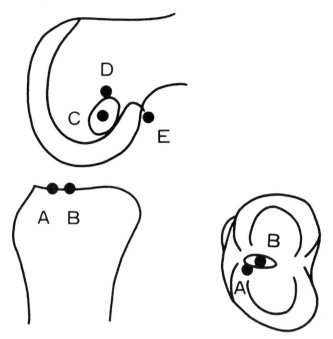

Fig 4–2.—Attachment sites used in study: A, anteromedial tibial; B, central tibial; C, central femoral; D, anterior femoral; E, over-the-top. The same 6 sites were located in each knee. (Courtesy of Muneta T, Yamamoto H, Sakai H, et al: *Am J Sports Med* 21:299-304, 1993.)

in flexion but not in near extension. Among the knees tested there was some variation in the relationship between length and force change and flexion angle for a given set of attachment sites.

Implications.—Intraoperative isometry measurements can indicate when an ACL graft is overloaded in flexion, but the change in length near extension may not reliably indicate the force on the graft.

▶ One of the important findings of this study is the amount of variability among the measurements taken using these 8 cadaveric knees. The authors were trying to determine the differences resulting from the different combinations of fixation holes that were used. However, they found that, although the force and length patterns for a given combination of holes were similar for most of the cadaveric knees tested, the force and length patterns for 1 or more knees did not follow the norm. They believe that the variability is caused in part by experimental error and in part by biological variability among the cadaveric knees. Their estimate as to the variability accounted for by experimental error is about 15%, leaving about 85% of the variability to be accounted for by biological differences among the cadaveric knees. The cadavers from which the knees were taken had a mean age of 63.9 years. Is it possible that age can cause part of that biological variability?—Col. J.L. Anderson, PE.D.

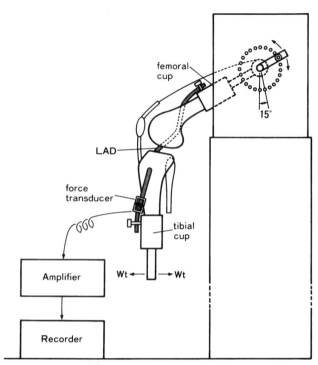

femoral
cup

15°

LAD

force
transducer

tibial
cup

Amplifier

Wt ← → Wt

Recorder

Fig 4–3.—Schematic of the examining setup: force detected by the buckle transducer in the reconstructed ACL was amplified with the dynamic strain amplifier and recorded by a pen recorder. (Courtesy of Muneta T, Yamamoto H, Sakai H, et al: *Am J Sports Med* 21:299–304, 1993.)

Roofplasty Requirements In Vitro for Different Tibial Hole Placements in Anterior Cruciate Ligament Reconstruction

Berns GS, Howell SM (Univ of California, San Diego, La Jolla; David Grant Med Ctr, Travis Air Force Base, Calif)
Am J Sports Med 21:292–298, 1993   139-94-4–3

Background.—When anterior cruciate ligament (ACL) graft impingement occurs, it can cause pain and graft failure. To determine the relationship of the ACL graft to the intercondylar roof as the knee is flexed and extended, measurements were made in 7 fresh-frozen cadaveric knees.

Methods.—The perpendicular force of the intercondylar roof against an ACL graft was measured by using a force transducer implanted in the intercondylar roof (Fig 4–4). The effect of varying the amount of roof removed was examined for 2 tibial hole positions: an anterior-eccentric hole and a customized hole aligned 4–5 mm posterior and parallel to the slope of the intercondylar roof in the extended knee. Graft tension was also measured. Load cycles were repeated with the roof force sensor

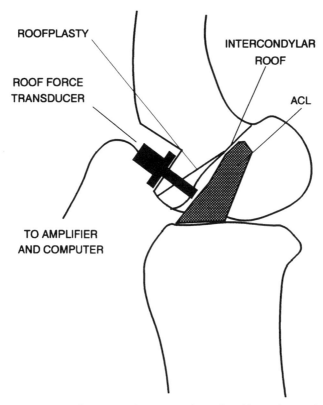

ROOFPLASTY

ROOF FORCE
TRANSDUCER

INTERCONDYLAR
ROOF

ACL

TO AMPLIFIER
AND COMPUTER

Fig 4–4.—A pressure transducer was used to measure the total roof force. The transducer was implanted perpendicularly to the intact roof after performance of a generous roofplasty. (Courtesy of Berns GS, Howell SM: *Am J Sports Med* 21:292–298, 1993.)

backed out in .8-mm increments, representing a corresponding increase in the amount of bone removal at roofplasty.

Results.—At all backout increments, the flexion angle at the roof-graft contact was consistently larger when the anterior tibial hole was used than when the customized hole was used. The anterior hole required an average of 4.6 mm of roof removal, compared with 1.3 mm of roof removal at the custom hole for zero graft impingement.

Conclusion.—A significant relationship was demonstrated between the placement of the tibial hole for ACL grafting and intercondylar force. The anterior-eccentric tibial hole placement required on average significantly more bone removal at roofplasty than did the customized tibial tunnel to produce zero graft impingement. This suggests that the amount of roofplasty performed should be determined intraoperatively and that the placement of the tibial hole will influence this decision.

▶ Although the authors do not report how often or what percentage of the time impingement of an ACL graft occurs, it is well understood that the clinical consequences of unrecognized graft impingement can be severe and include graft failure, extension deficit, chronic knee effusions, and pain. This study, done using fresh-frozen cadaveric knees, tried to determine the amount of roofplasty necessary to eliminate ligament graft impingement. It is unclear to me how closely this research, using cadaveric knees, can be related to surgery done on the knees of live patients.—Col. J.L. Anderson, PE.D.

Biomechanics of Intra-Articular and Extra-Articular Reconstruction of the Anterior Cruciate Ligament
Amis AA, Scammell BE (Imperial College, London)
J Bone Joint Surg (Br) 75–B:812–817, 1993   139-94-4–4

Background.—There are 2 main types of autogenous reconstruction of the anterior cruciate ligament (ACL): the intra-articular (IA) and the extra-articular (EA); at times a combination of the 2 methods (IA + EA) is used. The biomechanical properties of these reconstruction techniques were tested in a series of cadaveric knee reconstructions.

Method.—Extra-articular, intra-articular, and IA + EA reconstruction was done in 10 cadaveric knees after the ACL was ruptured by a rapid anterior drawer movement. The stability at each stage before and after rupture and reconstruction was tested by anterior drawer, Lachman, varus-valgus, and tibial rotation tests.

Results.—Normal stability was restored by the IA and the IA + EA reconstructions. The IA reconstruction alone restored normal stability on anterior drawer and tibial rotation testing. The EA reconstruction improved stability but did not return it to normal. The IA + EA reconstruction provided no additional stability over that achieved by an IA reconstruction alone.

Conclusion.—In a study of cadaveric knees, ACL rupture was caused by a rapid anterior drawer movement. This method of rupture suggests that great anterior instability can be produced without stretching the collateral ligaments. This casts doubt on their previously accepted role as secondary restraints after ACL rupture. For isolated ACL deficiency, there is no biomechanical basis for adding the EA procedure to an IA reconstruction and no basis for performing an EA reconstruction alone.

▶ This is another excellent study using cadaveric knees, and the last sentence of my comment made in Abstract 139-94-4–3 concerning the relationship between cadaveric knees and live knees still applies. This is especially true for this study because these cadaveric knees were obtained from elderly specimens with no benefit of stabilization by muscles. Regardless, as a clinical study it was well done and provides valuable clinical information concerning the apparent benefits of the IA method over the EA or the IA + EA methods.

The authors believe that this is the first study of its kind in which traumatic rupture of the ACL was the starting point. They also believe that, because their procedures caused "definite slackening" of the secondary restraint system to include the collateral ligaments and they found that the collateral ligaments were shown to have been stretched by the anterior tibial displacement, their research casts doubt on whether the collateral ligaments really are a part of the secondary restraint system. They believe that the implication is that the posterolateral and posteromedial capsuloligamentous tissues provide the secondary restraint to anterior drawer movement.—Col. J.L. Anderson, PE.D.

A Test for Eliminating False Positive Anterior Cruciate Ligament Injury Diagnoses

Draper DO, Schulthies S (Brigham Young Univ, Provo, Utah)
J Athletic Train 28:355–357, 1993   139-94-4–5

Introduction.—In a recent study in which physicians and physical therapists used the Lachman test to evaluate the anterior cruciate ligament (ACL), 30% of individuals lacking a ligament tear were told that they had a damaged ACL. A false positive test may occur when the posterior cruciate ligament (PCL) is damaged, leading the tibia to sag posteriorly onto the femur. When an anterior drawer or Lachman test is done, the tibia seems to move forward on the femur in conjunction with anterior instability.

The Alternate Lachman Test.—A false positive diagnosis of ACL injury may be ruled out by palpating the anterior joint margin with the knee supported in 30 degrees of flexion. Pressure is applied downward and forward on the posterior aspect of the proximal tibia. If the tibia moves on the femur 6 mm more than on the other side, an ACL lesion probably is present. Otherwise, any anterior tibial motion noted on the conventional Lachman test may be ascribed to a torn PCL. This may be confirmed by the posterior sag and posterior drawer tests.

Advantages.—The alternate Lachman test is done with the patient in a prone position, so that gravity will cause the tibia to remain in its normal position even if the PCL is damaged. Palpation of the joint line throughout the test allows an end feel to be readily detected.

▶ Rebman reported on the use of this test in 1988 (1). I have used it and found it to be a more accurate and easier method of evaluating ACL injuries. Most of my colleagues continue to depend on the Lachman test to evaluate ACL problems. I believe it is easier for the patient to relax in the prone position, and I am able to support the weight of the lower leg and to feel movement along the joint line more easily. If there is a torn PCL, gravity will not cause me to get a false positive anterior shift of the tibia on the femur.—F.J. George, A.T.C., P.T.

Reference

1. Rebman LW: *J Orthop Sports Phys Ther* 9:381, 1988.

Prospective Evaluation of the McMurray Test
Evans PJ, Bell GD, Frank C (Univ of Calgary, Alta: Univ of Toronto)
Am J Sports Med 21:604–608, 1993   139-94-4-6

Purpose.—The McMurray test is used clinically to diagnose meniscal tears. Although the test has been used since 1940, its validity has often been questioned. The accuracy and inter-examiner reliability of the McMurray test for meniscal tears were compared with arthroscopic findings.

Methods.—The McMurray test was performed on the knees of 104 patients undergoing elective arthroscopic knee surgery and on both knees of 60 medical students. Each knee was tested by 2 independent examiners. The test was recorded as positive if a thud was elicited during rotation of the knee or if a sensation mimicking the clinical symptoms was reported during manipulation of the knee.

Results.—Sixty-nine meniscal tears were found in 59 of the 104 knees (56%) examined by arthroscopy. Fifty-one knees had a positive McMurray test. A thud elicited on the medial joint line was the only significant sign to correlate with meniscal injury. The medial thud had a sensitivity of 16%, a specificity of 98%, and a positive predictive value of 83%. The test was not useful for lateral meniscal tears. The test had low inter-examiner reliability.

Conclusion.—The McMurray test is of limited use in the diagnosis of meniscal tears.

▶ This paper places the value of the McMurray test into its proper perspective. Specifically, it is a noninvasive, cost-effective examination that has both a high specificity and a high predictive value. With regard to its low sensitivity, we must conclude that that is what arthroscopy is for.—J.S. Torg, M.D.

The Quantitative Measurement of Normal Passive Medial and Lateral Patellar Motion Limits
Skalley TC, Terry GC, Teitge RA (Hughston Orthopaedic Clinic, PC, Columbus, Ga; Teitge Orthopaedic Clinic, Warren, Mich)
Am J Sports Med 21:728–732, 1993   139-94-4-7

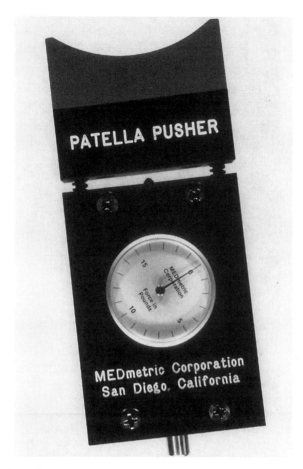

Fig 4–5.—The Patella Pusher, a handheld force gauge, was used to apply a displacement force to the patella. (Courtesy of Skalley TC, Terry GC, Teitge RA: *Am J Sports Med* 21:728–732, 1993.)

Objective.—The limits of normal medial and lateral passive patellar motion in extension and flexion were established in 67 high school athletes (43 male and 24 female) who were randomly chosen from among 1,340 who were having a preseason physical examination. The average age was 15 years.

Methods.—Patellar displacement was measured at knee flexion angles of 0 and 35 degrees, using both a handheld force gauge (Fig 4–5) and a manual technique (Fig 4-6). Two investigators performed the measurements under constant conditions.

Findings.—With the knee extended, passive patellar displacement averaged 9.6 mm medially and 5.4 mm laterally. In flexion, medial and lateral displacements averaged 9.4 and 10 mm, respectively. The limits of patellar motion did not correlate positively with demographic data or

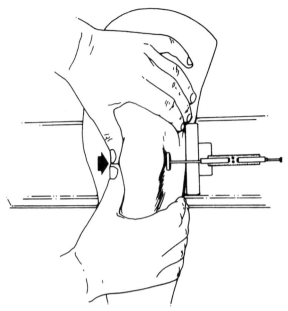

Fig 4–6.—Manual application of a displacement force to the patella. (Courtesy of Skalley TC, Terry GC, Teitge RA: *Am J Sports Med* 21:728–732, 1993.)

with the findings on physical examination. The 2 methods gave similar results, but more variable findings were obtained with the Patella Pusher on testing in flexion.

Suggestion.—When passive patellar mobility is examined, the examination should be done at both extension and 35 degrees of flexion.

▶ The authors believe that the passive medial and lateral patellar motion limits determined in this study of normal knees can provide reasonable clinical quantitative parameters of motion limits. Of note, the measurements from the mechanical handheld Patella Pusher force gauge were not as reproducible as a manually produced displacement.—J.S. Torg, M.D.

Endoscopic Extra-Articular Lateral Release
Chow JCY (Orthopaedic Clinic of Mt Vernon, Ill)
Arthroscopy 9:327–331, 1993   139-94-4-8

Background.—The current arthroscopic technique for lateral retinacular release requires cutting through the synovial membrane by electrocautery. To decrease the risk of hemarthrosis and reduce the amount of postoperative pain associated with a lateral release of the retinaculum, a less invasive extra-articular release has been designed.

Technique.—The procedure is performed with the patient under general anesthesia and using currently available endoscopic instrumentation. An uninflated tourniquet is applied to the affected thigh. The arthroscope is inserted through a portal located about 3 fingerbreadths proximal to the proximal pole of the patella. The main point of the new technique is that a slotted cannula assembly is passed between the synovium and the lateral retinaculum and that the synovial membrane does not have to be cut before the retinaculum can be released.

Outcome.—All 20 patients who underwent the new arthroscopic procedure were able to start rehabilitation exercises immediately after the procedure. At the follow-up visit 7–10 days after arthroscopic release, most patients had little postoperative pain and had regained knee joint motion.

▶ The authors describe an innovative approach to performing a lateral retinacular release. A description of this method has been published as a technical note. The definitive report must determine whether the technique is effective and reduces the number of complications associated with the arthroscopic lateral retinacular release.—J.S. Torg, M.D.

Principles and Decision Making in Meniscal Surgery
Newman AP, Daniels AU, Burks RT (Univ of Utah, Salt Lake City)
Arthroscopy 9:33–51, 1993   139-94-4-9

Background.—Once thought to be inconsequential and functionless, it is now understood that menisci are integral components of normal knee function. The basic science of menisci and clinical information on meniscal surgery were reviewed.

Basic Science.—Laboratory studies have demonstrated that the menisci are involved in many important functions, such as tibiofemoral load transmission, shock absorption, lubrication, and passive stabilization of the knee joint. Histologic and structural studies have shown that menisci are annular structures that can transmit and properly distribute load over the tibial plateau, facilitated mainly by the circumferential collagen fibers in the peripheral one third of the meniscus, in conjunction with their strong bony attachments at the anterior and posterior horns. According to biological research, meniscal healing occurs in 1 of 2 ways—through an intrinsic ability of the meniscal fibrochondrocyte to migrate, proliferate, and synthesize matrix, or through extrinsic stimulation by neovascularization.

Meniscal Surgery.—Animal and clinical studies indicate that degenerative changes commonly develop after meniscectomy. Therefore, surgeons have become more aggressive in conserving as much meniscal tissue as possible. Current treatments of meniscal tears are based on a thorough understanding of meniscal structure, biology, and function; they require familiarity with the basic principles of meniscal repair and

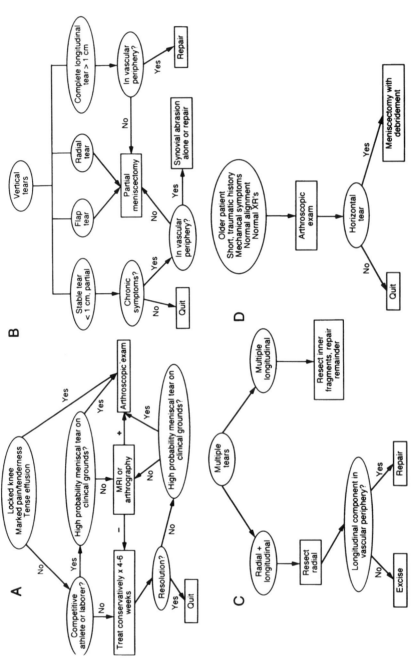

Fig 4–7.—Algorithm for treatment of meniscal lesions. **A,** decision to proceed to arthroscopy; **B,** management of vertical tears; **C,** management of multiple tears; **D,** management of horizontal tears. XR, roentgenogram. (Courtesy of Newman AP, Daniels AU, Burks RT: *Arthroscopy* 9:33–51, 1993.)

resection. The algorithm provided (Fig 4-7) can guide surgical decisions in different clinical situations.

Conclusion.—Treatment decisions in cases of meniscal lesions can now be based on sound mechanical and biological principles. Individual patient characteristics, such as age, activity level, and associated injuries, also need to be considered.

▶ This is an excellent comprehensive review of the principles of dealing with arthroscopic meniscal surgery. The original article is recommended reading for the interested reader.—J.S. Torg, M.D.

Arthroscopic Assessment of the Posterior Compartments of the Knee Via the Intercondylar Notch: The Arthroscopist's Field of View
Morin WD, Steadman JR (Naval Hosp, San Diego, Calif; Steadman-Hawkins Clinic, Vail, Colo)
Arthroscopy 9:284–290, 1993   139-94-4-10

Background.—Multiple views of the knee joint are essential to accurate arthroscopic assessment of all compartments. The adequacy of visualization, the limits of the arthroscopic field of view (FOV), and the potential blind spots at the periphery of the meniscocapsular junction during standard arthroscopic evaluation were investigated.

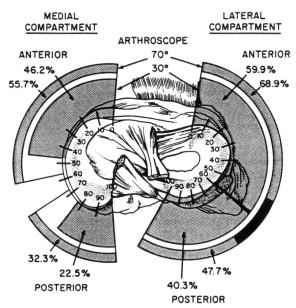

Fig 4–8.—Arthroscopic FOV for medial and lateral compartments, with 30-degree and 70-degree arthroscopes. (Courtesy of Morin WD, Steadman JR: *Arthroscopy* 9:284–290, 1993.)

Methods.—Five human cadaveric knees were used. Arthroscopy was performed through standard anteromedial and anterolateral portals. The posterior compartments were reached through the intercondylar notch. The FOV was maximized with a 30-degree and then a 70-degree arthroscope, and the farthest point of visualization was marked with a laser. The FOV was designated as a percentage of the total meniscocapsular periphery.

Findings.—The mean FOV was 100.2% with the 30-degree arthroscope and 116.6% with the 70-degree arthroscope. The entire periphery of the lateral meniscocapsular junction could be visualized in all knees with the 30-degree scope anteriorly in combination with the 70-degree scope posteriorly. Medially, the mean FOV was 68.9% and 88.1% with the 30- and 70-degree scopes, respectively. A blind spot, found in all knees, averaged 21.5% of the meniscocapsular periphery anteriorly with the 30-degree arthroscope and posteriorly with the 70-degree arthroscope (Fig 4–8).

Conclusion.—There is an arthroscopic blind spot in the posteromedial compartment viewed through the intercondylar notch. If abnormalities in the posteromedial compartment are suspected but not seen on initial arthroscopic evaluation, the arthroscopist must assess the blind spot through an accessory posteromedial portal.

Arthroscopic Visual Field Mapping at the Periphery of the Medial Meniscus: A Comparison of Different Portal Approaches

Tolin BS, Sapega AA (Univ of Pennsylvania, Philadelphia)
Arthroscopy 9:265–271, 1993   139-94-4–11

Background.—It has been found that the posteromedial compartment, especially the posterior horn of the medial meniscus, is a common source of diagnostic error in knee arthroscopy when access is restricted to anterior portals. The anatomical basis of this apparent technical limitation was investigated.

Methods.—Visible and blind zones of the posteromedial meniscal periphery were studied in 6 fresh knee specimens. The arthroscopic approaches used included a direct anteromedial frontal view with a 30-degree arthroscope (AM-30); anterolateral portal with a 30-degree arthroscope, transnotch view (AL-30); anterolateral portal, 70-degree arthroscope, transnotch view (AL-70); central portal, 70-degree scope, transnotch view (C-70); and posteromedial portal, 30-degree scope, direct rear view (PM-30).

Findings.—In all knees, only the anterior half or less of the total superior meniscosynovial junction length could be visualized with the AM-30 approach. The AL-30 enabled visualization of the posteriormost 16.4%; the C-70, 24.2%; AL-70, 31.6%; and the PM-30, 54.9% of the upper meniscal rim. Combined with the AM-30 visual field, the PM-30 approach

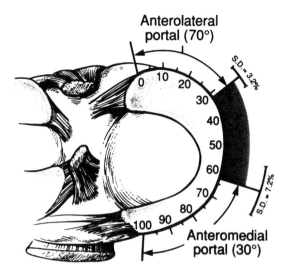

Anterolateral
portal (70°)

S.D. = 3.2%

0 10 20
30
40
50
60
70
80
100 90

S.D. = 7.2%

Anteromedial
portal (30°)

Blind Zone ■ = 32% (±10)

Fig 4–9.—Mean (± standard deviation [S.D.]) posterior visual field and blind zone with use of an anterolateral portal and a 70-degree arthroscope through the intercondylar notch, in combination with a frontal view of the medial meniscal periphery via an anteromedial portal with a 30-degree arthroscope. (Courtesy of Tolin BS, Sapega AA: *Arthroscopy* 9:265–271, 1993.)

provided the most thorough overall visualization of the superior meniscosynovial junction. The mean blind zone was only 8.4% between the anterior and posterior visual fields. The AL-30, C-70, and AL-70 approaches resulted in significantly greater areas of the meniscal rim being unseen (Figs 4–9 and 4–10).

Conclusion.—Visualization of the posteromedial meniscosynovial junction with direct frontal viewing is limited or impossible in many knees. A 70-degree arthroscope placed in the posteromedial compartment through the intercondylar notch will not permit complete assessment of the posteromedial meniscal periphery. Typically, it is blind to a 3- to 5-cm zone at the posteromedial corner.

▶ From these 2 papers (Abstracts 139-94-4–10 and 139-94-4–11), one can conclude that with regard to the evaluation of fresh-frozen human cadaveric knees there exists a small peripheral blind zone at the posteromedial corner. The authors do not clearly establish how this in vitro observation relates to the operative setting, where with adequate distraction and use of a probe, most if not all medial menisci may be adequately examined. Also, the authors have failed to discuss the possible complications resulting from routine use of a posteromedial portal.—J.S. Torg, M.D.

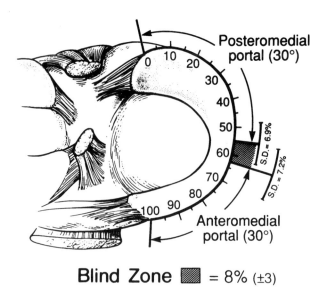

Blind Zone ▨ = 8% (±3)

Fig 4–10.—Mean (± standard deviation [S.D.]) posterior visual field and blind zone with use of a posteromedial portal and a 30-degree arthroscope, in combination with a frontal view of the medial meniscal periphery via an anteromedial portal with a 30-degree arthroscope. (Courtesy of Tolin BS, Sapega AA: *Arthroscopy* 9:265–271, 1993.)

Trephination of Incomplete Meniscal Tears

Fox JM, Rintz KG, Ferkel RD (Southern California Orthopedic Inst, Van Nuys)
Arthroscopy 9:451–455, 1993   139-94-4–12

Background.—Methods of promoting healing of meniscal lesions have been designed to help preserve important meniscal functions. One method involves trephination—the creation of vascular access channels by removing a core of tissue from the meniscal periphery to the tear, thus connecting a lesion in the avascular part of the meniscus to the peripheral blood supply. Experience with using arthroscopic trephination in treating incomplete meniscal tears was reviewed.

Patients.—Thirty patients underwent trephination of incomplete meniscal tears. The 25 men and 5 women were aged 19–65 years. Twenty-nine were available for reexamination.

Technique.—The procedure begins with diagnostic arthroscopic assessment of the knee under anesthesia. With the arthroscope in the inferolateral portal, the meniscus is probed from the inferomedial portal. The superior and inferior surfaces of the meniscus are probed with special attention to the area of the tear, to ensure that it does not extend to both meniscal surfaces. The edges of the tear are then freshened with a full radius resector or basket forceps, or both. An 18-gauge spinal needle bent to maneuver between the articular surfaces is used to puncture the meniscus from the inside out, extending from the inner rim and substance of the tear into the capsule, until multiple bleeding puncture sites are seen. This part of the procedure is performed without the tourniquet inflated so the vascularity after trephination may be better assessed.

Outcomes.—The outcomes of the procedure were good to excellent in 90% of patients and fair to poor in 10%. Twenty-one of the 24 patients (88%) who were athletically active before surgery returned to the same sport without limitations. Twelve percent changed their sport or resumed the original sport with limitations.

Conclusion.—Symptomatic incomplete meniscal tears can be treated by stimulating vascular channels. This procedure avoids the risk associated with tissue suturing and preserves the important functions of the meniscus. Overall outcomes were good to excellent in 90% of patients.

▶ This is an interesting report, prospective in nature and with apparent merit. The authors' failure to have a comparable control series renders the conclusion somewhat inconclusive. Also, pre- and postsurgical MRI studies would have been helpful in demonstrating the effect of the procedure.—J.S. Torg, M.D.

Arthroscopic Treatment of Meniscal Cysts

Ryu RKN, Ting AJ (Santa Barbara, Calif; Palo Alto, Calif)
Arthroscopy 9:591–595, 1993   139-94-4–13

Background.—The strong association between primary meniscal pathologic change and meniscal cyst formation has only recently been accepted, its validation attributable in no small part to use of the arthroscope as an investigative tool. Despite this key to the pathogenesis of cyst formation, our understanding of the process is incomplete. Treatment options generally involve cyst excision or decompression in combination with varying degrees of meniscectomy. A study was conducted to confirm the association between meniscal tears and cyst formation, to determine the ratio of medial to lateral cysts, and to assess the efficacy of arthroscopic cyst decompression.

Materials and Methods.—The 5-year study included data on 18 patients who had undergone arthroscopy and who had MRI-documented meniscal cysts. Patients were reexamined or interviewed at the time of the study. In each of the patients, a horizontal cleavage tear was observed, the leading edge of which was trimmed. The cyst opening was located by gentle pressure, which often ejected some cystic material. Openings were enlarged to 4–5 mm and the cysts were emptied.

Results.—Eight of the patients had medial cysts and 10 had lateral cysts. All complained of pain, and just over half had received a predisposing injury an average of 2.8 years earlier. After surgery, all patients returned to normal activity; 16 were asymptomatic, whereas 2 complained of occasional stiffness and effusions but did not consider themselves limited. To the date of publication, there were no recurrences.

Discussion.—Cyst formation may occur through a pumping action that involves the flow of synovial fluid along a tear line. The process of trimming the tear and enlarging the cyst's opening appears to be effective in treating this condition. The use of imaging techniques before surgery is recommended, because the cyst can be located and may indicate the region of the tear.

▶ The authors' conclusion that treatment of a meniscal cyst can be entirely arthroscopic is in keeping with my own experience.—J.S. Torg, M.D.

MR Diagnosis of Recurrent Tears in the Knee: Value of Intraarticular Contrast Material

Applegate GR, Flannigan BD, Tolin BS, Fox JM, Del Pizzo W (Valley Presbyterian Magnetic Resonance Ctr, Van Nuys, Calif; San Antonio Orthopedic Group, Tex; Southern California Orthopedic Inst, Van Nuys)
AJR 161:821–825, 1993   139-94-4–14

Objective.—Because routine MRI has not proved reliable in detection of recurrent meniscal tears after surgical resection, MR arthrography was

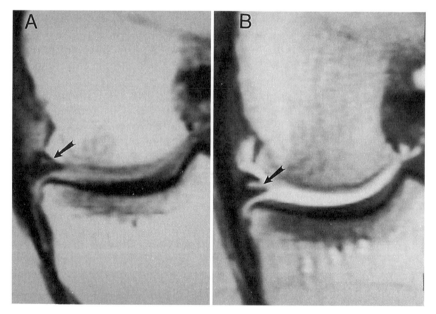

Fig 4–11.—**A,** coronal T1-weighted conventional MR image shows a meniscal remnant (*arrow*) with grade II intrameniscal signal intensity. **B,** coronal T1-weighted MR arthrogram shows a recurrent horizontal tear (*arrow*) extending to the superior articulating surface. (Courtesy of Applegate GR, Flannigan BD, Tolin BS, et al: AJR 161:821-825, 1993.)

evaluated in 37 patients who underwent either meniscal repair or resection. The patients, 19 women and 18 men aged 17-72 years, all had persistent or recurrent knee pain after surgery.

Methods.—Conventional MR studies included spin-echo T1-weighted and T2-weighted images and a 16-cm field of view. Magnetic resonance arthrography was performed by using 40-50 mL of a 1:100 saline solution of gadopentetate dimeglumine. Arthroscopy was performed shortly after the MR studies, and follow-up arthroscopic surgery was performed an average of 6½ weeks later. The conventional MR studies and MR arthrograms were reviewed separately and randomly, and the findings were compared with the arthroscopic appearances.

Results.—Conventional MRI revealed recurrent meniscal tears with a sensitivity of 69% and a specificity of 60%. Its negative and positive predictive values were 53% and 75%, respectively. Magnetic resonance arthrography was 89% sensitive and 86% specific and had negative and positive predictive values of 80% and 92%, respectively. A majority of postoperative menisci had undergone 25% to 75% resection; in these cases, MR arthrography was substantially more accurate (Fig 4–11). Magnetic resonance arthrography allowed detection of small meniscal remnants. Conventional MRI was insensitive when an effusion tracked into a meniscal tear.

Conclusion.—Magnetic resonance arthrography is a useful alternative to repeated arthroscopy in patients treated surgically for meniscal tear. Results of further studies with high-resolution pulse sequences will be of interest.

▶ The authors fail to identify how they confirmed that a defect in the inner rim of a postsurgical meniscus was, in fact, the cause of the patient's symptoms. If correct, then the authors further fail to identify the benefit of MR arthrography compared with routine arthrography. Routine arthrography is highly accurate for the detection of the morphology of the inner rim of a postsurgical meniscus. Routine arthrography also is one third the cost of MR arthrography. A routine knee arthrogram, including the anesthetic and analgesic preparation of the knee, can be performed in approximately 15–20 minutes.

According to this study, MR arthrography requires 60–90 minutes and, if fluoroscopy is not used, the MR is tied up for 30 minutes during the injection procedure. Additionally, the contrast used for MR arthrography is not approved for intra-articular use. It is interesting that the authors use an 18-gauge needle for MR arthrography when a 20- or 22-gauge needle is adequate for routine arthrography; this would imply that MR arthrography is both financially and physically more invasive than routine arthrography.—J.S. Torg, M.D.

An Evaluation of Pre- and Postoperative Nonsteroidal Antiinflammatory Drugs in Patients Undergoing Knee Arthroscopy: A Prospective, Randomized, Double-Blinded Study

Nelson WE, Henderson RC, Almekinders LC, DeMasi RA, Taft TN (Univ of North Carolina, Chapel Hill)
Am J Sports Med 21:510–516, 1993   139-94-4–15

Introduction.—Previous studies have suggested that nonsteroidal antiinflammatory drugs (NSAIDs) can reduce pain and enhance recovery after orthopedic operations, including arthroscopy. Preoperative knee pain is the most important determinant of postoperative knee pain, but it remains to be seen whether giving NSAIDs preoperatively could have a significant effect on postoperative pain.

Methods.—This prospective, randomized, placebo-controlled, double-blind study examined the effects of preoperative and postoperative NSAIDs in 67 patients undergoing knee arthroscopic surgery. The average patient age was 31 years, and most patients were recreational or competitive athletes. The 22 patients in group A received diclofenac, 75 mg twice daily, for 3–5 days preoperatively and for 7 days postoperatively. The 19 patients in group B received placebo before surgery and diclofenac afterward; the 26 patients in group C received placebo both before and after surgery. All patients could take codeine, if needed, after the operation. Subjective and objective outcome measures were analyzed, including isokinetic knee flexion and extension strength.

Results.—On the day after surgery, group C had higher pain scores than group A. This was the only time at which the 3 groups showed any significant differences in pain scores. Codeine requirements in the first 72 hours after surgery were lower in groups A and B than in group C (3 vs. 7 tablets). There were no significant differences in recovery of strength and function or in knee effusion, range of motion, and gait.

Conclusion.—The effectiveness of diclofenac in the immediate postoperative period after knee arthroscopy was documented. However, it does not appear to enhance recovery from the procedure. The most likely explanation for this lack of effect was the fast recovery time in the patient group studied.

Arthroscopy of the Knee: Ten-Day Pain Profiles and Corticosteroids

Highgenboten CL, Jackson AW, Meske NB (Orthopaedic Consultants, Dallas; Univ of North Texas, Denton)
Am J Sports Med 21:503–506, 1993   139-94-4–16

Background.—Although arthroscopic surgery has become a common procedure, particularly for knee injury, little has been written on patient pain, recovery, and rehabilitation after the procedure. Ten-day pain and analgesic use profiles of patients undergoing arthroscopic knee surgery were investigated with emphasis on whether the use of corticosteroids would significantly enhance these profiles.

Methods.—Sixty-eight patients who underwent arthroscopic surgery of the knee were assigned to experimental and placebo groups by random selection. Experimental group patients received the corticosteroid, methylprednisolone, in 4-mg tablet form. On 6 consecutive days they took 6, 5, 4, 3, 2, and 1 tablet orally per day. The control group took the placebo tablets with the same protocol. Both groups received the same prescription of analgesic for pain relief after surgery.

Results.—A positive prognosis was seen for most patients. Crutch use ranged from 0 to 10 days. Of the 45 patients who worked outside the home, only 16 had not returned to work after 10 days. Analgesic use and perceived pain levels were moderate on day 1 after surgery but had decreased by day 4. Six patients reported high pain scores on day 1, but by day 4 only 2 were still in significant pain. In terms of corticosteroid use, no differences in the recovery profiles were observed between the experimental and placebo groups. Contrary to observations in other studies, corticosteroids did not have a positive effect. This result may be attributable to the type of corticosteroids used, to the fact that they were administered postoperatively rather than intraoperatively, or to the fact that the trauma associated with the patients in the current study was less severe than that experienced by patients in previous studies.

Conclusion.—Most patients who underwent arthroscopic surgery of the knee reported moderate levels of pain on the first day after surgery. This pain had decreased by the fourth day. Analgesic use followed this pattern. Administration of corticosteroids did not produce any changes in the recovery profile, probably because of the limited pain, edema, and trauma experienced by patients in this study.

▶ Another consideration not adequately dealt with by these 2 papers (Abstracts 139-94-4–15 and 139-94-4–16) is that of the occurrence of possible side effects with use of the drugs.—J.S. Torg, M.D.

Effects of Intraarticular Morphine on Analgesic Requirements After Anterior Cruciate Ligament Repair

Joshi GP, McCarroll SM, McSwiney M, O'Rourke P, Hurson BJ (Cappagh Orthopedic Hosp and Mater Misericordiae Hosp, Dublin)
Reg Anesth 18:254–257, 1993   139-94-4–17

Background.—Pain after anterior cruciate ligament (ACL) reconstruction is severe and difficult to manage. The usual treatments, intramuscular or epidural opioids and local anesthetic infusion, may be highly toxic and provide only limited relief. Intravenous patient-controlled analgesia (PCA) is an expensive alternative. Intra-articular morphine injection after arthroscopic knee surgery provides extended analgesia, moderated by local mediators. The analgesic effects of intra-articular morphine injection after ACL repair were evaluated using a double-blind prospective design.

Methods.—Twenty males undergoing elective ACL repair were randomized to receive an intra-articular injection of either 5 mg of morphine in a 25-mL dilution or 25 mL of saline at the conclusion of surgery. After closure, morphine or saline was injected into the joint through a separate site. Immediately after surgery, patients received a loading dose of morphine (2–5 mg as an intravenous bolus) every 5 minutes until pain was controlled, followed by PCA (1–1.5 mg of morphine every 6 minutes). Pain was measured by a visual analogue scale ranging from 0 (no pain) to 10 (worst pain imaginable).

Results.—Patients treated with intra-articular morphine consumed significantly less total morphine (mean, 3.4 mg) compared with controls (mean, 73.5 mg). Postoperative pain scores were consistently lower in the morphine group, although between-group differences were not significant.

Conclusion.—Intra-articular morphine injection decreases the total dose of morphine needed to control pain after ACL repair. This local administration of morphine may reduce the toxicity of postsurgical analgesia and may permit effective pain management with less toxic agents such as nonsteroidal anti-inflammatory drugs. Future research should focus on this multimodal approach to postoperative pain management.

Postarthroscopy Analgesia With Intraarticular Bupivacaine/Morphine: A Randomized Clinical Trial
Allen GC, St Amand MA, Lui ACP, Johnson DH, Lindsay MP (The Pennsylvania State Univ, Hershey; Univ of Ottawa, Ont, Canada; Ottawa Civic Hosp, Ont, Canada)
Anesthesiology 79:475–480, 1993   139-94-4–18

Background.—Satisfactory analgesia after arthroscopic knee surgery can be achieved with intra-articular bupivacaine, but only for a few hours. In contrast, intra-articular morphine provides longer-lasting analgesia, but at a delayed onset. Because the time of onset and duration of action of these agents appear to complement each other, the combination of intra-articular morphine and bupivacaine should provide ideal analgesia after knee arthroscopy.

Study Design.—One hundred twenty outpatients, American Society of Anesthesiologists Physical Status I to II, underwent knee arthroscopy under general anesthesia with intravenous fentanyl, propofol, N_2O, O_2, and isoflurane. At the end of surgery, before tourniquet release, the patients received, in a random manner, intra-articular injections of .25% bupivacaine (group 1); 1 mg of morphine in saline (group 2); 2 mg of morphine in saline (group 3); or 1 mg of morphine in .25% bupivacaine (group 4). The volume injected was 30 mL, and all solutions contained 1:200,000 epinephrine. For postoperative analgesia, the patients received intravenous fentanyl and/or oral acetaminophen.

Outcome.—At 1-6 hours after arthroscopy, scores on the visual analogue pain scale (VAPS) and the McGill Pain Questionnaire were lowest in groups 1 and 4. Despite receiving a larger dose, group 3 had significantly greater VAPS scores than did group 2. At 24 hours, VAPS scores were lowest in groups 2, 3, and 4. Furthermore, patients in groups 1 and 4 required less supplemental analgesia for the first 12 hours, but no differences were observed between groups at 24 hours. There were no adverse effects to treatment.

Conclusion.—Intra-articular morphine, 1 mg in 30 mL of .25% bupivacaine with 1:200,000 epinephrine, may provide superior analgesia for up to 24 hours after knee arthroscopy, compared with bupivacaine or morphine alone.

▶ These 2 papers (Abstracts 139-94-4–17 and 139-94-4–18) support similar findings by Khoury et al. (1) and Joshi (2). Joshi also pointed out that the low levels of plasma morphine observed were a result of poor lipid solubility, which hampers its passage across the synovial membrane, thus increasing the effective half-life of the agent in the joint. Because the levels of plasma morphine are very low, this technique is safe and causes relatively few side effects.—J.S. Torg, M.D.

References

1. Khoury GF, et al: *Anesthesiology* 77:263, 1992.
2. Joshi GP, et al: *J Bone Joint Surg (Br)* 74-B: 749, 1992.

Complications of Arthroscopic Meniscal Repair
Austin KS, Sherman OH (New York Univ)
Am J Sports Med 21:864–869, 1993   139-94-4–19

Background.—The surgical repair of meniscal tears is associated with a wide range of risks and side effects, although the efficacy of the technique is generally accepted. Reports of the complication rate for arthroscopic meniscal repair have varied considerably. The specific complications of these repairs were examined.

Materials and Methods.—A total of 101 consecutive arthroscopic repairs of the meniscus performed between November 1984 and January 1991 were reviewed. Sixteen patients with concurrent anterior cruciate ligament (ACL) injury chose to receive meniscal repair without ACL reconstruction. The inside-out technique was used to repair most tears of the meniscus, with the outside-in technique being used for the most posterior tears. During the study, the postoperative care provided for these patients was changed: since 1989, full unrestricted motion without a brace has been allowed, and since 1990, weight-bearing has been allowed at earlier times after surgery, depending on the size of the meniscal tear.

Results.—Lateral meniscal tears were repaired in 23 patients and medial tears were repaired in 78. Sixty-five patients had associated injury to the ACL; in 15 cases the injuries were lateral and in 50 they were medial. Complications occurred in 18 patients: saphenous neuropathy and arthrofibrosis accounted for 13. Arthrofibrosis occurred only in the presence of concurrent or previous ACL injury, resulting in insufficient function. Five complications occurred in 36 cases of isolated meniscal tears (14%); all occurred with medial repairs. In the presence of ACL injury, the rate of complications increased to 20%. The complication rate for female patients was considerably higher than that for male patients (29% vs. 13%, respectively). Four cases of failed repair were examined; these all occurred before the aggressive weight-bearing protocol was implemented. Eight other patients required further surgery: 6 for adhesions, 1 to repair the saphenous nerve, and 1 for deep infection.

Discussion.—In repairing the meniscus, damage to the medial portion presents the greatest risk, with saphenous neuropathy being the most likely complication. Careful exposure of the capsule should minimize this risk, although it is believed this complication is sometimes unavoidable.

▶ The authors present a candid enumeration of complications associated with meniscal repair. The overall complication rate of 18% certainly gets our attention. However, it should be pointed out that virtually all of the reported complications either resolved spontaneously or had satisfactory outcomes after appropriate treatment.—J.S. Torg, M.D.

Popliteal Pseudoaneurysm After Arthroscopic Meniscectomy: A Report of Two Cases
Ritt MJPF, Te Slaa RL, Koning J, Bruijn JD (Reinier de Graaf Gasthuis, Delft, The Netherlands; Westeinde Hosp, The Hague, The Netherlands)
Clin Orthop 295:198–200, 1993   139-94-4-20

Purpose.—The advantages of arthroscopic diagnosis and treatment have led to their widespread use. Arthroscopy does have its complications, both minor and major, although there are few reports of their incidence. In 2 cases a popliteal artery pseudoaneurysm occurred as a complication of arthroscopic meniscectomy.

Case Report.—Man, 22, underwent arthroscopic partial meniscectomy for a bucket-handle tear of the lateral meniscus of the right knee sustained while playing volleyball. The tourniquet time was 37 minutes, and pedal pulses were normal after the procedure. The patient had progressive pain and swelling in the popliteal fossa during the next 3 weeks.

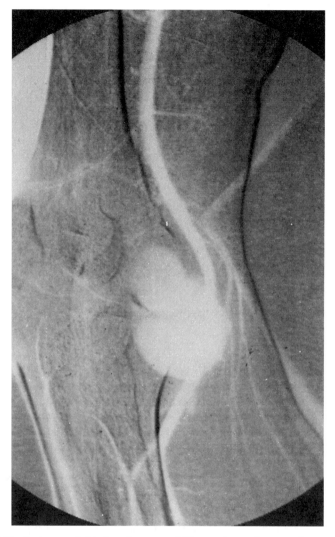

Fig 4–12.—Angiogram of right knee in man aged 22 years shows a large pseudoaneurysm of the popliteal artery. (Courtesy of Ritt MJPF, Te Slaa RL, Koning J, et al: *Clin Orthop* 295:198–200, 1993.)

On examination, he had a pulsatile popliteal mass but no signs of ischemia. Ultrasound revealed a mass communicating with the popliteal artery, and femoral angiography confirmed the suspicion of pseudoaneurysm with slight popliteal artery stenosis (Fig 4–12). Surgery revealed a .5-cm lesion on the ventral side of the artery (Fig 4–13), which required an autogenous short saphenous vein interposition graft to close. The patient recovered uneventfully. He had palpable pedal pulses and normal ankle blood pressure indices at 1-year follow-up.

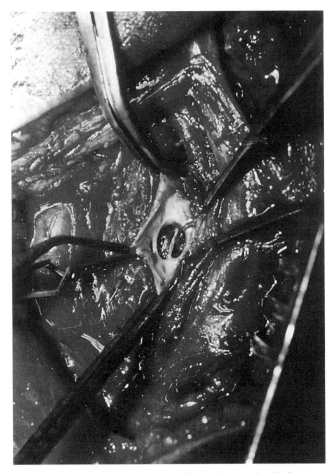

Fig 4–13.—Intraoperative photograph shows the defect in the ventral wall of the popliteal artery, causing the pseudoaneurysm. (Courtesy of Ritt MJPF, Te Slaa RL, Koning J, et al: *Clin Orthop* 295:198–200, 1993.)

Discussion.—Two patients were seen with the rare complication of popliteal artery pseudoaneurysm after arthroscopic meniscectomy. In a national survey by the Arthrosocpy Association of North America, 6 cases of penetrating vascular injuries to the popliteal artery were recorded among 118,590 arthroscopic procedures. These injuries call for early detection and resection or exclusion, followed by bypass grafting. Arthroscopic surgeons should be aware of the possibility of vascular sequelae and how to manage them.

▶ Vascular complications resulting from arthroscopic surgery are rare. Reported in a national survey were 6 cases of penetrating vascular injury to the popliteal artery that occurred in 118,590 arthroscopic procedures (1). Small reported 9 cases of penetrating trauma to the popliteal artery that occurred in 375,000 patients (2). The authors point out that although complaints may be minimal, pseudoaneurysms of the popliteal artery can result in limb-threatening ischemia caused by thrombosis or embolization. In view of the fact that the use of a tourniquet can be questioned, early recognition of arterial injury should avoid the development of late sequelae.—J.S. Torg, M.D.

References

1. DeLee JC: *Arthroscopy* 1:214, 1985.
2. Small NC: *Arthroscopy* 2:253, 1986.

"Bone Bruises" on Magnetic Resonance Imaging Evaluation of Anterior Cruciate Ligament Injuries
Graf BK, Cook DA, De Smet AA, Keene JS (Univ of Wisconsin, Madison)
Am J Sports Med 21:220–223, 1993   139-94-4–21

Background.—"Bone bruise" on MR assessment of anterior cruciate ligament (ACL) injuries is a finding that only recently has been studied. The incidence and location of bone bruises were determined in knees with ACL tears.

Methods and Findings.—Ninety-eight consecutive patients with clinically diagnosed ACL injuries underwent MRI of the knee. Forty-seven patients (48%) had focal signal abnormalities consistent with the diagnosis of a bone bruise. Seventy-one percent of the MR images obtained within 6 weeks of injury showed bone bruises. None of the scans obtained after this period demonstrated a bruise. The lesions tended to be located in the lateral compartment. Lesions were typically found in the middle one third of the lateral femoral condyle and the posterior one third of the lateral tibial plateau in the sagittal plane. No correlation was found between the presence or location of a bone bruise and articular changes or meniscal tears seen at surgery in 31 patients.

Conclusion.—The term "bone bruise" appears to be most descriptive of the signal characteristics, location, and resolution of this abnormality on MRI. The histology and clinical significance of bone bruises have yet to be determined.

▶ The characteristic bone bruise pattern demonstrated in association with ACL injuries is helpful in confirming an ACL injury when the MR injury pattern is equivocal. The specific bone bruise pattern also helps confirm the mechanism of injury. Subsequent to the publication of this article, fat-suppressed, fast-proton-density spin-echo sequences have been shown to be more sensitive to bone marrow edema; hence, the detection of subtle bone bruises is improved.—J.S. Torg, M.D.

Partial Meniscectomy and Anterior Cruciate Ligament Rupture in Soccer Players: A Study With a Minimum 20-Year Followup

Neyret P, Donell ST, Dejour D, Dejour H (Centre Hospitalier Lyon-Sud, Lyon, France)

Am J Sports Med 21:455–460, 1993   139-94-4–22

Background.—There have been many studies on the long-term effects of meniscectomy, and some have looked at anterior cruciate ligament (ACL) rupture. However, most studies involved heterogeneous groups of patients with a mixture of types of meniscectomy. Soccer players, who indulge in a sport that puts maximal demands on the knee, were evaluated. The long-term results of a rim-preserving meniscectomy were examined in players with intact and ruptured ACLs.

Method.—A retrospective evaluation of 77 soccer players with 91 affected knees that had undergone rim-preserving meniscectomy was carried out. The patients were divided into 2 groups: those with an intact ACL (group 1) and those with a concomitant ACL rupture (group 2). A minimum follow-up of 20 years was made, with an average follow-up of 27 years. Ninety percent of knees were studied clinically; the rest were evaluated by mailed questionnaire. Sporting level and knee function were recorded by the ARPEGE system.

Results.—Five years after surgery, 76% of group 1 patients were still playing soccer, compared with 52% of patients in group 2. Thirteen percent of group 1 had given up regular sports, as opposed to 28% in group 2. Eighty percent of group 1 patients had a good sporting assessment, 15% were average, and 5% were bad, compared with 62% good, 18% average, and 20% bad for group 2. By the time the patients averaged 53 years of age, 51% of group 1 had given up sports, whereas 76% had given up in group 2. Follow-up meniscectomies were carried out in 5% of group 1 compared with 32% of group 2. Operations for osteoarthritis were performed in 2% of group 1 compared with 16% of group 2. A greater degree of osteoarthritis was radiologically diagnosed in group 2. Functionally, 60% of group 1 knees were excellent at follow-up, compared with 9% of group 2 knees. A greater number of group 1 patients were still involved in sports, and 97% of group 1 patients were satisfied with their knees compared with only 74% of group 2.

Conclusion.—All patients in this study underwent rim-preserving meniscectomy; however, the outstanding factor influencing the long-term results was concomitant ACL rupture, which tended to render the knee unstable. Anterior tibial translation causes repetitive injury to the posterior structures. Therapeutic measures should be aimed at reducing the amount of anterior tibial translation by rigorous rehabilitation and cessation of sports or reconstruction of the ACL. For soccer players seen with an ACL rupture and a meniscal tear, the best course of treatment is ACL reconstruction.

▶ The value of this paper is the long-term follow-up in a homogeneous group of patients. Certainly, the conclusion that a soccer player with an ACL rupture and a meniscal tear should be offered a reconstruction is in keeping with current thinking. However, whether an ACL reconstruction will facilitate a return to activity as well as reverse the occurrence of degenerative changes must be addressed.—J.S. Torg, M.D.

Results of Meniscectomy in the Knee With Anterior Cruciate Ligament Deficiency
Hazel WA Jr, Rand JA, Morrey BF (Mayo Clinic and Found, Rochester, Minn)
Clin Orthop 292:232–238, 1993   139-94-4–23

Introduction.—Meniscal injuries commonly are seen in knees with acute tears in the anterior cruciate ligament (ACL). There is concern that meniscectomy in the knee with ACL deficiency may increase anterior tibial translation and symptoms of instability. To determine whether partial or total meniscectomy can be of value without cruciate reconstruction, the long-term results of arthroscopic treatment of meniscal tears in ACL-deficient knees were evaluated.

Patients and Methods.—Sixty-two patients with insufficiency of the ACL were treated by arthroscopic partial or total meniscectomy without ligament reconstruction. The average patient age at initial examination was 24 years; the mean interval from injury to surgical treatment of the meniscus was 4.8 years. Forty-seven knees had chronic instability and 16 had an acute injury. All but 8 of the injuries were sports-related. Both medial and lateral menisci were torn in 16 knees. Fifty-eight patients returned for examination at a mean of 4.3 years after arthroscopy.

Results.—The subjective results of treatment were favorable in 84% of patients; 81% of acute injuries and 85% of chronic injuries were improved. Although pain was significantly diminished at follow-up, 68% of patients reported some knee pain. The incidence of episodic locking was reduced from 51% before surgery to 3% postsurgery, but 52% of patients had episodes of giving way. One third of the patients used a brace some of the time. Thirty-four knees had objective findings of instability, and 35 patients were unable to return to sports because of symptomatic instability. Acute reinjury occurred in 27% of knees. Roentgenographic evidence of osteoarthrosis was present in 65% of knees. Six of 15 patients who underwent additional surgery had anterior cruciate reconstruction at an average of almost 5 years after the initial meniscectomy.

Conclusion.—Partial meniscectomy can provide symptomatic improvement of meniscal damage, although patients are unlikely to be able to return to their preinjury level of function. Thus, for active individuals with meniscal injury and ACL deficiency, the knee should also be stabilized.

▶ I will certainly agree that "meniscectomy without a stabilization procedure should be performed only infrequently in knees with deficient ACL." Although management of meniscal derangements by partial or total meniscectomy will initially alleviate most if not all of the symptoms in the ACL-deficient knee, the older literature demonstrates that 70% to 80% of these patients are able to return to previous levels of activity.

This paper points out that at a mean follow-up of 4.3 years, 65% of the knees demonstrated evidence of osteoarthrosis. On the basis of my own experience, I can only suggest that the authors obtain roentgenograms of these knees again at 10 years postmeniscectomy to fully appreciate the marked degenerative changes that occur. Of course, the other side of the coin is to document with long-term follow-up whether reconstruction of the ligament will prevent the progression of the degenerative changes.—J.S. Torg, M.D.

Arthroscopic Treatment of Anterior Cruciate Ligament Avulsion
Lubowitz JH, Grauer JD (Univ of California, Los Angeles)
Clin Orthop 294:242–246, 1993   139-94-4-24

Introduction.—Avulsion of the insertion of the anterior cruciate ligament (ACL) is more common in children, but it can also occur in adults. Conventional methods of treatment for ACL avulsion in adults may lead to stiffness because of prolonged immobilization or the morbidity of arthrotomy. Current arthroscopic techniques of percutaneous pinning still require cast immobilization. A new technique of arthroscopic reduction and internal fixation (ARIF) of ACL avulsion has been developed, and its use was illustrated in a case study.

Case Report.—Woman, 42, sustained a twisting injury to her left knee, with an audible pop, while skiing. Radiographs revealed a type IIIA avulsion of the tibial insertion of the ACL, which was confirmed by MRI. Closed reduction was unsuccessful, and the patient was brought to surgery.

The procedure was performed with the patient under general anesthesia. Arthroscopic examination showed obvious avulsion and superior displacement of the tibial insertion of the ACL, although the ligament itself was normal. After exsanguination and tourniquet application, the fracture was elevated and all soft tissue interposed between the fragments was removed. The tibial eminence fracture was then reduced with a probe and straight grasper. The fragment was temporarily fixed with 2 small guidewires. Two 3.5-mm, fully threaded, cannulated screws were placed via the anteromedial portal to secure the anatomical fixation (Fig 4–14). The leg was braced for 6 weeks, although 50% weight-bearing began at 3 weeks. The patient was walking by 6 weeks, and she had full active range of motion by 2 months. Two years after surgery the patient walked without a limp and had returned to Nordic skiing.

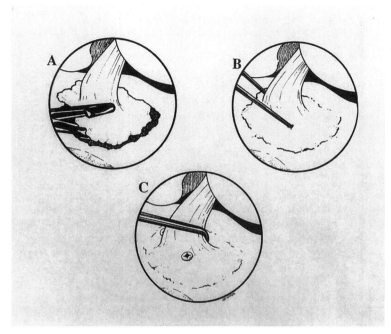

Fig 4–14.—**A,** type III avulsion of the tibial attachment of the ACL. The avulsed fragment is lifted from its underlying crater using an arthroscopic grasper. **B,** provisional fixation of the ACL avulsion fracture with guide pins. **C,** rigid anatomical fixation using 2 cannulated screws. A probe is used to check ACL tension. (Courtesy of Lubowitz JH, Grauer JD: *Clin Orthop* 294:242–246, 1993.)

Discussion.—A new technique of ARIF for ACL avulsion uses cannulated screws to provide rigid fixation while avoiding arthrotomy. It permits early mobilization and return to activity. In patients with significant interstitial damage, accurate reduction itself cannot restore knee stability; for these patients, ACL reconstruction should be considered. Proper tensioning of the ligament is another key consideration.

▶ Although not specifically stated, it is clear that avulsion fracture of the intercondylar eminence in the mature skeleton should be managed differently from those in the immature skeleton. Specifically, for optimum results in the adult, reduction and fixation are necessary. With the advent of arthroscopic technology, this can be done either by cannulated screws or transtibial suture. My own preference is the latter technique because of the technical ease with which it can be effected.—J.S. Torg, M.D.

Comminuted Tibial Eminence Anterior Cruciate Ligament Avulsion Fractures: Failure of Arthroscopic Treatment

Berg EE (Univ of South Carolina, Columbia)
Arthroscopy 9:446–450, 1993   139-94-4-25

Introduction.—Comminuted tibial eminence fracture with an anterior cruciate ligament (ACL) avulsion is considered an indication for surgery. Two adult patients with comminuted tibial spinal ACL avulsion fractures

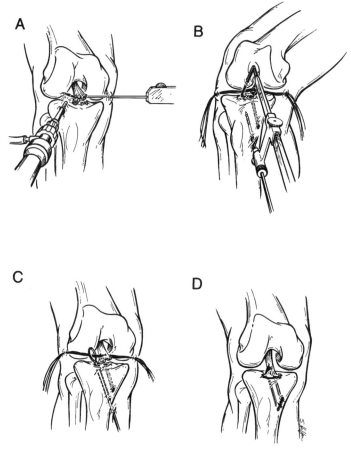

Fig 4–15.—A, a suture passer penetrates the ACL proximal to the avulsed tibial eminence. Four nonabsorbable sutures are thus placed in the ligament. **B,** just medial to the tibial tuberosity, a 3.5-mm-diameter Hoffman drill bit creates 2 holes in the proximal tibia. These tunnels are directed into the lateral and medial-most portions of the avulsion fracture bed. There should be ≥ 1 cm of metaphyseal cortex between the 2 drill holes. **C,** a suture passer or 24-gauge wire loop is advanced into each drill hole to snare the ligament sutures, which are then (**D**) pulled taut and individually tied over the tibial bone bridge. (Courtesy of Berg EE: *Arthroscopy* 9:446–450, 1993.)

that were fixed with a multiple suture technique performed arthroscopically were studied.

Technique.—A Rose suture passer is placed in the anteromedial portal and penetrates the ACL just proximal to the avulsed tibial bone (Fig 4-15, A). Four intraligamentous sutures are placed from posterior to anterior using a nonabsorbable braided suture. Through the anteromedial portal, a drill guide is placed in the most medial portion of the fracture bed (Fig 4-15, B). A 3.5-mm-diameter Hoffman drill bit is advanced into the proximal tibia. A second drill hole is fashioned in the most lateral portion of the fracture site. A Hewson suture passer is advanced through the drill holes (Fig 4-15, C), and ligament sutures are threaded and pulled through both tunnels. The knee is extended and the tibial eminence avulsion fractures are reduced to the fracture bed. The sutures should be tied individually (Fig 4-15, D). The patient is placed in a rehabilitative knee brace and begins partial weight-bearing.

Case Report.—Woman, 55, fell off a chair and injured her right knee. At 3 weeks after injury, her knee was locked in 20 degrees of fixed flexion. A radiograph demonstrated a tibial eminence fracture. At arthroscopy, the knee was comminuted into 3 fragments. The avulsed fractures were repaired as described above. The patient was then placed in a hinged cast brace for 8 weeks. She was seen 7 months later with a 20-degree flexion contracture with further flexion to 105 degrees. Radiography showed ectopic calcification. Two months later, arthroscopy was performed to lyse adhesions, and physical therapy was initiated. At 2-year follow-up, the patient's range of motion was 10–120 degrees.

Conclusion.—A minimally invasive arthroscopic suture repair for comminuted tibial spine avulsion fractures was performed in 2 adults. Although the repair was successful in restoring cruciate ligament stability and promoting fracture healing, arthrofibrosis and loss of knee joint motion occurred. A tibial eminence fracture is not a benign injury in an adult.

▶ It has been my experience that excellent results can be obtained by treating tibial eminence avulsion fractures using the described arthroscopic method. Perhaps the poor results reported with these 2 patients were caused by the fact that the first patient was kept in a hinged cast brace for 8 weeks because of a concomitant medial collateral ligament injury and the second patient did not comply with her postoperative rehabilitation program.—J.S. Torg, M.D.

Effect of Surgical Timing on Recovery and Associated Injuries After Anterior Cruciate Ligament Reconstruction
Wasilewski SA, Covall DJ, Cohen S (Sun Valley Sports Medicine, Idaho; Boston Univ)
Am J Sports Med 21:338–342, 1993   139-94-4-26

Purpose.—Arthroscopically assisted repair of the anterior cruciate ligament (ACL) followed by aggressive rehabilitation has gained wide acceptance. The effect of surgical timing on recovery from arthroscopic knee surgery was determined.

Methods.—Eighty-seven patients, aged 13–52 years, who underwent arthroscopic ACL reconstruction using a double semitendinosus graft comprised the study sample. The time from injury to surgery was used to classify the knee injuries as chronic, subacute, or acute. There were 41 knees with acute injuries, 14 with subacute injuries, and 32 with chronic injuries. Meniscal injury and its treatment were also coded. Postoperative knee motion, quadriceps strength, and stability were measured at 3, 6, 12, and 18 months.

Results.—Only 6.3% of knees with chronic injuries had normal menisci at operation vs. 28.6% of knees with subacute injuries and 29.3% of knees with acute injuries. Postoperative recovery of motion after acute knee injury was significantly less at all time points than after subacute or chronic injury. Recovery of quadriceps strength after repair of acute knee injuries was also slower. Postoperative knee stability was similar in all 3 groups. Reparable tears were found at operation in 37.8% of knees. Chondral lesions in the tibiofemoral joint were found in 17% of knees with acute injury, 7% with subacute injury, and 44% with chronic injury. Patellofemoral pain was present in 17% of the acute group, none of the subacute group, and 9.3% of the chronic group.

Conclusion.—Arthroscopically assisted ACL reconstruction performed within 6 months of knee injury does not jeopardize the knee. Recovery is significantly slower after acute ACL repair than after subacute or chronic repair.

▶ Shelbourne recently has reported a higher incidence of stiffness after acute ACL reconstructions with patellar tendon grafts (1). My own experience has been that with postoperative CPM, early weight-bearing as tolerated, and aggressive rehabilitation, stiffness and arthrofibrosis do not appear to be a problem.—J.S. Torg, M.D.

Reference

1. Shelbourne KD, et al: *Am J Sports Med* 19:332, 1991.

The Maquet Procedure: Effect of Tibial Shingle Length on Patellofemoral Pressures
Pan HQ, Kish V, Boyd RD, Burr DB, Radin EL (Henry Ford Hosp, Detroit; West Virginia Univ, Morgantown; Indiana Univ, Indianapolis)
J Orthop Res 11:199–204, 1993   139-94-4-27

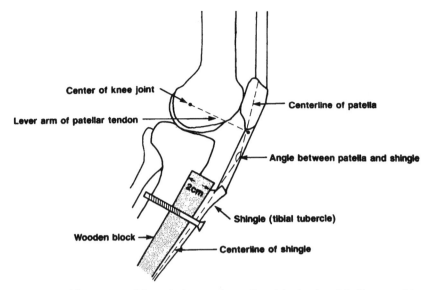

Fig 4–16.—Measurements of the angles between the patella and the shingle and the lever arm of the patellar tendon were taken before and after surgery. Wood blocks were used to simulate the bone grafts that are used in surgery to elevate the tendon. (Courtesy of Pan HQ, Kish V, Boyd RD, et al: *J Orthop Res* 11:199-204, 1993.)

Background.—When Maquet et al. proposed lowering the interarticular patellofemoral pressure by lengthening the lever arm of the patellar tendon, it appeared to be an ingenious biomechanical solution to the problem of symptomatic osteoarthrosis at this site. The procedure elevates the patellar tendon on the proximal tibia by anterior shingling up of the proximal tibial cortex from an attached distal base. The tubercle is raised anteriorly by at least 2 cm. The patellofemoral joint contact force is significantly lowered, but the operation has remained controversial for both clinical and biomechanical reasons.

Objective and Methods.—The influence of tibial shingle length on patellofemoral pressure was examined by recording contact pressure and area in 15 cadaveric knees at shingle lengths of 7 and 20 cm. The specimens were from 11 men and 4 women aged 25–75 years. Radiographs at 30 degrees of flexion were acquired before and after surgery (Fig 4-16), using wooden blocks to simulate bone grafts.

Observations.—The lever arm of the patellar tendon increased after all variations of the Maquet operation, but significantly only after 2 cm of elevation. With a short shingle and 2 cm of elevation, the angle between the patella and the shingle changed nearly 15 degrees, tipping the patella on its superior pole. Surgery with the short and long 2-cm elevated shingles significantly reduced the patellofemoral contact pressure by 27% and 36%, respectively. The patellofemoral contact area increased on knee flexion to between 15 and 30 degrees, and it did not decrease with elevation of the tibial tubercle.

Recommendation.—The Maquet operation for symptomatic osteoarthrosis of the patellofemoral joint is most effective when a long shingle is used and the tibial tubercle is elevated by 2 cm.

▶ These authors seem to have reconfirmed the benefits of the Maquet procedure, which was designed to lower the interarticular patellofemoral pressure by lengthening the lever arm of the patellar tendon. Other researchers had cast doubt on the procedure, but Pan et al. seem to think that previous investigators made modifications to the original procedure that may have caused the problems.—Col. J.L. Anderson, PE.D.

Arthroscopic and Histologic Analysis of Human Patellar Tendon Autografts Used for Anterior Cruciate Ligament Reconstruction
Rougraff B, Shelbourne KD, Gerth PK, Warner J (Indiana Univ, Indianapolis; Methodist Sports Medicine Ctr, Indianapolis, Ind; Methodist Hospital, Indianapolis, Ind)
Am J Sports Med 21:277–284, 1993   139-94-4-28

Purpose.—Experimental studies in animals have shown that a patellar tendon autograft, when used for the reconstruction of an anterior cruciate ligament (ACL), undergoes complete necrosis before peripheral cellular invasion and eventual ligamentization occur. Transplanted patellar autografts were examined in human beings.

Patients.—Twenty-three patients had ACL reconstruction for which the central one third of the patellar tendon was used as an autograft. They agreed to second-look arthroscopy with biopsy of the transplanted autograft at 3 weeks to 6.5 years after operation.

Results.—Arthroscopy and histologic analysis of the biopsy specimens revealed that ligamentization of transplanted patellar tendon autografts progressed through 4 stages. During the first 2 months after ACL reconstruction, there was a modest increase in the number of fibroblasts in the patellar tendon graft and in the metabolic rate. During the next 10 months, the number of fibroblasts in the graft increased dramatically, and the metabolic rate and the rate of neovascularity were high. For the next 2 years, the graft gradually became less cellular, less metabolically active, and less vascular. The ligamentization process was complete at 3 years after ACL reconstruction.

Conclusion.—Human patellar autografts, when used for ACL reconstruction, are viable as early as 3 weeks after operation and may not go through a necrotic stage. It takes approximately 3 years for complete ligamentization of the autograft.

An In Vitro Analysis of Patellofemoral Contact Areas and Pressures Following Procurement of the Central One-Third Patellar Tendon

D'Agata SD, Pearsall AW IV, Reider B, Draganich LF (Univ of Chicago)
Am J Sports Med 21:212–219, 1993   139-94-4–29

Introduction.—Patients in whom the central one third of the patellar tendon is used for reconstruction of the anterior cruciate ligament (ACL)-deficient knee may have patellofemoral pain. This is a complex problem that could result from a variety of physiologic and biochemical processes. Cadaveric knees were examined to determine the effects of harvesting the central one third of the patellar tendon on the patellofemoral contact areas and pressures.

Methods.—The central 10 mm of the patellar tendon in 5 cadaveric knees was removed, and isometric quadriceps forces were applied to produce about 30% of reported maximum voluntary knee extension moments. Pressure-sensitive film was used to make measurements for the normal knee, after graft removal, and after closure of the tendon, and to measure contact areas and pressures at 20–80 degrees of knee flexion.

Results.—Patellofemoral contact areas ranged from 1.6 cm² at 20 degrees of flexion to 3.0 cm² at 60 degrees. The range of average patellofemoral contact pressures was 1.9 MPa at 20 degrees of flexion to 3.0 MPa at 30 degrees. The 3 states tested showed no significant differences in average patellar contact area or pressure at any flexion angle.

Conclusion.—This experimental study suggests that patellofemoral contact area and pressure are unaffected by harvesting the central one third of the patellar tendon or by closure of the resulting gap in the tendon. The possible effects of postoperative biological processes or direct damage to the patellar articular surface, however, were not investigated.

Quadriceps Strength and Functional Capacity After Anterior Cruciate Ligament Reconstruction: Patellar Tendon Autograft Versus Allograft

Lephart SM, Kocher MS, Harner CD, Fu FH (Univ of Pittsburgh, Pa)
Am J Sports Med 21:738–743, 1993   139-94-4–30

Introduction.—The central one third of the patellar tendon is commonly used in reconstruction of the anterior cruciate ligament (ACL). However, harvesting of this portion of the patellar tendon is believed to be associated with reduced quadriceps strength and functional capacity. Quadriceps strength and functional capacity were retrospectively compared in athletes who had undergone ACL reconstruction using patellar tendon autograft vs. allograft.

Methods.—The subjects were 33 active men (mean age, 24 years) who had undergone ACL reconstruction a mean of 19 months previously. The reconstruction was done using patellar tendon autograft in 15 pa-

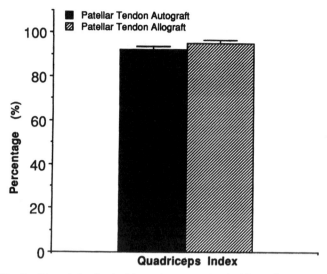

Fig 4–17.—Quadriceps index (involved leg peak torque, uninvolved leg peak torque at 60 degrees/sec) for patellar tendon autograft and allograft groups. *Horizontal lines* represent standard error (P >.05). (Courtesy of Lephart SM, Kocher MS, Harner CD, et al: *Am J Sports Med* 21:738-743, 1993.)

tients and allograft in 18; both groups completed an intensive rehabilitation program. The Cybex II isokinetic testing devices were used to assess quadriceps strength and power. Three specially designed functional performance tests and the hop test were used to assess functional capacity.

Results.—Quadriceps strength and power were no different between the 2 groups of patients, including peak torque measured at 60 and 240 degrees per second, torque acceleration energy at 240 degrees per second, and quadriceps index (Fig 4-17). Nor were there any significant differences in performance on the individual functional performance tests, the total functional performance test, or the hop index.

Conclusion.—These retrospective findings suggest that harvesting of the central one third of the patellar tendon for ACL reconstruction is not associated with reduced quadriceps strength or function in athletic, intensively rehabilitated patients. For these patients, patellar tendon allograft reconstruction offers no advantage over autograft reconstruction in terms of quadriceps strength and functional capacity.

Achilles Tendon Allograft Reconstruction of the Anterior Cruciate Ligament-Deficient Knee

Linn RM, Fischer DA, Smith JP, Burstein DB, Quick DC (Minneapolis Sports Medicine Ctr)
Am J Sports Med 21:825–831, 1993   139-94-4-31

Introduction.—The use of human tendon allografts for intra-articular anterior cruciate ligament reconstruction offers some advantages over autogenous tissue and synthetic materials. Because allograft reconstruction has not been widely practiced, patients were followed for 2–4 years to confirm that the outcomes were satisfactory.

Patients and Methods.—Thirty-five of 56 patients with anterior cruciate ligament deficiency who underwent intra-articular reconstruction using fresh-frozen Achilles tendon allografts were available for follow-up. Two thirds of the patients were males; 26 were between the ages of 15 and 29 years. Arthroscopy of the knee was conducted in all patients, followed by an open reconstructive procedure. The allograft was prepared by thawing in an antibiotic solution. Sutures in each end of the graft were used to apply 10 kg of tension, thereby prestretching the graft and allowing easy access for trimming, sizing, and tubing. After the graft was secured, a final check of the range of motion and a Lachman test were made. The goal of a progressive rehabilitation program was recovery to a full functional level at approximately 9 months postoperatively.

Results.—The objective clinical results in these 35 patients were quite good. All patients believed that the knee was better and most reported dramatic improvement. Objective measurements confirmed that effusion, synovitis, ligament laxity, and instability were reduced. Most patients recovered a good range of motion. Sixteen patients had further surgery for removal of ligament fixation screws and evaluation of the graft. Radiologic results were less favorable than clinical, arthroscopic, and biopsy results. Most patients had a significant size increase in femoral and tibial bone tunnels. Such enlargement appeared to occur early after operation and stabilize within 2 years. The etiology and clinical significance of these unexpected bone tunnel changes are unknown. Several patients with the largest bone tunnels competed in athletic activities.

Conclusion.—The clinical results of allografts should be expected to approach those of autografts. Because of the marked enlargement of bone tunnels after reconstruction of the Achilles tendon with allografts, this technique is recommended only as a salvage procedure or as an alternative to synthetic ligaments.

The Strength of the Central Third Patellar Tendon Graft: A Biomechanical Study
Cooper DE, Deng XH, Burstein AL, Warren RF (Cornell Univ, New York)
Am J Sports Med 21:818–824, 1993   139-94-4-32

Introduction.—Previous studies of bone–patellar tendon–bone (B-PT-B) composite grafts have been limited by small numbers, varying donor age, and difficulty with clamp fixation of the specimens. The work of Noyes et al. examined graft strength relative to anterior cruciate ligament strength in central third patellar tendon B-PT-B and medial B-PT-B composites that were substantially larger in width than grafts used in routine clinical practice. The biomechanical properties of the central third B-PT-B composite were evaluated, using more narrow grafts in both straight and twisted positions.

Methods.—Thirty-seven B-PT-B composite grafts were obtained from the knees of 21 human cadavers within 12 hours of death. The average age of the donors was 28 years. The specimens had been rejected for the purposes of allograft transplantation because of contamination or other contraindications. The composites were divided into 4 groups, 3 with 10 grafts (5 pairs) and 1 with 7 grafts from 6 donors. In group I, 10- vs. 15-mm wide grafts used without twisting were tested. Group II was a comparison of 10-mm wide grafts with and without twisting (90 degrees). Group III was a comparison of 10-mm wide grafts twisted 90 degrees and 10-mm wide grafts twisted 180 degrees. Group IV consisted of 10- vs. 7-mm wide grafts that were not twisted. Tests were carried out with a newly described potting technique and clamp system and a servohydraulic testing machine with an elongation rate of 5 cm/sec to approximate the rate of 100% per second reported previously.

Results.—The difference between the mean ultimate load in the 10- and 15-mm composites in group I was significant: 3,057 N vs. 4,389 N. Seven-mm wide composites (group IV) had a mean ultimate load of 2,238 N. Twisting the graft 90 degrees increased its strength, but further twisting to 180 degrees had no significant effect. For the entirety of B-PT-B composites, the mean maximal elongation was 17.88% as determined by clamp displacement to failure. Maximal elongation was not significantly affected by rotation.

Conclusion.—The findings of this cadaveric study suggest that the central one third of the patellar tendon graft is stronger than previously recognized. Thus, the use of grafts of narrow width (10 mm) in clinical practice seems to be justified and should prevent the potential complications of patellar fracture and graft impingement in the notch. Twisting the graft 90 degrees increases the ultimate tensile strength.

▶ These 5 papers (Abstracts 139-94-4-28 through 139-94-4-32) clearly reaffirm the bone–infrapatellar tendon–bone graft as the gold standard for anterior cruciate ligament reconstruction.—J.S. Torg, M.D.

Comparison of Perioperative Morbidity of Anterior Cruciate Ligament Autografts Versus Allografts
Saddemi SR, Frogameni AD, Fenton PJ, Hartman J, Hartman W (Med College of Ohio, Toledo)
Arthroscopy 9:519–524, 1993   139-94-4-33

Background.—Complications have been reported after anterior cruciate ligament (ACL) reconstruction with either autogenic or allogeneic bone–patellar tendon–bone grafts. Perioperative morbidity associated with ACL reconstruction with both types of grafts was examined in a retrospective study.

Methods.—Fifty patients with complete ACL tears underwent arthroscopic bone–patellar tendon–bone reconstruction followed by standard postoperative rehabilitation. Thirty-one autografts and 19 fresh-frozen, γ-irradiated allografts were used. Range of motion, swelling, thigh atrophy, and anteroposterior translation were recorded at 1, 2, 6, 12, 24, 52, and 104 weeks after surgery. Quadriceps and hamstring strength and endurance were tested at 24, 52, and 104 weeks.

Results.—The swelling, range of motion, atrophy, muscle strength and endurance, and stability were comparable for the allograft and autograft groups. One reconstruction in each group failed: The autograft failure had a 5.4-mm increase in anteroposterior translation with a positive Lachman test and positive pivot shift; the allograft failure involved the tibial attachment site. Two flexion contractures occurred in the autograft group; both resolved with arthroscopic débridement. Persistent anteromedial pain and pain at the tibial hardware site were reported by 1 patient in each group. Additional complications included a superficial wound infection in 1 autograft recipient and persistent idiopathic effusions in 2 allograft patients. A greater incidence of postoperative crepitus was found among autograft patients, but patellofemoral pain and mobility were comparable between the groups.

Conclusion.—Perioperative morbidity did not differ significantly between autogenic and allogeneic bone–patellar tendon–bone grafts for ACL reconstruction. Even at 2 years after operation, the grafts did not differ in muscle strength, atrophy, patellofemoral symptoms, and stability. The development of flexion contractures in 2 autograft patients may be significant and is currently under investigation.

Quantitative Evaluation After Arthroscopic Anterior Cruciate Ligament Reconstruction: Allograft Versus Autograft

Shino K, Nakata K, Horibe S, Inoue M, Nakagawa S (Osaka Rosai Hosp, Japan; Osaka Univ, Japan)

Am J Sports Med 21:609–616, 1993   139-94-4-34

Purpose.—Arthroscopic anterior cruciate ligament (ACL) reconstruction followed by advanced rehabilitation is almost always clinically successful. Postoperative knee function was measured at the most athletically active period after clinically successful arthroscopic ACL repair.

Patients.—Anterior laxity and thigh muscle power were measured in 92 patients who had undergone arthroscopic ACL reconstruction 18–36 months earlier. Only patients wtih unilateral ACL insufficiency without posterolateral instability were included in the analysis. Forty-seven patients (mean age, 20 years) received a fresh-frozen tendon allograft, and

45 patients (mean age, 23 years) underwent autogenous patellar tendon reconstruction. Anteroposterior ligament laxity of both knees was measured at 20–30 degrees of flexion using the Knee Instability Tester at 200–250 N of force. Quadriceps muscle strength was measured on the Cybex II dynamometer.

Results.—The ACL-reconstructed knees showed significantly more anterior laxity than the contralateral normal knees, regardless of which graft material was used. However, male patients in the allograft group tended to have smaller differences in anterior laxity between normal and operated knees than did female patients. Knees treated with allografts achieved better static anterior stability than autograft-treated knees. Recovery of quadriceps muscle strength was also significantly better with allograft-treated knees.

Conclusion.—An ACL-reconstructed knee with a clinically successful outcome may have subclinical deficits in ACL laxity and quadriceps muscle strength. Allograft-repaired knees appear to do better than autograft-treated knees.

▶ Saddemi et al. (Abstract 139-94-4–33) found the results of both autografts and allografts to be statistically similar for postoperative static stability and quadriceps strength. Shino et al. (Abstract 139-94-4–34), on the other hand, state that "although the statistical analysis between allograft and autograft patients of the same sex failed to prove that there was a significant difference in anterior laxity difference between the allograft and autograft groups, we did find that there was no statistical difference in each mechanical parameter between the involved and the contralateral knees except in the male subjects of the allograft group." They point out, however, that the older and less active patients received the autogenous grafts (thereby creating a bias) and that the 2 groups were not comparable in terms of age and activity level. Therefore, their conclusion that the allograft knees showed better results in terms of restored anterior static stability must be questioned.—J.S. Torg, M.D.

Morphologic Changes in the Human Patellar Tendon After Bone-Tendon-Bone Anterior Cruciate Ligament Reconstruction
Meisterling RC, Wadsworth T, Ardill R, Griffiths H, Lane-Larsen CL (St Croix Inst for Orthopaedic Research, Stillwater, Minn)
Clin Orthop 289:208–212, 1993   139-94-4–35

Background.—Arthroscopic reconstruction of the anterior cruciate ligament (ACL) by using the central one third of the patellar ligament as a bone–patellar tendon–bone (BTB) autograft is becoming the procedure of choice in competitive athletes. However, postoperative quadriceps weakness, patellofemoral pain, and infrapatellar contracture syndrome (IPCS) have been reported. Whether the patellar donor site could be causing these complications was investigated.

Methods.—Fifteen patients underwent MRI of both knees at a mean of 2.5 years after arthroscopic BTB ACL reconstruction. For comparison, 5 patients who underwent arthroscopic ACL reconstructions with a semitendinosus tendon graft were examined with MRI a mean of 4.1 years after operation. The length, width, and thickness of each patellar tendon were measured and the differences between the involved and uninvolved knees were calculated.

Results.—Among patients who underwent BTB ACL reconstruction, none of the differences between patellar tendon length, width, and thickness for involved and uninvolved knees reached statistical significance. Patellar measurements in these patients did not differ significantly from those in patients who had undergone ACL reconstruction with a semitendinosus tendon graft.

Conclusion.—Harvesting the central one third of the patellar tendon for arthroscopic ACL reconstruction does not appear to cause the observed postoperative complications.

Patellar Tendon Length Change After Anterior Cruciate Ligament Reconstruction Using the Midthird Patellar Tendon
Shaffer BS, Tibone JE (Georgetown Univ, Washington, DC; Kerlan-Jobe Clinic, Inglewood, Calif)
Am J Sports Med 21:449–454, 1993   139-94-4-36

Objective.—It has been suggested that harvesting of the middle one third of the patellar tendon as a graft for anterior cruciate ligament (ACL) reconstruction causes the remaining patellar tendon to contract and thus contributes to postoperative infrapatellar contracture syndrome. A prospective study was undertaken to determine whether patellar tendon length changes occur after the middle one third of the patellar tendon is harvested for ACL reconstruction.

Patients.—During a 6-month period in 1989, 36 patients aged 18–39 years underwent arthroscopic ACL reconstruction performed with autogenous patellar tendon (middle one third) and patellar and tibial bone blocks. By random assignment, the patellar tendon defect was closed in 18 patients and left open in the other 18 patients. Patellar tendon length was measured during surgery and on bilateral lateral knee radiographs obtained before surgery, within 2 weeks after operation, and at the 3- and 6-month postoperative follow-up visits. All radiographs were reviewed by the same examiner.

Results.—Of the 18 patients whose tendon defects were closed, 5 showed no change on intraoperative patellar tendon measurement, 6 showed shortening of 1 mm, and 7 had shortening of 2 mm. A comparison of preoperative and postoperative radiographs showed no changes in patellar tendon length greater than the measurement error. Patella baja did not develop in any patient.

Conclusion.—Use of a patellar tendon autograft for arthroscopic ACL reconstruction does not appear to result in significant patellar tendon shortening.

▶ These 2 papers (Abstracts 139-94-4–35 and 139-94-4–36) are at variance with previous reports in which harvesting the middle one third bone–infrapatellar tendon–bone for ACL grafting resulted in tendon shortening and patella baja. However, it is believed that the failure to observe patellar tendon shortening may be a result of the implementation of more early, aggressive rehabilitation programs.—J.S. Torg, M.D.

Deterioration of Patellofemoral Articular Surfaces After Anterior Cruciate Ligament Reconstruction
Shino K, Nakagawa S, Inoue M, Horibe S, Yoneda M (Osaka Rosai Hosp, Japan; Osaka Univ, Japan)
Am J Sports Med 21:206–211, 1993   139-94-4–37

Purpose.—Patellofemoral pain in the absence of radiographic findings is one of the most common postoperative complications compromising the outcome of primary repair of the anterior cruciate ligament (ACL). Whether postoperative knee symptoms can be attributed to degenerative changes on the articular surfaces of the patellofemoral joint was investigated.

Patients.—Second-look arthroscopy was performed in 187 patients, aged 15–46 years, who had undergone ACL repair in which either fresh-frozen allogeneic tendon or the central one third of the autogenous patellar tendon was used. The average time between primary ACL repair and arthroscopic reevaluation was 19 months. The second-look arthroscopic evaluation included examination of the cartilaginous lesions on the patellofemoral joint. The findings were compared with those recorded at the time of primary ACL reconstruction.

Results.—Of 181 evaluable knees, 93 (51%) had deteriorated, 74 (41%) had remained unchanged, and 14 (8%) had improved since primary ACL reconstruction. Most of the deteriorative changes were located around the central ridge of the patella. Multivariate analysis identified open surgery rather than arthroscopic reconstruction and use of an autogenous patellar tendon graft rather than a fresh-frozen allogeneic tendon graft as possible risk factors for postoperative deterioration. Only 2 patients had complained of serious anterior knee pain, demonstrating that the articular lesions found at second-look arthroscopy did not correlate with the symptoms.

Conclusion.—Patellofemoral deterioration after ACL reconstruction is a significant risk. The rate of postoperative joint deterioration can be reduced by avoiding open surgery and the use of patellar tendon grafts.

► Although statistical multivariate analysis showed the surgical approach using the conventional medial parapatellar incision and the central one third of the autogenous patellar tendon graft as possible risk factors for the deterioration of the patellofemoral articular surfaces, the chi-square analysis failed to demonstrate statistical significance. Also, in that the incidence of deterioration was 44% for the allograft group and 42% for the arthroscopically assisted cases, other factors must contribute to postoperative patellofemoral deterioration.—J.S. Torg, M.D.

Reconstruction of Old Anterior Cruciate Ligament Tears With a Dacron Prosthesis; A Prospective Study
Gillquist J, Odensten M (Univ Hosp, Linköping, Sweden)
Am J Sports Med 21:358–366, 1993   139-94-4–38

Objective.—Patellar tendon autografting generally is considered the treatment of choice for chronic ruptures of the anterior cruciate ligament (ACL), but problems may develop, including graft failure, poor tendon quality, and prolonged rehabilitation. Some of these problems can be avoided with the use of prosthetic ligaments, but they have their own disadvantages, including adverse host reactions, breakage, and infection. The risks and benefits of a Dacron ACL prosthesis were analyzed in a prospective series of 70 patients.

Patients.—The patients were all treated for chronic anterior instability by ACL reconstruction using a Stryker-Meadox Dacron prosthesis pretensioned to 60 N. Forty-nine percent of the patients had combined medial instability, 32% had failure of previous ACL surgery, and 37% had previous meniscectomy. Medial instability was managed at the time of the ACL reconstruction in 12 of 34 patients. Patients were followed for 5 years, with special attention to ligament survival and time from surgery at which half of the prostheses had failed.

Findings.—A synovial fistula required removal of the prosthesis at 8 months in 1 patient. At 5 years, an excellent result was achieved in 39% of the patients, a good result occurred in 16%, a fair result was achieved in 17%, and a poor result occurred in 3%. In addition, 23% of the prostheses ruptured. The proportion of results was similar at the 2-year follow-up, but the rupture rate was lower. Placement of the tibial tunnel in the anterior one third of the tibia increased the rupture rate ninefold, and co-existing nonrepaired medial instability increased it fivefold. When the ligament was perfectly placed in a patient with good medial stability and no previous ligament surgery, there were no ruptures. Stability gained at surgery was lost gradually, at a rate of 11.2% per year. The uninjured knee also lost 41% of its preoperative stability by 5 years, for a mean laxity difference of ± 2 mm. Subjective knee ratings of knee function were significantly improved throughout follow-up. The patients never reached their preinjury level of activity.

Conclusion.—There was a 45% rupture rate when the Dacron prosthesis was used as a salvage procedure in patients with chronic ACL ruptures. Technical factors play an important role in the results for all other patients. Implantation technique appears to be the most important factor in the success or failure of the reconstruction.

Dacron Ligament Reconstruction for Chronic Anterior Cruciate Ligament Insufficiency

Wilk RM, Richmond JC (Lahey Clinic Med Ctr, Burlington, Mass; Tufts Univ, Boston)
Am J Sports Med 21:374–380, 1993   139-94-4-39

Background.—Artificial ligaments initially were studied only in "salvage cases" for failed anterior cruciate ligament (ACL) reconstructions or as augmentation for autologous tissue reconstructions. Since then, their use has been expanded to primary ACL reconstruction. A prospective, multicenter study was undertaken to assess the efficacy and safety of a Dacron ACL prosthesis for reconstruction of ACL-deficient knees.

Methods.—Eighty-four patients entered the study and were followed for at least 5 years. Two groups of patients were studied: group 1, consisting of 50 patients with isolated ACL laxity; and group 2, 34 patients with a failed previous ACL surgery or combined laxity. Thirty patients were managed by reconstruction through drill holes in the tibia and femur, whereas the other 54 were managed by using the over-the-top position with the Dacron ligament wrapped in a strip of iliotibial band.

Results.—A 2-year failure rate of 20% increased to 36% at 5 years. Lysholm score improved from 61 at baseline to 90 at 2 years, decreasing somewhat to 86 at 5 years. Tegner activity levels increased from 3 at baseline to 5 at both the 2- and 5-year follow-up evaluations. Failure rates were not significantly different between groups 1 and 2—38% vs. 32%. There appeared to be a trend toward early failure in group 2. There was no significant difference in failure rate by surgical technique, although more patients who underwent over-the-top reconstruction had failure between 2 and 5 years.

Conclusion.—The Dacron ligament prosthesis can restore stability and improve function of the ACL-deficient knee, at least in the short term. The long-term function of these reconstructions remains uncertain. The prosthesis may be most useful in older, less active patients, and the use of drill holes through both the tibia and femur may be better for restoration of isometricity.

The Dacron Ligament Prosthesis in Anterior Cruciate Ligament Reconstruction: A Four-Year Review

Barrett GR, Line LL Jr, Shelton WR, Manning JO, Phelps R (Mississippi Sports

Medicine and Orthopaedic Ctr, Jackson; Millsaps College, Jackson, Miss)
Am J Sports Med 21:367–373, 1993   139-94-4-40

Purpose.—Dacron ligaments, although commonly used in knee reconstruction, are not without problems, most frequently persistent synovitis or foreign-body reactions. The intermediate-term results of Dacron ligament anterior cruciate ligament (ACL) reconstruction were assessed in 40 patients.

Patients.—The patients were 35 men and 5 women (mean age, 28.8 years) who were operated on during a 3-year period for chronic ACL deficiency. All patients received a Dacron ligament prosthesis with a modified MacIntosh over-the-top technique. The prosthesis was augmented with an iliotibial band. Although 30 of the patients had had a previous surgical procedure on their knee, only 7 had a previous ACL reconstruction. The patients were followed for a mean of 47.5 months.

Outcomes.—The average side-to-side arthrometer difference at follow-up was 1 mm. The Lysholm score improved from 65 to 89, and the Tegner activity level score improved from 3 to 5. At follow-up, the Lachman test result was negative in 75% of the patients and the pivot shift results were negative or trace in 95.1%. About 88% of the patients still reported mild knee pain during daily activities. The complication rate was 27.5%, including 5 patients with implant rupture and 2 patients who had their grafts removed. There were 5 cases of synovitis. Overall, 47.5% of the procedures were considered to have failed. When radiographic evidence of tracer separation was included as a criterion of failure, the failure rate increased to 60%. The results were worse in patients with multiple previous surgeries of any type.

Conclusion.—There were high complication and failure rates and suboptimal end results in patients undergoing Dacron ligament prosthesis ACL reconstruction. The results were especially poor in patients with previous damage to the secondary stabilizers or menisci. Patients—especially athletes—must understand the importance of these structures in the ultimate outcome of knee reconstruction.

▶ The 4- to 5-year failure rates of 45%, 60%, and 36% reported independently in these 3 papers (Abstracts 139-94-4–38 through 139-94-4–40), effectively relegate the Dacron ACL prosthesis to a historical note. Clearly, all inanimate material wears and eventually fails.—J.S. Torg, M.D.

Arthroscopically Assisted Reconstruction of the Anterior Cruciate Ligament With Use of Autogenous Patellar-Ligament Grafts: Results After Twenty-Four to Forty-Two Months

Buss DD, Warren RF, Wickiewicz TL, Galinat BJ, Panariello R (Minneapolis Sports Medicine Ctr; Hosp for Special Surgery, New York)
J Bone Joint Surg (Am) 75-A:1346–1355, 1993   139-94-4–41

Background.—Open arthrotomy with autogenous grafting of the central one third of the patellar ligament has achieved success rates as high as 90% in torn anterior cruciate ligament (ACL) repair. However, postsurgical complications include reduced joint mobility and patellofemoral pain. Arthroscopy requires minimal incisions and may facilitate identification of the optimal sites for graft attachment. The long-term results of arthroscopically assisted ACL reconstruction using an autogenous central patellar ligament graft were assessed.

Methods.—The records of the first 68 arthroscopic ACL reconstructions at the Hospital for Special Surgery between December 1985 and May 1987 were reviewed. Arthroscopy was used to diagnose the injury, repair meniscal lesions, obtain the graft, and reconstruct the damaged ACL. Range-of-motion rehabilitation began on the first postoperative day. Knees were protected by a hinged thigh-to-ankle brace; full weight-bearing resumed after 6 weeks. Follow-up 24–42 months postreconstruction included a patient-completed questionnaire, examination of the knee, stability testing, and radiographs.

Findings.—At the most recent follow-up (24–42 months postsurgery), the median ligament rating score was 93 (maximum, 100). The ratings were excellent in 44, good in 15, fair in 6, and poor in 3 knees. Patellofemoral joint symptoms were present in 18 knees. Sixty-three knees had full range of motion; only 2 knees required manipulation for loss of flexion. Up to 4 mm of anterior-posterior displacement was observed in 93% of the 56 patients who underwent KT-1000 arthrometric measurement for both knees. Changes in the Insall-Salvati patellar ligament–to-patella ratios did not correlate with patellofemoral joint pain.

Conclusion.—Arthroscopic ACL reconstruction is as effective as open operative techniques with minimal injury to the joint capsule and synovial membrane. Combined with early rehabilitation, arthroscopic ACL reconstruction decreases the likelihood of patellofemoral pain and loss of mobility.

Miniarthrotomy Versus Arthroscopic-Assisted Anterior Cruciate Ligament Reconstruction With Autogenous Patellar Tendon Graft

Shelbourne KD, Rettig AC, Hardin G, Williams RI (Methodist Sports Medicine Ctr, Indianapolis, Ind)
Arthroscopy 9:72–75, 1993   139-94-4–42

Objective.—The short-term results of anterior cruciate ligament (ACL) reconstruction in 2 groups of matched patients were compared. Group I underwent an arthroscopic-assisted procedure and group II was treated with traditional open miniarthrotomy reconstruction.

Patients and Methods.—The groups were matched for age, sex, injury chronicity, and number of previous knee surgeries. Each group was treated by a single surgeon, and all ACLs were reconstructed with autogenous patellar tendon. Postoperative rehabilitative protocols were similar for all patients and emphasized early motion, immediate full passive extension, and early weight-bearing activity. Follow-up data collected included length of hospitalization, pain medication requirements, range of motion at 1.5, 2.5, and 6 weeks postoperatively, KT-1000 measurements, and isokinetic evaluation scores.

Results.—With one exception, the operative data were similar for the 2 groups. Postoperative drainage output was significantly higher for group II than for group I (201 mL vs. 110 mL). Both groups were off crutches at approximately 2 weeks postoperatively and began running programs by 11 weeks. There was a tendency for group II patients to exhibit earlier recovery of motion. No significant differences were observed between the groups for average KT-1000 arthrometer measurements or isokinetic evaluation scores. One patient in each group had a superficial infection.

Conclusion.—The benefits of arthroscopic-assisted techniques are expected to occur primarily during the first 6 postoperative months. The findings suggest that either surgical technique—open or arthroscopic-assisted—will yield similar early clinical results in patients undergoing autogenous middle one third patellar tendon ACL reconstruction followed by an aggressive rehabilitation protocol. Although hospital stay is theoretically shortened or eliminated by using arthroscopic techniques, the first few postoperative days have been critical to successful rehabilitation.

▶ These 2 studies (Abstracts 139-94-4–41 and 139-94-4–42) both support the conclusion of Shelbourne et al. that "ACL reconstruction with midthird patellar tendon, performed by skilled surgeons using either open or arthroscopic-assisted techniques combined with an aggressive postoperative rehabilitation protocol will yield similar acceptable early clinical results."—J.S. Torg, M.D.

The Effect of Early Versus Late Return to Vigorous Activities on the Outcome of Anterior Cruciate Ligament Reconstruction
Glasgow SG, Gabriel JP, Sapega AA, Glasgow MT, Torg JS (Univ of Pennsylvania, Philadelphia)
Am J Sports Med 21:243–248, 1993   139-94-4-43

Objective.—The optimal timing of safe return to vigorous physical activity after anterior cruciate ligament (ACL) reconstruction has not been determined. The long-term effects of early (2–6 months) vs. late (7–14 months) return to cutting activities were evaluated in patients undergoing the procedure.

Patients and Methods.—Sixty-four of 186 ACL reconstructions performed between 1981 and 1987 met study criteria. None of the patients had osteochondral fractures, grade IV chondromalacia lesions, or severe varus instability at surgery. Reconstructions were performed using a distally attached median one third patellar tendon. All patients were given a long leg cast postoperatively and remained non–weight-bearing for 6 weeks. Quadriceps and hamstring isometrics were started at 6 weeks and full range of motion, isotonic quadriceps, and hamstring exercises at 8 weeks. Thirty-one patients returned to vigorous activity at a mean of 5 months (early, group 1) and 33 at a mean of 9 months (late, group 2) after ACL reconstruction.

Results.—The mean length of follow-up was 45 months for group 1 and 47 months for group 2. The groups were comparable in severity of injuries incurred and surgical procedures performed. The mean time to return to final range of motion differed significantly at 4.3 months for group 1 and 5.4 months for group 2. The groups did not differ significantly in the highest activity level returned to or in the incidence of reinjuries requiring reoperation. Clinical examination, KT-1000 arthrometer measurements, subjective evaluation, and Cybex testing results were similar after early and late return to activity.

Conclusion.—An early return to vigorous activity after ACL reconstruction does not increase a patient's risk of reinjury or result in less satisfactory long-term results than does a slower return to activity. Knee stability and the lack of giving way, the most significant subjective parameters at follow-up, were equally favorable in patients with early and late return to activity.

▶ It should be noted that early return to vigorous activity was achieved in this group despite the fact that the reconstruction was performed through a generous anterior arthrotomy incision. Also, an important conclusion of this study was that "A KT-1000 maximal manual excursion rather than a 20-pound anterior pull should be used to assess an AP laxity difference after ACL reconstruction."—J.S. Torg, M.D.

Arthroscopic Treatment of Symptomatic Extension Block Complicating Anterior Cruciate Ligament Reconstruction

Fisher SE, Shelbourne KD (Methodist Sports Medicine Ctr, Indianapolis, Ind; Indiana Univ, Indianapolis)
Am J Sports Med 21:558–564, 1993   139-94-4–44

Purpose.—Failure to regain full knee extension after anterior cruciate ligament (ACL) reconstruction is a common problem. Previous studies have implicated the intra-articular formation of excess fibrous tissue. The effectiveness of arthroscopic excision of this tissue in patients with persistent postoperative knee problems after open ACL was assessed.

Methods.—During a 7½-year period, 42 (4%) of 959 patients who had open ACL reconstruction required further surgical treatment because of persistent knee problems that had failed to respond to aggressive conservative therapy. The treatment consisted of arthroscopic examination of the knee and excision of hypertrophic fibrous tissue attached to the reconstructed ligament. All patients underwent aggressive postoperative rehabilitation therapy. Twenty randomly selected patients who had undergone ACL reconstruction and regained normal knee extension served as controls.

Results.—Thirty-five patients ranging in age from 14 to 39 years at the time of open ACL reconstruction were available for follow-up. The average interval between ACL surgery and arthroscopic treatment was 9 months. Resection of the impinging tissue and aggressive rehabilitation therapy significantly improved knee extension in all patients. Only 7 patients had some residual contracture. There were no new complications attributable to the arthroscopic resection, and none of the patients were dissatisfied with the outcome.

Conclusion.—Arthroscopic excision of the excess tissue that sometimes forms after ACL reconstruction and interferes with full knee extension will significantly improve the problem.

▶ Current thinking attributes symptomatic extension block after ACL reconstruction to the cyclops syndrome, as described by Jackson and Schaefer (1). This study indicates that a block to full extension can be caused by hypertrophic fibrous tissue attached to the reconstructed ligament and the roof of the intercondylar groove. Also, a fibrotic anterior fat pad, a bone protruding from the site of the tibial tunnel, or an inadequate notchplasty can be responsible for the extension block. It should be emphasized that surgical débridement is not considered complete until no further block to full extension can be demonstrated.—J.S. Torg, M.D.

Reference

1. Jackson DW, Schaefer RK: *Arthroscopy* 6:171, 1990.

The Effects of Sectioning of the Posterior Cruciate Ligament and the Posterolateral Complex on the Articular Contact Pressures Within the Knee

Skyhar MJ, Warren RF, Ortiz GJ, Schwartz E, Otis JC (San Dieguito Orthopaedic Med Group, Encinitas, Calif; Hosp for Special Surgery, New York)
J Bone Joint Surg (Am) 75–A:694–699, 1993   139-94-4-45

Introduction.—Both the need for treatment and the optimal type of repair of a torn posterior cruciate ligament are matters of controversy. Although some patients appear to do well clinically after such an injury, others experience pain whether they are treated operatively or nonoperatively. Damage of the articular cartilage probably is the most important factor contributing to a poor long-term prognosis. Cadaveric knees with intact and sectioned ligaments were measured to examine the effect of injuries to the posterior cruciate ligament and the posterolateral complex (the posterolateral capsule, the popliteus muscle and tendon, and the lateral collateral ligament) on articular contact pressures.

Methods.—Ten fresh-frozen knees were tested using film and a model that simulated non–weight-bearing resistive extension of the knee. The patients ranged in age from 54 to 69 years at the time of death. Measurements were repeated after sequential sectioning of the posterior cruciate ligament and the posterolateral complex.

Results.—Intact knees exhibited a 41% increase when the patellofemoral pressure at 15 degrees of flexion was compared with that at 90 degrees of flexion. This difference was also evident, although less pronounced (16%), after sectioning of the posterior cruciate ligament. Intact knees had a combined average pressure of 23.2 Pa. This value increased to 28.0 Pa with sectioning of the posterior cruciate ligament and to 34.8 Pa when the posterolateral complex was sectioned as well. Medial compartment pressure was significantly elevated after sectioning of the posterior cruciate ligament; the quadriceps load was most significantly elevated after combined sectioning of the ligament and the posterolateral complex.

Conclusion.—Results of the experimental studies coincided with, and may partially explain, the clinical findings associated with these ligamentous injuries. Patients with these tears or ruptures are at increased risk of damage to the articular cartilage of the patellofemoral and medial compartments. Physicians need to recognize the presence of combined injuries.

▶ This is an excellent bench study that helps explain the clinical findings associated with injuries to the posterior cruciate ligament and posterolateral complex. Of significance, the authors point out that "At the very least, preservation of the medial meniscus is important . . . to avoid diminished areas of contact between the tibia and the femur in the medial compartment of the knee joint."—J.S. Torg, M.D.

Intraarticular Abnormalities in Association With Posterior Cruciate Ligament Injuries

Geissler WB, Whipple TL (Univ of Mississippi, Jackson; Orthopaedic Research of Virginia, Richmond)
Am J Sports Med 21:846–849, 1993   139-94-4-46

Background.—Tears of the anterior cruciate ligament occur frequently, and their effects on the articular and meniscal cartilages have been well studied. However, tears of the posterior cruciate ligament (PCL) without other complications are relatively rare and less is known about their effects on the cartilage. Their management is controversial. Cases of isolated PCL tears were reviewed to learn more about their etiology, diagnosis, and their effects on the joint cartilage.

Materials and Methods.—Eighty-eight cases of uncomplicated PCL tears and their treatment were studied retrospectively. Damage to the cartilage was rated as grade I–IV, which described conditions ranging from minor blistering to exposed bone. The injuries were rated as acute or chronic, depending on whether the surgery followed the injury by less or more than 3 weeks.

Results.—Surgically significant articular cartilage defects occurred in 35% of patients with isolated PCL injuries. The patellofemoral articulation was the site most commonly involved, with nearly half the articular defects arising from this articulation. The PCL patients with chronic injury were more likely to manifest articular cartilage injury. The patella and lateral femoral condyle were most often affected in acute injury, whereas the patella and medial femoral condyle were most often affected in chronic injury. Meniscal tears were seen only slightly more often in chronic than in acute injury (36% vs. 27%, respectively). Lateral meniscal tears were associated with acute injury, but medial meniscal tears occurred more frequently in chronic injury and may be associated with accumulated insults.

Conclusion.—These findings support earlier reports that PCL injuries are likely to result in degenerative changes in the medial compartment.

▶ The problem with this study, as pointed out by the authors, is that the review is based on a biased patient population that was symptomatic enough to seek orthopedic care and consent to an arthroscopic operative procedure.—J.S. Torg, M.D.

Biceps Tendon Tenodesis for Posterolateral Instability of the Knee: An In Vitro Study

Wascher DC, Grauer JD, Markoff KL (Univ of California, Los Angeles)
Am J Sports Med 21:400–406, 1993   139-94-4-47

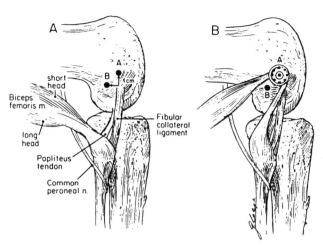

Fig 4–18.—Surgical technique for the biceps tenodesis. **A,** fixation points are located 1 cm anterior (*point A*) and proximal (*point B*) to the FCL attachment on the femoral epicondyle. **B,** completed tenodesis with use of the anterior fixation point. (Courtesy of Wascher DC, Grauer JD, Markoff KL: *Am J Sports Med* 21:400–406, 1993.)

Introduction.—Posterolateral instability of the knee frequently occurs in combination with injury to the anterior or posterior cruciate ligament. Surgical exploration reveals the arcuate ligament to be torn in most cases, and co-existing injury to the popliteus tendon is common. Delay in diagnosis often prohibits primary repair of the posterolateral structures. Biceps tendon tenodesis, a recently proposed surgical procedure for chronic posterolateral instability, was evaluated.

Methods.—The effects of biceps tendon tenodesis on internal-external and varus-valgus laxity were measured in fresh-frozen cadaveric knee specimens. The posterolateral structures and the fibular collateral ligament had been sequentially sectioned. The biceps tenodesis was performed according to a previously described technique (Fig 4–18), using 89 N graft tension and a fixation point located 1 cm anterior to the fibular collateral ligament's insertion on the femur.

Results.—The tenodesis was able to correct increased external rotation and varus laxity caused by sectioning of the posterolateral structures and fibular collateral ligament. The procedure overconstrained external tibial rotation at all flexion positions and varus angulation at 60 and 90 degrees of flexion. Internal rotation and valgus laxity were not affected. By eliminating the increased external rotation laxity in posterolateral instability, the biceps tenodesis should help correct this abnormal posterior subluxation of the lateral tibial plateau.

Conclusion.—Findings suggest that tenodesis of the biceps tendon has the potential to restore static laxity to the posterolateral-deficient knee. Initial overconstraint may be desirable because of concerns about the tenodesis stretching out in vivo. Long-term results are likely to depend on initial tendon strength and the effects of any tissue remodeling that may have occurred.

Posterolateral Knee Reconstruction Using Clancy Biceps Tenodesis: Surgical Technique
Bach BR Jr, Jewell BF, Dworsky B (Rush-Presbyterian-St Luke's Med Ctr, Chicago)
Am J Knee Surg 6:97–103, 1993   139-94-4–48

Introduction.—Numerous studies of the anterior cruciate ligament (ACL)-deficient knee have been published, but little information on the optimal treatment of posterolateral instability has been presented. The biceps femoris tenodesis technique described by Clancy in 1988 was described in detail, and the anatomical structure of the posterolateral knee and recent biomechanics/cutting studies of the posterior cruciate ligament (PCL) were reviewed.

Technique.—The knee is meticulously examined under anesthesia. A 6-in. incision based over the posterolateral aspect of the knee carries dissection through the subcutaneous tissues. Anterior and posterior flaps are created. With attention directed toward the more posterior dissection, the knee is flexed at approximately 30 degrees. The fibular head serves as an anatomical landmark throughout the procedure, and, in a modification of the Clancy technique, the common peroneal nerve is identified and dissected initially. To minimize any entrapment that may occur when the biceps femoris tendon is transferred anteriorly and

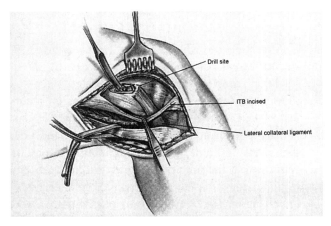

Fig 4–19.—The posterior intermuscular septum is incised. The posterior half of the iliotibial band (*ITB*) is retracted posteriorly, and the LCL is palpated and identified. Layer II fascia over the LCL is incised to allow better visualization. The vastus lateralis is retracted anteriorly. Soft tissues are débrided from the lateral supracondylar region. An osteotome or gauge is used to decorticate the femur adjacent and proximal to the LCL origin. (Courtesy of Bach BR Jr, Jewell BF, Dworsky B: *Am J Knee Surg* 6:97-103, 1993.)

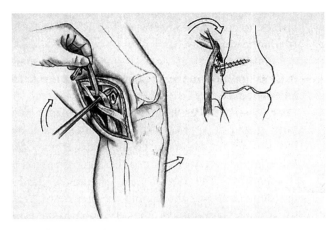

Fig 4–20.—A Cobb gauge is used to lever the tendon over the screw and spiked washer as the knee is extended. (Courtesy of Bach BR Jr, Jewell BF, Dworsky B: *Am J Knee Surg* 6:97–103, 1993.)

tenodesed, and thin fascia overlying the common peroneal nerve is released proximally and distally.

With the knee further flexed, the region of the lateral collateral ligament (LCL) is exposed (Fig 4–19). The goal of the surgical procedure is to transfer the biceps femoris tendon medial to the iliotibial band and secure this at the origin of the LCL. A 3.2-mm hole is drilled in the region of the origin of the LCL, placed slightly anteriorly, and a 6.5-mm AO screw of appropriate length is positioned along with a spiked washer. The actual transfer of the biceps tendon onto the screw and spiked washer post is one of the more difficult aspects of the surgical procedure (Fig 4–20). With the knee extended and the tibia in neutral rotation, the tenodesis is secured (Fig 4–21), and the knee is brought through a range

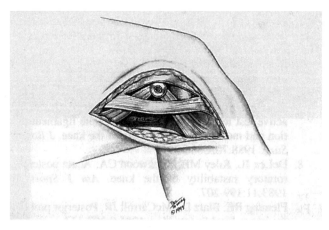

Fig 4–21.—The tenodesis is secured with the knee extended and the tibia in neutral rotation. The distal portion of the tenodesis parallels the LCL. (Courtesy of Bach BR Jr, Jewell BF, Dworsky B: *Am J Knee Surg* 6:97–103, 1993.)

of motion to make certain that the tendon will not subluxate or dislocate from the screw and spiked washer. To reduce hamstring spasm, the knee can be placed in 20–30 degrees of flexion in the early postoperative period.

Conclusion.—Injuries to the posterolateral structures of the knee are uncommon and can easily be missed. Overall evaluation and conclusions are difficult because the wide variety of associated pathologic conditions results in an extremely heterogeneous patient group. The Clancy biceps tenodesis procedure has had good short-term results in patients with a valgus or neutral anatomical alignment.

▶ These 2 papers (Abstracts 139-94-4–47 and 139-94-4–48) describe a previously unreported surgical technique for management of posterolateral instability of the knee that was originally performed by Clancy. What Wascher et al. and Bach et al. have in common with Clancy is that none of them have reported the results of this procedure. So once again we see the "sports medicine fast shuffle," which is to identify a problem, then describe a surgical solution, but not to bother with details like whether it works, is associated with complications, or will stand the test of time. Needless to say, this does not appear to be the way clinical science is supposed to work.—J.S. Torg, M.D.

Subjective Evaluation of Function Following Moderately Accelerated Rehabilitation of Anterior Cruciate Ligament Reconstructed Knees
Draper V, Ladd C (Knoxville Orthopedic Clinic, Tenn)
J Athletic Train 28:38–41, 1993   139-94-4–49

Background.—Surgical reconstruction and rehabilitation protocols for anterior cruciate ligament tears have become increasingly aggressive, leading to an earlier return to functional and sports activities. The timing of the return to motion, weight-bearing, and functional activities usually is dependent on objective measures, including range of motion, knee-arthrometer measures of ligament stability, and isokinetic measures of quadriceps and hamstring peaking torque and endurance. Patients' assessments of their knee functions have contributed to the decision to resume activity; to augment the objective measures, pain, sensations of mechanical abnormalities, and the patient's perception of knee stability were determined.

Method.—One hundred eighty patients who underwent a bone-patellar tendon–bone autograft reconstruction were rehabilitated in a moderately accelerated protocol (table). Fifty-eight patients who were at least 1 year postsurgery were surveyed to assess the long-term effects of early weight-bearing, immediate full motion, early incorporation of closed-chain activities, and early return to sports. The 58 patients responded to the Lysholm Knee Scoring Scale and a questionnaire regard-

Modified Accelerated Rehabilitation Program

Time After Reconstruction	Rehabilitation Activities
Pre-op (7–10 days)	QF and HS isometrics; SLRs (all planes); HS stretch; ROM (A,AAA and PROM); cryotherapy
2–3 days	Discharge from hospital, Prerequisites: 1) able to do SLR; 2) full extension; 3) 90° flexion desirable; 4) 20- to 30-lb weight-bearing, emphasis on heel-toe gait. Continue pre-op activities.
5–7 days	ROM-full extension; active assisted flexion; strengthening: E-stim and/or biofeedback-assisted SLRs, partial weight-bearing (heel-toe gait); patellar mobilization; outpatient physical therapy 2/wk to 3/wk
10–14 days	ROM (0°–90°); bicycle for ROM only; SLRs with weights; Continue pre-op activities
2–4 weeks	ROM (0°–120°); multi-angle (90°–45°) isometric QF workout on Kin-Com; hydrotherapy (SLRs, ROM, gait training)
4–6 weeks	ROM (0°–140°); full weight-bearing with crutches as tolerated (wean from crutches when normal gait is possible); closed chain activities: Nordic track, Stair-master, mini-squats, step-ups; passive mode concentric QF/HS exercise on KIN-COM (90°–45°); Isotonic PREs with light weights (90°–45°); bicycle for conditioning
6–12 weeks	Increase isotonic PREs (QF and HS curls, leg press, hip, calf raises); eccentric HS on Kin-Com; proprioceptive training
3–4 months	KT-1000 evaluation; velocity mode on Kin-Com for QF and HS; continued closed chain activity; Proprioceptive training; sport cord running in pool (forward/backward); continue PREs; light running allowed
4–6 months	Isokinetic evaluation at 60°/s and 180°/s; KT-1000; in a functional brace begin agility workouts and sport-specific activities
6–8 months	Return to athletics with functional brace

Abbreviations: QF, quadriceps femoris muscle; SLR, straight leg raise; PRE, progressive resistive exercise; HS, hamstring muscle; ROM, range of motion.
(Courtesy of Draper V, Ladd C: J Athletic Train 28:38–41, 1993.)

ing preinjury and postinjury activity levels, pain and stability ratings, and current activity.

Findings.—The preinjury activity level of the 58 patients surveyed was generally high, with 46% engaging in level 4 or 5 organized sports. Seventy-one percent of the patients returned to their preinjury activity level and 3% increased their activity. Pain ratings were low and stability ratings were good during both daily and recreational activities.

Conclusion.—The accelerated rehabilitation protocol encourages full weight-bearing at 2–3 weeks, eliminating crutches as early as 4 weeks and allowing a return to sports as early as 4 months. The patient's perception of knee function should be an integral part of the decision to resume preinjury levels of activity.

▶ We have accepted the moderately accelerated rehabilitation protocol for knees undergoing anterior cruciate ligament reconstruction. The prevention of knee flexion contractures and quadriceps extensor lag has made this type of program much easier on the patient and the entire rehabilitation team. Emphasis on closed-chain kinetic exercises speeds functional return and helps avoid patellofemoral problems in rehabilitation. In general, our athletes have not been returning to full activity in 4 months, but they usually are ready in 6–9 months (usually closer to 9 months than to 6).—F.J. George, A.T.C., P.T.

Biomechanical Effects of Functional Knee Bracing: Practical Implications
Vailas JC, Pink M (New Hampshire Musculoskeletal Inst, Manchester; Centinela Hosp, Inglewood, Calif)
Sports Med 15:210–218, 1993   139-94-4–50

Objective.—There is ongoing debate over the use of bracing in the anterior cruciate–deficient knee. Although subjective studies find that functional bracing offers some perceived benefit to the patient with an unstable knee, studies of its effects on athletic performance have yielded conflicting results. The wide variation in study methods has led to increased efforts to analyze the biomechanical effects of functional knee braces. The literature on the biomechanical effects of functional knee bracing was reviewed and an attempt made to identify some practical implications for its clinical use.

Brace Design.—Studies of brace design suggest that the bigger and stronger the patient and the more strenuous his or her sport, the heavier and more rigid the brace required. Heavy, rigid braces have also been suggested for patients whose injured leg has less than 80% of the quadriceps function of the uninjured leg. Although there are different types of hinge joint designs, the important consideration is its placement—the hinge should match the kinematic axis of rotation of the knee as closely as possible. Correct hinge placement is difficult enough, and it is complicated by the problem of slippage, which is the main complaint of patients with braces. The position of the hinge axis must be maintained by proper and rigid fitting, which provides a better match for the patient's knee motion.

Practical Implications.—The evidence suggests that functional knee bracing can play a useful role in the management of the patient with an anterior cruciate–deficient knee. The precise role will vary according to the patient's clinical signs and symptoms. Factors such as body weight, level of athletic competitiveness, and degree of functional instability must all be considered in prescribing a brace. The brace should fit properly, without moving up and down the knee. Custom braces fit better than off-the-shelf braces. Custom braces may feel more restrictive to the patient, but that may indicate that they are providing some mechanical protection. Shell-type braces have a greater biomechanical constraining effect and are more durable than strap-type braces.

Athletes with the greatest functional instability are the most likely to benefit from a more durable, custom-fitted, more rigid brace, usually a shell type. In contrast, athletes with minimal signs and symptoms may achieve better results with an off-the-shelf, strap-type brace. In this case, the functional results will be better if the patient has good leg strength with minimal clinical laxity, modified activities, and light body weight.

Summary.—This review concludes that functional knee bracing can play a role in the management of the athlete with an anterior cruciate-deficient knee. Bracing can be a key component of the comprehensive rehabilitation program, which emphasizes returning the strength of the injured leg to normal, activity modification, control of the body during sports participation, and patient awareness of the signs and symptoms of instability.

▶ There has been an ongoing controversy regarding the benefits of bracing the anterior cruciate–deficient knee. The authors have stressed the importance of hinge placement and fit of the brace to prevent slippage. They state, "Hinge position is more critical than hinge design as it pertains to matching the knee kinematics." Patient compliance is certainly related to comfort and lack of restriction. The durability and reliability of any brace are very important factors. There is nothing more frustrating than to have an athlete's brace break the day before a big event and experience the running around that must be done to get it repaired.—F.J. George, A.T.C., P.T.

Biomechanical Considerations in Patellofemoral Joint Rehabilitation
Steinkamp LA, Dillingham MF, Markel MD, Hill JA, Kaufman KR (Functional Rehabilitation and Sports Therapy, Palo Alto, Calif; Sports, Orthopedic and Rehabilitation Medicine Associates, Portola Valley, Calif; Univ of Wisconsin, Madison; et al)
Am J Sports Med 21:438–444, 1993   139-94-4-51

Introduction.—Patellofemoral joint arthritis, a problem frequently seen in orthopedic medical practices, can occur in patients of all ages and activity levels. There is considerable controversy regarding the proper rehabilitation of patellofemoral joint arthritis. Two means of strengthening the quadriceps—leg extension maneuvers and leg press exercises—were compared in a biomechanical study of 20 normal individuals.

Subjects and Methods.—The participants were 10 men and 10 women, aged 18-45 years. None had a history of patellofemoral joint injury or disease. The volunteers were trained in the proper use of the leg press and performance of the leg extension exercises. Quadriceps force, patellofemoral joint reaction force, and patellofemoral joint stress were determined at 0, 30, 60, and 90 degrees of knee flexion for both leg press and leg extension exercises.

Results.—All 3 parameters were significantly greater in leg extension exercise than in leg press exercise at 0 and 30 degrees of knee flexion. At 60 and 90 degrees of knee flexion, however, all 3 parameters were significantly greater in the leg press exercise. Knee moments for leg press exercise and leg extension exercise intersected at 50.7 degrees of knee flexion. Knee moments, patellofemoral joint reaction forces, and patellofemoral joint stress values were higher for men than for women during both exercises, a finding not duplicated in all studies.

Conclusion.—Because leg press maneuvers place minimal stress on the patellofemoral joint in the functional range of motion and simulate normal movement patterns, this type of rehabilitation exercise may be better tolerated by patients with patellofemoral joint arthritis. The authors' own empirical observations support this conclusion; many such patients have increased symptoms during leg extension. Although leg press exercise may not isolate the quadriceps, the quadriceps can be effectively strengthened without joint isolation. One limitation of this study is its failure to consider that because there is no patellofemoral articulation from 10 degrees of knee flexion to full extension, it is generally safe to strengthen in this range with any type of exercise. Thus, stress values in this range of motion may be inaccurate.

▶ We continue to search for the best method of increasing quadriceps strength with our patellofemoral joint patients. This remains one of the most difficult problems to solve in the training room. Exercising in the last 10–15 degrees of knee extension (terminal knee extension exercises) had been a major part of our program. However, in some patients even this exercise can cause an increase in symptoms. Our general goal is to increase strength in the oblique portion of the vastus medialis, decrease vastus lateralis activity, and stretch the lateral retinaculum. This is often not an easy goal to achieve and many different methods are attempted, from biofeedback to orthotics. We rely on closed-chain exercises and insist that the exercises always be pain-free. Please read Abstract 139-94-4-52 for more on this topic.—F.J. George, A.T.C., P.T.

Electromyographic Analysis of Exercises Proposed for Differential Activation of Medial and Lateral Quadriceps Femoris Muscle Components

Karst GM, Jewett PD (Univ of Nebraska, Omaha; Team Rehab, Clayton, Mo)
Phys Ther 73:286–299, 1993   139-94-4–52

Introduction.—A wide variety of exercise regimens are designed to strengthen the quadriceps femoris muscle (QF). Although gains in QF torque production are important, other considerations should enter into the choice of a rehabilitation program for patients with knee disorders. Whether active exercises combining hip adduction with knee extension activate medial components of the QF more than does knee extension alone was determined.

Subjects and Methods.—Twelve healthy adults, 6 men and 6 women, volunteered to take part in the study. None had current knee pathology. All exercises were performed with the right leg. The subjects performed quadriceps femoris setting (QS), straight leg raising (SLR), straight leg raising with the hip laterally rotated (SLR/LR), and straight leg raising combined with isometric hip adduction (SLR/ADD). After 5 repetitions of the QS exercise, the subjects sequentially performed 1 repetition each of the SLR, SLR/LR, and SLR/ADD exercises until a total of 5 repetitions of each SLR variation was completed. Sessions concluded with an additional 5 QS repetitions. During all variations of the SLR exercise, resistance was added by applying ankle weights equivalent to 5% of body weight. An external torque tending to adduct the hip was applied via a rope-and-pulley apparatus for the SLR/ADD exercise. Electromyographic activity was recorded from the oblique and longitudinal portions of the vastus medialis, vastus lateralis, and rectus femoris muscles.

Results.—For 10 of the subjects, the QS exercises elicited the greatest mean electromyographic activity in each of the single-joint QF components—oblique and longitudinal portions of the vastus medialis and the vastus lateralis. Neither SLR/LR nor SLR/ADD elicited greater relative activity of medial QF components than did QS or SLR. Thus, exercises requiring combined hip adduction and knee extension torques are not superior to the QS or standard SLR exercise in eliciting an increase in the relative activity of the medial components of the QF.

Conclusion.—These findings support and expand those of previous studies, demonstrating that QS exercises tend to elicit a greater degree of activity of the single-joint knee extensors than do SLR exercises. Isometric QS may be the treatment of choice in patients requiring QF strengthening in the fully extended knee position.

▶ The good news after reading this study is that quadriceps setting has been a part of our knee rehabilitation program. The bad news is that we have also been doing SLR with adduction in the hopes of eliciting more activity of the oblique portion of the vastus medialis, and this study refuted that theory. Please read Abstract 139-94-4–51.

Jenny McConnell wrote the commentary that appears after this study. She discourages the use of terminal knee extensor exercises and encourages a method of correcting the position of the patella by the use of tape and then doing specific muscle training exercises.—F.J. George, A.T.C., P.T.

5 Injuries of the Leg, Ankle, and Foot

The Role of Arthroscopy in the Assessment and Treatment of Tibial Plateau Fractures
Fowble CD, Zimmer JW, Schepsis AA (Boston City Hosp)
Arthroscopy 9:584–590, 1993   139-94-5-1

Background.—Tibial plateau fractures are relatively common injuries, but deciding on a specific plan of treatment is difficult. The results of arthroscopic treatment of tibial plateau fractures were compared with those of traditional open methods.

Methods.—Forty patients with tibial plateau fractures were seen at an inner-city hospital between January 1989 and August 1992. Twenty-three patients with certain fracture patterns—local compression or split compression fractures—were included in the study. Twelve patients were treated with arthroscopic reduction and percutaneous fixation (ARPF), and 11 had open reduction and internal fixation (ORIF).

Outcomes.—All reductions in the ARPF group were anatomical and remained fixed for at least 3 months after surgery. Only 55% of the ORIF group initially had anatomical reductions. One patient in the ORIF group had further loss of reduction on follow-up radiography. Iliac crest bone graft was used in 2 patients in the ARPF group and in 10 in the ORIF group. In the former group, the use of bone graft did not affect final outcome. The mean length of hospitalization after surgery was 5.4 days for ARPF-treated patients with isolated tibial plateau fractures and 10.3 days for ORIF-treated patients. The mean time to full weight-bearing in the ARPF and ORIF groups was 9 and 12.3 weeks, respectively. None of the patients had medial collateral ligament repairs. None of those in the ARPF group had valgus laxity after surgery. One patient in the ORIF group had residual instability, and 1 needed a cane to walk. All concomitant knee abnormalities were addressed and treated arthroscopically in patients in the ARPF group. Open reduction and internal fixation was associated with more frequent and more severe complications than ARPF.

Conclusion.—The outcomes of ARPF were superior to those of ORIF in this series. The length of hospitalization and time to full weight-bearing were shorter with the former treatment. The ARPF method was more effective in achieving the goals of joint congruity, stability, and angular alignment. The rates of anatomical reduction in the ARPF and

ORIF groups were 100% and 55%, respectively. Thus, in selected tibial plateau fractures, ARPF should be the treatment of choice.

▶ Of concern is the fact that the authors present a retrospective chart and roentgenographic review with an average follow-up of 6 months for both the ARPF and ORIF groups.—J.S. Torg, M.D.

Iliotibial Band Syndrome in Cyclists
Holmes JC, Pruitt AL, Whalen NJ (Western Orthopaedics, Denver; Western Orthopaedic Sports Medicine and Rehabilitation, Denver)
Am J Sports Med 21:419–424, 1993   139-94-5-2

Background.—Iliotibial band (ITB) syndrome, an overuse injury, results from repetitive friction of the ITB across the lateral femoral epicondyle. Thought to be indigenous to runners, it is now being seen in cyclists. The occurrence and treatments for this syndrome in cyclists were reviewed.

Patients.—Forty-seven male and 14 female cyclists were seen between 1985 and 1991 with complaints of atraumatic lateral knee pain associated with cycling. Both knees were affected in 8 patients. These patients were very active and competed often, some at the national and interna-

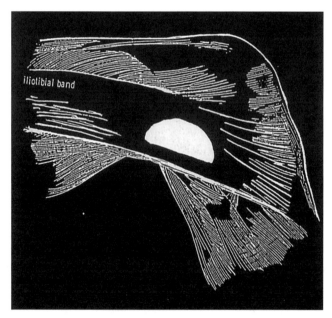

Fig 5–1.—Surgical excision of elliptical piece (2 cm × 4 cm) of distal posterior ITB. (From Holmes JC, Pruitt AL, Whalen NJ: *Am J Sports Med* 21:419–424, 1993. Courtesy of Insall JN: *Surgery of the Knee.* New York, Churchill Livingstone Inc, 1984.)

tional level. Complaints and physical findings indicating ITB syndrome included exquisite tenderness of the distal ITB over the lateral femoral epicondyle; a history of previously diagnosed ITB syndrome; complaints of a stabbing or burning pain or hot flash on the outside of the knee while cycling, frequently associated with loss of power; crepitus; localized swelling; and a snapping of the distal one third of the ITB over the lateral femoral epicondyle with knee flexion and extension. Also, 10 patients were found to have a tight tensor fascia lata complex proximally and distally on Ober's test.

Treatments.—Bicycle adjustments were directed mainly toward correcting misalignments between the cyclist and cycle observed during the examination. Training modifications were also recommended because high-resistance and high-mileage cycling have been postulated to contribute to irritation of the distal ITB. Cortisone injections were considered for cyclists with acute ITB syndrome who did not respond to initial treatment or for cyclists who wanted temporary relief for a race. Surgery was performed on patients whose symptoms failed to respond to prolonged nonoperative measures or previous surgery. Four had percutaneous release. In an open release-excision, performed on 21 cyclists, an ellipse of tissue measuring 4 cm at the base and 2 cm at the apex was excised (Fig 5–1).

Conclusion.—Iliotibial band syndrome in cyclists requires prompt treatment. Misalignments between cyclist and bicycle must be corrected or symptoms will persist. Surgery should be done only after extensive nonsurgical treatments have been unsuccessful. The surgical removal of abrading tissue of the distal posterolateral ITB from the lateral femoral condyle was safe and effective.

▶ The results of treatment have been noted. Fifty-seven percent of the cyclists responded to nonoperative treatment. Percutaneous release was successful in only 1 of 4 patients. Twenty-one patients underwent the open surgical release-excision described. Of these, 17 (81%) reported that they had returned to preinjury levels of cycling by 8 weeks postoperatively. Nine of the 21 developed "small" seroma in the incisions, which were attributed to the patients' rapid return to activity.—J.S. Torg, M.D.

Ischial Apophysis Injuries in Athletes

Kujala UM, Orava S (Helsinki Research Inst for Sports and Exercise Medicine; Hosp Meditori, Turku, Finland)
Sports Med 16:290–294, 1993   139-94-5-3

Background.—Chronic ischial tuberosity pain in the posterior thigh may result from a number of conditions, and the diagnosis and treatment of ischial tuberosity pain may be difficult even for sports medicine specialists. The clinical entities to be considered in the differential diagnosis of painful ischial tuberosity and the treatment modalities were reviewed.

Classification of the Injuries.—Sports injuries of the ischial tuberosity include apophysitis, adult tug lesion, unfused apophysis, or acute or old avulsions. The apophysis (traction epiphysis) is the site of origin or insertion of major muscles or muscle groups. Ischial apophysis includes the insertion of the hamstrings and the adductor magnus. The ossification rate of an ischial apophysis varies with each individual, but generally it is complete before age 25 years. Ischial apophysis commonly occurs at age 17–18 years, before the tuberosity has fused. Tug lesions, characterized by sclerosis in the insertion area, are sometimes seen in adults. Avulsions of the ischial tuberosity occur as a result of violent muscle contraction. The avulsion may or may not include a bony fragment visible on x-ray films. An insertional tendon rupture is also possible.

Treatment.—Apophysitis may be successfully treated with modification of activities and anti-inflammatory medication. Conservative treatment is also adequate for avulsions if they are diagnosed early. Surgery is recommended for total or near-total soft tissue hamstring muscle insertion rupture, dislocation of the apophysis, or bony avulsion of more than 2 cm. In a healed, old avulsion, excision of the excessive mass or poorly united fragment provides pain relief.

Conclusion.—Ischial tuberosity pain in athletes may result from several clinical entities, including apophysitis, adult tug lesion, unfused apophysis, or acute or old avulsions. Diagnosis determines the decision for conservative or surgical treatment. Conservative treatment is adequate for apophysitis and for avulsions that are diagnosed early. Surgery is recommended for total or near-total soft tissue hamstring muscle insertion rupture, dislocation of the apophysis, or bony avulsion of more than 2 cm. Surgical excision of the excessive mass or poorly united fragment in an old, healed avulsion can provide pain relief.

▶ The authors have presented a logical classification based on the anatomy of the different stress injuries that occur to the ischial tuberosity. I question the wisdom of an aggressive surgical approach to both total soft tissue hamstring muscle insertion ruptures and apophysis avulsions.—J.S. Torg, M.D.

Radiographic Imaging of Muscle Strain Injury
Speer KP, Lohnes J, Garrett WE Jr (Duke Univ, Durham, NC)
Am J Sports Med 21:89–96, 1993   139-94-5-4

Purpose.—Although muscle strain injuries of the lower extremity are very common and well recognized clinically, there is little information on their pathophysiology. These injuries appear to occur near the myotendinous junction and to be followed by inflammation and edema. Fibrosis begins as the inflammatory reaction resolves. Muscle strain injuries

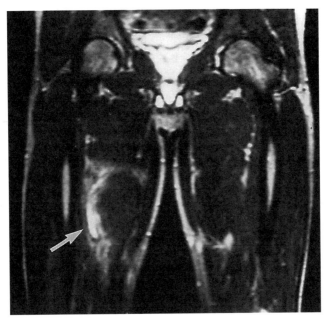

Fig 5–2.—T2-weighted coronal image (repetition time, 2,000 ms; echo time, 70 ms) of an adductor longus muscle strain. The *arrow* identifies edema, inflammation, and possible hemorrhage. (Courtesy of Speer KP, Lohnes J, Garrett WE Jr: *Am J Sports Med* 21:89–96, 1993.)

have been studied with CT and MRI for more than a decade; the findings are reviewed.

Methods.—Fifty athletes with acute muscle strains of the adductor, hamstring, quadriceps, or triceps surae muscles were studied. The average patient age was 28 years, and most injuries were studied within 2–4 days. The first 23 patients were studied by axial CT scanning. Since 1987, patients have been studied by axial, coronal, and sagittal spin-echo MRI.

Findings.—On MRI scanning, T2-weighted images were best for evaluation of muscle strain injuries (Fig 5–2). Both imaging methods localized the strain injury to a single muscle in a group of synergistic muscles. The muscles most vulnerable to injury seemed to be the adductor longus, rectus femoris, and medial head of the gastrocnemius. As predicted, disruptions occurred at the myotendinous junction. Fluid collecting at the site of the disruption subsequently dissected along the epimysium and subcutis. Significant injury was apparent in muscle tissue far away from the myotendinous junction on MRI, with signal changes consistent with edema and inflammation. Muscular atrophy, the development of fibrosis, and calcium deposition were all clearly seen on follow-up CT and MRI.

Conclusion.—Muscle strain injuries of the lower extremity can be detected on CT and MRI examination. They are found in characteristic locations and have characteristic imaging traits during both the acute and chronic stages. Uncharacteristic lesions can also be identified by CT and MRI for more thorough evaluation.

▶ This is an excellent study demonstrating the common muscle injury patterns affecting the lower extremity. Familiarity with the characteristic muscle and soft tissue injuries increases the clinical and MR diagnosis by enabling the appropriate MR study to be done, both with respect to the area to be included in the examination and also with the use of the appropriate techniques.—J.S. Torg, M.D.

MR Imaging in the Prognostication of Hamstring Injury: Work in Progress

Pomeranz SJ, Heidt RS Jr (Christ Hosp, Cincinnati, Ohio)
Radiology 189:897–900, 1993   139-94-5-5

Introduction.—The hamstring group of muscles may show alterations in signal intensity on MRI after trauma or inflammation. The morphological and signal alterations in the hamstring muscle complex were correlated with short-term prognosis and convalescence interval (CI) in professional athletes.

Methods.—Fourteen male athletes with a clinical diagnosis of hamstring strain were evaluated with a 1.5-T superconductive magnet operating at 63.86 MHz. All patients were studied within 8 days after the initial hamstring injury and their injuries categorized according to muscle group involved, percentage of cross-sectional area affected, location, and signal intensity on T1- and T2-weighted spin-echo images. The CIs for each athlete were determined by the ability to lift 60% of body weight at 60 degrees per second on a flexion/extension isokinetic strengthening device.

Results.—Six hamstring injuries were in the biceps femoris group, 5 were in the semimembranosus group, 2 in the quadratus femoris complex, and 1 in the semitendinosus group of muscles. Shorter CIs, equal to or less than 5 weeks, were seen in superficial muscle injuries and muscle belly injuries that involved small cross-sectional areas of the muscle. Athletes with complete transection; greater than 50% cross-sectional muscle involvement; ganglionlike fluid collections (long T1 and T2); hemorrhagelike signal intensity (short T1 and T2); distal myotendinous junction tears; and deep muscular tears had CIs of 6 weeks or more. The 2 cases of tendon transection or retraction were associated with CIs of 13 and 15 weeks. Proximal hamstring injuries resulted in chronic pain for up to 10 weeks even though the average CI for such injuries was less than 5.8 weeks.

Conclusion.—The evaluation of complete hamstring injuries with MRI can predict the CI in high-performance athletes. In the area of professional sports, such predictions have both economic and medical significance. Poor prognostic factors in hamstring injuries include rupture and retraction, hemorrhage, localized fluid collections, large cross-sectional area involvement, and tendinous/myotendinous junction rather than pure muscular proximal involvement.

▶ The authors identify that the more extensive the injury patterns seen on MRI, the longer the CI will be. It is not surprising that MRI confirms what one's grandmother already knows, i.e., the more severe the injury, the longer it takes to recover. This study also is not conclusive in that the number of athletes involved was small (14) and the decision to return the athlete to athletic endeavors was subjectively determined.—J.S. Torg, M.D.

Operative Versus Nonoperative Treatment of Achilles Tendon Rupture: A Prospective Randomized Study and Review of the Literature
Cetti R, Christensen S-E, Ejsted R, Jensen NM, Jorgensen U (Glostrup Univ, Denmark; Hφrsholm Hosp, Denmark; Kolding Hosp, Denmark; et al)
Am J Sports Med 21:791–799, 1993   139-94-5–6

Introduction.—Rupture of the Achilles tendon is treated both operatively and nonoperatively, generally in accordance with the preference of the orthopedic surgeon. The 2 types of treatment were compared in a randomized series of patients. The results were examined in light of an evaluation of the literature.

Patients and Methods.—The study group consisted of 156 patients with a diagnosis of acute total rupture of the Achilles tendon; 45 were excluded from analysis for a variety of reasons. The patients were treated from October 1982 to May 1984 at 8 hospitals in Denmark. Fifty-six were randomized to operative treatment and 55 were randomized to nonoperative management. The 2 groups were similar regarding age, sex, side and site of rupture, and work and sport activity. Most (83%) had sustained the rupture during sports. All patients in the operative treatment group wore a below-knee plaster cast with the foot in 20 degrees of plantar flexion for 6 weeks. They were not allowed to bear weight on the injured leg during this period. A similar cast was worn by the nonoperative group for 4 weeks. During the next 4 weeks, they were allowed to bear weight in a new cast with a heel applied with the foot in neutral position. Patients were reexamined 4 and 12 months after injury.

Results.—The operative and nonoperative groups did not differ significantly in mean period of hospitalization, mean duration of sick leave, symptoms at 4 months, or the incidence of rerupture and of major complications. There were significantly fewer minor complications in the nonoperative group. Results after 12 months were significantly different for 2 of the 5 symptoms recorded. Abnormal ankle movement occurred in 17.9% of the operative group vs. 47.3% of the nonoperative group; calf atrophy occurred in 39.3% of the operative group and 63.6% of the nonoperative group. At 12 months, the operative group had significantly fewer problems with pain, walking, or wearing shoes and were significantly more likely than the nonoperative group to resume sports at their preinjury level.

Conclusion.—The results of this prospective study were similar to the findings of a literature evaluation. Operative treatment was determined to be preferable to nonoperative treatment in patients with rupture of the Achilles tendon. However, because many of the outcomes measured were similar, nonoperative treatment is an acceptable alternative.

▶ The authors present an impressive prospective, randomized study dealing with the controversial question of operative vs. nonoperative treatment for Achilles tendon rupture. Importantly, they note that "The operatively treated patients had a significantly higher rate of resuming sports activities at the same level, a lesser degree of calf atrophy, better ankle movement, and fewer complaints 1 year after the accident." Also to be noted, in the operative treatment group there were 3 reruptures and 2 deep wound infections as compared with 7 reruptures, 1 second rerupture, and 1 extreme residual tendon lengthening in the nonoperative group. In view of the gratifying results being obtained with the current accelerated rehabilitation techniques, my own practice is to manage Achilles tendon rupture in the active individual operatively.—J.S. Torg, M.D.

Early Mobilization After Operative Repair of Ruptured Achilles Tendon
Saw Y, Baltzopoulos V, Lim A, Rostron PKM, Bolton-Maggs BG, Calver RF (Whiston Hosp Prescot, Merseyside, England; Univ of Liverpool, England; Walton Hosp, Liverpool, England)
Injury 24:479–484, 1993   139-94-5-7

Purpose.—The postoperative treatment of a ruptured Achilles tendon usually involves serial plastering and gradual dorsiflexion of the ankle. However, prolonged immobilization can cause a variety of complications. The benefits of early mobilization after surgical repair of a ruptured Achilles tendon were examined in a pilot study.

Patients.—Sixteen men and 3 women, 25-60 years of age, had surgical repair of a ruptured Achilles tendon. At 1 week after operation the plaster cast was removed, and gentle active dorsiflexion of the ankle with the patient in the sitting position was initiated. Active plantar flexion was not attempted yet. Between therapy sessions, the ankle was kept in the equinus plaster cast. Sutures were removed at 2 weeks. The foot was then placed in a lower-leg walker, which was removed at 8 weeks. All patients were reevaluated at a mean of 13.6 months after surgery.

Results.—Isokinetic measurement of maximum strength plantar flexion and dorsiflexion revealed normal values with an almost normal range of ankle movement in all patients. At 2 weeks after operation 2 patients had minor wound infection develop, which responded to antibiotic therapy. At follow-up, 15 of the 19 patients stated that they had returned to their preinjury level of activity. The 4 patients who had not achieved their preinjury status were between 5 and 8 months postsurgery. Tendon rerupture did not occur.

Conclusion.—Early mobilization after surgical repair of a ruptured Achilles tendon avoids the complications associated with prolonged immobilization, and it does not appear to increase the risk of tendon rerupture. This regimen is particularly suitable for athletically active individuals.

▶ This report on both the effectiveness and advantages of early mobilization after surgical repair of a ruptured Achilles tendon is in keeping with the findings of Carter et al. (1) as well as our own. We observed similar results with early motion and accelerated rehabilitation after repair using an experimental polylactic acid biodegradable device (2). One criticism of this study is that the protocol did not include a randomly selected control group.—J.S. Torg, M.D.

References

1. Carter TR, Fowler PJ: *Am J Sports Med* 20:459, 1992.
2. Glasgow S: The results of primary Achilles tendon repair with polylactic acid augmentation. Presented at the American Academy of Orthopedic Surgeons Annual Meeting, 1993.

Surgical Management of Exertional Compartment Syndrome of the Lower Leg: Long-Term Followup
Schepsis AA, Martini D, Corbett M (Boston Univ)
Am J Sports Med 21:811–817, 1993   139-94-5-8

Background.—Exertional or "chronic" compartment syndrome has become an increasingly recognized cause of exercise-induced pain in the lower extremity. However, there is some controversy surrounding exactly what the pressure criteria are for diagnosing this condition and how it should be treated. The long-term results of patients undergoing fasciotomy for exertional anterior and deep posterior compartment syndromes were investigated. Measurements of intracompartmental pressure for the establishment of a diagnosis in past studies were compared to pressure measurements found in this surgical series.

Method.—A total of 52 patients participated in the study. All had clinical pressure measurement that led to diagnosis of exertional compartment syndrome according to established criteria. Thirty-eight underwent surgical decompressive fasciotomy, and 28 were available for long-term follow-up. Of the 28, 18 patients had bilateral surgery, providing a total of 48 limbs to be investigated. The patients were divided into 2 groups: those with exertional anterior compartment syndrome comprised group 1, and those with exertional deep posterior compartment syndrome made up group 2. When followed up, patients completed a questionnaire based on their ability to return to former physical activities after surgery. The results were categorized as excellent, good, fair, and poor.

Results.—Most of the patients with chronic compartment syndrome met the 3 parameters proposed by Pedowitz et al. requiring 1 or more of the following conditions: a resting pressure of greater than or equal to 15 mm Hg, a 1-minute postexercise pressure of greater than or equal to 20 mm Hg, and a 5-minute postexercise pressure of greater than or equal to 20 mm Hg. Completing the questionnaire after treatment, 15 of the 16 patients with exertional anterior compartment syndrome (group 1) gave excellent results. All could return to full activity and were able to run an unlimited distance with no recurrence of symptoms at an average follow-up of 4.2 years. One patient in this group reported fair results and complained of numbness and some weakness in the foot. The results of surgery in group 2 were not as successful. Of the 12 patients with exertional deep posterior compartment syndrome, 5 reported excellent results, and 8 said they had good results. Four patients reported fair and 3 reported poor results.

Conclusion.—The established criteria appear to be the best measures for diagnosing exertional compartment syndrome. Patients treated surgically for exertional deep posterior compartment syndrome do not enjoy the high success rate of fasciotomy seen in patients treated for exertional anterior compartment syndrome. Further studies are required to establish the reasons for this discrepancy in outcome.

▶ This paper asks why patients treated surgically for exertional deep posterior compartment syndrome do not have the high success rate from fasciotomy that those with exertional anterior compartment syndrome do. It is pointed out that, although it is relatively easy to place the catheter in the anterior compartment, deep posterior compartment placement can be more difficult. The authors also question whether deep posterior compartment syndrome is a multifactorial problem. Thus, fasciotomy may not fully address the causes of the exertional pain. Hopefully, time will provide the answers to these problems.—J.S. Torg, M.D.

Muscle Hernia in a Recreational Athlete
Berglund HT, Stocks GW (Texas Tech Univ, Lubbock)
Orthop Rev 22:1246–1248, 1993   139-94-5-9

Background.—Muscle hernia is a relatively rare condition that often is asymptomatic. When it is painful, as can occur in physical activity, it may come to the attention of the clinician.

Case Report.—Woman, 26, had a painful mass on the calf muscle. She was a recreational athlete who had recently begun an exercise program. Physical activity, including weight-bearing, caused pain and swelling. The fascial margins could be palpated, although no bruits or circulatory problems were noted. After tumor, varicosity, phlebitis, and neurologic complications were excluded, conservative therapy was begun, consisting of support hose worn during activity. However, this was unsuccessful and the patient elected to undergo surgery. The peroneus longus muscle was herniated over a 1 × 2-cm area at the site where the superficial peroneal nerve exited. The hernia was treated with a longitudinal fasciotomy of the affected region. The patient returned to full weight-bearing as tolerated and recovered full and painless function.

Discussion.—Muscle hernias occur most often in the distal portion of the calf, often at the site where a vein or nerve passes through the fascia. This event may signify an inherited weakness of the region (constitutional hernia) or a traumatic injury (traumatic hernia). It is associated with muscle hypertrophy and fascial injury, such as a bullet wound. When a nerve exit is involved, strangulation may occur. Longitudinal fasciotomy is considered the safest form of treatment; fascial closure may result in compartment syndrome—if this procedure is attempted, the patient should be carefully observed after surgery.

▶ Although only a case report, this paper presents significant observations regarding a relatively uncommon problem. Specifically, symptomatic muscle hernias in the leg characteristically involve herniation of the peroneus longus muscle through the fascial hiatus transversed by the superficial peroneal nerve. In my own experience, this problem is successfully treated, as pointed out by the authors, by limited longitudinal fasciotomy. Characteristically, the symptoms are precipitated by physical activity, and muscle hernia should be included in the differential diagnosis of exertional leg pain.—J.S. Torg, M.D.

Decision Rules for the Use of Radiography in Acute Ankle Injuries: Refinement and Prospective Validation
Stiell IG, Greenberg GH, McKnight RD, Nair RC, McDowell I, Reardon M, Stewart JP, Maloney J (Univ of Ottawa, Ont, Canada)
JAMA 269:1127–1132, 1993   139-94-5-10

Background.—One of the most common reasons for ordering radiologic examination in the emergency department is acute ankle injury. To reduce the expense and waiting time involved in unnecessary ankle radiographs, clinical decision rules have been derived to aid the efficient use of radiology in acute ankle injuries. The original decision rules were prospectively validated and redefined.

Method.—The study was carried out in 2 stages in the emergency departments of 2 teaching institutions. The participants included 1,032 adults who came to the emergency department with pain or tenderness secondary to blunt ankle trauma caused by any mechanism of injury. The patients were assessed by attending emergency physicians for standardized clinical variables. The physicians classified the need for radiography according to the original (first stage) and the refined (second stage) decision rules. The decision rules were assessed for their ability to correctly identify the criterion standard of clinically significant fractures seen in the ankle or foot radiographic series. The original decision rules were refined by univariate and recursive partitioning analyses.

Results.—During the first stage, the original decision rules had sensitivities of 1.0 for identifying 121 malleolar zone fractures, and .98 for diagnosing 49 midfoot zone fractures. For interpretation of the rules in 116 patients, κ values were .56 for the ankle series rule and .69 for the foot series rule. Recursive partitioning of 20 predictor variables yielded refined decision rules for ankle and foot radiographic series. During the second stage, the refined rules had sensitivities of 1.0 for 50 malleolar zone fractures, and 1.0 for 19 midfoot zone fractures. The possible reduction in radiography is estimated to be 34% for the ankle series and 30% for the foot series. If the corresponding decision rule is "negative," the probability of fracture is estimated at 0% in both the ankle and foot series.

Conclusion.—Decision rules for the use of radiography in ankle injuries were prospectively validated and refined. The rules have been proven highly sensitive for diagnosing fractures and can reduce the use of radiography by 30%. Further studies will assess the effect of the ankle rules on clinical practice.

▶ The development of appropriate guidelines for the use of ankle radiography to reduce the waiting time for those patients who predictably will have normal radiographs and to reduce health care costs by elimination of needless radiography is admirable. Management of ankle injuries per the Ottawa guidelines, however, must be balanced by the development of United States guidelines regarding malpractice exposure.—J.S. Torg, M.D.

The Influence of an Ankle Orthosis on the Talar and Calcaneal Motions in Chronic Lateral Instability of the Ankle: A Stereophotogrammetric Analysis
Löfvenberg R, Kärrholm J (Univ Hosp of Umeå, Sweden)
Am J Sports Med 21:224–230, 1993   139-94-5-11

Background.—Although the ankle is often injured during sports, the mechanical properties and efficacy of external ankle support have not been studied as thoroughly as those of adhesive taping in patients with ankle injuries. The effect of an ankle brace on talar and subtalar mobility in patients with chronic lateral instability of the ankle was investigated.

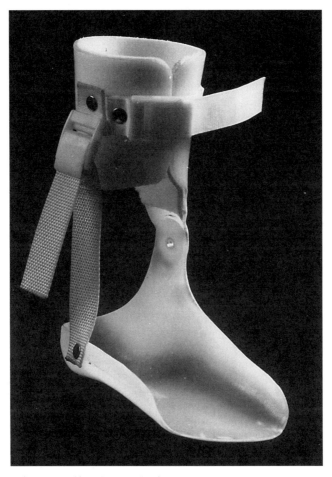

Fig 5–3.—The Strong ankle orthosis, made of a thermoplastic material, permits plantar and dorsal flexion by means of the medially situated hinge. The adjustable lateral strap counteracts the adduction. (Courtesy of Löfvenberg R, Kärrholm J: *Am J Sports Med* 21:224–230, 1993.)

Methods and Findings.—Fourteen ankles in 13 patients with symptoms of chronic lateral instability were included in the study. The mechanical support provided by a semirigid, polypropylene orthosis was tested using stereophotogrammetric analysis. Talar and calcaneal rotations were assessed with and without the Strong ankle orthosis (Fig 5–3) during manual adduction testing and adduction assessment with a predetermined torque of 5 N-m. When the orthosis was applied, there was a significant decrease in talar and calcaneal plantar flexion, internal rotation, and varus angulation.

Conclusion.—The Strong ankle orthosis, which significantly reduced talar and calcaneal plantar flexion, internal rotation, and varus angulation, may provide enough external support to prevent ankle sprains and protect ligament reconstructions.

▶ The authors conclude that the "polypropylene orthosis tested in this study significantly reduced talar and calcaneal plantar flexion, internal rotation, and varus angulation, which supports its use in clinical practice." They have failed to mention, however, whether this proposed use should be as prophylactic and/or functional brace. It would appear that before recommending widespread use of the device, a prospective, randomized clinical study should be performed to determine its efficiency.—J.S. Torg, M.D.

Longitudinal Rupture of the Peroneal Tendons
Bassett FH III, Speer KP (Duke Univ, Durham, NC)
Am J Sports Med 21:354–357, 1993   139-94-5-12

Introduction.—Injury to the peroneal tendons and their supporting structures can occur as a result of an ankle plantar flexion and inversion injury. During a 17-year period, 8 patients with longitudinal rupture of 1 of the peroneal tendons were treated. Motivated by the retrospective observations from these patients, the physicians conducted cadaveric studies to define more precisely the injury mechanism of the peroneal tendon longitudinal tear.

Patients.—In all patients, the injury was sustained as a result of plantar flexion–inversion ankle injury during sports. The lateral ankle sprain was successfully managed nonoperatively. However, the patients complained of persistent lateral ankle swelling, popping, and retrofibular pain at 7 days to 6 months after injury. All ankles were clinically stable, but palpable retrofibular popping occurred with active foot rotation. Peroneal tenograms were suggestive of peroneal tendon injury but were not specific enough to reveal the rupture. On exploration of the peroneal tendons, all patients had longitudinal tears measuring 1–3 cm; 5 involved the peroneal longus tendon and 3 involved the peroneal brevis tendon. All of the patients had excellent results during an average 7.9 years of follow-up.

Cadaveric Studies.—Fifteen cadaveric lower extremities were studied. With plantar flexion in the range of 15–25 degrees, tears of the tendon could occur as the peroneus longus impinged against the tip of the fibula and as the peroneus brevis impinged against the lateral wall of the peroneal groove or against the longus tendon.

Conclusion.—Longitudinal rupture of the peroneal tendon should be included in the differential diagnosis of persistent lateral ankle symptoms after a plantar flexion–inversion ankle sprain. The degree of plantar flexion may be the major determinant of the nature of injury, with the severity of the injury being determined by the magnitude of force.

▶ The surgical management of these patients is noteworthy. Each underwent exploration of the peroneal tendons under local anesthesia. With exposure of the superior peroneal retinaculum, the patient was then instructed to recreate the popping sensation by actively rotating the ankle. Subluxation of the tendons was not noted. The retinaculum was then incised and the tendons inspected. The peroneus longus was injured in 5 patients and the brevis in 3. Surgical treatment involved primary repair of the tendon defect. With an average follow-up of 7.9 years, all ankles were reported to have remained asymptomatic with the patients maintaining full athletic activity.—J.S. Torg, M.D.

Comparison of Inversion Restraint Provided by Ankle Prophylactic Devices Before and After Exercise

Martin N, Harter RA (Barry Univ, Miami Shores, Fla; Oregon State Univ, Corvallis)
J Athletic Train 28:324–329, 1993   139-94-5-13

Background.—Several recent studies have suggested that there are more effective ways of preventing ankle injuries than prophylactic ankle taping. Nevertheless, taping remains the most common form of prophylactic external ankle support in organized athletics. Three types of ankle prophylaxis for limiting inversion after dynamic loading—basketweave inversion ankle taping, a lace-up brace, and a semirigid orthosis—were compared.

Methods.—In the experiments, dynamic loads were imposed by repetitive walking at 4 mph and running at 9 mph on an 8.5-degree laterally tilted treadmill. In 4 separate sessions, 10 volunteers were videotaped while walking and running before and after 20 minutes of vigorous exercise. Biomechanical analysis of rearfoot motion was performed to determine the average maximum inversion angle for each form of ankle stabilization and for an unsupported control condition.

Results.—On comparison of the various ankle supports, significant differences in average maximum inversion angle were noted during both walking and running. There were also significant differences between the pre- and postexercise measurements at walking speed, between the semirigid orthosis and the control condition at both walking and running speed, and between the lace-up brace and the control condition at walking speed. Inversion restraint during dynamic loading was greatest with the semirigid orthosis, followed by the lace-up brace, ankle taping, and the control condition, in that order.

Conclusion.—Ankle taping cannot restrict inversion under dynamic loading conditions after a brief period of exercise. A semirigid orthosis is best at restricting inversion, although results are similar with a lace-up stabilizer. These findings do not support the continued use of closed basketweave ankle taping as a prophylactic measure in athletes.

▶ The authors state that the lace-up ankle stabilizer and the semirigid orthosis were similar in restricting inversion after exercise, and both were superior to taping. In my own experience involving patients with acute ankle sprains or athletes with unstable ankles who wish to participate, a combination of ankle taping with stirrups, figure eights, basketweave, and heel locks, along with a rigid orthosis, is the most effective means of preventing inversion sprains. I have not seen any studies on this combination of taping and bracing but have found it to be most effective.—F.J. George, A.T.C., P.T.

Syndesmosis Ankle Sprains: Diagnosing the Injury and Aiding Recovery
Taylor DC, Bassett FH III (Dwight David Eisenhower Army Med Ctr, Ft Gordon, Ga; Duke Univ, Durham, NC)
Physician Sportsmed 21:39–46, 1993   139-94-5–14

Background.—Syndesmosis ankle sprains are potentially disabling injuries that often appear benign on presentation. Diagnosis and treatment of this injury were discussed.

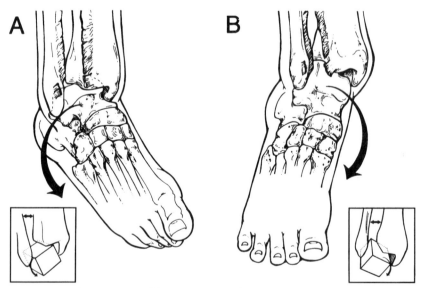

Fig 5–4.—Syndesmosis sprains of the ankle can result from either external (**A**) or internal (**B**) rotational forces. In either case, rotation of the cubelike talus (*inset*) forces a widening of the ankle mortise and damage to the syndesmosis ligaments. (Courtesy of Taylor DC, Bassett FH III: *Physician Sportsmed* 21:39–46, 1993.)

Mechanisms of Injury and Patient History.—External ankle rotation, a key finding in a patient's history, was long believed to be the mechanism of injury in syndesmosis ankle sprains. However, 1 team of researchers found that only 1 in 10 syndesmosis injuries was attributable to external rotation. Other possible mechanisms of injury include inversion and internal rotation, eversion and external rotation, and plantar flexion. Either internal or external rotation can cause the ankle mortise to widen (Fig 5–4). Patients must be asked about their ability to bear weight, as disruption of ankle mortise stability may prevent weight-bearing.

Diagnosis.—Commonly, a syndesmosis sprain appears benign with minimal swelling. The clinician should look for tenderness over the anterior inferior tibiofibular ligaments and tenderness extending proximally up the interosseous membrane. Less often, patients have tenderness over the posterior inferior tibiofibular ligament and transverse tibiofibular ligament. During a dorsiflexion maneuver, ankle range of motion typically is limited by pain. The squeeze test is also provocative. If the patient reports pain in the syndesmosis area when the clinician squeezes the fibula and tibia together at the midshaft, the test is positive. The external rotation stress test may also be useful. Gait examination can reveal difficulty in weight-bearing. In addition to these physical findings, imaging studies contribute to diagnosis.

Treatment.—Therapy is based on the grade of injury. Patients with grade 1 and 2 injuries should undergo aggressive functional rehabilitation. Patients with grade 3 injuries are referred to an orthopedic surgeon. Treatment of syndesmosis sprains often is frustrating because recovery time is prolonged.

Summary.—Syndesmosis ankle sprains are characterized by a rotational mechanism of injury, long recovery times, and often heterotopic ossification. Physical examination and imaging findings form the basis for diagnosis and injury grading. Treatments, based on the grade of the injury, include aggressive functional rehabilitation and surgical stabilization. If the ankle mortise is anatomically decreased and synostosis between the tibia and fibula is avoided, the long-term outcome can be good.

▶ This injury can be an athlete's and athletic trainer's nightmare. As the authors state, the initial symptoms and signs may often be benign, and the athlete is told he or she will probably be able to return to activity very soon, which is certainly not the case with this injury. Rehabilitation and return to activity are often prolonged and extended well beyond initial predictions.

All of the tests described by the authors should be done to make this very difficult diagnosis and to initiate proper treatment. We keep these injuries non–weight-bearing longer than usual and use a cuplike ankle brace to disperse the force when weight-bearing is allowed. Athletes, athletic trainers, and coaches must understand this is not a simple ankle sprain and return to activity may be delayed for a significant amount of time.—F.J. George, A.T.C., P.T.

Treatment of the Inversion Ankle Sprain: Comparison of Different Modes of Compression and Cryotherapy

Wilkerson GB, Horn-Kingery HM (Trover Clinic, Madisonville, Ky; 3rd Med Ctr/SGHY, Elmendorf AFB, Alaska)
J Orthop Sports Phys Ther 17:240–246, 1993   139-94-5-15

Background.—Inversion ankle sprain is a common injury in physically active people. Treatment has varied widely in the past, with relatively few studies addressing their comparative effectiveness. Recovery of function may be related to how well edema is controlled at the site of injury. The effects of 3 methods of application of cold and compression on recovery after an inversion sprain were compared.

Methods.—The study sample comprised 34 Air Force Academy cadets who had sustained a grade II inversion ankle sprain. Patients were assigned to 1 of 3 treatment methods, each incorporating an Air-Stirrup brace: uniform compression by elastic tape, focal compression with a U-shaped device, and focal compression with simultaneous cryotherapy. Function was assessed every day after injury using an 11-level, 100-point scale until a score of 90 was achieved.

Results.—No significant difference in time required to achieve 9 levels of function was noted in this small study sample. However, the 2 groups receiving focal compression appeared to achieve each level of function about 25% quicker than the group receiving uniform compression. The differences between the focal vs. uniform compression groups appeared to be greatest at the higher levels of function.

Conclusion.—These findings suggest that focal compression can result in quicker functional recovery than uniform compression in treatment of inversion ankle sprain. The use of a greater than usual frequency and duration of cryotherapy does not appear to confer any additional benefit.

▶ Athletic trainers have been using different types of focal compression and different types of adhesive and elastic tape for compression when treating acute inversion ankle sprains. It would take a very long study to incorporate all of the different methods that are used, and then I'm sure some would still be missed. It appears that the general concept of RICE (rest, ice, compression, and elevation) is a sound practice to follow. Whichever procedure is followed, comfort and ease of application for the injured athlete must certainly be considered.—F.J. George, A.T.C., P.T.

Development of Lower Leg Strength and Flexibility With the Strength Shoe

Cook SD, Schultz G, Omey ML, Wolfe MW, Brunet MF (Tulane Univ, New Orleans, La)
Am J Sports Med 21:445–448, 1993   139-94-5-16

Introduction.—The Strength Shoe is a modified athletic shoe designed to prevent the heel from striking the ground during exercise. A 4-cm thick rubber platform attached to the front half of the sole is said to increase the work done by the triceps surae muscle, intensifying training. In a prospective, randomized trial, the efficacy and safety of the Strength Shoe training regimen were tested.

Subjects and Methods.—The study participants were 12 intercollegiate track-and-field athletes who followed the regimen suggested by the manufacturers of the Strength Shoe for 8 weeks. Six of the athletes wore the Strength Shoe during workouts and 6 wore their usual training shoes. All participants continued with their usual training program as well; none had leg pain at the start of the study. Data on physical performance, strength, range of motion, and calf circumference were collected at baseline and at the end of the 8-week program by an observer who was blind to the shoe assignment.

Results.—Athletes who wore the Strength Shoe had no improvements in flexibility, strength, or performance on completion of the study. Neither group had a significant increase in calf circumference. Changes in range of motion, plantar flexion torque at 30 degrees/sec and 180 degrees/sec, and in dorsiflexion torque at both speeds were negligible or not significantly different between the 2 groups. There was a slight but nonsignificant advantage for wearers of the Strength Shoe in 40-yd dash and vertical leap performance. Four athletes who wore the Strength Shoe complained of shin splints and 1 had to leave the study because of severe anterior tibial pain.

Conclusion.—The Strength Shoe program is based on the controversial concept of plyometrics. According to proponents, exercising by rapid concentric contraction after a "prestretching" eccentric contraction develops a significantly greater amount of elastic energy in the activated muscle. Although the use of plyometrics may prove valuable in some settings, the Strength Shoe regimen offered no training benefit and was associated with increased anterior tibial pain.

▶ I agree with the authors' statement that "the Strength Shoe was found to provide no training benefit and was associated with increased anterior tibial pain. It may compound the risk of injury associated with plyometrics especially for the poorly conditioned athlete. Use of the Strength Shoe cannot be recommended as a safe, effective training method for development of lower leg strength and flexibility." I have treated severe Achilles tendon problems in 2 athletes who used these shoes for training. We recommend that our athletes not wear these shoes for training.—F.J. George, A.T.C., P.T.

Surgical Treatment of Freiberg's Infraction in Athletes

Sproul J, Klaaren H, Mannarino F (Wright State Univ, Dayton, Ohio)
Am J Sports Med 21:381–384, 1993   139-94-5–17

Background.—Freiberg's infraction has been well described, but its etiology remains uncertain. Nonoperative treatment including activity restriction, casting, the use of orthoses with metatarsal pads, and stiff-soled shoes may be effective in the early stages of the disease. Surgical treatment may include joint débridement, synovectomy, removal of loose bodies, metatarsal head resection, articular cartilage elevation and grafting, and metatarsal osteotomy. Experience with Freiberg's infraction was reviewed.

Patients.—The study population consisted of 8 female patients and 2 male patients (average age, 26.5 years) who underwent operation on 11 feet in the treatment of Freiberg's infraction. All patients were active athletically, and pain at the affected metatarsal head was limiting their sports activities. Two patients with 3 lesions recalled a specific trauma; 7 patients first experienced pain during sports-related running, and 1 patient reported the onset of symptoms with normal walking. Conservative treatment had failed in 8 patients. All operations were performed in an outpatient setting. Nine patients underwent metatarsophalangeal joint débridement and 1 had a metatarsal head resection. Follow-up ranged from 6 to 108 months.

Results.—After operation, 6 patients (7 feet) had no pain or restriction of activities, 1 patient had pain on prolonged standing, and 2 patients had occasional aching. All patients were able to return to their earlier level of sports participation. Follow-up radiographs showed no evidence of joint space narrowing or major arthritic changes. None of the patients regretted having had the operation.

Conclusion.—Early-stage Freiberg's infraction may be amenable to nonoperative treatment in some patients, but early operative treatment in selected patients with higher grade lesions may be more effective.

▶ The authors report consistent surgical findings of articular surface softening and irregularity with loosening of the dorsal 30% to 50% of the articular surface. Importantly, the volar articular surface was intact. Surgery consisted of partial resection of the dorsal half of the metatarsal head with removal of loose bodies, partial synovectomy, and removal of loose articular surface. The average follow-up of 39 months (range, 6–108 months) is noteworthy.—J.S. Torg, M.D.

Stress Fracture of the Proximal Phalanx of the Great Toe

Shiraishi M, Mizuta H, Kubota K, Sakuma K, Takagi K (Kumamoto Univ, Japan)
Foot Ankle 14:28–34, 1993   139-94-5–18

Purpose.—Although stress fractures of the metatarsal bones are common, they are rare in the proximal phalanx of the great toe. Three such cases in adolescents were discussed.

Case Report.—Girl, 12 years, was seen with pain in her right first metatarsophalangeal (MTP) joint. She was a volleyball player and had been training 2 hours per day, 6 or 7 days per week. She had mild swelling and pain with motion in the midportion of the joint, with tenderness at the center of the basal portion of the proximal phalanx of the great toe. She had no abnormalities of alignment.

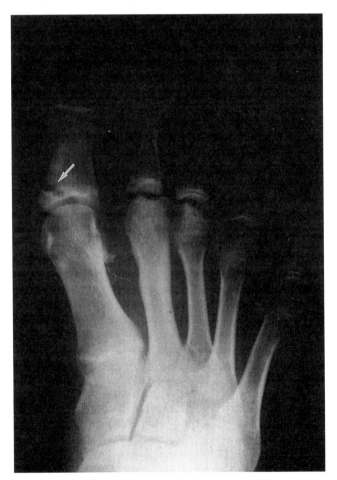

Fig 5–5.—In the radiograph taken at the initial examination of a 17-year-old female distance runner, an oblique fissure (*arrow*) was found in the medial side of the basal portion of the proximal phalanx. (Courtesy of Shiraishi M, Mizuta H, Kubota K, et al: *Foot Ankle* 14:28–34, 1993.)

Radiographic examination showed a longitudinal fissure in contact with the center of the epiphyseal line at the basal portion of the proximal phalanx. Training was stopped for 1 month, after which the radiographic fissure resolved nearly completely and the symptoms disappeared. The diagnosis of stress fracture of the proximal phalanx of the right great toe was made at this time. After shoes with shock-absorbent soles were prescribed, the patient was able to resume her previous level of training. The other 2 patients described in this study were a 17-year-old distance runner (Fig 5-5) and a 12-year-old soccer player.

Discussion.—Stress fracture of the proximal phalanx of the great toe may develop after repeated, forced dorsiflexion of the first MTP joint with changing steps. This diagnosis should be considered for athletes who engage in repeated running and jumping with pain of the first MTP joint and no history of trauma. Treatment is complete discontinuation of training.

▶ Stress fracture of the proximal phalanx of the great toe has rarely been reported in the literature (1, 2). However, it appears that this condition joins turf-toe, sesamoid disorders, medial plantar digital proper nerve syndrome, and hallux valgus in the differential of causes of pain in the first MTP joints in the athlete.—J.S. Torg, M.D.

References

1. Hulkko A, Orava S: *Int J Sports Med* 8:221, 1987.
2. Yokoe K, Mannoji T: *Am J Sports Med* 14:240, 1986.

Diastasis of Bipartite Sesamoids of the First Metatarsophalangeal Joint
Rodeo SA, Warren RF, O'Brien SJ, Pavlov H, Barnes R, Hanks GA (Hosp for Special Surgery, New York; New York Giants Football Team, Meadowlands, NJ; Camp Hill, Pa)
Foot Ankle 14:425–434, 1993   139-94-5-19

Background.—"Turf-toe," a traumatic injury of the capsule of the first metatarsophalangeal (MTP) joint, is common in football players and usually results from a hyperextension injury on artificial turf. Four cases of first MTP plantar capsular injury that involved bipartite or tripartite sesamoid bones and simulated the mechanism of injury and clinical findings of turf-toe were reviewed.

Patients.—The injuries occurred in 3 patients, 2 professional football players and 1 collegiate player. All patients sustained first MTP plantar capsular injury, with diastasis of a bipartite sesamoid (Fig 5-6). Three cases initially were managed with observation and protection of the joint, which resulted in progressive widening of the sesamoid fragments with associated pain and disability. Eventually they required resection of the distal fragment and repair of the plantar capsule. The remaining pa-

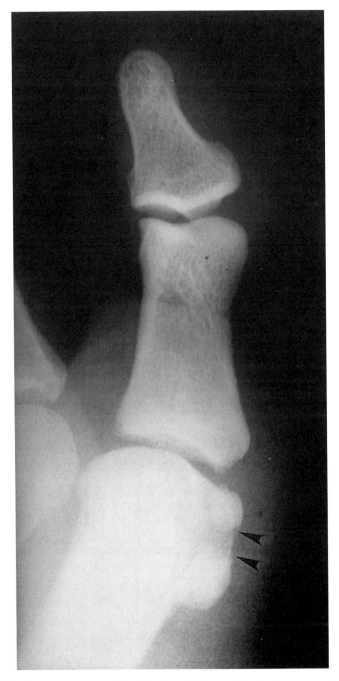

Fig 5–6.—Roentgenogram revealed a bipartite medial sesamoid with 3-mm separation between components, with no evidence of acute sesamoid fracture. (Courtesy of Rodeo SA, Warren RF, O'Brien SJ, et al: *Foot Ankle* 14:425–434, 1993.)

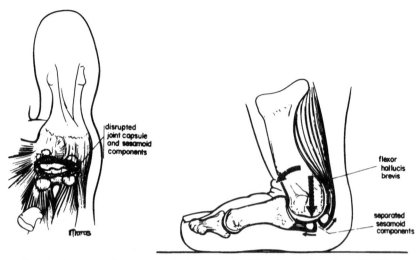

Fig 5–7.—Illustrations demonstrating the hyperextension injury causing disruption of the joint capsule and the resulting separation of the sesamoid components. (Courtesy of Rodeo SA, Warren RF, O'Brien SJ, et al: *Foot Ankle* 14:425-434, 1993.)

tient had acute repair of the medial retinaculum and capsule. All patients were able to return to full football participation.

Discussion.—Injuries of the sesamoid complex of the first MTP joint have not previously been included in reports of turf-toe. The finding of diastasis of the partite sesamoid supplies objective evidence of disruption of the plantar capsular mechanism (Fig 5-7). Stress radiographs can confirm this injury, which can be managed by acute retinacular repair if painful. It is believed that the term turf-toe should be reserved for hyperextension injuries to the first MTP joint in which there is disruption of the volar capsule proximal to the sesamoid.

▶ This article points out that there are few reports of traumatic injuries to the first MTP joint sesamoids in the literature. The differential diagnosis of sesamoid injuries reported in the athlete include stress fracture, acute sesamoid fracture, sesamoiditis, osteochondritis, chondromalacia of the sesamoid articulating surface, and flexor hallucis brevis tendinitis. As indicated, a diagnosis of diastasis of a bipartite sesamoid can be established by a dorsiflexion stress radiograph—J.S. Torg, M.D.

Second Metatarsophalangeal Joint Instability in the Athlete
Coughlin MJ (St Alphonsus Regional Med Ctr, Boise, Idaho)
Foot Ankle 14:309–319, 1993   139-94-5-20

Objective.—Nine athletes with second metatarsophalangeal (MTP) joint instability were studied. Areas of interest were the demographics

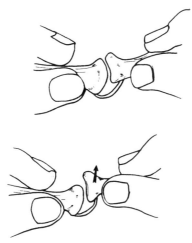

Fig 5–8.—Drawer sign used to diagnose instability of the second MTP joint. The proximal phalanx is grasped between the thumb and forefinger (*top*). With dorsal stress, plantar pain is elicited with MTP instability (*bottom*). (Courtesy of Coughlin MJ: *Foot Ankle* 14:309–319, 1993.)

associated with second MTP instability, the results of conservative and surgical treatment, and the value of a positive drawer sign as a predictive factor in the preoperative examination.

Patients and Methods.—Second MTP joint instability was bilateral in 2 patients. Seven toes underwent surgical reconstruction, and 4 were treated nonsurgically. The initial evaluation consisted of a physical examination, weight-bearing anteroposterior and lateral radiographs, and a drawer test (Fig 5–8). Patients were questioned regarding onset of pain, length of symptoms, and type and level of athletic activity. Surgery was recommended for patients with deformity or unrelenting pain. Conservative treatment consisted of a period of taping. Surgical patients were followed for an average of 20.4 months and nonsurgical patients for an average of 15 months.

Results.—The average duration of symptoms was 11 months. All patients reported an insidious onset of pain, at first isolated to the plantar aspect of the second MTP joint. Two patients had previously undergone a total of 5 forefoot surgeries. All had taken part in athletic activities at a high level and were prevented from participation by intractable metatarsalgia. Ten of 10 toes tested had a positive drawer sign. Radiographic examination revealed all second metatarsals to be excessively long in comparison to adjacent metatarsals. Three of the 4 toes treated nonsurgically had a good result. In the fourth case, the second MTP joint eventually dislocated, and the patient had a severe fixed hammertoe deformity develop. Two of the surgical patients rated their results as excellent, 3 as good, 1 as fair, and 1 as poor. Those with good results had mild pain with sports activity. The patient with a poor result had undergone several other forefoot operations and eventually had to have the second toe amputated.

Conclusion.—The single most useful clinical procedure in the initial evaluation of patients with suspected second MTP joint instability is the drawer test. A common finding was excess length of the second metatarsal compared with the first and third metatarsals. Early diagnosis and intervention may prevent progression to deformity and dislocation, but many patients may have to decrease their level of athletic activity.

▶ This is an interesting paper that is both well illustrated and well documented. What the authors have described as a "drawer sign" would more accurately be termed a second MTP joint Lachman's test.—J.S. Torg, M.D.

Overuse Ballet Injury of the Base of the Second Metatarsal: A Diagnostic Problem

Harrington T, Crichton KJ, Anderson IF (Royal North Shore Hosp, St Leonards, Australia; North Sydney Orthopaedic & Sports Medicine Centre, Crows Nest, Australia; Sports X-Ray Orthopaedic & Sports Medicine Radiology, Crows Nest, Sydney, Australia)
Am J Sports Med 21:591–598, 1993   139-94-5–21

Background.—Pain over the second metatarsal joint in ballerinas may be an indication of traumatic synovitis of the second tarsometatarsal joint or a stress fracture at the base of the second metatarsal. A prompt diagnosis is important because each condition requires a different course of treatment. Eight ballerinas were treated for pain over the second metatarsal joint.

Patients.—Eight ballerinas between 15 and 24 years of age complained of pain in the midfoot region that was worse en pointe and with jumps. Each dancer had a clinical examination, plain radiography, bone scanning, and MRI. All problems were unilateral.

Results.—Clinical examination, radiography, and scintigraphy did not differentiate bone stress from traumatic synovitis. A bone stress reaction at the base of the second metatarsal was demonstrated on MRI scans of 6 dancers (Fig 5–9), and a fracture line could be identified on 4 examinations. The other 2 dancers had normal MRI scans, and a diagnosis of traumatic synovitis was made by exclusion. Dancers with stress reactions were advised to rest and gradually return to dancing. Three ballerinas followed this advice and were symptom-free after 6–8 weeks of rest, and 3 dancers continued to dance against their physician's advice. The 2 dancers with traumatic synovitis were treated with nonsteroidal anti-inflammatory drugs and passive mobilization and were allowed to continue dancing; both became symptom-free within 6 weeks.

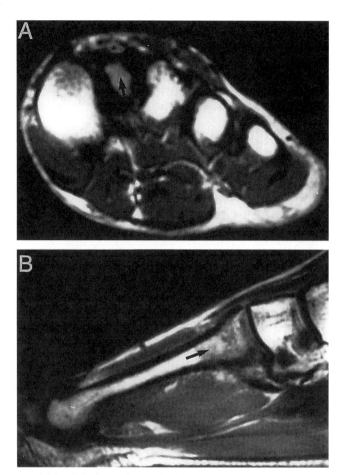

Fig 5–9.—Axial (**A**) and tilted sagittal T₁-weighted (**B**) MR images of a patient with marked decrease in bone marrow signal in the base of the second metatarsal (*arrows*), but with no visible fracture line. This area normally has identical marrow signal intensity to that in the adjacent metatarsals. The findings here are believed to represent bone stress or trabecular microfracture. (Courtesy of Harrington T, Crichton KJ, Anderson IF: *Am J Sports Med* 21:591–598, 1993.)

Conclusion.—The prompt differential diagnosis of pain and tenderness over the second metatarsal joint in ballet dancers shortens the course of treatment.

▶ The cost-effectiveness of an MRI to establish the diagnosis of a stress fracture at the base of the second metatarsal must be questioned.—J.S. Torg, M.D.

Tarsometatarsal Joint Injuries in the Athlete

Curtis MJ, Myerson M, Szura B (Union Mem Hosp, Baltimore, Md)
Am J Sports Med 21:497–502, 1993   139-94-5–22

Purpose.—A retrospective evaluation of the results of treatment of 19 consecutive patients who sustained athletic injuries to the tarsometatarsal (TMT) joint of the foot was provided.

Subjects.—The participants were 14 males and 5 females with a mean age of 25.5 years. Six patients were injured while playing basketball; 5 while running; 4 while sailboarding (Fig 5–10), and 4 during cricket, soccer, or gymnastics. The injuries resulted from a combined forced plantar flexion and rotation. Diagnosis was made on the basis of history and physical and radiographic foot examination. Tenderness across the foot was made worse by passive joint stress in plantar flexion or dorsiflexion, and by passive pronation and simultaneous abduction of the forefoot with the hindfoot held still by the examiner (Fig 5–11). Plain radiographs were examined for diastasis at the TMT joint or between the bases of the first and second metatarsals (Fig 5–12). Fluoroscopy was conducted to search for instability on stressing the articulation. There were first- and second-degree sprains in 9 patients, third-degree sprains in 3, avulsion fractures in 4, and type B2 lateral dislocation in 3 patients. Three

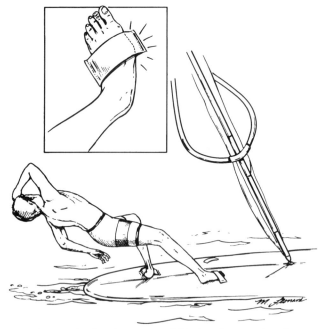

Fig 5–10.—Mechanism of sailboarding injury—a fall backward, causing forced equinus of the fixed forefoot. (Courtesy of Curtis MJ, Myerson M, Szura B: *Am J Sports Med* 21:497–502, 1993.)

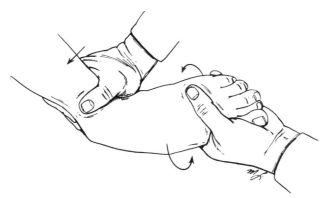

Fig 5–11.—The passive pronation and abduction test for injury at the tarsometatarsal joint. (Courtesy of Curtis MJ, Myerson M, Szura B: *Am J Sports Med* 21:497–502, 1993.)

patients were examined after more than 2 weeks had elapsed since the injury. Treatment was non–weight-bearing without immobilization in 2 patients, immobilization in a short leg cast in 9, and open reduction and internal fixation in 5 patients.

Results.—Patients were assessed clinically, functionally, and radiographically at a mean follow-up of 25 months. Three patients were unable to return to sports. Two of these 3 patients required orthoses to alleviate pain, and the other underwent arthrodesis of the TMT joint. The remaining patients returned to sports with a mean lag time of 4.1 months. Among the 9 patients with first- and second-degree sprains, 5 had an excellent result, 2 had a good result, and 2 had a fair result. There was no relation between method of treatment and results. Among the 7 patients with fractures or dislocations, 4 had excellent, 2 had fair and 1 had good results. The best results were achieved with open reduction and internal fixation.

Conclusion.—Injury to the TMT joint can occur during sports and can be associated with severe morbidity. Injuries should be analyzed by fluoroscopy for stability. Only stable injuries should be treated nonoperatively. Fracture dislocations, unstable fractures, and third-degree sprains could not reliably be treated nonoperatively but required open reduction and internal fixation for optimal functional return.

▶ This is an excellent paper that calls attention to the potentially devastating effects that injury to the TMT joint can have on the athlete. The recommendation that only stable injuries should be treated nonoperatively is sound. Also, "Third-degree sprains were indistinguishable from unstable fractures and fracture-dislocations in that good results were not reliably obtained by nonoperative treatment, and both classes of injuries seem to require open reduction and internal fixation for optimal return to function." The authors point out that anatomical reduction requires internal fixation, their prefer-

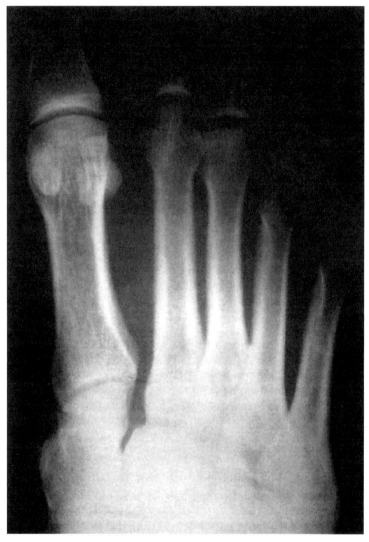

Fig 5–12.—Radiograph demonstrating diastasis of the second, third, and fourth metatarsal bases at the Lisfranc joint. (Courtesy of Curtis MJ, Myerson M, Szura B: *Am J Sports Med* 21:497–502, 1993.)

ence being a transarticular 3.5-mm AO cortical screw with fixation placed as a lag screw to maintain an anatomical reduction of the diastasis without compression of the articular surfaces.—J.S. Torg, M.D.

Stress Fractures of the Tarsal Navicular Bone: CT Findings in 55 Cases

Kiss ZS, Khan KM, Fuller PJ (Mercy Private Hosp, East Melbourne, Victoria, Australia; Olympic Park Sports Medicine Centre, Melbourne, Victoria, Australia; Sports Medicine Centres of Victoria, Ashwood, Australia)
AJR 160:111–115, 1993   139-94-5-23

Background.—Stress fracture of the tarsal navicular bone in athletes is an uncommon injury that is increasingly being diagnosed with the use of CT. However, there have been no reviews of the CT appearance of this injury in the radiology literature. The clinical and radiologic findings of 86 radiologically confirmed navicular stress fractures diagnosed at 5 Australian sports medicine clinics during 10 years were presented.

Patients.—The patients were 30 men and 24 women (mean age, 21 years) participating in a variety of sports at levels ranging from recreational to professional. Pain was a presenting symptom in all patients. Computed tomography scans of both feet were obtained for comparative purposes. All scans were reviewed for position, appearance, and extent of the fracture, which was measured on axial and coronal scans.

Findings.—The fractures, 53 of which were partial and 2 complete, involved the central one third of the proximal dorsal articular margin of the navicular. Of the partial fractures, 43 were linear (Figs 5–13 and 5–14), 5 were linear with a bone fragment, and 5 had rim defects with associated ossicles. All fractures were detectable in both planes, and two thirds measured the same distance in both. About half of the fractures measured between 10% and 50% the height of the bone. Follow-up scans showed dorsal cortical bridging in 3 of 8 fractures at 6 weeks and

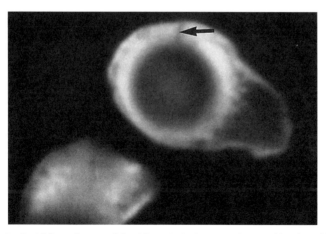

Fig 5–13.—Partial linear fracture of the right navicular bone in a 21-year-old male middle-distance runner who had signs and symptoms for 2 months. Axial CT scan shows a 3-mm sagittal fracture (*arrow*) of the middle one third of the proximal dorsal articular margin of bone. (Courtesy of Kiss ZS, Khan KM, Fuller PJ: *AJR* 160:111–115, 1993.)

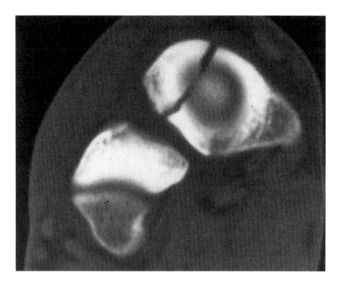

Fig 5–14.—Complete fracture of the right navicular bone in a 22-year-old female sprinter who had signs and symptoms for 6 weeks. Axial CT scan angled to the plane of the talonavicular joint shows a complete, undisplaced fracture curving slightly laterally from the middle one third of the dorsum of bone. In this plane, the normal proximal articular rim of navicular bone appears as a sclerotic ring. (Courtesy of Kiss ZS, Khan KM, Fuller PJ: *AJR* 160:111–115, 1993.)

firm cortical union in 32% of fractures at 4 months. There were 12 cases of nonunion, which demonstrated a persistent fracture gap and lack of cortical healing, Medullary cysts and cortical notching sometimes persisted after the fracture was completely healed (Fig 5–15).

Conclusion.—The CT appearance of stress fracture of the tarsal navicular bone was described. Computed tomography is useful for both diagnosis and follow-up of these injuries, although small fractures may be

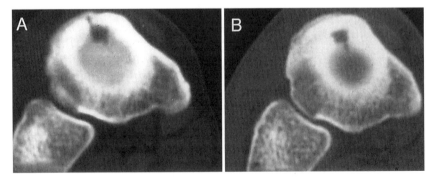

Fig 5–15.—Stages in healing of a partial fracture of the right navicular bone in a 23-year-old female sprinter. **A,** axial CT scan obtained 6 weeks after the foot was immobilized with a non–weight-bearing cast shows cortical bridging with a 5-mm residual cyst. **B,** axial CT scan obtained 13 months after **A** shows dense cortical healing with a persistent cyst and small cleft. The patient was asymptomatic at this time. (Courtesy of Kiss ZS, Khan KM, Fuller PJ: *AJR* 160:111–115, 1993.)

missed if the radiologist is unfamiliar with their appearance. The proximal articular surface of the navicular bone must be included in the scan, and appropriately high window and level settings must be used.

▶ The importance of positioning the foot correctly to demonstrate a tarsal navicular stress fracture on CT is appropriately emphasized. This point also is applicable to the MR examination. These fractures are symptomatic while they are partial and confined to the extreme proximal dorsal aspect of the navicular, and they can be missed, despite expensive imaging techniques, if the examination is not properly performed.—J.S. Torg, M.D.

Outpatient Percutaneous Screw Fixation of the Acute Jones Fracture
Mindrebo N, Shelbourne KD, Van Meter CD, Rettig AC (Methodist Sports Medicine Ctr, Indianapolis, Ind)
Am J Sports Med 21:720–723, 1993   139-94-5-24

Background.—The Jones fracture is a transverse fracture of the base of the fifth metatarsal occurring within 1.5 cm of the tuberosity. It usually occurs from indirect trauma during athletic activity, especially basketball and football. Treatment is usually cast immobilization, a non–weight-bearing period with crutches for a minimum of 6–8 weeks, and foot immobilization for up to 12 weeks. These time restraints are especially difficult for in-season or preseason athletes. Outpatient percutaneous screw fixation of acute Jones fractures has been recommended to minimize immobilization and non–weight-bearing time. The results of using outpatient treatment of acute Jones fractures in 9 varsity athletes were reviewed.

Outpatient Treatment.—Eight male athletes and 1 female athlete ranging in age from 17 to 22 years were treated for Jones fractures. All underwent outpatient percutaneous intramedullary screw fixation an average of 8 days after injury. Seven to 10 days after surgery, the patients began weight-bearing as tolerated with a CAM walker. Stationary bicycling, swimming, and use of the Stairmaster were allowed at 2–3 weeks. The athletes returned to running at an average of 5.5 weeks and to full competition at an average of 8.5 weeks. All fractures achieved clinical and radiographic union with no refracture or screw breakage.

Conclusion.—Outpatient percutaneous intramedullary screw fixation of acute Jones fractures had a high success rate and low morbidity. The 9 patients achieved solid union of the fracture with no refracture or screw breakage during an average follow-up of 2.5 years. The early weight-bearing at 7–10 days after surgery and short immobilization possible with this technique make it especially useful for in-season or preseason athletes. All patients studied had predictable healing and returned to full sports participation within 12 weeks.

▶ The authors' justification for percutaneous screw fixation of the acute Jones fracture is the apparent result of either their not having read or their not having understood our paper dealing with nonoperative management of this problem (1). Specifically, they erroneously state that using our recommended treatment for the acute Jones fracture—cast immobilization and non–weight-bearing with crutches—"Torg et al. achieved high healing rates (93%) in acute injuries. Some patients returned to full activities by 12 months after injury; others required a longer period." What we had reported was that of 15 acute fractures treated with non–weight-bearing, 14 healed in a mean of 7 weeks. It is interesting to note that in the Mindrebo series, "radiographic evidence of union was present at 6 weeks" and that they returned to full sports participation within 12 weeks. For this we need surgery?—J.S. Torg, M.D.

Reference

1.   Torg JS, et al: *J Bone Joint Surg (Am)* 66-A:209, 1984.

Plantar Fasciitis
DeMaio M, Paine R, Mangine RE, Drez D Jr (United States Navy, Oakland, Calif; Rehabilitation Services of Houston; Kentucky Rehabilitation Services, Ft Mitchell; et al)
Orthopedics 16:1153–1163, 1993   139-94-5-25

Epidemiology.—Plantar fasciitis may occur as a primary disorder or as a "final common pathway" caused by some other disorders. Among athletes, it is most frequent in sports involving running, in which about 10% of participants may be affected. Dancers, tennis players, and basketball players frequently have plantar fasciitis develop, as do individuals whose work entails prolonged weight-bearing. Fasciitis reportedly is more frequent in males, but this may reflect the types of work done or sports played. Most patients are older than age 40 years.

Pathomechanics.—The plantar fascia acts as a truss linking the tarsal bones with the ligaments of the foot. Increasing tension causes the fascia to stiffen. Weakness of the plantar flexors increases the load on both the muscles and the plantar fascia. A pronated subtalar joint everts the calcaneus and lengthens the plantar fascia, increasing its tension. Overloading is the most common injury pattern leading to plantar fasciitis; in the general population, it is most often secondary to excessive pronation or being overweight. In runners, excessive pronation and training errors are common findings. Chronic plantar fasciitis is characterized by microtears in the fascia near or at its insertion. Partial ruptures also are seen. Biopsy

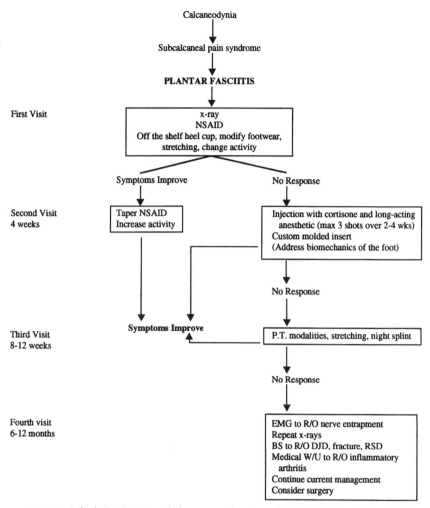

Fig 5–16.—Individualized treatment before surgery. (Courtesy of DeMaio M, Paine R, Mangine RE, et al: *Orthopedics* 16:1153-1163, 1993.)

specimens show changes consistent with fatigue failure, inadequate healing, and chronic inflammation.

Diagnosis.—Pain occurs at the medial aspect of the calcaneus and may radiate to the medial malleolus or even the sole. Often pain is noted in the morning. It typically occurs under the heel, especially medially, and is of gradual onset with no history of trauma. Bone spurs may be seen, but are not thought to cause plantar fasciitis. It is important to exclude systemic disorders (e.g., arthritis and sarcoidosis) as well as nerve entrapment syndromes.

Management.—An approach to treating plantar fasciitis is shown in Figure 5–16. Ice and electric muscle stimulation can relieve pain and inflammation, and nonsteroidal drugs may be helpful. Orthotics and shoe modification have proven to be effective measures. Runners should train on a relatively soft surface. In some patients, total rest is mandatory. Weight reduction may be indicated. Stretching of the Achilles tendon and plantar fascia may help restore normal foot mechanics. Other measures that may be helpful are steroid injections, ice massage, and use of a night splint. Surgery is considered only when all conservative measures have failed.

▶ This article is a comprehensive review of the subject. The authors point out that a surgical release of the plantar fascia is only rarely indicated. Reviewed are the numerous procedures described. Specifically, they include a limited release, a wide release of the Steindler type, and a wide release combined with release of the nerve to the abductor digiti quinti and excision of the heel spur. The authors also mention that stripping of the plantar fascia and the superficial plantar muscles from the calcaneus may destabilize the windlass mechanism in the supple pronated foot.—J.S. Torg, M.D.

Haglund's Disease in Athletes
Ghiggio P, Nobile G, Bronzo P (Ospedale Civile, Ivrea, Italy)
J Sports Traumatol 15:89–96, 1993   139-94-5-26

Background.—Heel pain is a frequent complaint in athletes. In young female athletes, particularly basketball players, volleyball players, and long-distance road runners, the cause of pain may be Haglund's disease. The effectiveness of surgery in treating this disorder was examined.

Method.—Eleven women aged between 17 and 24 years, who were competitively engaged in basketball, volleyball, and running participated in the study. All had posterior talalgia caused by Haglund's disease that had not responded to conventional treatments. The women underwent surgery involving bursectomy and resection of the superoposterior portion of the calcaneus. Care was taken to ensure that resection extended to the whole of the projecting calcaneal area, as far as the insertion of the Achilles tendon. This method of resection has been shown to avoid recurrence. All patients were followed up for 18 months.

Results.—Nine of the 11 women returned to competitive sport within 3–5 months of surgery. One patient had scar hyperplasia after 7 months, and another demonstrated calcification in the retroachillean recess. Postsurgical treatment included the usual medication, along with applications of cortisone and keratolytic agents. Ultrasound therapy and massage were used in 7 patients. On their return to sports, patients were encouraged to wear shoes with a soft back and a counter whose height would not lead to local rubbing.

Conclusion.—Haglund's disease is relatively common among young female volleyball and basketball players and long-distance runners. Generic pictures of achillodynia should, therefore, be carefully assessed in these athletes. The relationship between the calcaneus and the Achilles tendon should be determined, particularly when bursitis is present, through radiographic evaluation of departures from the normal angles. It is thought that chronic mechanical irritation causing friction between the tendon and the superoposterior surface of the calcaneus is the origin of Haglund's disease. In cases that cannot be resolved by conservative treatment, surgery is an alternative that must be carried out with close attention to the lines of calcaneal resection that run from the most anterior corner of the bursal process to the insertion of the Achilles tendon.

▶ I would describe the occurrence of Haglund's disease as rare, rather than "not uncommon." A reliable method of determining the presence of the problem as manifested by an excessive bursal projection is to determine Pavlov's pitch lines (1). The relatively protracted postoperative course of 3–5 months before return to competitive activities is noteworthy and is in keeping with my own experience.—J.S. Torg, M.D.

Reference

1. Pavlov H, et al: *Radiology* 144:83, 1992.

6 Biomechanics, Warm-Up, Strength, and Flexibility Training

Sport Biomechanics 2000
Zatsiorsky VM, Fortney VL (Pennsylvania State Univ, University Park)
J Sports Sci 11:279–283, 1993   139-94-6–1

Purpose.—Although predicting future developments in the sciences is at best an uncertain proposition, it is still useful to attempt such prognostication. The state of the art in sport biomechanics is forecast for the turn of the century in this report.

Methods and Equipment.—One important advance will be the availability of inexpensive, high-resolution video cameras designed specifically for use in measurement. These cameras will largely replace high-speed cinematography. Force-measuring equipment and telemetric electromyography systems will be affordable for smaller laboratories, and noninvasive methods for assessing the internal forces acting in the body will become available. Ultrasound and other nonoptical techniques will be used for registration of human movement, and portable devices to measure the biomechanics of sport will become available. Advanced digitization techniques will aid in the analysis of video data.

In research, there will be a shift toward the use of statistical methods, although their validity in the field of sport biomechanics will have to be defined. Research will use mathematical methods combining functional and stochastic approaches. New methods of analyzing nonrandom biomechanical curves—especially the methods of time and amplitude transformation—will also be developed. Software for biomechanical research will become more advanced and less expensive.

Research Directions.—An interdisciplinary research focus is predicted in such fields as motor control, muscle physiology, and morphology. More studies will combine biomechanical and motor control approaches and address muscle activity of the body from a biomechanical perspective. Models will be evaluated for studying the response of the body to vibration and impact, and fundamental studies in "statistical biomechanics" will emerge. Important areas for applied research will include the biomechanical basis of sports equipment, injury prevention, the biomechanical basis of conditioning and motor learning, and exercise machines. Biomechanical information from diverse sources will become more accessible in the form of review papers and/or monographs.

Discussion.—Some predictions were made for the near future of sport biomechanics. The time until the year 2000 is short and the authors are not sure that all of their predictions will become reality by that time.

▶ I include this paper for the benefit of anyone who wants to consider playing futurist along with these authors from 2 very prestigious research institutions (Pennsylvania State University and the Central Institute of Physical Culture in Moscow). These authors, together with their reviewers, realize that this is a very ambitious agenda to complete within 6 years and that all of the items in their paper probably will not be attained by the year 2000. However, the role of a futurist is to prepare us, which they have attempted to do.—Col. J.L. Anderson, PE.D.

The Relationships Between Isokinetic Peak Torque and Cross-Sectional Area of the Forearm Flexors and Extensors
Housh DJ, Housh TJ, Johnson GO, Chu W-K (Univ of Nebraska, Lincoln)
Isokinetics Exerc Sci 3:133–138, 1993   139-94-6–2

Background.—Most studies on the association between strength and muscle cross-sectional area (CSA) have been performed on the leg extensor muscles using anthropometry, CT scanning, or ultrasound. The results have shown great interindividual variability in strength per unit of muscle CSA. This variability may be partly attributed to the function of the muscle or muscle group involved, the type of strength testing used, or the technique used to estimate muscle CSA. Recently, MRI has been recommended over other techniques for determining muscle CSA. Magnetic resonance imaging was used to examine the relationships between the CSA of the flexors and extensors of the forearm and isokinetic peak torque at speeds of contraction from 0–300 degrees/sec.

Method.—Ten male volunteers underwent strength testing with the use of a calibrated Cybex II isokinetic dynamometer. Each performed 1 set of 3 maximal effort repetitions of flexion and extension of the dominant forearm at 0, 60, 120, 180, 240, and 300 degrees/sec. Magnetic resonance imaging was used to determine the CSA of the extensor and flexor muscles.

Results.—For the forearm flexors, there were significant correlations between muscle CSA and peak torque at 0, 60, and 120 degrees/sec. The relationships at slow, but not at faster, speeds of contraction may be related to the contributions of slow- and fast-twitch fibers to force production at various speeds of contraction. There were no significant correlations between muscle CSA and isokinetic peak torque at any speed of contraction for the forearm extensors.

Conclusion.—The only significant correlation between isokinetic peak torque and muscle CSA for the forearm flexors was at 0, 60, and 120 degrees/sec. There were no significant correlations between muscle CSA and isokinetic peak torque at any speed of contraction for the forearm extensors. These results were probably influenced by the contribution of primarily fast-twitch fibers to peak torque at fast speeds of contraction and the differences between the parallel fiber orientation of the forearm flexor muscles vs. the pennate fiber orientation of the extensor muscles.

▶ This study is an example of how improvement in accuracy of measurement may cause us to question some of the theories of the past that were formed through research methods using inaccurate measurements. For example, with MRI, these researchers were able to more accurately measure the muscle CSA. However, the true relationship between muscle CSA and strength is not settled because of questions still to be answered concerning the relative contributions of fast-twitch and slow-twitch muscle fibers, and the differences in the muscle architecture. I can remember that not too many years ago many of us were ready to accept as a truism that greater muscle CSA automatically meant greater strength. Would it have been helpful if these researchers had also considered the angle of peak torque at each of the testing speeds? See the study by Bemben and Johnson (Abstract 139-94-6–3) also included in this YEAR BOOK.—Col. J.L. Anderson, PE.D.

Reliability of the Biodex B-2000 Isokinetic Dynamometer and the Evaluation of a Sport-Specific Determination for the Angle of Peak Torque During Knee Extension

Bemben MG, Johnson DA (Univ of Oklahoma, Norman; Health and Fitness Inst, Concord, Calif)
Isokinetics Exerc Sci 3:164–168, 1993   139-94-6–3

Background.—Although some isokinetic dynamometers are in current use, some questions remain about the data they generate (e.g., the angle of occurrence for peak torque). This angle could have diagnostic importance because peak torque alone does not provide a complete evaluation. The reliability of the Biodex B-2000 isokinetic dynamometer and the use of the angle of peak torque as a diagnostic tool were examined.

Methods.—The subjects were 30 college-aged male volunteers. Ten were soccer players, 10 were baseball players, and 10 were nonathletes. They performed right and left isokinetic knee extension exercises at 60 and 450 degrees/sec on the Biodex B-2000 isokinetic dynamometer. The data generated were analyzed to determine whether there was a sport-specific angle at which concentric peak torque was generated during these exercises. Half of each group was tested twice to assess the reliability of the device. The subjects also underwent anthropometric measurements, including leg length, thigh circumference, and anterior and posterior thigh skinfolds.

Results.—There were no significant differences in peak torque or angle of peak torque for either leg between days. The 2 athletic groups demonstrated higher reliability coefficients, as did the slower isokinetic speed. Because peak torque and angle of peak torque were not significantly different among the 3 groups, the data were combined to compare the right and left legs. This comparison also showed no significant differences in peak torque and angle of peak torque. There appeared to be a specific joint angle at both speeds—17 degrees at the slower speed and 55 degrees at the faster speed—at which peak torque was generated, regardless of athletic activity or leg dominance.

Conclusion.—The Biodex B-2000 isokinetic dynamometer generally yields reliable data at slower speeds, even in nonathletes. Injury or potential for injury to the force-producing muscles of the upper leg may be seen in subjects who deviate from the angles of peak torque defined in this study. It may be possible to establish normative data for use in determining whether the angle of peak torque for a specific testing protocol is appropriate.

▶ Although the primary purpose of this study was to determine the reliability of a piece of equipment—the Biodex B-2000—the authors also were successful in demonstrating that peak torque appears to be speed-specific and not experience- or sport-specific. This means that it may be possible—after developing normative data for the angle of peak torque at various testing speeds—to use this technique in the diagnosis of injuries or in testing the extent of rehabilitation after surgery. Most rehabilitative protocols with which I am familiar use only peak torque when testing the extent of rehabilitation. A fairly common protocol for rehabilitation after knee surgery calls for the affected knee to return to within 10% of the peak torque of the unaffected knee. Maybe these authors are correct in suggesting that the angle of peak torque should also be considered.—Col. J.L. Anderson, PE.D.

Movement of the Axis of Rotation of the Glenohumeral Joint While Working on the Cybex II Dynamometer: Part I. Flexion/Extension
Walmsley RP (Queen's Univ, Kingston, Ont, Canada)
Isokinetics Exerc Sci 3:16–20, 1993   139-94-6-4

Introduction.—There is agreement that the dynamometer axis should be aligned with the joint axis during Cybex testing but not on what to do when there is considerable movement of the joint's axis of rotation. This occurs during active flexion-extension and abduction-adduction of the shoulder complex.

Objective and Methods.—Glenohumeral joint motion was analyzed in 9 normal male undergraduate students while they were performing flexion-extension of the shoulder on the Cybex isokinetic dynamometer. The Watsmart 3-dimensional digitizing system was used for kinesiologic

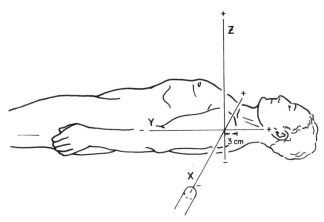

Fig 6–1.—Position of patient and X, Y, and Z axes around the glenohumeral joint. (Courtesy of Walmsley RP: *Isokinetics Exerc Sci* 3:16–20, 1993.)

analysis (Fig 6–1). Light-emitting diodes were placed at several sites while the subject exercised (Fig 6–2).

Results.—On average, the glenohumeral joint became elevated by 8 cm during exercise, representing 12.5% of the distance from the joint to the wrist. The subjects flexed their elbows to compensate for upward shoulder motion when retaining a hold on the Cybex handle. During arm extension, the shoulder was protracted and the elbow was straightened, bringing the glenohumeral joint back into alignment with the dynamometer axis.

Suggestion.—The value recorded by the Cybex data reduction computer should be lowered by 12.5%.

▶ This is another study by researchers who are on the lookout for possible measurement error that may be introduced by the measuring device.—Col. J.L. Anderson, PE.D.

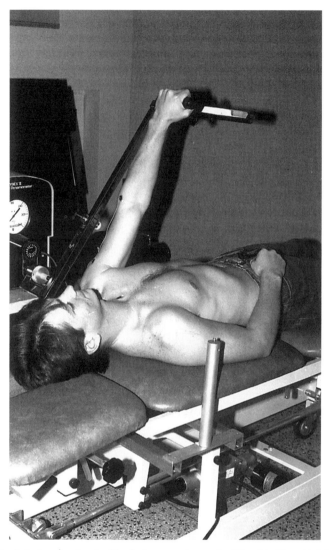

Fig 6–2.—Patient performing shoulder flexion-extension on the Cybex Machine with light-emitting diodes attached. (Courtesy of Walmsley RP: *Isokinetics Exerc Sci* 3:16–20, 1993.)

Influence of the Dynamometer Driving Mechanism on the Isokinetic Torque Angle Curve of Knee Extensors

Stam HJ, Binkhorst RA, van Nieuwenhuyzen JF, Snijders CJ (Univ Hosp Rotterdam, The Netherlands; Univ of Nijmegen, The Netherlands; Erasmus Univ Rotterdam, The Netherlands)

Clin Biomech 8:91–94, 1993   139-94-6–5

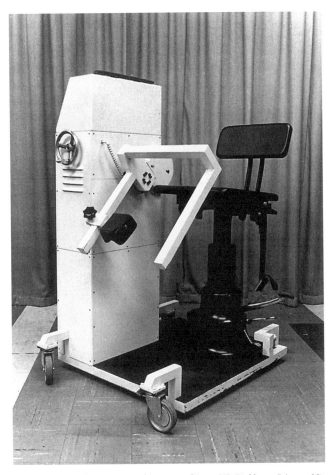

Fig 6–3.—The quadriceps dynamometer. (Courtesy of Stam HJ, Binkhorst RA, van Nieuwenhuyzen JF, et al: *Clin Biomech* 8:91–94, 1993.)

Background.—The isokinetic dynamometer is often used to estimate torque exerted by various muscle groups. A hydraulic system is used in passive devices such as the Cybex II, whereas in active isokinetic systems, an electric motor assures a constant velocity of the lever arm. Passive and active systems may yield torque angle curves of differing shape, thereby influencing maximal torque value and the point in the angular range of motion where torque is maximal.

Study Design.—The influence of the type of isokinetic drive mechanism on torque angle curves for the knee extensors was studied in 20 healthy young adults of both sexes. The subjects were tested alternately on an active device, the Quadriceps Dynamometer (QD) (Fig 6–3), and a passive dynamometer, the Cybex II.

Results.—The Cybex II produced higher values for mean maximum torque than did the QD in both male and female subjects. The difference—approximately 10%—was statistically significant. The Cybex II also produced higher values for maximal torque joint position in male subjects, but not in female subjects. The values of mean work produced by the 2 systems did not differ significantly. With the Cybex II, no torque was registered during the first part of the range of motion study, and torque subsequently built up rapidly. Mean torque values were higher for the Cybex II than for the QD in the second part of the angular range-of-motion study.

Implications.—The design of the dynamometer is a factor when muscle torque is measured with an isokinetic dynamometer. For the knee extensors, peak torque values may differ by as much as 10% when measured using an active vs. a passive system.

▶ These authors have done other researchers, especially neophytes, a service in pointing out that the design of measuring instruments will often affect the data output as much as or more than that variable being measured. Measurement error should always be expected, even when we may not understand it.—Col. J.L. Anderson, PE.D.

A Panning DLT Procedure for Three-Dimensional Videography
Yu B, Koh TJ, Hay JG (Univ of Iowa, Iowa City; Cleveland Clinic Found, Ohio)
J Biomech 26:741–751, 1993   139-94-6–6

Background.—The direct linear transformation (DLT) method frequently is used in biomechanical analysis to acquire 3-dimensional space coordinates from film and video records. When used to analyze events taking place over a large area, problems are encountered in constructing and transporting a control object of adequate size. Furthermore, image size and the accuracy of digitization both decline as the control volume becomes larger. The computed coordinates may not accurately depict those parts of an event that occur outside the control volume.

A Possible Solution.—In a new approach to 3-dimensional videography, panning cameras are used to analyze human motion, and on-site measurements are not required to specify camera positions. Several small single control volumes are combined to construct a large total volume. A regression equation (calibration equation) is developed for each single control volume to express each of 11 DLT parameters as a function of camera orientation. It then is possible to estimate the parameters from arbitrary camera orientations. Once the DLT parameters are known for 2 or more cameras and the 2-dimensional coordinates are obtained, it is possible to compute the desired 3-dimensional spatial coordinates.

Validation.—Five single control volumes in a total control volume of $24.4 \times 2.44 \times 2.44 \text{ m}^3$ were used to determine how the position of the

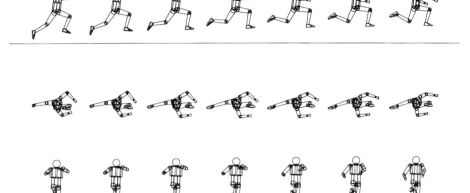

Fig 6–4.—Three-dimensional wire-frame diagram of step flight phase of the triple jump (from top to bottom: side, overhead, and rear views). The body positions depicted indicate qualitatively the validity of the results obtainable with panning DLT method. (Courtesy of Yu B, Koh TJ, Hay JG: *J Biomech* 26:741–751, 1993.)

single control volume affects the accuracy of the computed 3-dimensional space coordinates. In 4 instances, the error from using a linear calibration equation was significantly greater than that associated with the use of a quadratic calibration equation. When the quadratic equation was used, the position of the single control volume did not significantly influence the mean error in computed 3-dimensional coordinates. Panning reduced the mean error in computed 3-dimensional coordinates from 22 to 17 mm. An analysis of the flight phase of a triple jump (Fig 6–4) affirmed that this approach is potentially applicable to many types of human motion analysis.

Applications.—The panning DLT procedure has so far been used to analyze long and triple jumps in track and field. It may, however, prove useful in analyzing a wide range of activities including running, hurdling, javelin throwing, gymnastics, cross-country skiing, speed skating, swimming, and base running.

▶ When I did my first biomechanical analysis in 1966, we worked with only 2 dimensions and I wondered about panning and how to do my computations. Now, with 3-dimensional cinematography and digitizing through automation, we are moving in a direction that will allow us to analyze more complicated movements and be more accurate in our computations. However, there still will be great variability between and among subjects; we must develop our procedures to the point at which we can analyze the performance of each athlete or subject and compare the data with data taken earlier for each individual, rather than with some hypothetical mean taken from a number of subjects. When we get to that point, I think we will really be able to assist the coach and/or practitioner.—Col. J.L. Anderson, PE.D.

Amplitude and Frequency Measures of Surface Electromyography During Dual Task Elbow Torque Production
Caldwell GE, Jamison JC, Lee S (Univ of Maryland, College Park)
Eur J Appl Physiol 66:349–356, 1993   139-94-6–7

Background.—Task-specific motor units are seen within the muscles controlling the elbow, as documented by studies of motor unit recruitment thresholds. Frequency-based measures of electromyography have shown great promise in the characterization of recruitment strategies. Both amplitude- and frequency-based measures of electromyography were used to explore the activity patterns of certain arm muscles during different 1- and 2-df elbow torque production tasks.

Methods.—Fourteen subjects were tested while performing various combinations of isometric tasks: maximum voluntary contraction (MVC) flexion and MVC supination, both with a targeted torque of 0 in the second df; MVC flexion with targeted MVC supination (FS); and MVC supination with targeted MVC flexion (SF). Data were collected on flexion and supination torque, as were electromyography data from electrode pairs on the brachioradialis (BRAD), biceps brachii short head, and medial and lateral aspects of biceps brachii long head. Analysis of covariance models with planned contrasts were used to analyze median power frequency and root mean square amplitude under steady-state torque conditions.

Results.—The root mean square showed a significant main effect for task, but median power frequency did not. The root mean square response was significantly increased in the dual MVC tasks of FS and SF compared to the single MVC tasks of flexion and supination. Alterations in root mean square data were not associated with any frequency changes, suggesting a different underlying recruitment/rate coding scheme for dual-df than for single-df tasks. Both median power frequency and root mean square demonstrated task-by-site interactions, with the 3 biceps sites showing different responses to the flexion and supination tasks than the BRAD site.

Conclusion.—Evidence of task specificity was found at the 4 electrode sites studied. Synergy between the biceps and BRAD is not fixed, and flexor equivalence of the elbow is not maintained under all torque task conditions. The findings of this study may support the notion of motor unit task groups.

▶ These authors believe that their evidence of task specificity among the 4 electrode sites studied at least partially refutes the contention that surface electrodes are inadequate for detailed studies of muscle activation. However, they recognize that the restrictions in data interpretation leave open several possible explanations of their findings and agree that there is a need for more work on the exact nature of muscle task specificity using other methodologies.—Col. J.L. Anderson, PE.D.

The Influence of Air Temperature on the EMG/Force Relationship of the Quadriceps
Bell DG (Defence and Civil Inst of Environmental Medicine, North York, Ont, Canada)
Eur J Appl Physiol 67:256–260, 1993   139-94-6–8

Background.—The change of muscle electric activity required for a contraction in a cold air environment has not been established. The relationship of electromyography (EMG) and force was investigated in both a cold and a hot air environment and the results were compared with the EMG/force relationship at room temperature.

Methods.—Ten healthy subjects performed a criterion task of 5 isometric contractions at 10%, 25%, 50%, 75%, and 100% maximal voluntary contraction. Each subject performed the task 5 times during 1.5-hour exposures at 10°C, 23°C, and 40°C. Electromyographic signals from the rectus femoris and the forces associated with the contractions were recorded on FM tape and digitized at a 2,000-Hz sampling rate.

Results.—Regression analysis revealed that the 40°C curve differed significantly from both other curves, producing less EMG for the same force. At 60 and 90 minutes, the 10°C curve differed significantly from the 23° curve, with less EMG for the same force. Over time, the 23°C and 40°C curves did not change; the 10°C curve increased gradually, becoming significant at 60 and 90 minutes. The temperature of the skin over the quadriceps stabilized within 15 minutes in the hot environment but took 60 minutes to stabilize in the cold condition.

Conclusion.—The quadriceps EMG/force relationship measured using surface electrodes is influenced by ambient temperature. The differences may result from fluid shifts within the muscle, changes in conduction velocity within the muscle, sweating, or a combination of these factors. Estimating effort in adverse environments using an equation derived in control conditions requires careful calculation.

▶ This study points out certain conditions of temperature that anyone using surface electrodes for making EMG measurements must be aware of. Hot or cold temperatures may significantly alter the measurements. What about fine wire electrodes inserted into the muscles? Will hot or cold temperatures significantly alter the EMG measurements taken using Chafine wire electrodes?—Col. J.L. Anderson, PE.D.

Electromyogram Spectrum Changes During Sustained Contraction Related to Proton and Diprotonated Inorganic Phosphate Accumulation: A ^{31}P Nuclear Magnetic Resonance Study on Human Calf Muscles

Laurent D, Portero P, Goubel F, Rossi A (Université Joseph Fourier, Grenoble, France; Université de Technologie de Compiègne, France)
Eur J Appl Physiol 66:263–268, 1993   139-94-6-9

Background.—The mechanism of the decrease in mean power frequency during isometric contractions has not been clearly identified. Although ^{31}P nuclear MR spectroscopy has been used to monitor levels of inorganic phosphate, phosphocreatinine, adenosine triphosphate, and intracellular pH during muscle contraction, these signals have not been synchronized with electromyographic (EMG) frequency spectra. Electromyographic spectrum changes and proton and diprotonated forms of inorganic phosphate accumulation were measured simultaneously during isometric contraction.

Methods.—Five healthy volunteers performed a sustained isometric contraction at 70% of maximal voluntary contraction until exhaustion. The surface coils of a supraconducting magnet were positioned against the calf muscles. The EMG surface electrodes were applied to the gastrocnemius medialis muscle.

Results.—During isometric contraction, the concentration of phosphocreatinine declined to 25% of baseline and the intramuscular content of inorganic phosphate increased; the concentration of adenosine triphosphate did not change. Intracellular pH decreased to 6.75 after 5 minutes of exercise. By exhaustion, the diprotonated inorganic phosphate/sum total phosphorus ratio had increased significantly (by 650%) and moderate, continuous intracellular acidosis had developed. The change in intracellular pH was correlated with an average 167% rise in proton concentration. Intracellular pH did not correlate with the inorganic phosphate/phosphocreatinine ratio, which is the index of the "energy state." Mean power frequency decreased consistently over time. Significant relationships were established between the decrease in mean power frequency and proton accumulation.

Conclusion.—The EMG power spectrum changes during isometric contraction may be linked to metabolic parameters of muscle fatigue. These changes may be partially explained by a variation in electric activity related to fiber-type recruitment under the inhibitory influence of diprotonated forms of inorganic phosphate.

▶ The investigators designed this experiment to test whether changes in EMG activity during sustained isometric contraction could be related to metabolic data. The author could find no indication that others had made simultaneous measurements of EMG frequency spectra and ^{31}P nuclear MR spectroscopy.—Col. J.L. Anderson, PE.D.

Estimation of Muscle Forces About the Wrist Joint During Isometric Tasks Using an EMG Coefficient Method

Buchanan TS, Moniz MJ, Dewald JPA, Rymer WZ (Rehabilitation Inst of Chicago; Northwestern Univ, Chicago)

J Biomech 26:547–560, 1993   139-94-6-10

Background.—Because most major human joints are traversed by multiple muscles, many with similar mechanical moments, summary force equations are underdetermined. The system is said to be mechanically redundant with more unknowns than there are independent equations to solve them. Investigators have developed equivalent muscle methods, muscle stress methods, optimization methods, and quasi-determinate

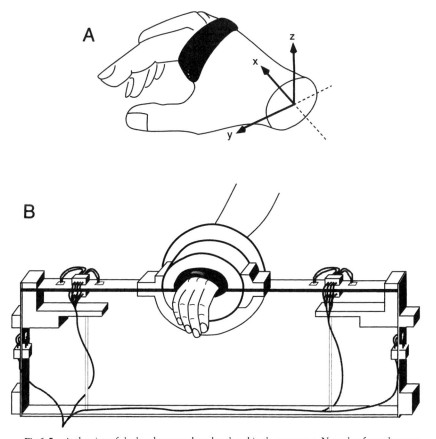

Fig 6–5.—A, drawing of the hand cast ready to be placed in the apparatus. Note that from the coordinate system used in the study, wrist torques measured were in the y − z plane. **B,** the three-dimensional load cell apparatus. Forces can be measured in flexion/extension, radial/ulnar deviation, and supination/pronation. (Courtesy of Buchanan TS, Moniz MJ, Dewald JPA, et al: *J Biomech* 26:547–560, 1993.)

methods to reduce the complexity of this problem. Alternatively, the co-efficient method develops estimates of muscle force by relating muscle electromyogram (EMG) data to muscle mechanical moments through the summary moment balance equations. The EMG coefficient method was used to estimate individual muscle forces for the wrist, and the results were compared with force estimates derived for directions in which determinate solutions are possible.

Method.—Electromyograms were recorded from 5 muscles acting at the wrist during a series of isometric contractions in flexion, extension, ulnar deviation, and radial deviation. The EMG signals and the necessary anatomical data were used to estimate individual muscle forces (Fig 6-5, A and B). In 1 of the 5 subjects, complete anatomical parameters were estimated by MRI reconstruction of muscle moment arms and lines of muscle action. Signal processing techniques and intensive subject training were used to reduce the errors associated with variability in the EMG signals. The EMG-based force estimates were validated by evaluations at torque directions in which no mechanical redundancy existed. A Monte Carlo simulation was performed to determine the error bounds of the force-EMG coefficients.

Results.—The individual muscle forces at the wrist can be estimated with considerable accuracy without assuming any control strategy. The coefficient method can be successfully used to obtain estimates of muscle forces in the wrist over a range of forces, specifically those in which linear force-EMG relationships apply. Physiologic parameters—such as muscle volumes, moment arms, and centroid lines of action—were obtained from MRI slices with very simple techniques.

Conclusion.—The EMG coefficient method predicted relatively accurate forces for the wrist muscles. In this study, the wrist muscles were not directly measured for comparison, but the repeatability of the results and the outcome of the Monte Carlo simulations suggest that the force estimates are reliable. One disadvantage is that the sensitivity of the method required signal processing techniques and intensive subject training to reduce the errors associated with variability in the EMG signals. Future work will determine whether the method can be used in highly redundant joint systems.

▶ Here is another excellent study that needs to be replicated using women as subjects. Our work at West Point has shown a significant difference between men and women in wrist and grip strength.—Col. J.L. Anderson, PE.D.

Myo-Electric Signals From Two Extrinsic Hand Muscles and Force Tremor During Isometric Handgrip

Löscher WN, Gallasch E (Landesnervenklinik Salzburg, Austria; Univ of Graz, Austria)
Eur J Appl Physiol 67:99–105, 1993   139-94-6-11

Objective.—The myoelectric signs of muscle fatigue and the isometric force tremor of 2 extrinsic hand muscles were investigated during isometric power grip. Most previous work in this area was performed on a single muscle of an agonistic group or in an agonist heterogeneous muscle group.

Methods.—Eight healthy, right-handed subjects—4 men and 4 women aged 26–31 years—participated in the experiments. The muscles examined were the extensor digitorum communis (extensor) and the flexor digitorum superficialis (flexor). The subjects were seated on a chair, with the proximal two thirds of the forearm fixed to an armrest and the wrist joint and hand unsupported. An isometric handgrip dynamometer measured grip force by the hand muscles. The myoelectric signal was recorded using electrodes placed over the flexor and extensor muscles; a special load cell recorded isometric force tremor. Four subjects started the experiments with their left hand and 4 with their right hand. Contractions were performed at 20%, 40%, 60%, and 80% of maximal voluntary contraction (MVC).

Results.—The decrease of mean power frequency with duration of contraction was greater in the left extensor muscle than in the left flexor muscle. No differences were observed in the decrease in mean power frequency with duration of contraction between the right extensor and flexor muscles. There was no change in isometric force tremor root mean square during contractions at a given contraction level. Isometric tremor amplitude increased from 20% to 60% of MVC and decreased at higher contraction levels. In the left hand, tremor amplitude was higher at all contraction levels except 60% of MVC.

Conclusion.—The myoelectric signals of both extrinsic hand muscles demonstrated mean power frequency and amplitude changes throughout a 20-second isometric handgrip. The number of these changes depended on the contraction level, and flexors and extensors exhibited subtle differences. Isometric force tremor amplitude, however, did not change throughout the contractions but was dependent on contraction level and left- or right-handedness. The dominant and nondominant hands appear to differ in fatigability and muscle fiber composition. Flexors and extensors also show metabolic and muscle fiber differences.

▶ I am pleased to see this study of grip strength. For those of us involved in athletics, grip strength is a very important topic for which we do not see enough studies. For example, much of what many of us think is a lack of upper-body strength in women is really the result of a lack of grip strength. I am certain that we will find the same thing with men if we do a few studies concerning grip strength in men.—Col. J.L. Anderson, PE.D.

The Influence of Electrode Position on Bipolar Surface Electromyogram Recordings of the Upper Trapezius Muscle

Jensen C, Vasseljen O, Westgaard RH (Norwegian Inst of Technology, Trondheim, Norway)

Eur J Appl Physiol 67:266–273, 1993   139-94-6-12

Background.—The midpoint between the seventh cervical vertebra and the acromion is the recommended bipolar surface electrode position for measuring shoulder muscle load. However, electromyographic (EMG) amplitude depression has been reported at this position. The relationship between the central depression in the upper trapezius EMG signal and the EMG amplitude variation was investigated in 10 healthy volunteers.

Methods.—The subjects performed maximal shoulder elevations with the arm in vertical, abducted, and flexed positions, and underwent a dynamic movement test. The myoelectric signal was recorded along the length of the right upper trapezius muscle using a 16-channel bipolar array electrode. The signal was integrated with a .2-second time resolution.

Results.—On the EMG amplitude profile, a plateau spanning at least 5 electrodes was located 10% to 30% of the distance from the midpoint, and a dip occurred halfway between the acromion and C7. The midpoint dip was displaced by 90-degree arm abduction or flexion. The mean EMG-force curve at the plateau appeared linear. At low contraction levels, dip and lateral EMG levels on the force curve increased faster and were higher compared with EMG levels at the plateau. On the movement test, median EMG activity revealed a dip similar to but slightly displaced from the dip in the maximal amplitude profile. At low contraction levels, the relative EMG levels at the most lateral electrodes approached those in the dip position.

Conclusion.—When using bipolar surface electrodes with a 2-cm interelectrode distance, a center position 2 cm lateral to the midpoint between C7 and acromion provides good repeatability and high signal yield.

▶ These authors used 5 women and 5 men as subjects in this study. The mean percentage differences between the male and female subjects were as follows: body mass mean of the 5 women was 75.8% of the 5 men; body height mean of the women was 93.1% of the men; the C7-to-acromion distance mean of the women was 87.4% of the men; and the mean force of the women was 78.1% of the mean force of the men. Although in this study these mean differences between men and women may not mean anything, there are some studies in which we must pay attention to various gender differences.—Col. J.L. Anderson, PE.D.

Myo-Electric Fatigue Manifestations Revisited: Power Spectrum, Conduction Velocity, and Amplitude of Human Elbow Flexor Muscles During Isolated and Repetitive Endurance Contractions at 30% Maximal Voluntary Contraction
Krogh-Lund C, Jørgensen K (Danish Acoustical Inst, Lyngby, Denmark; Univ of Copenhagen)
Eur J Appl Physiol 66:161–173, 1993 139-94-6–13

Background.—Earlier studies of myoelectric fatigue were focused on neuromotor regulatory mechanisms, whereas more recent studies have

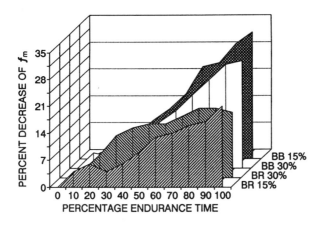

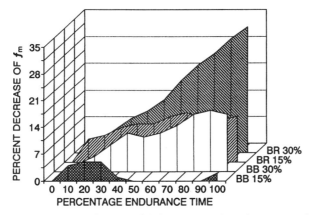

Fig 6–6.—Percentage of median frequency (fm) decreases over the endurance time of the BR and the BB muscles contributed by factors unrelated to (**upper part**), or directly reflecting conduction velocity changes (**lower part**), as documented in the present 30% maximal voluntary contraction (MVC) study and in the 15% MVC study of Krogh-Lund and Jørgensen (1992). Similar fill patterns indicate similar muscles and loads in both parts of the figure; it should be noted, however, that muscles and loads have been shown in different orders in both parts of figure to make viewing easier. (Courtesy of Krogh-Lund C, Jørgensen K: *Eur J Appl Physiol* 66:161-173, 1993.)

stressed the importance of local metabolic processes and disordered homeostatic mechanisms. Electromyographic (EMG) changes have been related to the synchronization and grouping of motor unit firing and to a reduced velocity of propagation of the action potential.

Objective and Methods.—An EMG study was carried out in 10 young men who performed static endurance contraction exercise at a moderate level. Isometric elbow flexion was performed at 30% of maximal voluntary contraction at an elbow angle of 135 degrees. The surface EMG was recorded from the brachioradialis (BR) and biceps brachii (BB) muscles.

Observations.—At the point of exhaustion, the conduction velocity of the BR muscle had declined by 33% from an initial level of 4.3 m/sec, about twice as much as that of the BB. The respective median frequency reductions were 50% and 43% (Fig 6-6). The root-mean-square amplitude of the BR and BB muscles increased by 150% and 120%, respectively. When further sets of endurance contractions were performed at 5-minute rest intervals, the relative conduction velocity decreased in direct proportion to the endurance time, and the reduction in median frequency varied with the conduction velocity.

Interpretation.—This study fails to support a causal relationship between a decrease in conduction velocity, signifying impaired fiber excitability, and the force failure characteristic of the exhausted state.

▶ These authors had 2 objectives in conducting this research. The first was to investigate the EMG of the elbow flexor muscles during a moderate load level of 30% maximum voluntary contraction to see whether the relative median frequency variation reflected changes in the conduction velocity. They also thought that the existence of a predictive interdependency between the myoelectric parameters and the functional state of the muscles could be shown by the performance of a series of endurance contractions separated by 5-minute intervals. Second, by cross-correlation of EMG recordings of fatigue and exhaustion, they planned to demonstrate instantaneous variations in conduction velocity. They expected that during the series of contractions the conduction velocity alterations would indicate any possible causal relationship between fiber excitability and the force failure of exhaustion. Although their data were unable to support a causal relationship, that in no way diminishes the excellence of this work.—Col. J.L. Anderson, PE.D.

Differences in Activation Patterns in Elbow Flexor Muscles During Isometric, Concentric and Eccentric Contractions
Nakazawa K, Kawakami Y, Fukunaga T, Yano H, Miyashita M (Natl Rehabilitation Centre for the Disabled, Tokorozawa City, Japan; Univ of Tokyo)
Eur J Appl Physiol 66:214–220, 1993   139-94-6–14

Objective.—Few studies have examined the activation pattern in elbow flexor muscles during various types of muscle contraction. The relative

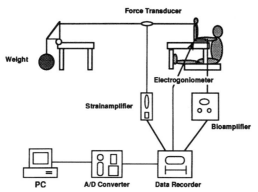

Fig 6–7.—Diagram of the experimental setup. *Abbreviation: PC,* personal computer. (Courtesy of Nakazawa K, Kawakami Y, Fukunaga T, et al: *Eur J Appl Physiol* 66:214–220, 1993.)

activation of the biceps brachii (BB) and brachioradialis (BR) muscles was compared during 3 different types of contraction.

Study Design.—Eight healthy male subjects (mean age, 25.5 years) were studied while performing concentric, eccentric, and isometric contractions against the same load. The experimental setup is diagrammed in Figure 6-7. Isometric contractions were performed at elbow angles of 10, 45, and 90 degrees. Electromyographic (EMG) recordings were made using bipolar surface electrodes, and the relative activation was estimated as the quotient of mean EMG activities.

Findings.—The BR muscle was activated more in concentric contractions than during eccentric contractions, especially at more extended elbow angles. At elbow joint angles of 0 to 60 degrees, the BR/BB activity ratio of concentric contractions was significantly greater than during eccentric contractions. During isometric and eccentric contractions, the BR/BB at flexed joint angles tended to exceed those at extended angles. No angle-dependent changes in BR/BB were noted during concentric elbow flexion. The patterns of the EMG power spectra associated with various types of contraction differed for the BR and BB muscles.

Conclusion.—The way in which the elbow flexor muscles are activated varies with the pattern of muscle contraction. It is simplistic to regard the elbow flexors as a single functioning unit during different types of contraction.

▶ These authors have replicated the work of others showing that during isometric contractions the activations pattern between the BR and the BB muscles varies with the amount of extension of the elbow. As the elbow angles toward extension, the activation of the BB muscle increased much more than the activation of the BR muscle. Past research has shown that the mechanical advantages of all elbow flexor muscles decreases with the extension of the elbow joint, with a smaller decrease for the BB muscle. In eccentric elbow flexions, the relative activation of the BR muscle increased as the elbow joint was flexed, but there was no angle-dependent variation in the BR muscle activation during concentric elbow flexions. The authors believe this implies that during concentric contractions the BR muscle is activated more intensely than for other contraction patterns. The question this poses may be as follows: Is it conceivable that the increased BR muscle activity during the concentric contractions may be strongly influenced by signals from a higher center? I wonder what the results would be if fine wire electrodes rather than surface electrodes were used to replicate this study?—Col. J.L. Anderson, PE.D.

Muscle Force as Affected by Fatigue: Mathematical Model and Experimental Verification
Hawkins D, Hull ML (Univ of California, Davis)
J Biomech 26:1117–1128, 1993   139-94-6–15

Background.—During activities over an extended period, the forces generated by the muscles, or the fibers within the muscles, may be re-

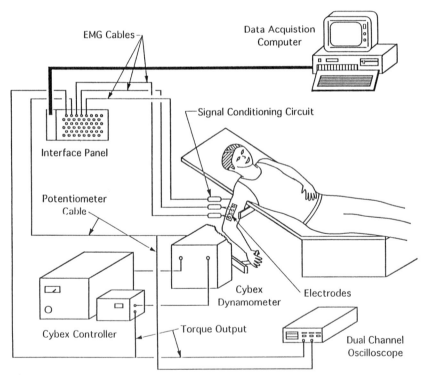

Fig 6–8.—The subject/equipment setup used in the elbow extension study. Elbow moments were determined from data recorded using a Cybex dynamometer. Joint angles were determined from potentiometer data. Levels of triceps muscle activation were recorded using surface electrodes. (Courtesy of Hawkins D, Hull ML: *J Biomech* 26:1117–1128, 1993.)

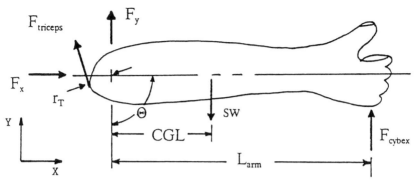

Fig 6–9.—A free body diagram of a patient's forearm. The triceps muscle force ($F_{triceps}$) and the weight of the forearm (SW), multiplied by their respective moment arm lengths to the elbow joint center, create a torque about the elbow. During an isometric test, this torque is balanced by the torque generated by the force (F_{cybex}) acting on the hand. (Courtesy of Hawkins D, Hull ML: *J Biomech* 26:1117–1128, 1993.)

duced as a result of fatigue. The effect of fatigue on muscle force production is not clearly understood. Although comprehensive mathematical muscle models are available, they have not been used to model the effects of fatigue. An empirical expression describing fatigue was incorporated into a muscle model. The muscle model includes variables of muscle length, shortening velocity, neural activation, and muscle architecture.

Study Plan.—The model assumes that a muscle is composed of a combination of slow-twitch, fast-twitch oxidative-glycolytic, and fast-twitch glycolytic fiber types. Muscle force is calculated as the sum of individual fiber forces determined on the basis of fiber kinematics and activation information. Fiber force is modified using previously reported indices of fatigue. An elbow extension study on 10 male volunteers was used to validate the modeled fatigue relationship for maximal effort activities (Fig 6–8). The triceps brachii forces generated during isometric and dynamic fatigue tests were determined by the muscle model and by a direct approach based on rigid-body dynamic analysis (Fig 6–9).

Results.—The triceps forces generated by the muscle model and the direct approach were not significantly different for times either less than 50 seconds for the isometric tests or greater than 40 seconds for the dynamic tests.

Conclusion.—A modeled fatigue relationship was tested in an elbow extension study that included isometric and dynamic fatigue conditions. Triceps force was computed using the muscle model and a direct approach based on rigid-body dynamic analysis. The modeled fatigue relationship predicted muscle force during most of the time intervals in the isometric and dynamic fatigue tests.

▶ As far as I know, this is the first attempt to incorporate a derivation of muscle fatigue into a comprehensive model for predicting muscle force.

Other investigators have developed models to predict muscle force, but none of those models account adequately for the contraction history effect of fatigue. This is an excellent study that needs to be replicated using more subjects.—Col. J.L. Anderson, PE.D.

Relationship Between Isokinetic Average Force, Peak Force, Average Torque, and Peak Torque of the Shoulder Internal and External Rotator Muscle Groups

Perrin DH, Tis LL, Hellwig EV, Shenk B (Univ of Virginia, Charlottesville; Georgia State Univ, Atlanta; Cedarville College, Ohio; et al)
Isokinetics Exerc Sci 3:85–87, 1993   139-94-6-16

Background.—Isokinetic dynamometry may quantify a muscle's capacity to generate work (the product of the force and distance of a muscle contraction) or power (the time required to produce work). Work and power may be predicted from peak torque; however, whether peak and average force and torque measures are interchangeable has not been determined. The relationship among concentric and eccentric peak and average force and torque of the shoulder rotator muscles was investigated.

Methods.—Thirty-three men with no history of injury to the nondominant shoulder girdle complex performed at least 3 maximal concentric and eccentric test contractions using internal and external rotator muscle groups. The nondominant side was tested with the shoulder at 90 degrees of abduction and the arm in the frontal plane. Peak force and torque values were obtained from the highest point in the strength curves; average values were calculated using the entire curve. Correlation matrices were generated to determine the relationship between peak force, average force, peak torque, and average torque.

Results.—Correlations between concentric external rotation measures were consistently high, ranging from .86 to .97; correlations for most eccentric external rotation measures ranged from .94 to .99; for concentric internal rotation, from .86 to .96; and for eccentric internal rotation, from .55 to .97. The relationships between internal rotation peak torque and average force, peak force, and average torque were somewhat lower, ranging from .55 to .59.

Conclusion.—Average and peak force and torque are probably valid measures of human muscular performance. However, damp, ramp, preload, and range of motion of the isokinetic assessment may confound the interchangeability of these parameters.

▶ These authors believe that the major finding of this investigation is that there is a strong relationship between most of the isokinetic measures of peak and average force and torque. They state that this suggests that peak torque, average torque, peak force, and average force are probably all valid isokinetic measures. However, because most manufacturers of isokinetic equipment have built in either a damp, preload, and/or ramp feature, the measures of peak and average force and torque can be confounded. The authors report that the use of a damp feature affects assessment of peak torque, and the use of a static preload affects measurement of average force or torque. To make isokinetic assessments, there must be consistency with respect to different manufacturers' equipment. Additional research is needed to further examine the relationships among various isokinetic parameters in various muscle groups, while considering the range of motion and skill levels of the various subjects.—Col. J.L. Anderson, PE.D.

Torque/Velocity Properties of Human Knee Muscles: Peak and Angle-Specific Estimates
Caldwell GE, Adams WB III, Whetstone MR (Univ of Massachusetts, Amherst; Univ of Maryland, College Park)
Can J Appl Physiol 18:274–290, 1993   139-94-6–17

Background.—The force/velocity characteristics of human muscle in vivo usually are examined by the maximal-effort torque/angular velocity (T-AV) characteristics at a joint. Angle-related variation may be removed by normalizing peak torque to the isometric maximum at that angular position. The T-AV relationship of both knee flexors and extensors was established and compared using angle-specific, peak, and normalized peak methods. To determine whether the peak method gives erroneous results, the T-AV relationships from the angle-specific and peak methods were used to assess the ratio of flexor-to-extensor torque at different angular velocities.

Method.—In 8 men, the angle-specific, peak, and normalized peak methods were compared in isovelocity knee flexion and extension at velocities between 50 and 250 degrees per second.

Results.—The peak and normalized peak methods produced more similar torque/velocity results when compared with the results yielded by the angle-specific method. Both the peak and the angle-specific methods demonstrated that the relative flexor/extensor ratio increased slightly with velocity. The variation attributable to differences in angle at which peak torques occur was very small.

Conclusion.—In this study, the torque declined with increased shortening velocity regardless of the calculation method used. The peak and normalized peak methods gave more similar results than the angle-specific method. The angle-specific method of describing human T-AV relationships is prevalent, but a conceptual flaw concerning contractile component velocity is a source of variability that affects the shape of the desired relationship. The comparative strength of antagonistic muscle groups should be assessed at specific angular positions. Muscular imbalance could be assessed by comparing muscular torque capabilities at specific angles throughout the joint range of motion. Another assessment method for muscular imbalance is a systematic exploration of all physiologic and mechanical phenomena that contribute to the expressed muscular torques.

▶ This is an excellent investigation that must be studied in its entirety for one to fully understand the results. This study should be replicated using women as subjects to see whether the results will be similar.—Col. J.L. Anderson, PE.D.

The Axes of Rotation of the Knee
Hollister AM, Jatana S, Singh AK, Sullivan WW, Lupichuk AG (Harbor-UCLA Med Ctr, Torrance, Calif)
Clin Orthop 290:259–268, 1993   139-94-6–18

Introduction.—Knee motion presumably takes place about a variable flexion/extension (FE) axis perpendicular to the sagittal plane and also a longitudinal rotation (LR) axis. Accordingly, a mechanical device was used to locate the FE and LR axes in fresh anatomical specimens.

Methods.—Observations were made on 6 specimen knees. A mechanical device, the axis finder, served to locate the FE and LR axes. The axis sites were documented by conventional roentgenography in 3 planes and also by MRI.

Results.—Movement of points on the LR axis produced circular, planar paths about the fixed FE axis. Magnetic resonance imaging in planes perpendicular to the FE axis revealed a circular profile for the femoral condyles. The FE axis, which was constant, was directed from anterosuperiorly on the medial side of the knee to posteroinferiorly on the lateral side. The axis passed through the origins of the medial and lateral collateral ligaments and was superior to the point where the cruciate ligaments cross. The LR axis was anterior to the FE axis.

Significance.—The presence of 2 fixed axes of knee motion that are offset from each other leads to the valgus and external rotation associated with knee extension. Knee motion itself consists of pure rotation about the fixed axes. Motion about each axis includes components of FE, internal-external rotation, and varus-valgus. The design of prostheses and braces, models for gait, methods of calculating forces, and reconstructive surgical methods are all based on a changing horizontal FE axis.

▶ This excellent study appears to update and possibly correct work done by other investigators concerning the functioning of the knee joint. It indicates that motion of the human knee occurs about 2 fixed, nonorthogonal axes. The authors believe that because prostheses, braces, models for gait, calculations of forces, and reconstructive surgery are based on a changing horizontal flexion/extension axis, the implications of this study are profound. Further studies to replicate these data are necessary.—Col. J.L. Anderson, PE.D.

A Stochastic Model of Trunk Muscle Coactivation During Trunk Bending

Mirka GA, Marras WS (Ohio State Univ, Columbus)
Spine 18:1396–1409, 1993   139-94-6–19

Background.—Occupation-related low back disorders are increasingly common in the industrialized world. Results of numerous studies suggest a link between injury during heavy work and the biomechanical stresses placed on the spine. Traditional biomechanical models of the spine assume that external moments imposed about the spine are countered by the activity of the trunk musculature. The large number of muscle groups within the trunk, however, means that there are an infinite number of possible combinations of muscle forces that can satisfy the biomechanical balance requirement for a given condition. A stochastic (probabilistic) model of trunk muscle activation was therefore developed.

Methods.—The first part of the study consisted of experimental data collection. Five male college students, all without a history of low back disorder, performed a variety of exertions using trunk muscles. Subjects had surface electrodes applied to their skin before being secured in the apparatus used to control the position, motion, and torque of each trial. The data on trunk muscle activity obtained from these experiments became the foundation on which the stochastic simulation model was based.

The Stochastic Model.—The model, based on a simulation of the experimentally derived data, predicted the possible combinations of time-dependent trunk muscle coactivations that could be expected given a set of trunk-bending conditions. The magnitude and variability of the spine reaction forces were estimated when simulated muscle activities were used as input to an electromyographically assisted biomechanical model. Thus, the range of spinal loads expected with a specific task could be assessed. Each lifting activity was found to result in significant variability in muscle activities. The variability in trunk muscle force had little effect on spinal compression variability but a considerable influence on both lateral and anteroposterior shear forces. A validation study was performed with 2 different male subjects, 1 similar to the original 5 subjects and 1 who was significantly larger and stronger. The model's overall predictive ability—82.4%—was not significantly diminished by use of a subject different in size and strength from the original experimental group. The success rate was 83.1% for the similar subject and 81.8% for the larger subject.

Conclusion.—It is possible to predict the range of electromyographic activities that would be expected during a trunk-bending task, given adequate knowledge of the trunk motion and external loading conditions.

The model developed could aid in an understanding of the muscle system activities and spinal loading associated with low back disorders.

▶ This research received the 1993 Volvo Award in Biomechanic Studies. This is an excellent study, not only because of the quality of the research design, but also because it addresses one of the most significant injury problems in our society today. We need considerably more research to help us understand the biomechanics of the back and spine and how to prevent injuries as well as treat them. I am certain that prevention through proper exercise is a great part of the answer. The exercises should be directed specifically toward maintaining the muscle tone of the back musculature as we age and keeping a reasonable balance between the strength of the back and the hamstring muscles. One successful and relatively simple method that I have tried is called the Backmate procedure.—Col. J.L. Anderson, PE.D.

Trunk Extensor Endurance and Its Relationship to Electromyogram Parameters
van Dieën JH, Oude Vrielink HHE, Housheer AF, Lötters FBJ, Toussaint HM (Inst of Agricultural Engineering, Wageningen, The Netherlands; Vrije Universiteit, Amsterdam)
Eur J Appl Physiol 66:388–396, 1993   139-94-6–20

Background.—Patients with low back pain display impaired trunk extensor muscle function and early myoelectric manifestations of muscle fatigue. However, the exact relationship between electromyographic (EMG) changes and trunk extensor muscle performance has not been determined. The role of muscle performance and EMG parameters of the trunk extensor muscles in the development of fatigue was investigated.

Methods.—Nine healthy male subjects with no history of low back pain performed continuous isometric trunk extensions at torque levels of approximately 25% and 40% of maximal voluntary contraction in 2 sessions 6 weeks apart. The EMG signals were recorded from different parts of the left and right erector spinae muscles: the longissimus thoracis, iliocostalis lumborum, multifidus, and latissimus dorsi.

Results.—The EMG amplitude increased during both tests in all subjects and in all parts of the erector spinae muscles. The greatest increase and variability occurred in the latissimus dorsi muscle, followed by the iliocostalis muscle. Generally, the mean power frequency of the parts of the erector spinae muscles demonstrated fairly consistent decline. The trend was most marked in the multifidus muscle and least marked in the latissimus dorsi. The time constants of the exponential change of EMG amplitude and mean power frequency were associated with endurance time. The use of both EMG parameters appeared to more accurately predict endurance than did relative force. The time constants of the mean power frequency changes of the multifidus and longissimus muscles appeared to be good predictors of endurance time. The consistency of EMG spectrum shift appeared to coincide with reduced variability of the activation of the involved muscle.

Conclusion.—The time constant of the exponential curves describing EMG parameter changes during isometric trunk extension at moderate torque levels appears to be a good predictor of endurance.

▶ Although the time constant of the exponential curves describing EMG parameter changes during isometric trunk extension at moderate torque levels appears to be a good predictor of endurance, someone must translate this into useful and practical information so that practitioners can use this information to learn how to prevent and treat low back pain. What are the best exercises to use to safely improve the endurance of the erector spinae muscles? I have been using 2 methods that are effective for most people—the Backmate procedure and the Bally Life Circuit back extension machine.—Col. J.L. Anderson, PE.D.

A Combined Finite Element and Optimization Investigation of Lumbar Spine Mechanics With and Without Muscles
Goel VK, Kong W, Han JS, Weinstein JN, Gilbertson LG (Univ of Iowa, Iowa City)
Spine 18:1531–1541, 1993   139-94-6–21

Introduction.—Various approaches to the study of the role of muscles in the biomechanics of the lumbar spine have been used over the years. However, there has yet to be a comprehensive description of the exact role of muscles in protecting the ligamentous spine. A combined finite element (FE) and optimization method was used to address the question of the muscles' effects on the biomechanics of the lumbar spine.

Methods.—A 3-dimensional, nonlinear, FE model of a ligamentous L3–4 motion segment (LIG model) was designed. A separate, biomechanical optimization-based force model was also designed to predict the forces in muscles and disk across this motion segment in an individual holding a 90-N load in his hands, with the spine flexed 30 degrees and the knees straight. The resultant predicted muscle forces were then incorporated into the FE model as nodal forces to simulate the muscle action (MUS model). The predicted responses from the MUS FE model were then compared to those of the LIG FE model subjected to an equivalent load for various biomechanical parameters.

Findings.—When muscular forces were added by way of the MUS model, anteroposterior translation and fixation rotation in the motion segment decreased in comparison to the LIG model predictions. The finding of reduced displacement in the sagittal plane suggested that the muscles lent stability to the ligamentous segment. The addition of muscular forces also decreased stress in the vertebral body and intradiskal pressure, as well as other important biomechanical factors. Still, load-bearing of the facets was increased compared with the ligamentous model, suggesting that facets play an important role in load transmission in the normal, intact spine.

Conclusion.—Through the use of LIG and MUS FE models, the authors have provided quantitative data on the stabilizing effects of muscles on the mechanics of the ligamentous spine. The findings support and provide a scientific explanation for the proposed "degenerative cascade" concept, as well as supporting the observation that facet osteoarthritis may follow disk degeneration. Muscle strength appears to be vital in maintaining spinal function.

▶ This research is exciting to me because it appears to verify what we have come to realize through our exercise prescription; that is, people with low back pain can be helped if they follow a prescribed exercise regimen designed to strengthen the erector spinae muscles and stretch the hamstring muscles.—Col. J.L. Anderson, PE.D.

Transfer of Lumbosacral Load to Iliac Bones and Legs: Part 2. Loading of the Sacroiliac Joints When Lifting in a Stooped Posture
Snijders CJ, Vleeming A, Stoeckart R (Erasmus Univ, Rotterdam, The Netherlands)
Clin Biomech 8:295–301, 1993   139-94-6–22

Background.—The largest muscles of the human body attach to the pelvis, resulting in considerable load transfer. The forces generated by the back muscles on the spine and the iliac bones theoretically contribute to the load transferred by the sacroiliac joints. The few studies of the biomechanics of the pelvis have not addressed the problems of sacroiliac joint stability in relation to posture. It is known that substantial loads are imposed on the lumbar spine when lifting in a stooped position. A biomechanical model of load transfer by the sacroiliac joints in relation to posture was developed (Fig 6–10). The model was verified by anatomical studies and by load application to volunteers. Magnetic resonance imaging verified the geometry in vivo.

Loading Modes.—The transfer of lumbar load to the pelvis in a stooped posture can take place in 2 ways. In 1 loading mode, the ligament and muscle forces that act on the sacrum raise the tendency of the sacrum to flex in relation to the hip bones. In a second loading mode, the ligament and muscle forces act on the iliac crests, raising the tendency of the sacrum to shift in caudal direction in relation to the hip bones. In both loading modes, a self-bracing mechanism comes into action to prevent shear in the sacroiliac joints. When a load is lifted while in a stooped position, the force raised by gravity acts in a plane perpendicular to the spine and the sacrum becomes of interest. In this situation, a belt may contribute to the stability of the sacroiliac joints.

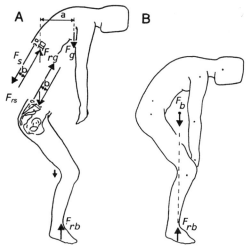

Fig 6–10.—**A,** to estimate the magnitude of forces in the back, a cross-section is made in the lumbar area for construction of a free-body diagram of the upper part of the body. **B,** in forward-bent posture, the center of gravity of the whole body is situated above the feet. The weight of the part of the body above the cross-section is F_g with its point of application near the armpit. The equilibrium of the forces in a vertical direction is obtained by the reaction force F_{rg} in the spine, which is equal in magnitude to F_g. Both forces form a couple, which acts clockwise with moment $F_g a$. To obtain equilibrium of moments, the resultant back muscle for (F_s) and its reaction force in the spine (F_{rs}) form an anticlockwise moment with lever arm b. This simplified model is often used to elucidate the heavy load on the lumbar spine, which is the consequence of the large ratio a/b in a forward-bent position. In this study, forces from muscles, ligaments, and gravity (F_s) were consistently drawn together with their reaction forces (F_{rs}) in the respective joint. This yields a configuration of couples of forces, giving a clear distinction of each contribution to joint load. (Courtesy of Snijders CJ, Vleeming A, Stoeckart R: *Clin Biomech* 8:295–301, 1993.)

Conclusion.—A biomechanical model of load transfer by the sacroiliac joints in relation to posture was developed. When a load is lifted in a stooped position, the force raised by gravity acts in a plane perpendicular to the spine and the sacrum. A self-bracing mechanism comes into action to prevent shear in the sacroiliac joints. The special belts, such as those used by weight lifters, may have a beneficial effect by contributing to the stability of the sacroiliac joints.

▶ This is an excellent, thoughtful biomechanical study of the pelvis and what happens when we lift heavy loads in a stooped position. It is well known that heavy loads are placed on the lumbar spine and the load must be transferred to the pelvis. These authors look at 2 ways for this transfer to take place. One way concerns ligament and muscle forces that act on the sacrum, raising the tendency of the sacrum to flex in relation to the hip bones. The other concerns ligament and muscle forces acting on the iliac crests, raising the tendency of the sacrum to shift in caudal direction in relation to the hip bones. The authors report that both loading modes deal with a self-bracing mechanism that comes into action to prevent shear in the sacroiliac joints. The insight into these interrelationships may make it possible to supplement training programs for muscle strength and coordination in the prevention and treatment of low back injuries.—Col. J.L. Anderson, PE.D.

The Relationship Between EMG Activity and Extensor Moment Generation in the Erector Spinae Muscles During Bending and Lifting Activities

Dolan P, Adams MA (Univ of Bristol, England)
J Biomech 26:513–522, 1993   139-94-6-23

Purpose.—Workers who perform frequent and heavy lifting are at increased risk of disk prolapse and low back pain in general, prompting attempts to measure and regulate compressive forces on the lumbar spine. Most of these forces come from the erector spinae, but electromyographic (EMG) measurements are difficult to apply to dynamic movements. In an attempt to come up with a simple method of estimating compressive forces on the lumbar spine, the effects of different variables on the EMG-extensor moment relationship in the erector spinae muscles were investigated.

Methods.—This relationship was assessed under both isometric and concentric conditions. A full-wave rectified and averaged EMG signal was recorded from skin-surface electrodes located over the belly of the erector spinae muscles at the T10 and L3 levels and compared with measurements of extensor moment. The overall curvature (θ) and the rate of change of curvature ($d\theta/dt$) of the lumbar spine in the sagittal plane were measured by using the 3-Space Isotrak system to assess the effects of muscle length and contraction velocity.

Results.—There was a linear association between extensor moment and EMG activity during isometric contraction. The "gradient" and "intercept" of this relationship depended on the subjects' lumbar curvature at the time of testing. The EMG signal (E) during concentric contraction was higher than the isometric signal (E_0) for a given torque. The relationship between these 2 signals was $E_0 = E/(1 + Ad\theta/dt)$, where $A = .0014$ exp, or $.045P$, and $P =$ percentage of lumbar flexion. The EMG data corrected by this equation for the effect of contraction velocity could then be used, together with the results of the isometric calibrations, to calculate the extensor moment generated by the erector spinae muscles during bending and lifting.

Conclusion.—A relatively simple equation is presented for calculating extensor moment generation in the erector spinae, which can be used to figure the compressive forces acting on the lumbar spine. The technique used in this study may fill the need for a simple method of measuring spinal loading in the workplace, and it may find applications in other areas of biomechanics as well.

▶ These and other researchers have shown that during normal lifting, the erector spinae muscle group exceeds all of the other trunk muscles in contributing to executing a lift. It is well known that the erector spinae muscles are the strongest of the back muscles. With low back pain being one of the most prevalent and costly injuries within the workforce, we must continue to study its causes and how to prevent it. At West Point, we have found that low back pain can be prevented, and can usually be treated, by strengthening the erector spinae muscles and stretching the hamstring muscles. I have tried both procedures, through the Backmate procedure and using the Bally Life Circuit back extension machine, and found them to be highly beneficial in preventing and/or treating low back pain.—Col. J.L. Anderson, PE.D.

Joint Moments and Muscle Activity in the Lower Extremities and Lower Back in Lifting and Lowering Tasks
de Looze MP, Toussaint HM, van Dieën JH, Kemper HCG (Vrije Universiteit, Amsterdam)
J Biomech 26:1067–1076, 1993   139-94-6-24

Objective.—Although a number of studies have addressed mechanical loading on the body during lifting, relatively few have examined the opposite act: lowering. The difference in mechanical loading between the 2 actions may be associated with different static and dynamic factors, with different implications for musculoskeletal disorders. Lifting and lowering were compared in terms of the associated mechanical loading of the lower extremities and back.

Methods.—Eight male volunteers repetitively lifted and lowered a 15.3-kg barbell in 2 different sessions: knee flexion was allowed in 1 session and not allowed in the other. Movement of the ankle, knee, hip, and lumbosacral joints was estimated, and the electromyographic (EMG) activity of various leg and back muscles was measured during lifting and lowering motions.

Results.—The differences between the 2 actions were comparable in the 2 sessions, with good agreement between the joint moment curves during lifting and the time-reversed moment curves during lowering. Lowering was associated with slightly lower peak moments, with peak lumbar moments being about 5% lower. Differences in acceleration profiles at the center of gravity of the body-load complex accounted for these slight differences. In contrast, the average EMG activity of the 7 muscles measured during lowering was about 69% of that measured in lifting. The difference appeared to result from the primarily concentric muscle action involved in lifting vs. the primarily eccentric action of lowering. Intermuscular coordination appeared similar in the 2 techniques.

Conclusion.—The actions of lifting and lowering produce approximately equal joint moments in the lower extremities and lower back. However, the forces are distributed over a significantly smaller cross-sectional area of active muscle during lowering. Thus, lowering may actually increase the risk of musculoskeletal injury, especially in individuals who underestimate its biomechanical stress.

▶ These authors suggest that lowering an object may increase the risk of musculoskeletal injury to the lower back compared with lifting the same weight. From a biomechanical perspective, I believe it is generally agreed that it is easier to lower any weight than it is to lift the same weight. It appears obvious to me that the reason is gravity. In lowering an object, it is only necessary to control the object as gravity does the work of lowering it. Why would it be necessary to exert more force in working with gravity than working against it? Why should the risk of injury be greater? I doubt that estimating mechanical stress has anything to do with it.—Col. J.L. Anderson, PE.D.

Trunk Muscle Geometry and Centroid Location When Twisting
Tsuang YH, Novak GJ, Schipplein OD, Hafezi A, Trafimow JH, Andersson GBJ (Natl Taiwan Univ, Taipei; Rush-Presbyterian-St Luke's Med Ctr, Chicago)
J Biomech 26:537–546, 1993   139-94-6–25

Background.—A number of epidemiologic investigations have linked twisting activities to low back pain, presumably because of the mechanical effects of twisting on the spine. The prediction of lumbar spine loading in biomechanical models requires more accurate data on the moment arms and cross-sectional areas of the trunk in asymmetric postures. Magnetic resonance imaging was used to investigate the trunk muscles of the lumbar region in different postures.

Methods.—Five healthy male volunteers were scanned in neutral and in 2 twisted postures. A computer-aided design digitizing system was used to measure the position of the trunk muscle centroids and the muscles' cross-sectional areas on the transverse MRI scans at 1-cm intervals from L2 to S1. The muscle centroids from successive sections were connected to create muscle lines of action. For each disk level, changes in cross-sectional areas and displacements in centroids were estimated in a 3-dimensional coordinate system and the local 2-dimensional coordinate system.

Results.—The 3-dimensional coordinate system demonstrated displacements of all muscle centroids during twisting, with alterations in the locations and orientations of all muscle lines of action. In contrast, the 2-dimensional coordinate system showed displacement of only the centroids of 4 abdominal muscles, most of which occurred in the first 25 degrees of twisting. Greater displacement was noted high in the lumbar spine, with changes in moment arms as high as twofold. The cross-sectional area changed significantly only in the abdominal oblique muscles (AOM), with increased area of the right AOM ipsilateral to the side of twisting, whereas the area of the left AOM was decreased.

Conclusion.—During twisting motions, significant changes are noted in the moment arms, cross-sectional areas, and muscle lines of action of the trunk musculature. The data suggest that the abdominal muscles move independently and the other trunk muscles follow the lumbar spine. These findings will have to be taken into account when measuring loading of the lumbar spine in biomechanical models.

▶ This ambitious study was designed to show how trunk twisting might contribute to low back pain. The authors used biomechanical modeling of the lumbar spine to explore the causes of low back pain. They believe that the positions and cross-sectional areas of the muscles are 2 of the more important parameters when calculating the internal forces and movements acting on the lumbar spine. However, regardless of the cause of low back pain, our work has shown that, in most cases, procedures to strengthen the erector spinae muscles through back extension are usually beneficial in helping to relieve the pain and prevent its recurrence.—Col. J.L. Anderson, PE.D.

Variability of Knee Moment Arms in the Frontal and Sagittal Planes During Normal Gait
Svensson OK, Weidenhielm L (Karolinska Inst, Stockholm; St Görans Hosp, Stockholm)
Clin Biomech 8:59–65, 1993   139-94-6-26

Background.—The reduced moment arm during gait after surgery may be analyzed indirectly by assessing the knee moment. However, body weight and walking speed may influence the results of this assessment. Use of the moment arm by itself may diminish the impact of walking speed. The utility and variability of a new measure—the length of the moment arm at the knee joint in the frontal and sagittal planes during normal gait—was evaluated.

Methods.—Ten healthy volunteers with no lower extremity joint symptoms walked at a free cadence while wearing their own shoes. Gait was analyzed by using a force platform and 2 video cameras, 1 trained on each plane. One subject underwent gait analysis on 5 consecutive days.

Results.—Mean midstance moment arm length in the frontal plane was 48 mm when the trials were performed minutes apart. Mean moment arm length for peak knee moment was 63 mm. In the sagittal plane, peak moment arm lengths demonstrated very high variability; trials done minutes apart demonstrated less variability than those done days apart for 10 of 15 parameters. The frontal plane variability of trials done minutes apart was always less than the variability of trials done days apart. The smallest variability in the trials performed at 1-minute intervals occurred in the external hip peak and midstance moments and the external knee peak and midstance moments. In the sagittal plane, the least variability occurred in the external peak and midstance dorsiflexing moments about the ankle. Variability was high in all ankle moments in the frontal plane and peak moments about the hip and knee in the sagittal plane.

Conclusion.—This new method is useful for studying changes in hip and knee moments and knee moment arms in the frontal plane. The variability demonstrated in healthy subjects indicates that care should be taken when evaluating changes in hip and knee moments in the sagittal plane and the ankle in the frontal plane.

▶ We should remember this about all biomechanical analyses: We will usually find significant variability among subjects. The means computed from a number of subjects may not fit any one of the subjects exactly. Care should always be taken when attempting to relate research data to any one individual.—Col. J.L. Anderson, PE.D.

Quadriceps Angle and Rearfoot Motion: Relationships in Walking
Kernozek TW, Greer NL (Univ of Minnesota, Minneapolis)
Arch Phys Med Rehabil 74:407–410, 1993   139-94-6–27

Introduction.—As more women participate in athletics, their incidence of lower extremity injuries, especially to the knee and ankle, increases. The angle of pull of the quadriceps muscle (q-angle) is greater in

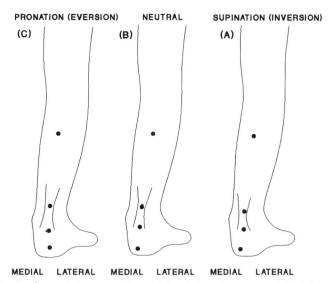

Fig 6–11.—Rearfoot angle is measured by examining the inversion-everson of shank throughout the stance phase of the gait cycle. **A,** at heel strike, the subtalar joint is in a supinated position, defined as a positive rearfoot angle. **B,** after heel strike, the rearfoot passes through a neutral position that is a 0-degree angle. **C,** the subtalar joint continues to evert during the stance phase, creating a negative rearfoot angle. This eversion is used to describe the amount of pronation that occurred. As foot contacts the ground, the rearfoot moves through a period of supination to pronation and back to supination at toe off. (Courtesy of Kernozek TW, Greer NL: *Arch Phys Med Rehabil* 74:407-410, 1993.)

women than in men (17 degrees vs. 14 degrees) and an excessive q-angle may predispose to injury. Any q-angle of more than 15–20 degrees is commonly regarded as pathologic. There is evidence that the q-angle is related to rearfoot motion.

Methods.—The relationship between q-angle and rearfoot motion during walking was studied in 20 healthy women. The subjects were videotaped with 2 cameras, 1 behind and 1 in front, as they walked barefoot at a speed of 1.5 mph on a treadmill. They were then videotaped in calibrated stance and chosen stance, and their leg length, hip width, and arch index were measured. The Peak Performance Motion Measurement System was used to digitize and analyze all data (Fig 6–11). The subjects' q-angles and rearfoot angles were averaged over 5 trials.

Findings.—The mean maximum pronation was −7.88 degrees and the mean total rearfoot motion was 8.2 degrees. The mean static rearfoot angle was −3.45 degrees in chosen stance and −2.4 degrees in calibrated stance. The mean dynamic q-angle was 16.13 degrees at heel strike and 16 degrees at midstance, whereas the mean static q-angle was 18.32 degrees in chosen stance and 17.42 degrees in calibrated stance. Mean hip width was 26 cm, mean leg length was 86 cm, and mean arch index was .23 cm². Rearfoot motion variables correlated poorly with both static and dynamic q-angle variables, as well as with anthropometric variables. Maximum pronation did correlate positively with the static rearfoot angle in calibrated stance, and all static q-angle measurements correlated positively with dynamic q-angle variables. Leg length showed a slightly better correlation with all q-angles than did hip width, and this explained 11% of the observed variance in static q-angle in calibrated stance.

Conclusion.—These results suggest there is little relationship between q-angle and rearfoot motion. There is no apparent association between increased static or dynamic q-angles and greater maximum pronation or total rearfoot motion during the stance phase of gait, nor does hip width appear to be significantly related to the q-angle.

▶ These authors recognize that women participating in athletics appear to be more susceptible to injuries, especially to the knees and ankles. At West Point, we have discovered that when men and women participate in similar physical training, women are significantly more likely to sustain injuries than are men. A few years ago, we did not have enough information to recognize the injury differences between men and women because there were not enough data from valid studies. Today, we know that there is a significant difference in injury history between men and women, but we do not know why. We do not know whether the differences can be explained because of social factors (girls/women do not begin athletic participation as early as boys/men) or because of biomechanical factors explained by anatomical or physiologic differences. This is an area that is ripe for study.—Col. J.L. Anderson, PE.D.

Interrelationships Between Mechanical Power, Energy Transfers, and Walking and Running Economy

Martin PE, Heise GD, Morgan DW (Arizona State Univ, Tempe; Louisiana State Univ, Baton Rouge; Univ of North Carolina, Greensboro)
Med Sci Sports Exerc 25:508–515, 1993   139-94-6–28

Background.—Most biomechanical studies of economy (steady-state aerobic demand for a given submaximal walking or running speed) have focused on the relationship between aerobic demand and specific descriptors of selected events or phases of the gait cycle. The associations observed have, in general, not been strong. A number of analytic procedures have been used to estimate mechanical work, energy, and power output during locomotion, but mechanical expressions cannot account for isometric muscle contributions during gait.

Objective and Methods.—The relationships among aerobic demand, kinematic and kinetic-based estimates of mechanical power output and energy transfer, and the total body angular impulse (sum of net joint moments integrated over time during a stride) were examined in 14 healthy men who walked at a rate of 1.69 m/sec. Sixteen recreational male runners were studied when running at a rate of 3.35 m/sec. The subjects exercised on a treadmill and also over ground.

Findings.—Economy tended to be more consistent during walking than during running, as reflected both by the range of oxygen consumption and by the coefficient of variation in walking economy. Nevertheless, aerobic demand correlated with expressions of power at a generally similar level during the 2 forms of exercise. Correlations between running economy and measures of mechanical power ranged from moderate to poor. Similar results were obtained when correlating the metabolic equivalent of economy (gross aerobic demand multiplied by its thermal equivalent, normalized to body mass) with the mechanical descriptors. Most measures of mechanical power correlated positively with aerobic demand. Subjects who exercised more economically tended to exhibit lower mechanical power.

Conclusion.—The measures often used in gait analysis—including mechanical power, energy transfer, and angular impulse—explain only a small part of the normal intersubject variability in aerobic demand at a given walking or running speed.

▶ These young researchers have discovered once again the difficulties in modeling the movements of the human body, even when the movements are artificially simplified by considering only 2 dimensions.—Col. J.L. Anderson, PE.D.

Vertical Forces and Plantar Pressures in Selected Aerobic Movements *Versus* Walking
Thompson DL, Hatley MR, McPoil TG, Cornwall MW (Northern Arizona Univ, Flagstaff)
J Am Podiatr Med Assoc 83:504–508, 1993   139-94-6–29

Background.—The high incidence of lower extremity injuries associated with high-impact aerobic dance prompted the introduction of low-impact aerobics. The vertical forces and plantar pressures in selected low- and high-impact aerobic movements vs. walking were investigated.

Methods.—Ten subjects, aged 19–29 years, participated in the study. They were asked to walk and to perform 4 aerobic movements over a force and pressure platform. As each subject performed all 5 activities, peak plantar pressure and peak vertical force data were obtained 3 times for the dominant leg.

Findings.—Peak vertical forces on the lower extremities were significantly less during the low-impact aerobic movements than during the high-impact movements. There were no differences between peak vertical forces during walking and during low-impact aerobic movements. Peak plantar pressures for walking did not differ significantly from those in any of the 4 aerobic movements.

Conclusion.—Peak vertical forces acting on the lower extremities are significantly greater during the 2 high-impact aerobic movements studied than in the low-impact movements. Additional research is needed to determine the effect of different aerobic floor surfaces and shoe cushioning properties.

▶ Aerobic dance has been a popular form of exercise for about 25 years. Vigorous aerobic dance, also called high-impact aerobic dance, has been the cause of significant injuries. Consequently, low-impact aerobic dance was developed to reduce the injuries for both instructors and students. The authors of this study used the force platform to measure the vertical forces produced in high-impact aerobics, low-impact aerobics, and walking. As might be expected, the vertical forces were greater for high-impact aerobics and not significantly different for low-impact aerobics and walking. All of the subjects in this study were women. Whether the results are the same if men are involved should also be examined. Our work at West Point indicates that women are more susceptible to overuse impact injuries than are men when both men and women are running under the same conditions. Because of the floor surface (wrestling mats), we have few, if any, overuse injuries in our high-impact aerobic exercise classes.—Col. J.L. Anderson, PE.D.

Muscular Control of the Ankle in Running

Reber L, Perry J, Pink M (Kerlan-Jobe Orthopaedic Clinic, Inglewood, Calif; Centinela Hosp Biomechanics Lab, Inglewood, Calif)
Am J Sports Med 21:805–810, 1993   139-94-6–30

Background.—Half of all running injuries involve musculotendinous problems below the knee. Defining the pathophysiologic processes of these injuries requires a thorough knowledge of the basic biomechanics of running. An electromyographic (EMG) study was conducted in an attempt to describe the firing patterns of the muscles controlling the ankle during running in recreational and competitive distance runners.

Methods.—The patients all ran at least 15 miles/wk and had been injury-free for at least 3 months. They were studied at 3 paces of running, with EMG monitoring of the activity of the gastrocnemius, soleus, peroneus brevis, tibialis posterior, and tibialis anterior muscles by means of fine-wire electrodes. The EMG data were synchronized with the 4 phases of running by high-speed cinematography.

Results.—The posterior muscles demonstrated peak firing activity during the midstance phase. These muscles contracted eccentrically to control ankle dorsiflexion as the center of gravity passed over the ankle; they did not appear to supply power for pushoff. The tibialis anterior muscle was found to fire above the fatigue threshold through 85% of the time during stride, whereas no other muscle fired at this level for more than 50% of the time. Peroneus brevis muscle activity increased dramatically with increasing pace.

Conclusion.—These EMG data suggest that many common running injuries may result from muscular fatigue or overuse of improperly trained muscles. They may prove useful in designing a rational, sport-specific exercise program for runners. The high sustained level of activity of the tibialis anterior muscle may account for its frequent injury in runners. The peroneus brevis muscle appears to have an important role in increasing the pace of running.

▶ The authors of this excellent study used subjects who ran at least 15 miles per week. I wonder whether these data will also hold up for people who are not runners but are required to run, e.g., trainees in the Army or new cadets at West Point. Also, what are the possible gender differences, if any? These authors included 2 female runners within the 15 subjects. Was that because they were certain that there were no gender differences? Our experience with training young men and women indicates that significantly more women will experience injuries such as shinsplints and stress fractures during early training. If we can determine how to prevent these injuries, significant time and money will be saved. This is more critical at this time when all of the military services are considering common training for both men and women.—Col. J.L. Anderson, PE.D.

Function of Mono- and Biarticular Muscles in Running

Jacobs R, Bobbert MF, van Ingen Schenau GJ (Vrije Universiteit, Amsterdam)
Med Sci Sports Exerc 25:1163–1173, 1993   139-94-6-31

Background.—The muscle stretch-shortening cycle refers to a successive occurrence of lengthening and shortening of muscles. Previous studies have suggested that monoarticular muscles are chiefly concerned with the generation of positive work, whereas biarticular muscles control the distribution of net moments and work produced at the joints. Monoarticular muscle inactivity has been noted during cycling, but it is not known whether the same inactivity is present in stretch-shortening cycle activities in which the environment provides the work required for lengthening. For example, in running, the quick stretch of plantar flexors on landing is followed immediately by active shortening in the pushoff. The function of leg muscles during stretch-shortening cycles in fast running was investigated.

Method.—Movement pattern, ground reaction forces, and electromyography (EMG) were recorded for a single stance phase in 7 elite male runners (Fig 6–12). Rough estimates of muscle force, obtained by shifting the EMG curves +90 ms, were correlated with origin-to-insertion velocity. Active state and internal muscle behavior were estimated using a Hill-type muscle model applied for the soleus and gastrocnemius. The

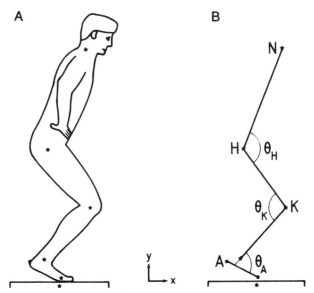

Fig 6–12.—**A,** positions of landmarks applied to the skin of the patient and to the force platform; **B,** definition of angles in joints. N, H, K, and A indicate neck, hip, knee, and ankle, respectively. θ_H, θ_K, and θ_A indicate angles in hip, knee, and ankle joints, respectively. (Courtesy of Jacobs R, Bobbert MF, van Ingen Schenau GJ: *Med Sci Sports Exerc* 25:1163–1173, 1993.)

muscle model simulates internal muscle behavior on the basis of measured EMG and kinematics as a function of time.

Findings.—There were high correlations between estimates of muscle force and origin-to-insertion velocity time curves for monoarticular hip, knee, and extensor muscles. For biarticular muscles, the correlation coefficients were low. The model results showed that the active state of the gastrocnemius was high during the increase of origin-to-insertion length. The active state of the soleus was low during the start of increase of origin-to-insertion length and rose to a plateau when lengthening ended and shortening started. The activation of the soleus may be a compromise between minimizing energy dissipation and using the stretch-shortening cycle optimally. The net plantar flexion moment during running reached a value of 302 Nm, 158% higher than the peak value for maximal jump and 127% higher than peak value for sprint pushoffs. The higher mechanical output in running compared with jumping could be ascribed to the use of the stretch-shortening cycle in running. The higher values for running compared with sprinting may lie in a difference in muscle stimulation.

Summary.—In this study of running, there were high correlations between estimates of muscle force and origin-to-insertion velocity time curves for monoarticular muscles and low correlation coefficients for biarticular muscles. The muscle model predictions demonstrated that the CNS appears to use the advantages of the stretch-shortening cycle. The proposed distinction between monoarticular muscles active in positive work and biarticular muscles responsible for the regulation of the net moments about the joints appears to be only a global distinction.

▶ We must always be careful with such a homogeneous group as elite runners if we want to compare the experimental group with the population as a whole. From the global viewpoint, these findings are satisfactory, but if we want to make them more predictive in a more specific way, the experimental group must be more heterogeneous and selected somewhat randomly.—Col. J.L. Anderson, PE.D.

Kinetics of the Lower Extremities During Drop Landings From Three Heights
McNitt-Gray JL (Univ of Southern California, Los Angeles)
J Biomech 26:1037–1046, 1993   139-94-6-32

Background.—There is a high incidence of soft tissue and bone injuries to the lower extremities of athletes participating in landing activities. One of the most challenging landings comes after the execution of a complex gymnastic skill during competition. Visual conditions and the configurations of the segments before contact may compromise the landing. Additionally, performance guidelines require bringing the velocity of the body to zero with a single placement of the feet. Even with all these constraints, the majority of gymnast landings do not result in injury. The landing preferences of gymnasts and recreational athletes were systematically examined by comparing the kinetics of drop landings performed from 3 heights. The variables representative of the demand placed on the muscles responsible for controlling flexion and dissipating the load were net joint moments and the work done on the extensor muscles of the ankle, knee, and hip.

Method.—The segment motion and ground reaction forces were acquired simultaneously using high-speed film and a force plate. The ground reaction force and kinematic data were used to calculate the joint reaction forces and net joint moments during landing.

Results.—The extensor joint moments peaked earlier after contact with increases in velocity. As impact velocity increased, the temporal sequence of events remained the same, although the time of the peak occurred earlier after contact. The magnitude of the extensor joint moments significantly increased when encountering progressively higher impact velocities. The work done on the extensor muscles of the ankle, knee, and hip was also significantly greater as impact velocity increased in both the gymnasts and recreational athletes. The gymnasts had significantly larger ankle and hip peak extensor moments across velocities than the recreational athletes.

Conclusion.—The kinetics of drop landings change with increases in impact velocity. There was a temporal consistency in kinematic and kinetic events across velocities and groups, although the gymnasts and recreational athletes responded differently to increases in impact velocity. The gymnasts dissipated the loads at contact by using larger ankle and hip extensor moments at higher impact velocities, whereas the recreational athletes used greater degrees of hip flexion. The increase in peak ankle and hip extensor moments used by gymnasts may help maintain balance during competitive gymnastics. The recreational athletes may be unable to produce large extensor moments at the ankle or hip during landings from great heights.

▶ The author used only 6 male gymnasts and 6 male recreational athletes in this study and recognizes that those numbers are too small to apply the results in a universal manner. Another concern is that there were no women included in this investigation. Here at West Point, we have found that there are significant differences in the way female recreational athletes perform during drop landings and the way male recreational athletes perform under similar circumstances. I tend to attribute that to the way they are reared and the greater experience males have when they are growing up. I have not seen any studies comparing male and female competitive athletes, but I intuitively believe they will be more similar in their performance than are the recreational athletes.—Col. J.L. Anderson, PE.D.

Eccentric Muscle Performance of Elbow and Knee Muscle Groups in Untrained Men and Women

Griffin JW, Tooms RE, Vander Zwaag R, Bertorini TE, O'Toole ML (Univ of Tennessee, Memphis)
Med Sci Sports Exerc 25:936–944, 1993   139-94-6-33

Introduction.—Eccentric muscle activity appears to be essential for many everyday activities, yet many aspects of eccentric muscle performance are unclear. There is a particular need for knowledge of expected torque-velocity relationships and eccentric-concentric (CONC) relationships between the sexes as well as between various muscle groups. There are also significant data regarding the relationship of eccentric torque to angular velocity.

Methods.—The maximal voluntary eccentric and CONC capacity of the knee and elbow muscles was studied in a group of 90 healthy, untrained subjects. The 50 women and 40 men ranged in age from 21 to 67 years. The average torque was measured at angular velocities of 30 degrees/sec and 120 degrees/sec from the knee flexor (KF), knee extensor (KE), and elbow flexor (EF) muscle groups unilaterally. Measurements were made by using an isokinetic protocol that included gravity compensation.

Results.—All muscle groups and both sexes showed similar torque-velocity relationships. The eccentric average torque did not change as a function of velocity, and the CONC torque decreased with increasing angular velocity. For women, eccentric torque was greater than CONC torque in both the upper and lower extremity muscle groups. The eccentric/CONC ratios were higher for KE and EF than for KF in both sexes. All muscle groups showed an increasing magnitude of eccentric-CONC differences with increasing angular velocity. For both types of contractions, the men showed higher KF/KE and EF/KF torque ratios than the women.

Conclusion.—This study documents similar torque velocity patterns for eccentric and CONC actions for both sexes in the muscle groups tested. Eccentric torque is greater than CONC torque in women than in men, and the KE and EF muscle groups show a greater capacity for eccentric than for CONC activity in both sexes. These data will be useful in the interpretation of isokinetic testing in untrained adults, as well as in guiding training and rehabilitation programs.

▶ This is an excellent, very comprehensive study that must be read in its entirety for anyone to fully comprehend the amount of data these researchers have generated. Some of the information is not surprising when compared with the work of others. However, a number of these findings call into question some past research or present new information that must be taken seriously. The high quality of this work makes it a study to which we should all pay attention. The authors' findings that women demonstrate greater eccentric relative to CONC capacity than men in upper as well as lower extremity muscle groups may be the beginning of an explanation for the physiologic performance differences between men and women. However, determining the significance of these gender differences to performance must await further studies.—Col. J.L. Anderson, PE.D.

Slow Force Recovery After Long-Duration Exercise: Metabolic and Activation Factors in Muscle Fatigue
Baker AJ, Kostov KG, Miller RG, Weiner MW (Univ of California, San Francisco; California Pacific Med Ctr, San Francisco)
J Appl Physiol 74:2294–2300, 1993   139-94-6-34

Introduction.—Both metabolic and nonmetabolic factors may be involved in the decline in expected force or power output that characterizes muscle fatigue. Studies using brief periods of maximal voluntary contractions (MVCs) have indicated alterations in intracellular metabolites, whereas nonmetabolic factors appeared to play a role in fatigue during longer-duration protocols. The roles of metabolic and nonmetabolic processes in fatigue caused by short-duration exercise (SDE) and long-duration exercise (LDE) protocols were investigated.

Methods.—Seventeen healthy volunteers, 13 men and 4 women, took part in the study. The exercise protocols used were relatively brief and produced similar levels of moderate fatigue. Fatigue, defined as a decrease in MVC force, was induced by isometric contractions of the ankle dorsiflexor muscles. Short-duration exercise consisted of 2 minutes of sustained MCV. The limb was made ischemic to limit oxidative metabolism and to produce a rapid onset of fatigue. Long-duration exercise consisted of 15–20 minutes of nonischemic intermittent maximal contractions to produce a gradual decrease in force. Potential mechanisms of fatigue were studied after exercise and during fatigue from measurements of voluntary, twitch, and tetanic forces. Intracellular metabolites were monitored with ^{31}P-nuclear MR spectroscopy.

Results.—After SDE, fatigue closely correlated with increased inorganic phosphate [P_i]. Approximately 5 minutes after completion of this exercise protocol, both force and [P_i] recovered. Force (voluntary, twitch, and tetanic) recovered more slowly after LDE. Although subjects exhibited significant fatigue beyond 15 minutes after exercise, recovery of [P_i] was not slowed. Neither exercise protocol had any significant effect on electromyographic signals.

Conclusion.—The findings of this study suggest that most of the fatigue from SDE may be attributable to metabolic inhibition of contraction. With LDE, however, there may be a long-lasting nonmetabolic component to fatigue that acts beyond the cell membrane at the level of excitation-contraction coupling. Previous studies have also suggested that impaired excitation-contraction coupling plays a role in the production of long-duration, low-frequency fatigue.

▶ For the purpose of this investigation, the authors used SDE that consisted of 2 minutes of sustained MVC. They defined LDE as 15–20 minutes of intermittent contractions. The authors found that differences in intracellular metabolites resulted from SDE when compared with LDE. For instance, SDE produced a moderate increase in [P_i] as compared with LDE. However, the recovery of [P_i] was not as fast after SDE compared with LDE, although the recovery of force was slower after LDE when compared with SDE. There was no significant difference in recovery of pH when SDE was compared with LDE.—Col. J.L. Anderson, PE.D.

Torque History of Electrically Stimulated Human Quadriceps: Implications for Stimulation Therapy
Lieber RL, Kelly MJ (Univ of California, San Diego; San Diego State Univ, Calif)
J Orthop Res 11:131–141, 1993   139-94-6-35

Objective.—Muscle strengthening is a primary goal of functional neuromuscular electric stimulation (NMES). The time course of knee extension torque was measured in human quadriceps muscles during the transcutaneous application of NMES.

Methods.—Six groups of 15 normal individuals aged 21–35 years were stimulated. Stimulation frequencies of 10, 30, and 50 Hz were combined with duty cycles of 50% and 70%. The subjects were seated in a customized testing apparatus (Fig 6–13) and initially performed a series of maximum voluntary contractions using visual feedback from the chart-recorder. This was followed by 30-minute stimulation sessions.

Results.—The degree of decrease in torque relative to the baseline value differed significantly with both stimulation frequency and the duty cycle. These factors did not themselves interact to a significant degree. Increasing either the frequency or duty cycle led to a more marked reduction in torque. Nevertheless, torque-time integrals, representing total activity, did not differ significantly. Total activity corresponded to approximately 7–14 maximum voluntary contractions. Average torque during stimulation was greatest with the 50 Hz/50% combination and least for the 10 Hz/70% group.

Conclusion.—During transcutaneous NMES, a smaller number of longer lasting contractions led to the highest muscle tension. The absolute levels of torque reached by using NMES are relatively low compared with those produced by voluntary muscular activity.

▶ These authors found that the absolute levels of torque reached by using NMES were relatively low compared with those produced by voluntary con-

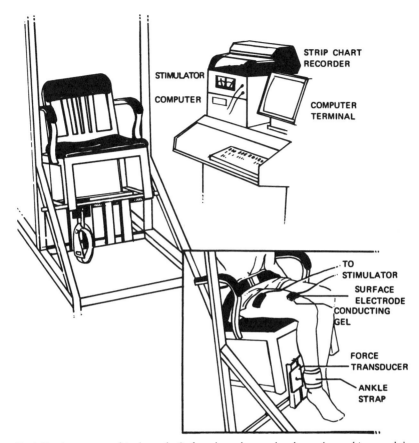

Fig 6–13.—Apparatus used in the study. Surface electrodes are placed over the quadriceps and the ankle is attached to a strap that is connected to a strain gauge (*inset*). Stimulation parameters, timing, and data acquisition are controlled by a computer. (Courtesy of Lieber RL, Kelly MJ: *J Orthop Res* 11:131–141, 1993.)

traction. However, one of our faculty members visited Russia and allowed the scientists at their athletic training institute to demonstrate on him how they use electric stimulation to produce extremely strong contractions of the muscles. Although he was not told how strong the electric stimulation was, he told me that it was very uncomfortable and the contractions produced were very strong. I assume the Russians would not use the most powerful electric stimulation on a visitor, so what they use on their athletes must be something else. Now, however, we should be in a position to get the Russians to share with us more information about their training methods.—Col. J.L. Anderson, PE.D.

Injured Athletes' Attitudes and Judgments Toward Rehabilitation Adherence

Fisher AC, Hoisington LL (Ithaca College, NY; Cornell Univ, Ithaca, NY)
J Athletic Train 28:48–54, 1993   139-94-6–36

Background.—Compliance with treatment, including injury rehabilitation regimens, is very complex. More than 200 variables may influence a patient's adherence to prescribed treatments. Formerly injured and rehabilitated athletes were questioned about factors presumed to affect sport injury rehabilitation adherence.

Methods.—Thirty-six athletes were given the Athletic Injury Rehabilitation Adherence Questionnaire. Results were compared with previously obtained data on athletic trainers' attitudes and judgments toward injury rehabilitation compliance. The 60-item questionnaire had 7 scales: the athletic trainer's influence, environmental effects, athlete's personality, pain tolerance, self-motivation, goals and incentives, and significant others. Four open-ended questions regarding successful and unsuccessful rehabilitation were also included.

Findings.—To the athletes, factors significant in rehabilitation adherence were good rapport and communication between the athletic trainers and injured athletes; support from athletic trainers and coaches; the athlete's self-motivation; and the convenience, accessibility, and flexibility of the rehabilitation facility and staff. Generally, the responses of the athletes and the athletic trainers were similar. Differences were in the areas of self-motivation, pain tolerance, education regarding injury and rehabilitation exercises, and degree of realistic feedback. Athletes' answers to open-ended questions stressed the importance of rapport, communication, and support. Athletes clearly did not like athletic trainers' threats and scare tactics.

Conclusion.—Athletes' responses on this questionnaire generally mirrored the responses of the athletic trainers. A primary factor in athletes' adherence to treatment is athletic trainer–athlete rapport. Although athletes' self-motivation seems to be more important than athletic trainers believed, it alone is not enough to ensure adherence in all cases.

▶ Many factors influence an injured athlete's compliance with rehabilitation programs. In this study, it was noted that athletes and athletic trainers agree on which are the most important factors. Athletic trainers who are looked upon as caring and supportive will achieve better compliance from their athletes. Good rapport with injured athletes is very important. Athletes believe that self-motivation plays an important role in their rehabilitation. They also believe that "the convenience, accessibility and flexibility of the rehabilitation facility and staff" are important. Student athletes have significant demands put on their time schedule and an accommodating athletic training staff and facility will play an important role in their rehabilitation.—F.J. George, A.T.C., P.T.

Enhancing Athletic Injury Rehabilitation Adherence
Fisher AC, Scriber KC, Matheny ML, Alderman MH, Bitting LA (Ithaca College, NY)
J Athletic Train 28:312–318, 1993   139-94-6-37

Introduction.—Successful rehabilitation is based on a partnership between the athletic trainer and the athlete. Athletes must understand the nature of their injury and its treatment as well as the outlook. They need help in dealing with uncertainty as well as feelings of guilt, anger, and loss of control. It is important that the athlete be able to do something about his or her condition.

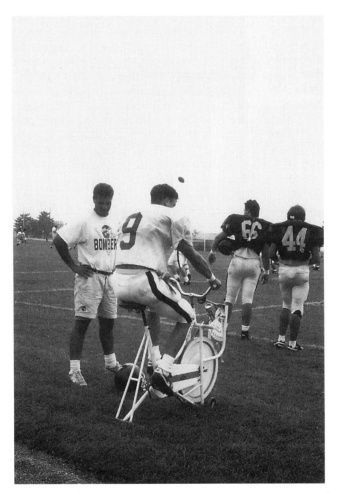

Fig 6–14.—Injured athlete using a bicycle ergometer on the practice field. (Courtesy of Fisher AC, Scriber KC, Matheny ML, et al: *J Athletic Train* 28:312–318, 1993.)

Education and Communication.—Athletes differ in how much information they wish to have. Training in preventing relapses should begin at an early stage. Adherence with management must be viewed as an ongoing process, not an all-or-nothing phenomenon. When asked by the athlete how long he or she can expect to be inactive, it is appropriate to ask in turn how prepared the athlete is to work at rehabilitation. The outcome of rehabilitation depends not merely on the athlete's character, but to an important degree on the quality of the healing environment created by how the trainer and athlete interact. It is important at all times for the trainer's responses to be specific, clear, detailed, and simple, and for the trainer to repeat important information when appropriate. Oral and written material should be used together. The trainer should be well acquainted with the position the athlete plays, the athlete's role on the team, and the upcoming schedule of events.

Support, Goal-Setting, and Progress.—The trainer can marshall support for the injured athlete from coaches and teammates. Using a bicycle ergometer or resistive equipment on the practice field will limit the psychosocial distance between the athlete and the sports environment (Fig 6–14). Treatment should be criteria-based; it is helpful to the athlete if specific functional progressions serve as criteria for return to participation. Goal attainment should be recorded on a regular basis. Goals may have to be reassessed. The athlete should feel some responsibility to his or her teammates and coaches as well as to himself or herself. Threats and ultimatums are not very constructive.

▶ In this article and the previous one (Abstract 139-94-6–36), the point was made that neither threats nor ultimatums should be a part of the athletic trainer's approach to an injured athlete; they are only counterproductive. In this article, the authors stress how important it is to know the injured athlete and the athlete's status on the team. Communication with the athlete and coach are very important. Another good idea I plan to incorporate into my rehabilitation program is to bring a stationary bike and other portable rehabilitation equipment to the playing field. The injured athlete will thus maintain some aerobic fitness and will feel more a part of the team. It can be quite devastating to an injured athlete's psyche to stand by, day after day, just watching his or her teammates hard at practice.—F.J. George, A.T.C., P.T.

Contribution of Rectus Femoris and Vasti to Knee Extension: An Electromyographic Study
Salzman A, Torburn L, Perry J (Rancho Los Amigos Med Ctr, Downey, Calif)
Clin Orthop 290:236–243, 1993   139-94-6–38

Background.—Few electromyogram (EMG) studies have related the movement of the 5 components of the quadriceps muscle during isometric knee extension to knee- and hip-angle variations. Activity of the individual quadriceps components may be measured by an intramuscular

EMG. The contribution of the rectus femoris and the 4 vasti to knee extension during maximal isometric contraction was investigated.

Methods.—Eleven normal volunteers without a history of knee injury or knee pathology participated in the study. The EMG signals were measured through fine-wire electrodes inserted into the vastus medialis oblique, vastus medialis longus, vastus lateralis, vastus intermedius, and rectus femoris. Each subject performed a 5-second maximal, voluntary isometric knee extension with the hip at 0, 40, and 80 degrees of flexion and with the knee at 15 or 60 degrees of flexion. The subjects rested for 4 minutes between contractions.

Results.—The EMG activity did not differ statistically significantly among the different muscles at any position tested, and the mean composite EMG for all vasti did not differ significantly from that of the rectus femoris. The greatest intersubject variability in EMG intensity occurred in the vastus lateralis. The coefficient of variation was greater for this muscle than for the other 4 muscles. For each of the 5 muscles, the mean EMG activity was highest at 40 degrees of hip flexion and 15 degrees of knee flexion. In all subjects, knee extension torques were significantly greater at 60 degrees of knee flexion than at 15 degrees of knee flexion in all 3 hip positions. Hip position did not significantly affect knee extension torque at 60 degrees of knee flexion.

Conclusion.—The vasti do not work in isolation from the rectus femoris during maximal knee extension. Because the vasti and rectus femoris were all active during each maximal isometric knee extension test, they may be strengthened in many different positions. Forty degrees of hip flexion and 15 degrees of knee flexion may be the most effective position for strengthening, because this position produced the greatest amount of EMG activity. Finally, maximal isometric knee extension torque depends on both the knee and hip position only when the knee is in a low range of flexion.

▶ Is it intuitively obvious that the position that causes muscles to produce the greatest amount of EMG activity is also the most effective position for strengthening the muscle? What about over the full range of movement? Are isometric contractions more effective in producing strength over the full range than isotonic movements? I agree with the authors; this requires more study.—Col. J.L. Anderson, PE.D.

Comparison of Tibiofemoral Joint Forces During Open-Kinetic-Chain and Closed-Kinetic-Chain Exercises
Lutz GE, Palmitier RA, An KN, Chao EYS (Mayo Clinic and Found, Rochester, Minn)
J Bone Joint Surg (Am) 75-A:732–739, 1993   139-94-6-39

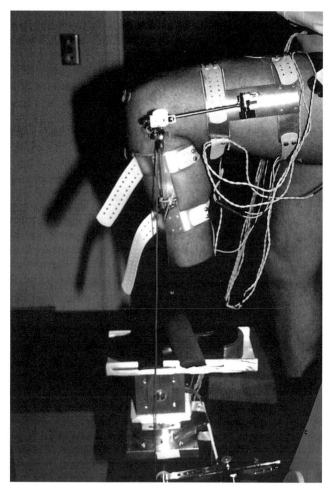

Fig 6–15.—Photograph of a patient being tested while mounted on the loading platform during closed-kinetic-chain leg-press exercise with use of a modified Cybex-II dynamometer and the 3-component load-cell and torque sensor. (Courtesy of Lutz GE, Palmitier RA, An KN, et al: *J Bone Joint Surg (Am)* 74-A:732–739, 1993.)

Background.—Two types of strengthening exercises are used to rehabilitate the knee. In closed-kinetic-chain exercises such as the squat and leg-press, the foot is fixed and motion at the knee joint is accompanied by motion at the hip and ankle joints. In open-kinetic-chain exercises such as leg extension and the leg-curl, the foot is mobile and motion at the knee is independent of motion at the hip and ankle joints. To adequately protect the operated knee, it is necessary to precisely estimate the strain on the anterior cruciate ligament during various types of strengthening exercise.

Moving?

I'd like to receive my *Year Book of Sports Medicine* without interruption.
Please note the following change of address, effective:

Name: _____

New Address: _____

_____

City: _____ State: _____ Zip: _____

Old Address: _____

_____

City: _____ State: _____ Zip: _____

Reservation Card

Yes, I would like my own copy of *Year Book of Sports Medicine*. Please begin my subscription with the current edition according to the terms described below.* I understand that I will have 30 days to examine each annual edition. If satisfied, I will pay just $64.95 plus sales tax, postage and handling (price subject to change without notice).

Name: _____

Address: _____

City: _____ State: _____ Zip: _____

Method of Payment
○ Visa   ○ Mastercard   ○ AmEx   ○ Bill me   ○ Check (in US dollars, payable to Mosby, Inc.)

Card number: _____ Exp date: _____

Signature: _____

LS-0909

*Your *Year Book* Service Guarantee:

When you subscribe to the *Year Book*, we'll send you an advance notice of future volumes about two months before they publish. This automatic notice system is designed to take up as little of your time as possible. If you do not want the *Year Book*, the advance notice makes it quick and easy for you to let us know your decision, and you will always have at least 20 days to decide. If we don't hear from you, we'll send you the new volume as soon as it's available. And, of course, the *Year Book* is yours to examine free of charge for 30 days (postage, handling and applicable sales tax are added to each shipment.).

BUSINESS REPLY MAIL

FIRST CLASS MAIL   PERMIT No. 762   CHICAGO, IL

POSTAGE WILL BE PAID BY ADDRESSEE

Chris Hughes
Mosby-Year Book, Inc.
200 N. LaSalle Street
Suite 2600
Chicago, IL 60601-9981

NO POSTAGE
NECESSARY
IF MAILED
IN THE
UNITED STATES

BUSINESS REPLY MAIL

FIRST CLASS MAIL   PERMIT No. 762   CHICAGO, IL

POSTAGE WILL BE PAID BY ADDRESSEE

Chris Hughes
Mosby-Year Book, Inc.
200 N. LaSalle Street
Suite 2600
Chicago, IL 60601-9981

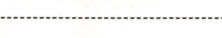

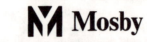

Dedicated to publishing excellence

Objective.—The tibiofemoral joint forces were analyzed during open-kinetic-chain and closed-kinetic-chain exercise in 5 healthy subjects, 4 men and 1 woman. Their mean age was 29 years.

Methods.—A Cybex-II isokinetic dynamometer was used as a loading apparatus, with a foot-plate mounted on top of a torque and load-cell attached to the machine (Fig 6–15). Maximum isometric contractions were performed at 30, 60, and 90 degrees of knee flexion. Electromyograms were recorded from the quadriceps and hamstring muscles. A 2-dimensional biomechanical model was used to calculate the tibiofemoral shear and compression forces.

Results.—Closed-kinetic-chain exercise produced significantly lower posterior shear force than did open-kinetic-chain extension exercise at all knee angles. In addition, it produced significantly less anterior shear force than did open-kinetic-chain flexion exercise, except at 30 degrees of knee flexion. The reduced shear forces were a result of a more axial orientation of applied force as well as muscular co-contraction. Only at 30 degrees of knee flexion did closed-kinetic-chain exercise produce significantly more tibiofemoral compression force. An analysis of electromyographic recruitment patterns showed that closed-kinetic-chain exercise produced more muscular co-contraction at the same angles at which open-kinetic-chain exercise produced minimal co-contraction.

Implication.—These findings support the use of closed-kinetic-chain exercise rather than open-kinetic-chain exercise in rehabilitation after injury or reconstruction of the anterior cruciate ligament.

▶ I can remember that not too many years ago we were all using isometric open-kinetic-chain exercises in rehabilitation after surgery for reconstruction of the anterior cruciate ligament. However, the scientific rationale provided by the results of this study seems compelling. I must say, however, that in our program I do not remember that we had any or many problems in rehabilitation using isometric open-kinetic-chain exercise.—Col. J.L. Anderson, PE.D.

Cryotherapy and Sequential Exercise Bouts Following Cryotherapy on Concentric and Eccentric Strength in the Quadriceps
Ruiz DH, Myrer JW, Durrant E, Fellingham GW (West Virginia Univ, Morgantown; Brigham Young Univ, Provo, Utah)
J Athletic Train 28:320–323, 1993   139-94-6–40

Purpose.—Studies of the effects of cryotherapy on strength have mainly addressed isometric contractions and have given conflicting results. If there are any strength deficits after the application of cold, they could affect the athlete's performance if he or she is allowed to return to competition. The immediate effects of cryotherapy on concentric and eccentric quadriceps strength were defined and the effects of sequential bouts of exercise and the delayed effects of cryotherapy on strength were examined.

Methods.—The 2-stage study included 19 young male wrestlers who participated in 4 sequences in randomly assigned order: ice and exercise, ice and rest, no ice and exercise, and no ice and rest. A kinetic communicator was used to gather data on concentric and eccentric quadriceps strength before exercise, immediately after treatment, and 20 and 40 minutes after treatment.

Results.—Immediately after 25 minutes of cryotherapy to the right quadriceps, both concentric and eccentric strength were reduced significantly. Cryotherapy had a significant delayed effect on eccentric but not concentric strength. Recovery of eccentric strength was unaffected by exercise, whereas recovery of concentric strength was significantly enhanced by exercise.

Conclusion.—Athletes who undergo cryotherapy immediately before competition may have decreased strength and, therefore, decreased ability to perform. Moderate exercise may help hasten postcryotherapy decrements in concentric strength. Further studies are needed to clarify the differences between concentric and eccentric strength in delayed response to cryotherapy and exercise.

▶ Very often we see an athlete remove an ice pack from an injury and immediately return to participation. This study indicates that a warm-up period may be necessary before the athlete has attained full strength. It also indicates that moderate exercise helped the recovery of concentric but not eccentric strength values. Since reading this study, I have not allowed an athlete to return to activity immediately after using an ice pack.—F.J. George, A.T.C., P.T.

Biomechanical Principles of Resistance Training
Lander J (Life College)
ICA Review May/June:35–39, 1993   139-94-6–41

Objective.—In discussing the biomechanical principles of resistance training, the author considers 3 topics: exercising the right muscles, training in the most efficient manner, and the effect of technique on safety.

Appropriate Muscles.—A knowledge of kinesiology, the application of anatomy to exercise science, can tell you what muscles you are working. A burning sensation in a muscle, for example, may just indicate fatigue rather than that the muscle is being trained for size or strength. In contrast, certain exercises may be accomplishing the goals of training even though they may not "feel" that way. Many exercises are prone to "technique abuse," including the low-lat-pull, or rowing. If done improperly, this exercise may involve little effort from the muscles it is designed to train: the upper back, the back of the shoulder, and the latissimus dorsi.

Training Efficiently.—Newton's 3 laws of motion can be applied to weight training. When lifting a bar, for example, the "inertial" forces that may increase or decrease the "effective weight" of the bar must be considered. The athlete must perform as explosively as possible on the way up, then lower the bar in a slow, smooth, and methodical manner. The maximal effort involved in lifting allows the bar to weigh more and less according to the strong points and weak points of the muscles, whereas the slow movement involved in lowering lessens the inertial forces at the bottom of the lift. Bars that are rather light in weight should also be lifted in a slow and smooth manner so that the bar will not become ballistic.

Technique and Safety.—The use of proper technique is the single most effective means of avoiding traumatic injury. Because sloppy technique occurs when fatigue increases, the last few repetitions of each set require special concentration and the use of a spotter. Chronic injuries resulting from poor technique are even more insidious. Individuals who perform resistance training should know how to read the body's obvious warning signals and respond to them before they become chronic problems of even greater importance.

▶ The author stresses the importance of using proper technique to prevent injury. Athletes must be coached and supervised in using proper strength training techniques just as they are on the field or court. Too often they are left on their own, competing in maximal lifts against one another and ending up with an injury. A good strength coach is a valuable asset to an athlete's training program. They are knowledgeable individuals who can instruct and supervise an athlete's conditioning program. Beware of noncertified individuals who claim to be training gurus. They often cause more harm than good.—F.J. George, A.T.C., P.T.

Strength Training and the Immature Athlete: An Overview
Metcalf JA, Roberts SO (George Mason Univ, Fairfax, Va; Lovelace Med Ctr)
Pediatr Nurs 19(4):325–332, 1993   139-94-6–42

Background.—It is estimated that at least 20 million children participate in competitive sports each year. Most earlier studies advised against weight training for young athletes because their developing bones and muscles are vulnerable to injury. However, recent studies have shown that properly supervised weight training in prepubescent and adolescent athletes produces important strength gains. The benefits and safety considerations of resistance training in young athletes were examined.

Review.—The methods of resistance training used in the above-cited studies included isometrics, free weights, weight machines, sport activities, and calisthenics. Although the data showed that resistance training in young athletes does increase strength, other factors also affect the outcomes of an athletic training program. These factors include the child's gender, age, percentage of lean body mass, and plasma hormone levels. To minimize the risk of injury in children who participate in resistance training programs, the following recommendations have been proposed: obtain medical clearance; provide proper supervision at all times; do not allow children to exercise unless the weight training facility is safe for them; never allow children to perform single maximal lifts or sudden explosive movements; do not allow competition with other children; teach children how to breath properly during exercise movements; never allow the use of broken or damaged equipment; encourage the intake of plenty of fluids before, during, and after exercise; and ensure that children tell their coach, parent, or teacher when they feel tired or when they have been injured. Power lifting or competitive lifting to determine the maximum amount of weight a child can lift is contraindicated.

Conclusion.—Proper strength training improves the athletic performance of immature athletes and reduces their risk of injury to vulnerable growing bones and muscles.

▶ Should young children lift weights to increase strength and improve performance? Only if they do so with proper and constant supervision and instruction. That is much easier said than done. Too often the instruction and supervision of young athletes are totally inadequate. The author has listed safety considerations and principles of resistance training for young athletes. These must be closely adhered to if the experience is to be safe and beneficial.—F.J. George, A.T.C., P.T.

Abdominal Muscle Training in Sport
Norris CM (Norris Associates, Altrincham, Cheshire, England)
Br J Sports Med 27:19–27, 1993   139-94-6–43

Introduction.—Abdominal strengthening exercises are popular in both fitness training and sport. Such exercises can be dangerous to the spine, however, if performed incorrectly. Several commonly used abdominal exercises were studied, and factors affecting their safety and effectiveness were examined.

Abdominal Muscles.—Four major muscles make up the abdominal wall—the rectus abdominis, external oblique, internal oblique, and transversus abdominis. The rectus abdominis flexes the trunk by approximating the pelvis and ribcage. In twisting actions, the external oblique rotates the trunk to the opposite side and the internal oblique rotates it to the same side. Both the internal oblique and transversus protect the inguinal canal and are continuously active in standing. The iliopsoas is also included in the discussion because of its effect on the lumbar spine during trunk exercise; its function is mainly hip flexion, with slight adduction.

Kinesiologic Analysis.—The trunk curl, consisting of flexion of the trunk without hip flexion, can impose extra stress on the oblique abdominals if the trunk is rotated. In a sit-up exercise, the abdominal muscles may be too weak to fix the pelvis of subjects in poor physical condition. In such cases, the iliopsoas can pull the lumbar spine into dangerous hyperextension. When foot fixation is used during a sit-up, greater hyperextension will occur and, thus, an increased likelihood of injury to the lumbar spine. Because of stress on the lumbar spine, severely deconditioned subjects should choose the trunk curl exercise over the bent-knee sit-up. The leg lowering movement and the bench-lying pelvic raise are modifications of the straight leg raise that reduce stress on the lumbar spine. An imbalance of strength and/or flexibility between the various trunk and hip muscles often occurs. Such an imbalance is associated with an alteration of pelvic tilt and a reduction in range of spinal flexion.

Recommendations.—Rapid, full change flexion exercises on the lumbar spine are not advised because of their potential to stress the posterior structures excessively. Such stress may ultimately lead to hypermobility and facet degeneration. Abdominal muscle training should reflect the requirements of a particular sport and an athlete's individual needs. Neither the sit-up performed with foot fixation nor the bilateral straight leg raise are recommended. A midrange lumbar position is desirable during exercise, and the use of proprioceptive training during balance activities is beneficial.

▶ The author cautions us that some exercises designed to strengthen abdominal muscles may be dangerous to the spine. For a number of years we have been using a bent-knee curl-up as our basic abdominal strengthener. We have found this exercise to be a safe and very effective abdominal strengthener. This was reported in the YEAR BOOK OF SPORTS MEDICINE in 1989, 1991, and 1992. The following is a summarization of how the exercise is performed.

1. The athlete lies supine with the knees bent and the feet flat on the floor (hook lying position).
2. The arms are folded across the upper chest.
3. The lower back is flat (pelvic tilt).
4. A curl-up or partial sit-up is done and held for a count of 6. The shoulders are raised about 12 in. off the floor. The chin is brought to the chest in a curling motion.

There are related abstracts and figures in the 1989, 1991, and 1992 YEAR BOOK OF SPORTS MEDICINE (1–3). —F.J. George, A.T.C., P.T.

References

1. 1989 YEAR BOOK OF SPORTS MEDICINE, pp 221–222.

2. 1991 YEAR BOOK OF SPORTS MEDICINE, pp 325–330.
3. 1992 YEAR BOOK OF SPORTS MEDICINE, pp 291–292.

The Warm-Up Procedure: To Stretch or Not to Stretch. A Brief Review
Smith CA (Cape Town, South Africa)
J Orthop Sports Phys Ther 19:12–17, 1994   139-94-6-44

Introduction.—It is an unwritten law of exercise among both elite and casual exercisers that a warm-up is essential for the success of any exercise program. Stretching is widely considered to be an important part of the pre-exercise warm-up, necessary to promote fitness, assure flexibility, and prevent injury. Many authorities recommend stretching before exercising, but some believe that it can do more harm than good and that stretching itself may cause injury.

Physiology of Stretching.—The muscle spindle that is attached to intrafusal and extrafusal muscle fibers is sensitive to active or passive stretch and helps to control the dynamic length of the muscle. Stretch receptors in the tendons are sensitive to tension and help prevent overstretching. There is evidence that both muscles and tendons act viscoelastically in response to stretch. Stretching a single muscle or a group of muscles appears to promote relaxation and lower tension in the muscle-tendon unit, allowing further stretching.

Method.—Ballistic stretching entails repeated bouncing movements in the lengthened position of the muscle; there is a risk of injury because muscle tension is increased. Static stretching involves a slow stretch that is held for up to 1 minute. The inverse stretch reflex comes into play, permitting further lengthening and greater flexibility. Proprioceptive neuromuscular facilitation applies the concepts of reflex activation and inhibition through a "contract-relax" procedure. A similar technique, termed "reciprocal relaxation," involves contraction of the agonist muscle at the end of the antagonist's range.

A Proposed Routine.—A program of stretching suitable for the activity in question should be part of the warm-up; it should last at least 15 minutes and be repeated after exercising. Slow static stretching is best, lasting 15–20 seconds and avoiding bouncing movements. Stretching should end short of pain. Each muscle group is stretched 3–5 times. Agonists and antagonists and both extremities are stretched alternately. A routine that is enjoyable will not become unduly burdensome.

► The author refers to some basic principles of stretching that should be adhered to. To avoid injury, only warm muscles should be stretched and ballistic-type movements should be avoided. Stretching should not put extreme pressure on any joint or tendon attachments. The goal of stretching should be to increase the length of the *muscle*. Stretching at the end of a workout can be beneficial and have a carry-over effect for the next workout. A slow static stretch held for 20 seconds and repeated 3 times is considered to be a safe and effective method of stretching.—F.J. George, A.T.C., P.T.

Review of the Afferent Neural System of the Knee and Its Contribution to Motor Learning
Nyland J, Brosky T, Currier D, Nitz A, Caborn D (Univ of Kentucky, Lexington)
J Orthop Sports Phys Ther 19:2–11, 1994   139-94-6-45

Background.—The traditional approach to rehabilitation has paid little attention to the functional influences of afferent neural structures and their contribution to motor learning. Closed-kinetic-chain functional training uses the afferent neural system of the knee, providing a more effective means of rehabilitating an injured or reconstructed knee.

Closed-Kinetic-Chain Functional Training.—The lower extremity kinetic chain is made up of the hip, knee, and ankle joints. A closed kinetic chain exists when the terminal joint of several successively arranged joints meets with external resistance, restricting its free motion. Closed-kinetic-chain functional training involves functional exercise activities that are in agreement with this definition. Through the synchronous recruitment of hip, knee, and ankle musculature, closed-kinetic-chain functional training makes use of the specificity-of-training principle. This principle implies that patients who include closed-kinetic-chain functional training during rehabilitation should perform more effectively. Recent studies have shown closed-kinetic-chain functional training to be the only method of reproducing the concurrent shift of antagonistic, biarticular muscle groups that occurs during the simultaneous hip, knee, and ankle actions of locomotion. Closed-kinetic-chain functional training also permits the problem-solving component of motor learning to create situations that gradually approximate actual sports performance.

The progression from slow, unresisted activities to quick movements against resistance brings engram patterning of the motor planning region of the cerebral cortex. Engram patterning, in turn, promotes neural adaptations (improved agonistic muscle recruitment, antagonist muscle inhibition, and motor unit recruitment synchronization). These adaptations are encouraged by the integration of afferent neural input, such as that provided by the mechanoreceptors of the knee. If clinicians progressively alter specific movement tasks and environments, thereby altering overall afferent neural system input, they can facilitate task-specific adaptations in efferent neural system activity. These adaptations take place as the motor planning region of the cerebral cortex integrates and modulates widely ranging stimuli to produce coordinated task-specific locomotor synergies. Sensorimotor adaptability is essential for posture control and for the control of movement within a given posture.

Conclusion.—The afferent neural system of the knee is of great importance in rehabilitation. The intricate relationship that exists between peripheral mechanoreceptors found in the inert and contractile tissues of the knee should not be ignored during treatment planning. Traditional rehabilitation methods do not effectively exploit afferent neural input from the knee or make full use of motor learning concepts. Closed-kinetic-chain functional training allows for task-specific applications, speed/intensity manipulation, and easy incorporation of motor learning concepts.

▶ Closed-kinetic-chain exercises have become a big part of most rehabilitation programs. Many of us started using these exercises without sufficient scientific data to support their acceptance. Abstracts such as this add supporting evidence to our use of these exercises and should encourage further experimentation in this area. Recently, we have moved to these types of exercises in our upper extremity rehabilitation program and in our low back stabilization program. In most cases, our final goal is to return the athlete to normal function or a previous level of function. Why not incorporate exercises that will achieve this goal?—F.J. George, A.T.C., P.T.

Electromyographic Evaluation of Closed and Open Kinetic Chain Knee Rehabilitation Exercises

Graham VL, Gehlsen GM, Edwards JA (Ball State Univ, Muncie, Ind)
J Athletic Train 28:23–30, 1993   139-94-6–46

Background.—Recently, authorities have advocated using closed-kinetic-chain knee rehabilitation exercises. The main reason for using these exercises is that they produce less anteroposterior shear force at the knee joint than traditional open-kinetic-chain exercises. The electromyographic (EMG) activity ratio of quadriceps to hamstrings in several exercises was investigated.

Methods and Findings.—Ten female student athletes were studied while performing unilateral one quarter squats, leg extensions, lateral step-ups, and movements on the Fitter, Stairmaster 4000, and slideboard. Electromyographic surface electrodes were placed over the biceps and rectus femoris muscles. Data were obtained from 3 trials. Baseline EMG activity was used to calculate the percentage of maximum EMG activity in each exercise. Significant differences among exercises were noted for range of motion, maximum angle, percent of maximum contraction, time of contraction, and total EMG.

Conclusion.—When choosing an exercise regimen for individuals with anterior cruciate ligament injury, clinicians need to consider safety (minimizing anteroposterior shear forces) and the efficacy of the exercise in strengthening appropriate muscle groups. The closed-kinetic-chain exercises studied resulted in minimal anteroposterior shear forces at the knee joint. These exercises seem to be appropriate and effective for improving quadriceps and hamstring strength. The exercise program needs to be monitored closely to increase range of motion and resistance as tolerable for the individual to achieve the best results. Selecting an effective combination of exercises is equally important.

▶ As I stated after Abstract 139-94-6–45, we have been searching for scientific data to support our switch to closed-chain exercises. This study indicates that closed-chain exercises are safer for anterior cruciate ligament rehabilitation programs because they produce less anteroposterior shear on the knee than do conventional exercises. These exercises do improve quadriceps and hamstring strength. However, we have included resistance and weight training closed-chain exercises to improve their effectiveness.—F.J. George, A.T.C., P.T.

Squat Board
O'Neil GD, Malacrea RF, Brenner JW (Princeton Univ, NJ)
J Athletic Train 28:31–33, 1993   139-94-6–47

Background.—Closed-kinetic-chain exercise—such as squats, lunges, step-ups, and heel raises—plays a major role in early lower extremity rehabilitation. Compared with open-kinetic-chain exercise, closed-kinetic-chain exercise facilitates a tricontraction of knee-stabilizing muscles, elicits a variety of muscle contractions in 1 movement, and places less strain on the anterior cruciate ligament. The squat board was developed to permit overload at certain sites while avoiding the problems of awkward positioning and potential for injury that can result with free weights, elastic tubing, and elastic bands.

The Squat Board.—The squat board is an exercise platform constructed of a 36 × 46 × .75-in. plywood top over a 2 × 4-in. baseframe. Rubber tubes attach to a waist belt and to the squat board. Differing lengths of rubber tubing permit a regular progression of resistance, with a change from longer to shorter lengths as rehabilitation progresses. The waist belt places resistance directly below the center of gravity, eliminating stress on the upper extremity and torso (Fig 6–16). Athletes perform squats, lunges, step-ups, and heel raises on the squat board.

Conclusion.—The squat board, used with a waist belt and rubber tubing, is an excellent, inexpensive piece of equipment for closed-kinetic-chain exercise. Athletes can use the squat board as a daily training tool because the different lengths of rubber tubing offer increasing resistance. The squat board permits overloads at appropriate sites with the simplicity of an exercise platform, the versatility of rubber tubing, and the convenience of a waist belt.

▶ As I stated after Abstract 139-94-6–46, some type of resistance must be added to closed-chain exercises if they are designed to increase strength. The squat board is an ideal apparatus for achieving resistance when doing

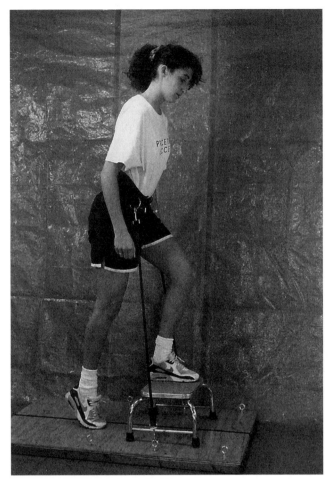

Fig 6–16.—Front step-ups on the squat board. (Courtesy of O'Neil GD, Malacrea RF, Brenner JW: *J Athletic Train* 28:31-33, 1993.)

closed-chain exercises. It is safe, inexpensive, and effective. It should be a part of most closed-chain lower extremity rehabilitation programs.—F.J. George, A.T.C., P.T.

The Role of Limb Torque, Muscle Action and Proprioception During Closed Kinetic Chain Rehabilitation of the Lower Extremity
Bunton EE, Pitney WA, Kane AW, Cappaert TA (American Rehabilitation Network, Southgate, Mich; Eastern Michigan Univ, Ypsilanti)
J Athletic Train 28:10–20, 1993   139-94-6–48

Background.—In the past decade, isokinetic exercises have become the treatment of choice for lower limb rehabilitation. However, closed-kinetic-chain exercises appear to have advantages over open-kinetic-chain exercises. The differences between these exercises and the role of limb torque, muscle action, and proprioception during rehabilitation were analyzed.

Kinematic Chains.—"Kinematic chain" refers to a series of links in a mechanical system. In human beings, it is a combination of successively linked motor segments. In closed-chain movements, the extremity is fixed in a kinematic system, and a predictable pattern of motion in other segments occurs. Open-chain systems consist of end segments freely moving in space, not necessarily resulting in predictable movement from another segment.

Limb Torque.—Segmental torque elements are transmitted through the distal extremity to the subtalar joint. In the closed chain, the subtalar joint acts as a torque converter of the lower leg and attenuates transverse plane rotation. Open-chain exercises allow much of the torque produced by the quadriceps to be absorbed by the patellofemoral joint. Closed-chain exercises reduce patellofemoral joint forces.

Muscle Action.—The dynamics of muscle action enable complex, unconscious acceleration and deceleration of the lower limb during locomotion in the sagittal, frontal, and transverse planes. Weight, terrain, joint hypermobility and hypomobility, and ground reaction forces influence these tasks. Limb abnormalities can markedly influence gait performance. In closed-chain exercises, muscle actions can be significantly affected and result in abnormal compensations.

Proprioception.—In theory, a closed-kinetic-chain progression of slow to faster motions against resistance results in CNS engram patterning when the emphasis is on precision of movement. If open-chain progression is used when the development of muscle strength and girth is essential and the proprioceptors are neglected, patients may complain of the knee or ankle giving out, even though noticeable gains in strength and size are achieved. Proprioception is very important in a rehabilitation program.

Conclusion.—The ultimate goal of closed-chain exercise is to improve proprioception, thereby building lower extremity stability when an unpredictable change in direction or speed occurs. The CNS must be held accountable for controlling external forces if movements are to be performed accurately. Proprioception, therefore, plays an integral part in rehabilitation.

▶ Proprioception plays a major role in rehabilitation programs. The need for increasing proprioception-type exercises brought about, for many of us, our first uses of closed-chain exercises. Our initial goal in using closed-chain exercises was to improve proprioception. We later expanded their use to improve range of motion and strength. We often encounter a strong ankle with normal range of motion and no joint laxity, yet the athlete complains of frequent episodes of the ankle giving out. The problem is, in many cases, loss of proprioception. Specific closed-chain exercises must be done to regain the lost proprioception.—F.J. George, A.T.C., P.T.

Effect of a Lateral Step-Up Exercise Protocol on Quadriceps and Lower Extremity Performance

Worrell TW, Borchert B, Erner K, Fritz J, Leerar P (Univ of Indianapolis, Ind)
J Orthop Sports Phys Ther 18:646–653, 1993   139-94-6–49

Introduction.—Some authors recommend closed-kinetic-chain exercises as a more functional and appropriate alternative to open-kinetic-chain exercises. However, a review of the literature reveals few research data on the effects of closed-kinetic-chain exercise on the performance of the quadriceps muscles and the lower extremity.

Methods.—This study sought to determine the effect of a lateral step-up exercise program on isokinetic quadriceps peak torque and various lower extremity activities. These activities were leg press, maximal step-up repetitions at 125% of body weight (Fig 6–17), hop for distance, and

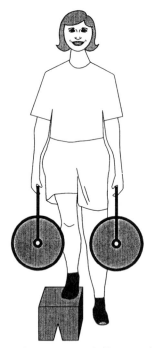

Fig 6–17.—Lateral step-up exercise for training period. (Courtesy of Worrell TW, Borchert B, Erner K, et al: *J Orthop Sports Phys Ther* 18:646-653, 1993.)

6-m timed hop. Twenty volunteers followed a 4-week lateral step-up exercise protocol; another 18 subjects served as controls.

Results.—Performance on the leg press, step-up exercises, hop for distance, and hop for time all improved significantly in the exercise group, with no significant increase in isokinetic quadriceps peak torque. During the 4-week exercise period, the weight used for the step-up exercise increased as repetitions decreased and step-up work remained unchanged. The control subjects showed no significant change in any of the variables studied.

Conclusion.—This research study suggests that lower extremity performance in healthy subjects is improved by a 4-week regimen of closed-kinetic-chain exercise. These improvements occur with no significant change in isokinetic quadriceps peak torque. The latter finding is an important one, as isokinetic values are commonly used in deciding on return to functional activity.

▶ Here are more scientific data to support the use of closed-kinetic-chain exercises. These studies are a must, especially when they address a problem such as an increase in function with no apparent change in isokinetic quadriceps peak torque. As the author states, many of us use isokinetic testing to determine levels of achieved rehabilitation. On-the-field testing must be done before a return to high-level activity can be approved.—F.J. George, A.T.C., P.T.

Control of Whole Body Balance in the Frontal Plane During Human Walking
MacKinnon CD, Winter DA (Univ of Toronto; Univ of Waterloo, Ont, Canada)
J Biomech 26:633–644, 1993   139-94-6-50

Background.—Maintaining balance and posture while walking constitutes a complex problem in motor control. Frontal plane balance is especially difficult. The narrow base of support in the single support phase mandates precise control of the trajectory of the center of mass (CM). Maintaining frontal plane balance entails regulating the balance of the head, arms, and trunk about the supporting hip, as well as balancing the total body CM about the supporting foot. Pelvic lateral tilt is an important determinant of gait, but how it is regulated remains uncertain.

Objective.—A whole body inverted pendulum model was used to study the mechanisms of balance control about the supporting hip and foot in the frontal plane during gait. Regulation of the CM trajectory was broken down into the contributions of active muscle moments, passive joint accelerational moments, and gravitational moments. Four normal men aged 21–32 years were studied in 10 sessions of natural walking. Thirty-one reflective markers served to define a whole body model. Marker coordinates were acquired by using 3 synchronized video cameras to record sagittal and frontal views. Two force platforms were used to record ground reaction forces.

Findings.—Whole body balance was maintained when the CM passed medially to the supporting foot, thereby creating an ongoing state of dynamic imbalance shifted toward the center line of the plane of progression. Acceleration of the CM medially resulted primarily from a gravitational moment about the supporting foot. The degree of acceleration was determined at the time of initial contact when the new supporting foot was placed lateral to the horizontal site of the CM. The trunk and swing leg remained balanced about the supporting hip through active hip abduction, which acted counter to a significant destabilizing gravitational moment. The lateral flexors of the spine regulated the posture of the upper trunk.

Implications.—The balance and posture of the whole body in the frontal plane are precisely regulated by an interactive control system in which the key is how the supporting foot is placed relative to the horizontal site of the CM. Erroneous foot placement is corrected either at the supporting subtalar or hip joints, which work synergistically. The supporting foot and hip muscles interact in a way that permits varying strategies for maintaining balance.

▶ As I began to read this study, the thing that caught my attention was ". . . this study demonstrated that whole body balance and posture in the frontal plane is precisely regulated by an interactive, hierarchical control system. Control over the lateral trajectory of the CM is achieved by regulating the angular rotation of the whole body CM about the base of support and the trunk CM about the hips during single support."

It made me think of a friend of mine, aged 83 years, who had just experienced what was considered a minor stroke. The only way you could even tell he had had a stroke was that he had difficulty maintaining his balance, especially during the first step or two, as he began to walk. This was painful for me to watch because he had been such an active, athletic person. Obviously, his gait had been significantly affected by the stroke and there appears to be little that can be done. Maybe a better understanding of this study will one day lead us to be able to help people like my friend.—Col. J.L. Anderson, PE.D.

7 Women, Children, Aging, Osteoporosis, and Osteoarthritis

Elbow Flexion Strength Curves in Untrained Men and Women and Male Bodybuilders

Tsunoda N, O'Hagan F, Sale DG, MacDougall JD (McMaster Univ, Hamilton, Ont, Canada)

Eur J Appl Physiol 66:235–239, 1993   139-94-7-1

Background.—Isometric strength training can modify the shape of the strength curve, possibly because of increased muscle mass. The elbow-flexor bulge associated with a short muscle length may alter muscle fiber alignment relative to the line of pull of the tendons, impairing force production. Elbow flexion strength curves were compared in 15 untrained women, 18 untrained men, and 11 male bodybuilders to determine the impact of elbow flexor size on the strength curve.

Methods.—Elbow flexion isometric strength was measured during 2 or 3 maximal contractions at 7 joint angles: 75, 90, 105, 120, 135, 150, and 165 degrees. The order of joint angle testing was randomized.

Results.—Peak torque varied significantly among the various joint angles, and the groups differed from each other at all joint angles. At the summits of the composite strength curves, the peak torque of the bodybuilders was 2.6 times greater than the peak torque of the women, and the peak torque of the untrained men was 1.9 times greater than that of the women. The joint angle affected torque differently in the 3 groups. The strength curve peaked at a 120-degree joint angle in both male groups, but it peaked at 90 degrees in the women. The decline in torque between 120 degrees and 75 degrees was marked for men but minimal for women. Thus, small joint angles favored the women, whose 75-degree peak torque value was 61% of untrained men's peak torque value and 49% of the bodybuilders' value. However, women's relative performance declined at larger joint angles, so the corresponding percentage values dropped to 49% and 37% at 120 degrees, and 47% and 33% at 165 degrees.

Conclusion.—Elbow flexion strength curves differ significantly between men and women: men have a greater decline in torque at the smallest joint angles and the peak of their strength curve occurs at a larger joint angle. These differences are believed to result from the larger muscles in men, which cause impaired torque production at short muscle lengths.

▶ These authors have identified some differences among the 3 experimental groups of this study: untrained men, male bodybuilders, and untrained women. I doubt that any of us are surprised that the elbow flexion peak torque favors the bodybuilders, the untrained men, and the untrained women in that order. However, it is somewhat of a surprise that there was a difference between men and women in the angle at which the summit of the strength curve occurred because other researchers have found no such difference. First, we must determine whether other researchers can replicate these results and then study why there are differences between men and women and what the differences mean for physiologic performance.—Col. J.L. Anderson, PE.D.

Isokinematic Muscle Mechanics in Four Groups of Women of Increasing Age
Stanley SN, Taylor NAS (Univ of Otago, New Zealand; Univ of Wollongong, Australia)
Eur J Appl Physiol 66:178–184, 1993   139-94-7–2

Background.—The reduction in muscle strength that occurs gradually with age may predispose the elderly to injury. In elderly women, reduced muscle strength has been observed at several angular velocities, although changes in dynamic agonist/antagonist muscular function are not well documented. The impact of age on changes in dynamic torque and work and power changes in knee extension and flexion was investigated.

Methods.—Six angular velocities of extension and flexion, ranging from 60 degrees per second to 400 degrees per second, were measured in 15 women in their third decade of life, 5 women in their fourth decade, 9 women in their sixth decade, and 6 women in their seventh decade. Data were collected on 2 separate occasions within 5 days of each other.

Results.—At each angular velocity, knee extensor and flexor peak torque values were significantly higher in both younger groups, compared to either of the older groups. Peak torque values did not differ significantly between the 2 younger groups. Peak torque was significantly greater in the sixth-decade group, compared to the seventh-decade group, for knee extensors but not for knee flexors. The decrease in extensor torque was greater than the decrement in flexor torque. The peak torque angle for extension and flexion occurred earlier in the range of motion in the younger groups than in either of the older groups; however, peak flexion occurred significantly earlier in the third-decade group compared with the other groups. Knee extensor and flexor work and power were significantly greater in the younger groups than in the older groups at each angular velocity. Mean knee flexor/extensor ratios for work and power revealed a greater loss of flexor function with increasing age.

Conclusion.—Aging is associated with a differential loss of function that is proportionately greater in the flexors. It is hypothesized that type II fiber loss or atrophy, or both, may account for these observations and that the shift in flexor peak torque angle observed in the fourth-decade subjects may be an early marker for this functional change. If correct, age-related functional changes in women may be apparent as early as the fourth decade.

▶ These are interesting results. We should collect more data, using many more subjects, within each of the age decades. Also, although within the limits of this study it appears that age-related functional changes in women may be apparent within the fourth decade, we should ask how long those functional changes can be delayed through exercise programs and how vigorous the exercise programs need to be.—Col. J.L. Anderson, PE.D.

Dietary Fat and Sports Activity as Determinants for Age at Menarche
Merzenich H, Boeing H, Wahrendorf J (German Cancer Research Ctr, Heidelberg, Germany)
Am J Epidemiol 138:217–224, 1993   139-94-7–3

Objective.—An early age at menarche is a risk factor for breast cancer. Diet may be an important factor in determining the onset of puberty and age at menarche, which is delayed by malnutrition. The effects of diet and other suspected lifestyle factors, such as sports participation, on the age at menarche were investigated.

Methods.—The subjects were 261 girls aged 8–15 years drawn from a German cross-sectional nationwide nutrition survey (Nationale Verzehrsstudie [NVS]) of 22,000 randomly selected subjects who completed a 7-day food and activity record. One hundred sixty-seven girls who had

---

Multivariate Age-Adjusted Estimates of Relative Risk (RR) for Onset of Menarche, With 95% Confidence Intervals (CIs), for Fat Intake Assessed at NVS (1985–1988) and for Physical Activity and Percentage of Body Fat by Questionnaire (1988–1989)

Variables	2nd quartile		3rd quartile		4th quartile		Two-sided *p* for trend
	RR	95% CI	RR	95% CI	RR	95% CI	
Energy-adjusted fat intake (NVS)	1.1	0.56–1.99	1.3	0.71–2.32	2.1	1.10–3.95	0.03
Physical activity (hours/week) (questionnaire)	0.7	0.42–1.22	0.4	0.21–0.69	0.3	0.12–0.51	<0.0001
% of body fat (questionnaire)	2.4	1.22–4.69	2.6	1.39–4.99	4.0	2.11–7.47	<0.0001

(Courtesy of Merzenich H, Boeing H, Wahrendorf J: *Am J Epidemiol* 138:217–224, 1993.)

not reached menarche and who provided complete response to a subsequent questionnaire were followed for 2 years or until menarche. The questionnaire requested information regarding their mother's age at menarche and the subject's health and dietary history, anthropometric measurements, regular sports activities, and nutritional habits. Adiposity was estimated by the body mass index and the Mellits and Cheek formula.

Findings.—Analysis of the NVS data suggested that increasing energy-adjusted fat intake was associated with increased changes of early menarche, but that hours spent in sports activities were unrelated to age at menarche. Analysis of the questionnaire-derived data from the prospective study found no association between energy-adjusted intake of fat and other nutrients with age at menarche. Menarche did appear to be delayed in girls who spent more time in sports activity. Early age at menarche was related to the anthropometric indicators of increasing body weight, body mass index, percentage of body fat, hip and leg circumference, and especially to breast circumference.

On analysis of only those girls with concordant results on the 2 sets of questionnaires, increased fat intake was associated with earlier age at menarche and increased sports participation with delayed menarche. A multivariate model accentuated the univariate effects of energy-adjusted fat intake, physical activity, and percentage of body fat (table). Age at menarche was unrelated to the mother's age at menarche, socioeconomic factors, breast-feeding, childhood diseases, medical and dietary history, and vitamin supplementation.

Conclusion.—The metabolically interrelated factors of fat intake, sports activity, and body fat percentage are independently associated with age at menarche. Dietary factors affecting onset of menarche may be expected to appear as risk factors for breast cancer as well. It is possible that the effect of fat intake on breast cancer risk is an indirect one, operating via age at menarche.

▶ The prospective data, which were obtained from girls who had not reached menarche at the time of the NVS study, do not support a role for energy-adjusted fat intake in affecting age of menarche. Only when discordant results for the NVS study and the prospective study were eliminated and the NVS data were used in the analysis does fat intake assume a significant role. Although some may accept the authors' justification for combining data from 2 dissimilar studies, it still raises a question as to the validity of the conclusions. More persuasive are the data for physical activity, body weight, body mass index, and circumference of the limbs. Nevertheless, it is an interesting hypothesis and should be tested in another population using a more stringent experimental design.—B.L. Drinkwater, Ph.D.

Hormone Anabolic/Catabolic Balance in Female Endurance Athletes
Lindholm C, Hirschberg AL, Carlström K, von Schoultz B (Karolinska Inst,

Stockholm; Huddinge Univ, Sweden)
Gynecol Obstet Invest 36:176–180, 1993   139-94-7–4

Objective.—The mechanism underlying the high incidence of menstrual dysfunction in some female athletes is unknown. The purpose of this study was to acquire a more complete understanding of anabolic/catabolic hormonal balance in female athletes and to examine differences between athletes with and without menstrual irregularities.

Study Plan.—Circulating levels of androgenic/anabolic and catabolic steroids, as well as growth hormone, insulin-like growth factor I, and insulin, were measured in 13 women who were middle-distance/long-distance runners. Five of them had been amenorrheic for 3 months or longer; 4 were oligomenorrheic; and 4 had regular periods. The runners trained for an average of 11 hours per week. Fifteen sedentary, regularly menstruating women were matched with the runners for age and body weight. Two blood samples were taken at 15-minute intervals in the morning after an overnight fast.

Findings.—The runners, as a group, had significantly higher basal cortisol levels than the control women, and the difference was more marked in those with irregular or absent menses (table). Levels of free cortisol were elevated in oligomenorrheic athletes, who also had lower

Serum Concentrations of Steroids, Steroid-Binding Proteins, and Peptide Hormones in Controls and Athletes

	Controls	Athletes total	oligoamenorrhoic
Subjects	15	13	9
Testosterone, nmol/l	1.2±0.1	1.2±0.1	1.1±0.1
SHBG, nmol/l	42.5±3.0	36.4±3.5	32.4±2.8*
NST, pmol/l	19.5±1.8	20.4±1.7	19.0±1.9
A-4, nmol/l	5.3±0.3	5.2±0.4	4.7±0.3
DHA, nmol/l	17.6±1.1	19.7±1.7	19.0±1.5
DHAS, nmol/l	4385±370	3618±377	3607±497
Cortisol, nmol/l	324±17	426±38*	454±46†
Transcortin, µg/ml	32.8±1.6	36.3±1.9	35.9±2.4
Free cortisol index, nmol/l	24.6±2.8	35.2±5.0	39.1±6.3*
GH, µg/l	7.0±1.8	6.0±1.6	4.2±0.9
Insulin, mIU/l	5.8±0.4	5.8±0.4	5.4±0.5
IGF-1, µg/l	296±19	287±22	265±26
TSH, mIU/l	1.1±0.1	1.1±0.2	1.1±0.2
Albumin, g/l	43.4±0.5	43.0±0.7	43.9±0.7

Note: Values are means ± SEM.
* $P < .05$, between controls and athletes.
† $P < .01$, between controls and athletes.
(Courtesy of Lindholm C, Hirschberg AL, Carlström K, et al: *Gynecol Obstet Invest* 36:176–180, 1993.)

sex hormone–binding globulin (SHBG) levels than control women. Amenorrheic athletes had the lowest SHBG levels. In the overall study population, cortisol and SHBG levels correlated negatively, but there was a positive correlation between the levels of growth hormone and 4-androstene-3,17-dione. Hormone levels were not correlated with anthropometric data.

Implications.—Menstrual irregularity in these female athletes was related to a lower body mass index, less body fat, and more marked endocrine abnormalities. Their anabolic state, however, appeared to be normal. Possibly the reduced SHBG levels observed in oligomenorrheic athletes are part of a compensatory mechanism intended to maintain stable androgenic/anabolic activity. Hypercortisolism, however, leads to an anabolic/catabolic imbalance that features a predominantly catabolic state.

▶ Elevated cortisol levels in oligomenorrheic athletes have been reported in several previous studies as well. However, whether hypercortisolism plays a role in the etiology of the menstrual irregularities in athletes or is merely a consequence of the changes in the reproductive cycle is unknown. Also of concern is the possibility that the high cortisol levels may be contributing to the bone loss experienced by many oligomenorrheic/amenorrheic athletes. The conclusion of the authors—that the severity of menstrual irregularities in this group of athletes is related to body mass index and body fat—should not be interpreted as a statement of cause and effect. There are a number of studies in the literature demonstrating that low body weight or fat is not a prerequisite for either oligomenorrhea or amenorrhea.—B.L. Drinkwater, Ph.D.

Calcium Supplementation and Bone Mineral Density in Adolescent Girls

Lloyd T, Andon MB, Rollings N, Martel JK, Landis JR, Demers LM, Eggli DF, Kieselhorst K, Kulin HE (Pennsylvania State Univ, Hershey; Procter and Gamble Co, Cincinnati, Ohio)
JAMA 270:841–844, 1993   139-94-7–5

Background.—It is currently recognized that high peak bone mass may be the most effective prophylaxis against osteoporosis. As such, interest in diet, exercise, and lifestyle factors, and how each impact on bone growth and subsequent maintenance in children and young adults has increased. The effect of calcium supplementation on bone acquisition in white female adolescents was evaluated.

Patients and Methods.—A total of 94 girls with a mean age of 11.9 years at study entry were enrolled in this randomized, double-blind, placebo-controlled study. All participants were within 80% to 120% of ideal weight for height, were not taking routine medication, did not have any medical conditions known to affect bone development, and did not have

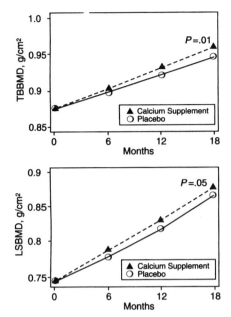

Fig 7–1.—Longitudinal model fit for the 2 study groups for total body bone mineral density (TBBMD) and lumbar spine bone mineral density (LSBMD) is shown for the 18-month study. The *P* values shown are for the differences in linear terms. (Courtesy of Lloyd T, Andon MB, Rollings N, et al: JAMA 270:841-844, 1993.)

any known dietary disorders. Forty-six participants were randomly assigned to calcium supplementation, and were instructed to take 250 mg of calcium citrate malate per day. The remaining 48 girls were assigned to a placebo group. Bone mineral density and bone mineral content of the lumbar spine and total body were measured via dual-energy x-ray absorptiometry, and calcium excretion was measured via 24-hour urine specimens. Measurements were taken at baseline and every 6 months thereafter for a total of 18 months. Prospective 3-day diet records were also completed at baseline and then every 6 months throughout the study.

Results.—The entire study group had an average daily intake of 960 mg of calcium from dietary sources, with supplemented participants receiving, on average, an additional 354 mg of calcium per day. Greater increases of lumbar spine bone density, lumbar spine bone mineral content, and total body bone mineral density were noted for supplemented participants as compared with controls, at 18.7% vs. 15.8%, 39.4% vs. 34.7%, and 9.6% vs. 8.3%, respectively (Fig 7–1). In addition, supplemented individuals had greater 24-hour urinary calcium excretion, at 90.4 vs. 72.9 mg/day for controls.

Conclusion.—Significant increases in total body and spinal bone density were achieved by increasing daily calcium intake from 80% of the recommended daily allowance to 110% via supplementation with calcium citrate malate. During adolescent growth, this yearly bone gain increase of 24 g equals an additional 1.3% of acquired skeletal mass per year, which may aid in preventing future osteoporotic fracture.

▶ Good news! When 12-year-old girls took calcium supplements for 18 months, bringing their daily calcium intake to over 1,300 mg, they gained bone mass. The gain, by some measures, was up to 5%. We once thought that bones in women reach peak mass by age 20. However, a study of 156 college-aged women in Omaha found that those who work out and get lots of calcium build bones until age 30 (1). Another relevant study, of 980 women in California aged 50–98 years, found that lifetime coffee drinkers tend to have weaker bones, but only if they drink no milk (2). For your bones, ladies, one daily glass of milk can easily override two cups of coffee. Cappuccino, anyone?—E.R. Eichner, M.D.

References

1. Recker RR, et al: *JAMA* 268:2403, 1992.
2. Barrett-Connor E, et al: *JAMA* 271:280, 1994.

Nalmefene Enhances LH Secretion in a Proportion of Oligo-Amenorrheic Athletes

McArthur JW, Turnbull BA, Pehrson J, Bauman M, Henley K, Turner A, Evans WJ, Bullen BA, Skrinar GS (Boston Univ; Boston City Hosp; USDA Human Nutrition Research Ctr on Aging)
Acta Endocrinol 128:325–333, 1993   139-94-7–6

Background.—It has been hypothesized that women participating in vigorous exercise have periodic elevations in endogenous opioid tone, which may play a role in exercise-associated menstrual dysfunction. The effects of orally administered nalmefene, an effective congener of naloxone, on luteinizing hormone (LH) secretion in oligomenorrheic athletes vs. nonathletes were evaluated.

Methods.—The subjects were 9 female athletes (mean age, 26.1 years) who had 0–1 menstrual periods per year, and 5 nonathletic women who were normally ovulating and menstruating. The subjects were studied in a clinical research center on 2 occasions; on 1 occasion, they received a single 20-mg dose of nalmefene; on the other, they received placebo. Levels of LH in blood were evaluated every 10 minutes for 6 hours before and 6 hours after treatment. Subjects were considered responders if their peak area under the curve after treatment exceeded their pretreatment area under the curve for LH by more than 1.96 SD. The subjects recorded any side effects experienced on the day of the study and for 5 days thereafter.

Results.—Five of the 9 athletes and 1 of the 5 controls had a significant LH response to nalmefene. The difference in response to the 2 treatments was significant in the oligomenorrheic group but not the control group. Response to nalmefene was not associated with mileage run the day before testing, habitual exercise pattern, percent of ideal body weight, basal levels of LH, or incidence of side effects. Luteinizing hormone pulses demonstrated a significantly higher amplitude after nalmefene treatment. Some of the athletes but none of the controls had some symptoms similar to those of narcotic withdrawal 1–4 hours after nalmefene treatment and again 12–18 hours later.

Conclusion.—Some athletes who are oligomenorrheic have increased serum levels and amplitude of LH pulses, as well as symptoms of narcotic withdrawal, in response to opioid receptor blockade with nalmefene. Thus, these athletes appear to have at least transient increases of heightened hypothalamic opioid tone. Almost all studies of hypothalamic amenorrhea have shown heterogeneous LH pulse patterns after naloxone administration.

▶ The inability to detect any significant differences between the oligomenorrheic (no. = 9) and eumenorrheic (no. = 5) groups in either the frequency or amplitude of LH pulses may well have been the result of the small sample size. Although recruitment of women for a study involving a pelvic examination and serial sampling of blood during a 12-hour period may be difficult, this study once again illustrates the importance of determining the sample size required to achieve adequate power to detect significant differences. The significant difference in the amplitude of LH pulses from preinfusion to postinfusion of nalmefene in the combined groups appears to be a result of lower preinfusion values (9.7 vs. 15.6 postinfusion) in this trial than in the placebo trial (15.3 vs. 15.4 postinfusion) rather than a response to the nalmefene. Although the purpose of the study was to determine whether endogenous opioid tone was greater in women who exercise vigorously, the selection of oligomenorrheic women as the active subjects adds the confounding factor of menstrual status to that of activity.—B.L. Drinkwater, Ph.D.

Spine and Total Body Bone Mineral Density in Amenorrheic Endurance Athletes

Rutherford OM (St Mary's Hosp Med School, London)
J Appl Physiol 74:2904–2908, 1993   139-94-7-7

Background.—Women who participate in sports that require intense endurance training often have menstrual abnormalities and amenorrhea. This hypoestrogenic state could lead to bone loss and to increased risk of osteoporosis. On the other hand, weight-bearing exercise is known to increase bone mass and might compensate for the low estrogen state of these female athletes. Body fat, lumbar spine, and total body and re-

Group Bone Mineral Density Values for Each Skeletal Site

	Lumbar Spine	Total Body	Arms	Legs	Total Spine	Trunk	Pelvis
Eumenorrheic Group	1.180 ($\pm$0.02)	1.166 ($\pm$0.01)	0.967 ($\pm$0.02)	1.231 ($\pm$0.02)	1.129 ($\pm$0.02)	0.925 ($\pm$0.01)	1.118 ($\pm$0.02)
Amenorrheic Group	1.071** ($\pm$0.02)	1.118 ($\pm$0.02)	0.905* ($\pm$0.02)	1.207 ($\pm$0.02)	0.972**** ($\pm$0.02)	0.857* ($\pm$0.02)	1.048 ($\pm$0.03)

Values are means $\pm$ SE given in g/cm^2. Significantly different from group that was eumenorrheic.
* $P < .05$.
** $P < .01$.
**** $P < .0001$.
(Courtesy of Rutherford OM: J Appl Physiol 74:2904–2908, 1993.)

gional bone mineral densities (BMDs) were compared in 31 elite runners and triathletes who were amenorrheic or eumenorrheic. Medical, training, and dietary histories were elicited by questionnaire.

Subjects.—The study group consisted of 31 top-class female athletes, 17 of whom were triathletes and 14 of whom were long-distance runners. The women who were eumenorrheic (group E) consisted of 7 triathletes and 9 runners. The women who were amenorrheic (group A) consisted of 10 triathletes and 5 runners.

Methods.—Bone mineral density of the lumbar spine and total body—including total spine, pelvis, trunk, arms, and legs—were measured using dual-energy x-ray absorptiometry. Results for each site were expressed as BMD and as a percentage of age- and weight-matched reference data from the Lunar database of 1,000 healthy British women.

Findings.—There was no significant difference in percentage body fat between group E and group A. There was no significant difference in amount of time spent training or in calcium intake between these 2 groups. The age of menarche was significantly later in the women of group A, and they had a greater incidence of stress fractures. Group A had a significantly lower lumbar spine BMD when compared with group E and to the reference data. There was no significant difference between group A and group E for total body BMD. Group A had significantly lower arm, trunk, and total spine BMDs when compared with group E (table). Group A athletes had significantly higher arm and leg densities but lower total spine densities than the reference data. Group E had higher densities than the reference group at all sites except the spine. A stepwise multiple regression analysis revealed that the only significant predictor of lumbar spine BMD was menstrual status.

Conclusion.—Loss of menses in endurance athletes can cause a decrease in BMD. However, because of their weight-bearing training regimens, these women can compensate and achieve normal to above normal BMDs at all skeletal sites, with the exception of the spine. Therefore, the effect of back exercises on BMD should be investigated among elite athletes who are amenorrheic.

▶ Two other studies (1, 2) have used dual-energy x-ray absorptiometry technology to examine BMD at skeletal sites other than the spine, and both report significant differences at most sites measured. Although it may seem reassuring that amenorrheic women in this study have normal or above normal bone density in regions other than the spine, Myburgh et al. found significant differences between amenorrheic and eumenorrheic athletes at the same sites. The reason for the discrepancy between the 2 studies may lie in the selection of subjects or in the use of different dual-energy x-ray absorptiometry machines. Rutherford's sample included elite triathletes and runners whereas subjects in the Myburgh et al. and Rencken et al. studies were primarily runners.

It may be premature to conclude that weight-bearing exercise can offset the negative effect of low estrogen levels on bone. We don't know what will happen when these athletes decrease their current levels of activity. In postmenopausal women, bone density gained through increased activity is lost when the activity ceases.—B.L. Drinkwater, Ph.D.

References

1. Myburgh KH, et al: *Med Sci Sports Exerc* 25:1197, 1993.
2. Rencken M, et al: *J Bone Miner Res* 8:S254, 1993.

Elevated Plasma Low-Density Lipoprotein and High-Density Lipoprotein Cholesterol Levels in Amenorrheic Athletes: Effects of Endogenous Hormone Status and Nutrient Intake
Friday KE, Drinkwater BL, Bruemmer B, Chesnut C III, Chait A (Univ of Washington, Seattle)
J Clin Endocrinol Metab 77:1605–1609, 1993   139-94-7-8

Introduction.—Concern that adverse changes in lipid and lipoprotein levels may occur in hypoestrogenic female athletes prompted a study of the interactive effects of hormone levels, exercise, and diet in 24 hypoestrogenic amenorrheic female athletes and 44 other athletes with normal menstrual function. A majority of both groups were runners. Blood samples were obtained at weekly intervals during a 1-month period. Dietary intake was estimated from a 3-day dietary record.

Findings.—Amenorrheic women had higher plasma levels of cholesterol, including both low-density lipoprotein (LDL) and high-density lipoprotein (HDL) fractions, and triglycerides than did the eumenorrheic athletes (table). More than 90% of amenorrheic women had HDL cholesterol levels above the population median (Fig 7–2). Two thirds had

Serum Lipids, Lipoproteins, and Apolipoproteins (Apos)

	Amenorrheic		Eumenorrheic		P
	Mean ± SEM	n	Mean ± SEM	n	
Cholesterol (mmol/L)	5.47 ± 0.17	24	4.84 ± 0.12	44	0.003
(mg/dl)	(212 ± 6)		(187 ± 5)		
Triglyceride (mmol/L)	0.75 ± 0.06	24	0.61 ± 0.03	44	0.046
(mg/dl)	(66 ± 6)		(54 ± 3)		
VLDL cholesterol	0.36 ± 0.04	24	0.30 ± 0.02	44	NS
(mmol/L) (mg/dl)	(14 ± 1)		(12 ± 1)		
LDL cholesterol	3.16 ± 0.15	24	2.81 ± 0.09	44	0.037
(mmol/L) (mg/dl)	(122 ± 6)		(109 ± 4)		
HDL cholesterol	1.95 ± 0.07	24	1.73 ± 0.05	44	0.007
(mmol/L) (mg/dl)	(75 ± 3)		(67 ± 2)		
HDL_2 cholesterol	0.84 ± 0.06	24	0.68 ± 0.04	44	0.02
(mmol/L) (mg/dl)	(32 ± 2)		(26 ± 2)		
HDL_3 cholesterol	1.11 ± 0.03	24	1.05 ± 0.03	44	NS
(mmol/L) (mg/dl)	(43 ± 1)		(41 ± 1)		
LDL/HDL cholesterol ratio	1.7 ± 0.1	24	1.7 ± 0.1	44	NS
Apo AI (mg/dl)	167 ± 4	24	162 ± 4	42	NS
Apo AII (mg/dl)	30 ± 1	24	29 ± 1	42	NS

(Courtesy of Friday KE, Drinkwater BL, Bruemmer B, et al: *J Clin Endocrinol Metab* 77:1605-1609, 1993.)

LDL cholesterol levels above the median. In the amenorrheic women, levels of HDL and HDL_2 cholesterol correlated positively with peak estradiol and peak prolactin levels. The only substantial dietary difference was a lower fat intake by the amenorrheic athletes.

Implications.—Female athletes who are amenorrheic and who have elevated plasma LDL cholesterol and triglyceride levels might be considered at increased risk of premature atherogenic changes. However, increased levels of HDL and HDL_2 cholesterol and a favorable LDL/HDL cholesterol ratio may neutralize the risk of cardiovascular disease in this group.

▶ The potential negative consequences that decreased endogenous estrogen levels may have on plasma lipoprotein cholesterol raise another concern about the effect of prolonged amenorrhea on the health of the amenorrheic athlete. Although the increased levels of HDL_2 cholesterol in the amenorrheic group and the same LDL/HDL cholesterol ratio as that of the eumenorrheic athletes might suggest that the effect of training offsets the negative effect of decreased estrogen on total and LDL cholesterol and triglycerides, this remains to be seen. The long-term effect of the hypoestrogenic state on the cardiovascular health of the amenorrheic athlete is an area of research that should receive more attention.—B.L. Drinkwater, Ph.D.

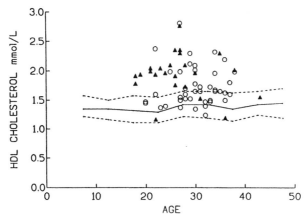

Fig 7–2.—Amenorrheic (*triangles*) and eumenorrheic (*circles*) athlete plasma HDL cholesterol values compared with the Lipid Research Clinic population studies age-adjusted median (*solid line*), 25th and 75th percentiles (*dashed line*). (Courtesy of Friday KE, Drinkwater BL, Bruemmer B, et al: *J Clin Endocrinol Metab* 77:1605–1609, 1993.)

The XY Female in Sport: The Controversy Continues

Hipkin LJ (Univ of Liverpool, England)
Br J Sports Med 27:150–156, 1993   139-94-7-9

Background.—Recent Olympic Games have been accompanied by much press coverage on the controversy and confusion over sex tests for women wishing to compete. The focus of the controversy was on the eligibility of XY females with androgen insensitivity to compete in women's events. The process of sex differentiation and its abnormalities were examined, with an emphasis on conditions in which the secretion of biologically active testosterone may confer an advantage in women's sports events.

Normal Sexual Development.—The complex process of sexual differentiation begins in the early embryo and is completed at puberty with the development of secondary sex characteristics. Human beings have 46 chromosomes, made up of 22 pairs of autosomes and 2 sex chromosomes—XX or XY.

Nonvirilized XY Females.—Nonvirilized females with an XY chromosome constitution have no evidence of androgen activity. There are 2 main subtypes: pure XY gonadal dysgenesis and complete androgen insensitivity. Complete, pure XY gonadal dysgenesis is characterized by amenorrhea and sexual infantilism with eunuchoidism and lack of breast development. Persons with complete androgen insensitivity have a feminine appearance and external female genitalia. The tissues, however, are insensitive to androgen.

Virilized XY Females.—There are several subgroups of females with an XY chromosome constitution or genotype and some ambiguity of external genitalia with some signs of virilization at puberty. These include partial androgen insensitivity, incomplete XY gonadal dysgenesis, mixed or asymmetric gonadal dysgenesis, defects in testosterone biosynthesis, and 5α-reductase deficiency.

Discussion.—Sex verification testing is done to assure that women in sports are competing on an equal basis. Genetic testing using the traditional sex chromatin pattern or detection of the male-determining gene of the Y chromosome does not distinguish only individuals who would have an unfair competitive advantage. Theoretically, nonvirilized women would compete on an equal basis, whereas virilized women, because the excessive endogenous testosterone secreted is biologically active, would have an unfair advantage.

Gender Verification in Competitive Sports
Simpson JL, Ljungqvist A, de la Chapelle A, Ferguson-Smith MA, Genel M, Carlson AS, Ehrhardt AA, Ferris E (Univ of Tennessee, Memphis; Karolinska Inst, Stockholm; Univ of Helsinki; et al)
Sports Med 16:305–315, 1993   139-94-7–10

Background.—In 1960 at the Rome Olympic Games, the International Amateur Athletics Federation (IAAF) established rules of eligibility for female athletes. Gender verification by physical examination, begun in 1966, was replaced by sex chromatin testing by buccal smear at the 1968 Olympic Games in Mexico City. In sex chromatin analysis, genetic females (46, XX) show a single X-chromatin mass that males (46, XY) do not. Sex chromatin analysis for gender verification proved unreliable and was replaced by another laboratory-based gender verification test, polymerase chain reaction (PCR)–based testing of the SRY gene at the 1992 Winter Games at Albertville.

The fundamental argument against all laboratory-based tests is that only chromosomal sex is analyzed and anatomical and psychosocial status are not considered. Female athletes may be unfairly excluded because of congenital abnormalities that convey no added advantage in sports. In January 1991, the IAAF abandoned gender verification testing but proposed a medical examination to establish satisfactory physical status for competition. A second IAAF working group in 1992 suggested that physical examination was unnecessary for femininity certification. As of May 1992, screening for gender is no longer undertaken at IAAF competitions. The current use of routine urine testing to exclude doping involves observation of voiding by an official. This official observation makes it unlikely that males could masquerade as females.

International Olympic Committee Practice.—The International Olympic Committee (IOC) has not yet abandoned laboratory testing for gender verification. The PCR testing for the presence of SRY to identify those with the Y chromosome was introduced at the Winter Olympics in

1992. Many have argued against the IOC decision that, the low error rate notwithstanding, the molecular method is a test for DNA sequence, not a test for sex or gender. The sensitivity and specificity of PCR testing remains unproven but its use is still included in the IOC position.

▶ The original purpose of "gender verification" was to prevent males from masquerading as females and competing as women in sporting events. Abstracts 139-94-7–9 and 139-94-7–10 discuss some of the problems encountered with the techniques used to determine the sex of the athlete but differ in their approach to the topic. Hipkin (Abstract 139-94-7–9) describes a number of conditions that can occur during the process of sex differentiation that may or may not confer an advantage in sport. The implication is that although the athlete may be a phenotypic female, any condition that leads to virilization should be grounds for disqualification. The term "femininity testing" is introduced in the discussion at the end of this paper. This, of course, moves into the area of psychosocial characteristics and is far afield from the original intent of identifying men posing as women.

The review article by Simpson et al. (Abstract 139-94-7–10) provides a broader perspective, not only detailing the history of sex testing in competitive sports but also the inadequacies of the tests. Although the IAAF has recognized that laboratory gender verification tests are inappropriate, the IOC continues to require them in spite of scientific and medical advice that they be discontinued.—B.L. Drinkwater, Ph.D.

Intrinsic Risk Factors for Exercise-Related Injuries Among Male and Female Army Trainees
Jones BH, Bovee MW, Harris JMcA III, Cowan DN (United States Army Research Inst of Environmental Medicine, Natick, Mass)
Am J Sports Med 21:705–710, 1993   139-94-7–11

Background.—Army recruits and other active individuals often sustain injuries related to physical training, but little is known about the causes of such training injuries. Only the risk factors of gender, age, and past physical activity have been identified. The relationship between a number of other factors and injuries to male and female recruits was examined.

Methods.—Potential risk factors were investigated in 310 army trainees enrolled in a prospective study. One hundred eighty-six women and 124 men were followed through 8 weeks of basic training. Seventy-one percent underwent an initial army physical training test.

Findings.—Women had a significantly higher incidence of time-loss injuries than men. These incidence rates were 44.6% and 29%, respectively. During training, the 50% of men who were slower on the mile run had more time-loss injuries—29% vs. 0%. Similarly, slower women had a greater risk of time-loss injuries than did faster ones—38.2% vs. 18.5%.

Men with histories of inactivity and with higher body mass index had a higher risk of injury, as did the shortest women.

Conclusion.—Among army trainees, female gender and low aerobic fitness are risk factors for training injuries. Gender may, in fact, be less important than the lower fitness level of the female recruits. Factors such as previous activity level and stature may affect women and men differently. High body mass index is a risk factor among men.

▶ Perhaps the most interesting aspect of this study is that it replicates previous studies in identifying intrinsic risk factors associated with training injuries in the military, which suggests that the army has done nothing to mitigate those factors since the earlier studies. Although the authors conclude that female gender is a risk factor, they also point out that the cause may be the lower fitness level of the female recruits rather than sex per se. Fitness is also a risk factor for the men, as is body mass index. An exercise physiologist reading this paper would probably conclude that the army should pay more attention to planning training programs that will increase fitness but decrease the incidence of injuries. The finding that 77% of the injuries to men and 88% of those to women involved the lower extremity certainly provides a clue to where appropriate changes might be made.—B.L. Drinkwater, Ph.D.

Effect of the Different Phases of the Menstrual Cycle and Oral Contraceptives on Athletic Performance
Lebrun CM (Univ of British Columbia, Vancouver, Canada)
Sports Med 16:400–430, 1993   139-94-7-12

Introduction.—The female athlete in her reproductive years may be influenced by the variations in endogenous estradiol and progesterone of a regular menstrual cycle or the exogenous synthetic hormones of oral contraceptives.

Cycle Fluctuations.—In surveys on the menstrual cycle and performance, 37% to 63% of female athletes did not report any cycle phase detriment, whereas 13% to 29% reported an improvement during menstruation. The best performances were reported in the immediate postmenstrual days with the worst performances during the premenstrual interval and the first few days of menstrual flow. Premenstrual symptoms such as fluid retention, weight gain, mood changes, and dysmenorrhea were associated with decreased performance. The premenstrual and menstrual periods have been associated with an increase in traumatic musculoskeletal injuries and an adverse effect on neuromuscular coordination, manual dexterity, judgment, and reaction time for complex tests.

Studies using estradiol and progesterone levels to confirm ovulation have not found significant differences in either maximal or submaximal exercise responses across the cycle. Conflicting evidence has demonstrated both a slight decrease in aerobic capacity and an enhancement of endurance performance during the luteal phase. The high progesterone levels during the luteal phase and pregnancy enhance ventilatory responsiveness to hypoxia and hypercapnia. Although this increased ventilatory response may be detrimental for nonathletic women, elite female athletes have reported no effect on performance.

Oral Contraceptives and the Female Athlete.—The lower dosages of oral contraceptives currently used have diminished their effects on female athletes, and the overall benefits probably outweigh any slight effects on physiologic function. Oral contraceptives have been associated with a slight decrease in maximal aerobic capacity and maximum oxygen uptake and a limited detrimental effect on isometric endurance. Combined estrogen and progestin oral contraceptive formulations increase cardiac output more than progestin-only formulas. The augmented stroke volume may increase oxygen delivery to the tissues, thereby benefiting performance.

Conclusion.—The effect of the menstrual cycle and oral contraceptives on female athletes is subject to a large degree of interindividual variability. The normal menstrual cycle may cause subtle physiologic variations in vascular volume dynamics, ventilation, thermoregulation, and substrate metabolism with little effect on actual athletic performance. Oral contraceptives may have undesirable effects on aerobic capacity and muscle strength and endurance. Further investigation is needed in both areas.

► A brief synopsis of this extensive review of the influence of endogenous and exogenous steroid hormones on athletic performance cannot do justice to the author's critical analysis of the literature. Readers who are interested in this topic should read the original article. What will immediately become apparent is the scarcity of well-designed prospective studies of how a commonly prescribed pharmaceutical agent—oral contraceptives—influences the physiology and athletic performance of young women. The author rightly points out that the wide individual differences among women in response to changes in the hormonal milieu in the normal menstrual cycle may also occur in response to the exogenous hormones. Although the effect of either endogenous or exogenous hormones may have a minimal effect on the athletic performance of most women, they may severely disrupt the performance in others.—B.L. Drinkwater, Ph.D.

Influence of the Menstrual Cycle and Oral Contraceptives on Thermoregulatory Responses to Exercise in Young Women

Grucza R, Pekkarinen H, Titov E-K, Kononoff A, Hänninen O (Polish Academy of Sciences, Warsaw, Poland; Univ of Kuopio, Finland)
Eur J Appl Physiol 67:279–285, 1993   139-94-7-13

Background.—The basal body temperature of women fluctuates during the menstrual cycle. Previous reports of how the fluctuation in basal body temperature influences thermoregulatory reactions to endogenous and exogenous heat loads have been contradictory. Changes in the thermoregulatory response to exercise on a cycle ergometer at 50% maximal aerobic power ($\dot{V}O_{2max}$) in a moderate environment (24°C, 50% relative air humidity) were examined during the luteal and follicular phases of the menstrual cycle in 10 women not taking oral contraceptives (NP) and 10 women using oral contraceptives (P).

Method.—The women were tested for maximal aerobic capacity in the climatic chamber the day before each standard submaximal exercise test to determine the appropriate workload for each phase of the menstrual cycle. Rectal, mean skin, and mean body temperatures, and heart and sweat rate were measured during the 45-minute exercise at 50% $\dot{V}O_{2max}$ in both follicular and luteal phases of the cycle.

Findings.—The NP women had a higher temperature threshold and larger gains for sweating in the luteal phase compared with the follicular phase. The dynamics and the whole period for sweating were greater in the luteal phase than in the follicular phase in NP women. In the NP group, rectal, mean skin, and mean body temperatures and heart rate increased significantly more in the follicular phase than in the luteal phase. The $\dot{V}O_{2max}$ did not differ either between phases of the menstrual cycle or between the 2 groups of women tested. The P group also showed an upward shift of rectal temperature threshold for sweating in the luteal phase.

Conclusion.—In NP women, the thermoregulatory system was affected during the luteal phase by a greater rectal temperature threshold for sweating and gains in sweating. The P women also showed an upward shift of rectal temperature threshold for sweating in the luteal phase but no phase-related differences in the gains of sweating. The thermoregulatory response to exercise appeared more uniform in the P women.

▶ There have been a number of studies designed to determine if and how the menstrual cycle affects the thermoregulatory response to exercise. Results have varied, and there is as yet no clear consensus on how important cycle phase might be in a woman's ability to tolerate exercise in a hot environment. In this paper, the thermal load was largely endogenous, brief, and did not challenge the thermoregulatory system to any extent. What was interesting and novel was the finding that oral contraceptives moderated the differences in response between the phases of the cycle but had no marked effect on the overall response.—B.L. Drinkwater, Ph.D.

Adherence to ACOG Guidelines on Exercise During Pregnancy: Effect on Pregnancy Outcome

Zeanah M, Schlosser SP (Univ of Montevallo, Ala; Samford Univ, Birmingham, Ala)
J Obstet Gynecol Neonatal Nurs 22:329–335, 1993   139-94-7–14

Background.—The guidelines of the American College of Obstetricians and Gynecologists (ACOG) for safe exercise during pregnancy have the stated goal of ensuring a safe and healthy pregnancy for most women. However, a number of questions remain regarding the relationship of these guidelines to pregnancy outcome, including whether they constitute a legal standard of care. The level of adherence of pregnant women to these guidelines on pregnancy and the effects of nonadherence on pregnancy outcome were examined in a retrospective survey.

Methods.—One hundred seventy-three women at 2 national physical fitness conferences who had exercised regularly during pregnancy were surveyed. Ninety-one percent had also exercised regularly before their pregnancy. The subjects responded to a 35-item questionnaire regarding their exercise program during pregnancy, including its frequency, duration, and intensity. The duration and intensity of exercise through the third trimester were the independent variables for assessment of pregnancy outcome.

Findings.—The response rate was 81%. Eighty-three percent of the responders knew about the ACOG guidelines, and 53% reported adhering to them. Pregnancy complications necessitated discontinuation of exercise in 13%, all of whom were excluded from further analysis. Eighteen women reported exercising at a heart rate of more than 150 beats per minute through the third trimester, and 37 reported exercising for longer than 40 minutes into the third trimester. These groups showed no significant difference in maternal weight gain, fetal birth weight, or gestational age of the newborn from women with more moderate levels of exercise. Women in the long-duration and moderate-intensity groups did have significantly fewer cesarean deliveries. There were no significant differences in the proportion of women from each group who delivered on time or more than 7 days early or late.

Conclusion.—Exercising in excess of the ACOG guidelines does not appear to have any adverse effects on maternal or fetal health for women who exercised regularly before conceiving and who have uncomplicated pregnancies. Women appear more likely to learn about the ACOG guidelines from exercise instructors than from their physicians. The findings suggest it may be desirable to revise the guidelines to allow women more opportunities to pursue appropriate levels of exercise during pregnancy.

▶ This paper was based on responses to a questionnaire rather than a laboratory study. However, it should be remembered that these responses came primarily from women who had been physically active before pregnancy, that women who experienced complications were eliminated from the data analysis, and that the majority of women decreased their activity during the third trimester. Most disturbing was the news that only 16% of the women had learned of the ACOG guidelines from their physicians; the others heard of the guidelines from fitness instructors or had read about them.

NOTE: A 1994 revision of the 1985 ACOG guidelines is now available.—B.L. Drinkwater, Ph.D.

Effects of Maternal Aerobic Fitness on Cardiorespiratory Responses to Exercise
Pivarnik JM, Ayres NA, Mauer MB, Cotton DB, Kirshon B, Dildy GA (Baylor College of Medicine, Houston; Texas Children's Hosp, Houston)
Med Sci Sports Exerc 25:993–998, 1993   139-94-7–15

Introduction.—Few data have been gathered on the acute exercise responses of endurance-trained women who continue their physical activity throughout pregnancy. A study was performed to determine whether aerobically fit pregnant women have an enhanced cardiorespiratory response to exercise compared to sedentary pregnant women.

Subjects and Methods.—Ten physically active pregnant women and 6 pregnant sedentary controls took part in the study. All were nonsmokers, between 20 and 35 years of age, and had no obstetric or medical complications. The women were prospectively studied during pregnancy between 24 and 26 weeks and 35 and 37 weeks of gestation and at 12 weeks post partum. On each of these occasions the groups were compared at rest (Table 1) and during 15 minutes of submaximal steady-state cycle exercise (Table 2) performed at a heart rate of 135–140 bpm. Indirect calorimetry was used to measure volumes and fractional concentrations of expired gases. Cardiac output was estimated via CO_2 rebreathing.

Results.—Both during pregnancy and post partum, resting heart rate was less in the physically active women than in the sedentary women whereas stroke volume was significantly higher at rest in active women. For all subjects, resting heart rate and cardiac output values were significantly lower and systemic vascular resistance was significantly higher at 12 weeks post partum compared with values during pregnancy. Active women were able to accomplish more work on the cycle ergometer at the same exercise heart rate as the sedentary women. Therefore, caloric expenditure during exercise, alveolar ventilation, and cardiac output responses to exercise were all significantly greater in physically active women. Ratings of perceived exertion during exercise did not, however, differ between the active and sedentary groups.

Conclusion.—Women who are aerobically fit at the start of pregnancy and continue to exercise maintain their cardiorespiratory advantages throughout pregnancy and into the post partum period.

TABLE 1.—Selected Mean (± SD) Cardiorespiratory Variables Measured at Rest

	25 wk		36 wk		12 PP	
	PA	SED	PA	SED	PA	SED
HR (b·min⁻¹)	# 71 ± 6	94 ± 7	# 80 ± 10	98 ± 8	# 63 ± 7*	80 ± 8*
SV (ml·b⁻¹)	# 83 ± 13	57 ± 9	# 77 ± 14	55 ± 13	# 84 ± 16	59 ± 14
Q̇ (l·min⁻¹)	5.8 ± 0.8	5.4 ± 0.8	6.0 ± 1.0	5.4 ± 1.3	5.3 ± 1.0*	4.8 ± 1.3*
a-v O₂diff (ml O₂·100 ml⁻¹)	4.4 ± 0.5	5.2 ± 0.6	5.0 ± 0.5	5.7 ± 1.7	5.5 ± 1.4	5.0 ± 1.4
MAP (mm Hg)	84 ± 7*	85 ± 7*	92 ± 8	93 ± 12	91 ± 5	96 ± 16
SVR (dyne·s·cm⁻⁵)	1121 ± 215	1236 ± 238	1177 ± 167	1387 ± 359	1373 ± 285*	1661 ± 587*
V̇O₂ (ml·min⁻¹)	256 ± 32	279 ± 44	302 ± 37	298 ± 65	280 ± 45	230 ± 47*
V̇E (l·min⁻¹)	10.6 ± 1.4	12.5 ± 2.2	13.4 ± 2.5	13.9 ± 3.1	11.0 ± 1.9*	10.0 ± 2.2*
V̇T (l·br⁻¹)	0.67 ± 0.12	0.69 ± 0.13	0.74 ± 0.14	0.80 ± 0.14	0.62 ± 0.15*	0.52 ± 0.15*
RR (br·min⁻¹)	17 ± 4	18 ± 1	19 ± 4	17 ± 2	18 ± 4	19 ± 7
V̇A (l·min⁻¹)	5.5 ± 0.9	6.5 ± 1.7	7.4 ± 1.2	8.2 ± 2.2	5.2 ± 1.5*	4.4 ± 1.3*
V̇E/V̇O₂	41.5 ± 4.5	44.6 ± 1.2	44.5 ± 6.5	46.8 ± 3.3	39.7 ± 7.5	44.7 ± 8.5
V̇E/V̇CO₂	50.2 ± 4.7	54.2 ± 4.9	50.2 ± 5.5	49.7 ± 3.8	51.6 ± 10.2	58.2 ± 12.7
VD/VT	0.38 ± 0.04	0.39 ± 0.05	0.36 ± 0.04	0.34 ± 0.04	0.43 ± 0.09*	0.43 ± 0.08*

Abbreviations: MAP, mean arterial pressure; PA, physically active; Q̇, maternal cardiac output; RR, respiratory rate; SED, sedentary; SVR, systemic vascular resistance; V̇$_A$, alveolar ventilation; V̇CO₂, carbon dioxide production; V̇$_D$/V̇$_T$, dead space/tidal volume ratio; V̇$_E$, minute ventilation; V̇O₂, oxygen consumption; V̇O$_{2max}$, aerobic capacity; V̇$_T$, tidal volume.
* Significantly different from that in other gestational ages ($P < .01$).
# Significant difference between PA (no. = 10) and SED (no. = 6) subjects ($P < .01$).
(Courtesy of Pivarnik JM, Ayres NA, Mauer MB, et al: *Med Sci Sports Exerc* 25:993–998, 1993.)

TABLE 2.—Selected Mean (± SD) Cardiorespiratory Variables During Submaximal Cycle Exercise

	25 wk PA	25 wk SED	36 wk PA	36 wk SED	12 PP PA	12 PP SED
HR (b·min^{-1})	138 ± 3	139 ± 3	138 ± 7	138 ± 4	139 ± 3	142 ± 1
SV (ml·b^{-1})	104 ± 15 #	70 ± 10	100 ± 16	74 ± 10 #	101 ± 12 #	76 ± 9
$\dot{Q}$ (l·min^{-1})	14.4 ± 2.2 #	9.6 ± 1.4	13.8 ± 1.9	10.2 ± 1.4 #	14.1 ± 1.5 #	10.8 ± 1.1
a-v O_{2diff} (ml O_2·100 ml^{-1})	10.1 ± 1.6	8.9 ± 1.3	10.2 ± 1.7	9.5 ± 1.3	10.9 ± 0.7	9.6 ± 1.1
MAP (mm Hg)	99 ± 9	102 ± 10	104 ± 3	105 ± 10	102 ± 4	107 ± 13
SVR (dyne·s·cm^{-5})	533 ± 67 #	828 ± 150	589 ± 83	795 ± 107 #	564 ± 65	773 ± 146
$\dot{V}O_2$ (ml·min^{-1})	1447 ± 256 #	862 ± 182	1388 ± 224	966 ± 152 #	1532 ± 192	1043 ± 177
$\dot{V}_E$ (l·min^{-1})	47.6 ± 12.0 #	34.1 ± 5.2	46.5 ± 10.6	38.7 ± 5.6 #	44.6 ± 7.1	38.5 ± 8.9
$\dot{V}_T$ (l·br^{-1})	1.71 ± 0.38 #	1.35 ± 0.40	1.68 ± 0.36	1.43 ± 0.30 #	1.71 ± 0.23	1.37 ± 0.26
RR (br·min^{-1})	29 ± 8	26 ± 5	29 ± 7	28 ± 5	27 ± 5	28 ± 4
$\dot{V}_A$ (l·min^{-1})	36.8 ± 10.9 #	23.5 ± 5.6	35.7 ± 9.2	29.2 ± 5.5 #	34.4 ± 5.2	27.5 ± 6.7
$\dot{V}_E/\dot{V}O_2$	32.7 ± 4.3	39.9 ± 2.9	33.3 ± 3.5	40.2 ± 2.1 #	29.4 ± 5.9*	36.9 ± 5.9*
$\dot{V}_E/\dot{V}CO_2$	33.7 ± 4.3	41.1 ± 5.3	34.6 ± 3.6	39.0 ± 2.4 #	29.7 ± 4.0*	35.7 ± 3.4*
$\dot{V}_D/\dot{V}_T$	0.20 ± 0.04	0.27 ± 0.06	0.20 ± 0.04	0.22 ± 0.07 #	0.19 ± 0.05	0.25 ± 0.04
RPE (units)	13.0 ± 1.1	13.2 ± 1.7	12.6 ± 1.3	13.5 ± 1.8	12.9 ± 2.0	13.0 ± 3.6

Abbreviations: MAP, mean arterial pressure; PA, physically active; $\dot{Q}$, maternal cardiac output; RPE, rating of perceived exertion; RR, respiratory rate; SED, sedentary; SVR, systemic vascular resistance; $\dot{V}_A$, alveolar ventilation; $\dot{V}CO_2$, carbon dioxide production; $\dot{V}_D/\dot{V}_T$, dead space/tidal volume ratio; $\dot{V}_E$, minute ventilation; $\dot{V}O_2$, oxygen consumption; $\dot{V}O_{2max}$, aerobic capacity.
* Significantly different from that in other gestational ages (P < .01).
# Significant difference between PA (no. = 10) and SED (no. = 6) subjects (P < .01).
(Courtesy of Pivarnik JM, Ayres NA, Mauer MB, et al: Med Sci Sports Exerc 25:993–998, 1993.)

▶ This paper provides additional evidence that women with uncomplicated pregnancies who exercise before pregnancy can continue to exercise throughout pregnancy without harm to themselves or to the fetus. This is essentially the conclusion reached by 6 established investigators in the field who reviewed recent studies in this area (1). However, it should be noted that the women in this study voluntarily reduced the intensity of their activity (i.e., a run to a walk) or changed the type of activity (i.e., running to swimming) during the third trimester.—B.L. Drinkwater, Ph.D.

Reference

1. McMurray RG, et al: *Med Sci Sports Exerc* 25:1305, 1993.

Thermoregulation of Pregnant Women During Aerobic Exercise on Land and in the Water
McMurray RG, Katz VL, Meyer-Goodwin WE, Cefalo RC (Univ of North Carolina, Chapel Hill)
Am J Perinatol 10:178–182, 1993   139-94-7–16

Background.—Maternal hyperthermia during the first trimester has been associated with adverse fetal development. However, temperature regulation by pregnant women during exercise has not been well studied. To avoid core temperature elevation, some experts are recommending exercise in water for pregnant women who wish to exercise. In this study, the thermoregulatory responses of pregnant women were compared while doing exercise of similar intensity both on land and in water.

Subjects.—Seven women in their 25th to 26th week of singleton pregnancy who were aged 26–35 years and who were active but not involved in a regular exercise program participated in this study. The subjects underwent a submaximal cycle ergometer test to determine maximal aerobic power ($\dot{V}O_{2max}$) at 70% of predicted heart rate maximum. They then underwent, in random order, a 20-minute session of land exercise and a 20-minute session of exercise while immersed in 30°C water. The exercises in water and on land were completed at a similar metabolic rate.

Results.—The mean skin temperature was significantly lower during water trials than during land trials. Exercise increased core temperature, with a greater increase during land trials (Fig 7-3) of half a degree Celsius.

Conclusion.—In pregnant women of average fitness, exercise on land at about 70% of maximal heart rate for 20 minutes can be performed without hyperthermia. Exercise in the water is even less likely to increase core temperature.

▶ There is nothing surprising in finding less thermal stress while exercising in cool water rather than on land, but qualifying the difference for a given percentage of maximum heart rate provides helpful guidance to those recom-

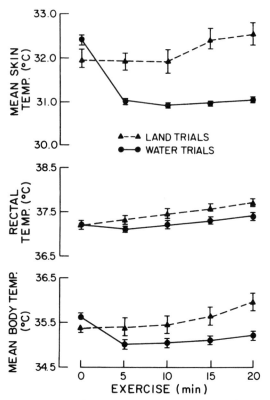

Fig 7–3.—Rectal, mean skin, and mean body temperature responses of pregnant women during 20 minutes of exercise at 70% of their maximal heart rate on land and in 30°C water (mean ± SEM). P < .05 land vs. water trials for all 3 measures. (Courtesy of McMurray RG, Katz VL, Meyer-Goodwin WE, et al: *Am J Perinatol* 10:178–182, 1993.)

mending water exercise to pregnant women. However, the comparisons would have been more meaningful if the authors had included information about the ambient temperature and humidity of the land environment as well as the temperature of the water.—B.L. Drinkwater, Ph.D.

A Spherical Model Analyzing Shoulder Motion in Overhand and Side-arm Pitching

Yoshikawa G-i (Shiga Univ of Medical Science, Japan)
J Shoulder Elbow Surg 2:198–208, 1993   139-94-7–17

Background.—Accurate measurement of shoulder movement during pitching is essential for prevention of "baseball shoulder." Three-dimensional image analysis was used to assess pitching motions.

Methods.—Thirty amateur baseball pitchers with an overhand pitching style and 5 with an underhand pitching style threw an overhand and un-

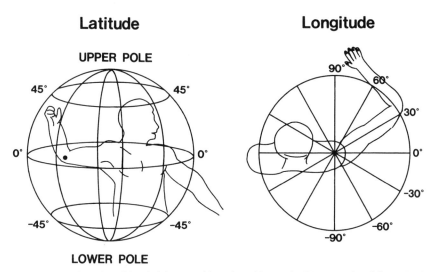

Fig 7–4.—Spherical model and definition of latitude and longitude. (Courtesy of Yoshikawa G-i: *J Shoulder Elbow Surg* 2:198–208, 1993.)

derhand fastball. High-speed video cameras photographed each pitch from 2 perpendicular directions. The visual images were analyzed and input into a computer that calculated the 3-dimensional movements of the shoulder joint. A spherical model was devised to represent shoulder joint movements, with the shoulder as the center of the sphere (Fig 7–4). The latitude and longitude of the elbow position were determined and regarded as the elevation angle and circumduction angle.

Results.—In all subjects, shoulder motion and time course differed little between pitching methods, although regression analysis revealed individual variations in both parameters. For the overhand throw, the upper arm was continuously slowly elevated for up to .16 seconds before the throw, peaking at a latitude above 0 degrees around −.25 seconds. Subsequently, latitude returned to 0 degrees and the arm began to elevate again, leading to ball release. Sidearm throw produced a similar curve. In the longitude time course for an overhand throw, the upper arm slowly moved backward for up to .17 seconds, then began to move forward until it reached an equilibrium lasting from .03 seconds before ball release to .02 seconds after ball release.

Discussion.—These findings may have useful clinical ramifications. Pitching shoulder motion evolves over time, beginning in childhood. A chronological study using image analysis is indicated to determine whether the learned shoulder motion can be changed by changing pitching style.

▶ These authors suggest that pitching shoulder motion evolves over time, beginning in childhood. I tested one 5-year-old boy and biomechanically compared his pitching style with the style of a great major league pitcher, Whitey Ford. There were significant similarities in style with only the coordination of the 2 styles demonstrating much difference. The coordination, which comes with years of practice, is what leads to the development of the most effective and efficient summation of forces. The summation of forces is a major determinant of ball velocity.—Col. J.L. Anderson, PE.D.

Decreased Physical Activity in Pima Indian Compared With Caucasian Children
Fontvieille AM, Kriska A, Ravussin E (Natl Inst of Diabetes and Digestive and Kidney Diseases, Phoenix, Ariz; Univ of Pittsburgh, Pa)
Int J Obes 17:445–452, 1993   139-94-7–18

Background.—Few cross-sectional and longitudinal studies have examined the likely role of physical activity in the development of obesity in children. In this study, the relationship between physical activity and body composition was investigated in Pima Indian (a group highly prone to obesity) and white children.

Patients and Methods.—A total of 43 Pima Indian and 42 white children participated. The ages of the subjects were 9.9 and 9.7 years, respectively. There were 22 male and 21 female Indian children and 21 male and 21 female white children. A list of typical leisure-time sporting activities was established, and children were asked to report how much time they had devoted to each activity during the past week and the past year. In addition to these estimations of physical activity, details about time spent playing outside and watching television or videos were also collected. Anthropometric and body composition measurements were obtained from each child, and information collected from the children was compared with that obtained from a parental questionnaire, which was completed when the child was not in the room.

Results.—Pima Indians were taller than whites (mean, 143 vs. 137 cm), heavier (mean, 48.6 vs. 32.9 kg), and fatter (mean, 39% vs. 24% fat). Compared with white girls, Pima Indian girls had participated in significantly less past-week and past-year sport leisure activity and had spent significantly more time watching television or videos. In addition, Pima Indian boys had participated in significantly less past-week sport leisure activity than white boys, and past-year sport leisure activity correlated negatively with body mass index and percentage body fat in Indian boys. Similar correlations were not noted in Indian girls, possibly because of their very low activity levels. In white children, time spent watching television positively correlated with waist/thigh ratio, and a positive correlation between television watching and percentage body fat was found in white girls. No association between measures of obesity and television viewing were noted for Pima Indians.

Conclusion.—It is suggested that decreased physical activity and increased television viewing may facilitate the development of obesity in Pima Indian children.

▶ In this cross-sectional study of the roots of obesity, Pima Indian children, compared with white children, were fatter, were less physically active, and watched more TV. Although such a study cannot determine cause and effect, the data at least tie the presence of obesity to decreased physical activity and increased television watching, suggesting practical ways to prevent or reduce obesity in kids. Presumably, when we turn off the TV, our kids will jump up, run a mile, and read Hamlet. A 55-year follow-up shows us that being overweight in adolescence predicts a broad range of adverse health effects in adulthood that are largely independent of adult weight (1). Prior studies also suggest that too much TV promotes obesity—and hypercholesterolemia—in kids (2, 3), and that parents can boost physical activity in their kids by playing with them and taking them to games (4).—E.R. Eichner, M.D.

References

1. Must A, et al: N Engl J Med 327:1350, 1992.
2. Dietz WH, Gortmaker SL: Pediatrics 75:807, 1985.
3. Wong ND, et al: Pediatrics 90:75, 1992.
4. Sallis JF, et al: Am J Dis Child 146:1383, 1992.

Leisure Time Physical Activity in the Young: Correlation With Low-Back Pain, Spinal Mobility and Trunk Muscle Strength in 15-Year-Old School Children
Salminen JJ, Oksanen A, Mäki P, Pentti J, Kujala UM (Turku Univ, Finland; Univ of Jyväskylä, Finland; Turku Regional Inst of Occupational Health, Finland; et al)
Int J Sports Med 14:406–410, 1993   139-94-7–19

Introduction.—Both sedentary behavior and a high level of physical activity may be harmful to spinal structures and result in back pain in the young. Moderate physical activity or training, however, may help to protect against low back pain (LBP). The prevalence of LBP was studied in 1,503 boys and girls aged 15 years, and structural abnormalities, spinal mobility, and trunk muscle strength were compared in those with and without LBP.

Methods.—A survey on LBP administered to the students had a 91.6% response rate, and the results indicated that the prevalence of continuous or recurrent LBP was 7.8%. A case-control study was carried out with a randomized sample of 40 affected children and 40 asymptomatic controls matched for sex, age, and school class. The subjects were interviewed regarding their leisure time activity and were examined for mobility and muscle strength.

Results.—Among the total sample, 32 subjects (42%) reported regular physical activity at least 3 days a week. A nearly equal percentage of boys (38.2%) and girls (38.1%) participated in no regular activity. Weight, height, and body mass index were similar in the active and sedentary groups. Those with a low level of leisure time physical activity, however, had an increased incidence of LBP compared with the more active children (73.7% vs. 42.1%). Four of the 7 tests of mobility correlated with leisure time physical activity. In the passive group, abdominal muscle strength was diminished and endurance strength of the back muscles was significantly decreased.

Conclusion.—A low frequency of physical activity appears to increase a young person's risk for LBP. Although there is some evidence that an extremely high level of physical activity can be harmful to the lower back, participation in sports as a leisure time activity has positive effects on spinal mobility and trunk muscle strength in both boys and girls.

▶ This article emphasizes that, regarding LBP in children, exercise can be a 2-edged sword. In other words, although excessive physical activity in the weight-loading, rotational, or back-arching sports can predispose to LBP from spondylolysis, too little physical activity can predispose to LBP from decreases in spinal mobility and in strength of back and abdominal muscles. In boys and girls, one risk factor for LBP seems to be sloth.—E.R. Eichner, M.D.

Weighing the Risks: Strength Training for Children and Adolescents
Tanner SM (Univ of Colorado, Denver)
Physician Sportsmed 21:105–106, 109–110, 114, 116, 1993
139-94-7–20

Background.—Strength training by children and adolescents in preparation for rigorous sports competition is becoming increasingly popular. However, unsupervised training and improper technique can cause significant injury to the immature musculoskeletal system of growing children.

Findings.—It has long been assumed that girls and prepubertal boys would not benefit greatly from strength training because of insufficient circulating androgens. However, more recent studies have shown that a properly designed strength training program can significantly improve strength in this age group. Although injuries associated with strength training in children have been reported, most injuries result from misused weight equipment belonging to others or from using incorrect techniques during supervised weight training. Such injuries do not usually occur in well-conducted programs. There is recent evidence that strength training in children may actually provide some resistance to injury, but long-term studies on whether strength training affects or damages bone growth are not available.

Conclusion.—A well-supervised program of progressive strength training can safely increase the strength of most children and adolescents and improve their athletic performance.

Recreational Weight Lifting and Aortic Dissection: Case Report
Schor JS, Horowitz MD, Livingstone AS (Univ of Miami, Fla)
J Vasc Surg 17:774–776, 1993   139-94-7-21

Objective.—In the absence of predisposing factors, patients younger than age 40 years rarely have aortic dissection. Type I, or ascending, aortic dissection has been reported in young weight lifters, but descending,

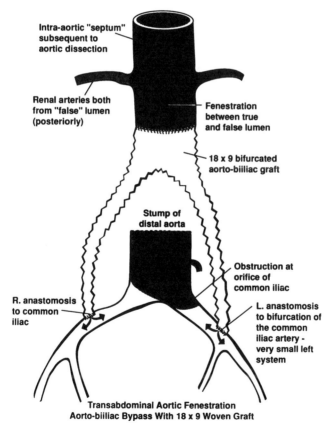

Fig 7–5.—Transabdominal aortic fenestration by use of aortobiiliac bypass with an 18 × 9 mm woven graft. (Courtesy of Schor JS, Horowitz MD, Livingstone AS: *J Vasc Surg* 17:774–776, 1993.)

or type III, dissection has not. Dissection in young weight lifters may be an increasingly common phenomenon.

Case Report.—Man, 18, with a known small muscular ventricular septal defect complained of claudication in the left buttock and leg after walking a short distance. Questioning revealed that he had felt a sharp, tearing pain in his chest and back during weight lifting. He had a blood pressure of 180/90 mm Hg, with a 30 mm Hg gradient between his arms and legs. He had a systolic murmur over the precordium, with diminished femoral and distal pulses.

The ventricular septal defect was unchanged on cardiac catheterization. The patient had aortic dissection beginning just distal to the left subclavian artery, with no aneurysmal dilation of the thoracic aorta. There was a double lumen to the abdominal aorta, the true lumen being anterior and giving rise to the celiac and superior mesenteric arteries, and the false lumen being posterior and serving as the origin of the renal arteries. Flow to the left iliac system was greatly reduced on Doppler flow studies, and an obstructive clot was seen at the area of the aortic bifurcation on MRI.

Via a nonthoracic approach, the patient underwent transabdominal aortic fenestration with aortobiiliac bypass using an 18 × 9 mm bifurcated knitted Dacron graft (Fig 7-5). Postoperatively, persistent hypertension was well controlled with nifedipine. Renal flow study showed perfusion of both kidneys, and distal pulses were palpable on day 8, when the patient was discharged. One month later, the patient's blood pressure was well controlled and he was completely free of symptoms of claudication.

Discussion.—This is the first reported case of descending aortic dissection occurring during weight lifting. In this case, chronic dissection manifested by iliac artery occlusion resulted in claudication of the buttock and leg. Weight lifting appears to be a major cause of aortic dissection; more cases similar to this one may be seen as more individuals take up weight lifting as a form of exercise.

▶ These companion articles (Abstracts 139-94-7–20 and 139-94-7–21) convey reassurance and caution regarding weight lifting by young people. Abstract 139-94-7–20 is a practical overview of strength training for boys and girls. It ponders potential dangers—low back pain, growth plate damage, aggravation of hypertension, blackouts—and expected benefits—increased strength and performance, as well as increased resistance to injury. It considers pros and cons of both free weights and machines. In simple terms, based on information from the American Academy of Pediatrics, it tells how to go about strength training. In agreement with a recent article on strength training in prepubescent boys (1), it concludes that most children can benefit from a supervised strength training program.

Abstract 139-94-7–21 reports a rare event—descending aortic dissection—that may have stemmed from weight lifting, which has been linked to ascending aortic dissection in subjects with cystic medial degeneration. No prior case of descending aortic dissection has been tied to weight lifting, but this patient had mild cystic medial necrosis. The authors warn that a new entity may be emerging: aortic dissection in young weight lifters. Let's hope not.—E.R. Eichner, M.D.

Reference

1. 1991 YEAR BOOK OF SPORTS MEDICINE, pp 307–308.

Kinematics of Recovery From a Stumble
Grabiner MD, Koh TJ, Lundin TM, Jahnigen DW (Cleveland Clinic Found, Ohio)
J Gerontol 48:M97–M102, 1993   139-94-7-22

Background.—Accident-related injuries among elderly patients most often result from falls during locomotion and stair climbing or descent. Several musculoskeletal and neuromotor risk factors for falls have been identified. Systematic analysis of the effects of perturbations during locomotion and requisites for recovery from a fall may enable development of clinical evaluations that identify persons at risk for falling. Recovery from an anteriorly directed stumble was analyzed in a biomechanical investigation.

Methods.—Seven healthy, active young male subjects walked along a walkway in a laboratory, and a mechanical obstacle in the floor was raised periodically to induce a stumble. Each subject performed 6 control trials without the obstacle and 6 trials in which the obstacle was used.

Results.—A substantial increase in post-stumble trunk flexion angle was observed. Maximum trunk flexion after the perturbation was significantly associated with preperturbation walking velocity. The differences between conditions for maximum knee flexion angle and maximum hip flexion angle were significant, although neither increase was significantly associated with preperturbation walking velocity. The maximum hip flexion velocity and maximum knee extension velocity did not differ significantly; increases in these parameters did not relate significantly to preperturbation walking velocity.

Conclusion.—Recovery from a stumble requires lower extremity muscular power and the ability to regain control of the flexing trunk. Identifying the primary elements of control during perturbed locomotion may advance understanding of the relationship between specific age-related performance deficits and some types of falls. The results from this study provide a starting point for further experimental biomechanical analysis of the mechanical and neuromotor factors associated with recovery from stumbles.

▶ These authors used younger subjects in studying recovery from a stumble because it would be too dangerous to use elderly subjects with this experimental design. However, knowing that recovery from a stumble requires lower extremity muscular power and the ability to regain control of the flexing trunk is of value while we continue to study other aspects of the stumble phenomenon. For instance, it seems to me that exercise programs for the aging population would indicate that any stumble prevention program should include exercise to strengthen the leg muscles, especially the leg flexor, and to strengthen the rector spinae and abdominal muscles.—Col. J.L. Anderson, PE.D.

Effects of Motor Unit Losses on Strength in Older Men and Women
Doherty TJ, Vandervoort AA, Taylor AW, Brown WF (Univ of Western Ontario, London, Canada; New England Med Ctr, Boston)
J Appl Physiol 74:868–874, 1993   139-94-7–23

Introduction.—The reduction in muscle mass and strength that occurs with aging may in part be the result of loss of α-motor neurons. A previous study found a substantial reduction in maximal isometric twitch force in older individuals that correlated well with a reduced number of motor units as estimated by an electrophysiologic technique. This study differs in its use of proximal muscles instead of the extensor digitorum brevis muscle. The latter is supplied by the common peroneal nerve, which is prone to injury and can show signs of denervation in younger subjects.

Methods.—Forty-four adult volunteers took part in the study. Twenty (10 women and 10 men) ranged in age from 60 to 81 years and 24 (9 women and 15 men) were between the ages of 21 and 38 years. All subjects were active and free of neurologic disease. Spike-triggered averaging was used to estimate the number of motor units in the biceps brachii and brachialis muscles. Electrophysiologic recordings were made on a computerized electromyographic system. The numbers of motor units present were estimated by dividing the amplitude of the maximum compound muscle action potential of the biceps brachii and brachialis muscles by the mean surface-recorded single motor unit action potentials (S-MUAPs) amplitude. Also recorded were the maximum isometric twitch contraction (MTC) and maximum voluntary contraction (MVC) of the elbow flexors.

Results.—The estimated numbers of motor units were reduced by 47% in older subjects relative to younger subjects (mean, 189 vs. 357). In contrast, the sizes of the S-MUAPs were significantly larger in older subjects. Age-associated reductions in the MTC and MVC were also observed; these differences were significant, although they were less dramatic than the reduction in motor units. Both young and older subjects had a considerable range in the peak-to-peak amplitudes of the S-MUAPs.

Conclusion.—Men and women older than 60 years have approximately one half the number of motor units of young adults in the biceps brachii and brachialis muscles. This age-related change is reflected by reductions in the maximal M-potential amplitude and an increased mean S-MUAP amplitude. Thus, the reduced contractile strength of older active persons appears to be secondary to losses of motor units. Older men and women exhibited similar reductions in strength.

▶ We need a controlled longitudinal study to determine what effect physical exercise, both moderate and vigorous, will have on the aging process. We all believe intuitively that we can significantly slow the aging process through exercise, but there are few controlled studies that we can point to that will show this.—Col. J.L. Anderson, PE.D.

The Physical Condition of Elderly Women Differing in Habitual Physical Activity
Voorrips LE, Lemmink KAPM, Van Heuvelen MJG, Bult P, Van Staveren WA (Wageningen Agricultural Univ, The Netherlands; Univ of Groningen, The Netherlands)
Med Sci Sports Exerc 25:1152–1157, 1993   139-94-7-24

Background.—Physical activity in old age can help sustain muscle mass, bone density, maximal oxygen uptake capacity, motor performance, grip strength, reaction time, and flexibility. A study of elderly women was undertaken to determine whether levels of physical activity corresponded with overall physical fitness.

Method.—On the basis of responses to a physical activity questionnaire, 100 women aged 60–80 years were divided into tertiles of active, intermediate, or least active. Nineteen women from the active tertile (highly active), 15 from the intermediate tertile (moderately active), and 16 from the least active (sedentary) tertile completed a battery of physical fitness tests and a questionnaire to evaluate subjective fitness and health. The physical fitness tests included peak expiratory flow, flexibility of the shoulder joint, flexibility of the hip and spine by a sit-and-reach test, balance, reaction time, grip strength, manual dexterity, and endurance. Data were also collected on height, body weight, and systolic and diastolic blood pressure.

Results.—The more physically active elderly women had better results than the least active on body weight, body mass index, endurance, and flexibility of hip and spine. There was a significant Pearson correlation coefficient between body weight and test results for diastolic and systolic blood pressure; flexibility of the hip, spine, and shoulder; grip strength; and endurance (table). The women's subjective evaluation of their physical fitness and health corresponded with the measured data.

Conclusion.—As hypothesized, habitually physically active elderly women had better results on physical fitness tests than less active women. The differences in body weight and body mass index, flexibility

Characteristics and Physical Fitness of Elderly Women With
Different Levels of Habitual Physical Activity

	Sedentary $\bar{x} \pm SD$ (N=16)	Moderately Active $\bar{x} \pm SD$ (N=15)	High Active $\bar{x} \pm SD$ (N=19)	P *
Age (yr)	72.1 ± 4.3	71.9 ± 3.9	70.8 ± 4.4	0.63
Height (cm)	163 ± 6	162 ± 7	162 ± 6	0.71
Weight (kg)	81 ± 11[a]	69 ± 13[b]	65 ± 9[b]	<0.05
BMI (kg·m^{-2})	30.5 ± 5.3[a]	26.5 ± 4.4[b]	24.9 ± 3.8[b]	<0.05
Blood pressure (mm Hg)				
Systolic	162 ± 27	154 ± 33	145 ± 20	0.17
Diastolic	87 ± 11	84 ± 14	78 ± 10	0.10
Lung function				
Peak-flow (l·min^{-1})	306 ± 117	353 ± 90	361 ± 92	0.25
Reaction time (ms)	247 ± 71	230 ± 33	235 ± 39	0.63
Grip strength (kgf)				
Dominant hand	26.9 ± 4.1	26.2 ± 4.4	25.6 ± 4.1	0.67
Nondominant hand	25.6 ± 3.6	24.7 ± 4.6	22.9 ± 5.5	0.23
Flexibility				
Hip and spine (cm)	22.9 ± 8.9[a]	30.1 ± 11.6[a,b]	35.2 ± 8.7[b]	<0.05
Shoulder (angle,°)	41.3 ± 3.9	40.8 ± 5.3	39.3 ± 7.2	0.56
Manual dexterity (s)	46.8 ± 4.2	46.1 ± 4.6	45.9 ± 5.0	0.42
Balance (s)	26 ± 2	25 ± 2	27 ± 2	0.06
Walking (25 m trajects)	12.1 ± 8.9[a]	22.0 ± 9.9[b]	26.6 ± 10.1[b]	<0.05

Note: Groups with the same superscript ([a,b]) are not significantly different from each other.
* P value for group effect (analysis of variance).
(Courtesy of Voorrips LE, Lemmink KAPM, Van Heuvelen MJG, et al: Med Sci Sports Exerc 25:1152–1157, 1993.)

of the hip and spine, and endurance on the walk test were significantly better for the more active women. Trends were observed for blood pressure, peak expiratory flow, and balance. The participants' subjective evaluation of their physical fitness and health corresponded with the measured results.

▶ Although reports like this are very encouraging for older women who are *already* active, long-term prospective studies of the effect of physical activity on these and other important fitness variables are needed to prove that sedentary women can benefit by increasing their level of activity. These authors attempted to recruit only healthy women for their study, but there may be subtle differences in health that determine one's decision to adopt an active or a sedentary lifestyle.—B.L. Drinkwater, Ph.D.

Physical Fitness as a Predictor of Mortality Among Healthy, Middle-Aged Norwegian Men
Sandvik L, Erikssen J, Thaulow E, Erikssen G, Mundal R, Rodahl K (Central Hosp of Akershus, Nordbyhagen, Norway; Natl Univ Hosp, Oslo, Norway;

Ullevaal Hosp, Oslo, Norway; et al)
N Engl J Med 328:533–537, 1993   139-94-7–25

Background.—It has been suggested that physical activity is an independent predictor of mortality from cardiovascular causes, but the issue remains controversial. The authors of this study previously reported that poor physical fitness in apparently healthy men aged 40–59 years was associated with increased mortality from cardiovascular causes during the next 7 years. The 16-year follow-up data are presented here.

Methods.—The original study population consisted of 2,014 healthy Norwegian men aged 40–59 years who entered the prospective study between 1972 and 1975. All men underwent comprehensive baseline evaluation, including conventional coronary risk factor assessment and physical fitness testing on a cycle ergometer. Men with existing cardiovascular disease were excluded from the study. Participants were divided into 4 fitness quartiles according to individual fitness level, with quartile 1 denoting the lowest fitness level and quartile 4 the highest.

Results.—After an average follow-up of 15.9 years, 271 men had died, 143 of them (52.8%) of cardiovascular disease. Of those who died, 61 were in the lowest fitness quartile, 45 were in quartile 2, 26 were in quartile 3, and 11 were in the highest fitness quartile. The relationship between physical fitness and mortality from cardiovascular causes began to appear only after 5 years (Fig 7–6). There was a graded difference in mortality from cardiovascular causes between men in quartiles 2 and 3 and those in quartile 4. After adjustment for age and smoking status,

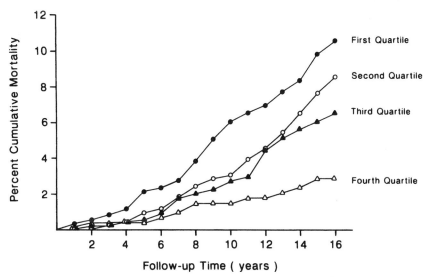

Fig 7–6.—Cumulative age-adjusted mortality from cardiovascular causes during 16 years of follow-up, according to fitness quartile. (Courtesy of Sandvik L, Erikssen J, Thaulow E, et al: *N Engl J Med* 328:533–537, 1993.)

overall mortality and mortality from cardiovascular causes were both lowest among men in fitness quartile 4.

Conclusion.—Physical fitness in healthy middle-aged men appears to be a graded, independent, long-term predictor of mortality from cardiovascular causes and is also associated with lower mortality from any cause.

▶ The unadjusted 7-year cardiovascular risk ratio (4.8 when comparing quartiles 1 and 4) is of an order similar to that previously reported by Blair and associates (1). Plainly, it is better to be fit than unfit. The authors concluded that physical fitness was an independent risk factor as a result of 3 multivariate analyses. The first statistical model adjusted their cardiovascular mortality data for age and smoking status; using this model, the risk in quartile 4 was only 30% of that in quartile 1 (relative risk .30). After further adjustment of mortality rates for serum lipids, blood pressure, resting heart rate, vital capacity, body mass index, level of physical activity, and glucose tolerance, the relative risk changed only slightly to .41. The risk ratio for all-cause mortality, using this more extensive model, was .54.

Although it is tempting to infer that physical fitness exerts a protective effect that is independent of physical activity (for example, some effect related to an inherited difference of body build), it is also possible that the measurement of physical activity is sufficiently crude that it only accounts for a fraction of the true activity-related variance in the mortality statistics, and that a determination of physical fitness provides a better measure of the same variable.—R.J. Shephard, M.D., Ph.D.

Reference

1. Blair S, et al: JAMA 262:2395, 1989.

Cycling: Longevity in the Winners of the Tour de France
de Mondenard J-P (Chennevières-Sur-Marne, France)
Médecine du Sport 66:103–110, 1992   139-94-7-26

Purpose.—Numerous authors have studied the life span of competitive athletes, but none of the studies found that competitive athletes live longer than the general population. A 1986 study comprising 17,000 elderly individuals reported that regular physical exercise decreases morbidity and mortality. Specifically, those who regularly rode a bike gained at least 2 years by age 80 years when compared with those who only occasionally rode a bike or did not ride bikes at all. Whether this benefit was also evident among winners of the Tour de France (TF) was analyzed.

Methods.—The records of all cyclists who won the TF between 1903 and 1990 were analyzed. Available data included the TF winners' date of birth, year when they won the TF, total number of days per year spent in competitive cycling, length of each TF course in kilometers, difficulty of the racing course, cycling pace, total kilometers raced per year, and age at death.

Results.—The average life span of TF winners for the entire study was 60.1 years. The life expectancy for French men ranged from 47 years in 1900 to 60 years in 1946 to 72.3 years in 1988. When accidental deaths were excluded, the average life span of TF winners increased to 67.1 years between 1930 and 1990. When only the years before World War II were considered, the overall average life span of TF winners increased to 63.9 years and increased further to 74.6 years when accidental deaths were excluded. For all analyses, the life span of TF winners was significantly shorter than that of the general population. An analysis of journals and news items identified the following risk factors for a decreased life span among professional cyclists: inadequate rest periods during races; not enough time between racing events; too many racing days per year; financial incentives; and abuse of corticosteroids, anabolic steroids, amphetamines, and other performance-enhancing aids.

Conclusion.—Professional cyclists who regularly participate in long-distance racing are at increased risk of a shortened life span.

▶ The TF is the cardiorespiratory endurance sport par excellence, and one might anticipate that any favorable effect of athletics on longevity would be seen among competitors in this event. However, in practice, the analysis is clouded by several factors: the need to accumulate data over a long period when the longevity of sedentary individuals was increasing rapidly; doping (which has been rampant in this and other cycling competitions); fatal road accidents; and retirement from cycle racing after only 10–20 years of involvement. In fact (and in keeping with current thinking), a much greater extension of life span is obtained from the use of a bicycle in ordinary daily living.—R.J. Shephard, M.D., Ph.D.

Prediction of Mortality and Morbidity With a 6-Minute Walk Test in Patients With Left Ventricular Dysfunction

Bittner V, for the Studies of Left Ventricular Dysfunction Investigators) (Univ of Alabama, Birmingham)
JAMA 270:1702–1707, 1993   139-94-7–27

Background.—Optimal clinical management of congestive heart failure (CHF) requires some reliable means of assessing the severity of symptoms, degree of left ventricular dysfunction, prognosis, and response to therapy. Some simple, noninvasive method of assessment is needed that can predict morbidity and mortality in patients with various causes and severity of CHF. This study examined the value of a 6-minute walk test—a self-paced submaximal exercise test widely used in the assessment of patients with chronic respiratory disorders—as a prognostic indicator in patients with left ventricular dysfunction.

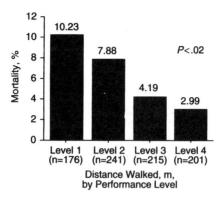

Fig 7–7.—Mortality (%) as a function of performance level (based on distance walked). Mortality decreased as performance on the 6-minute walk test improved. (Courtesy of Bittner V, for the Studies of Left Ventricular Dysfunction Investigators: *JAMA* 270:1702–1707, 1993.)

Methods.—The study included a stratified random sample of 898 patients from the Studies of Left Ventricular Dysfunction Registry, all with either radiologic evidence of CHF, an ejection fraction of no more than .45, or both. All patients had a complete clinical evaluation, including a 6-minute walk test. In this test, the patient was to cover as much ground as possible on a 30.5-m (100-ft.) marked course in a corridor. Patients were allowed to rest but were instructed to resume walking as soon as they felt they could. The distance walked was measured to the nearest meter. Any symptoms experienced during the walk were recorded for each patient.

Results.—During a mean follow-up of 242 days, 6.2% of the patients died and 30.3% required hospitalization. About 9% required hospitalization because of CHF. Overall, 13.7% either died or were hospitalized as a result of CHF. The likelihood of death was 10.23% in the patients with the poorest 6-minute walk test results compared to 2.99% for those with the best results (Fig 7–7). Chances of being hospitalized were 40.91% vs. 19.9%, whereas chances of being hospitalized for CHF were 22.16% vs. 1.99%, respectively. The distance walked in the 6-minute test was as strong and independent a predictor of death and hospitalization as ejection fraction on logistic regression analysis.

Conclusion.—For patients with left ventricular dysfunction, the 6-minute walk test appears to be a strong, independent predictor of morbidity and mortality. The test is easy to administer, inexpensive, noninvasive, and safe. It may be especially useful in identifying mildly to moderately symptomatic patients at greater risk of events, and possibly in monitoring the disease and its response to therapy.

▶ Simple walking tests are popular as a means of evaluating sick or elderly patients, as they appear less risky than a more formal laboratory evaluation. This study shows that a simple walking test gives approximately as much prognostic information as a much more costly determination of ejection fraction. However, it can also be inferred that neither test is particularly helpful. After allowance for other variables, the risk ratios of a poor walking speed are 1.5 for death and 2.6 for CHF; although there are significant intergroup differences, either type of test gives relatively limited insight into the likely prognosis of the individual patient.—R.J. Shephard, M.D., Ph.D.

Balance Improvements in Older Women: Effects of Exercise Training

Judge JO, Lindsey C, Underwood M, Winsemius D (Univ of Connecticut, Farmington)

Phys Ther 73:254–265, 1993   139-94-7–28

Background.—Elderly individuals who have decreased lower extremity strength are at increased risk for falling. A vigorous program of lower extremity strengthening, walking, and postural control exercises may improve the single-stance balance of healthy elderly women and reduce their risk of falling.

Methods.—Twenty-one healthy women aged 62–75 years were assigned to a treatment or a control group. The 12 women in the former group received combined training and the 9 in the latter group had flexibility training. The treatment group met 3 times per week and exercised

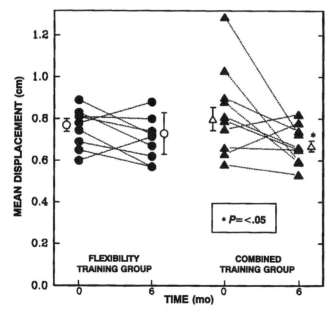

Fig 7–8.—Individual and group balance testing results for mean displacement of center of pressure in single-stance (3 upright and 3 forward-leaning trials) sampled for 8 seconds. The mean results (± standard error) (*open symbols*) precede and follow individual measurements (*filled symbols*). (Courtesy of Judge JO, Lindsey C, Underwood M, et al: *Phys Ther* 73:254–265, 1993.)

using knee extension and sitting leg press machines, walked briskly for 20 minutes, and performed postural control exercises, including simple tai chi movements. The control group did postural control exercises every week.

Findings.—After training, participants' double-stance measurements were unchanged. The mean displacement of the center of pressure in single stance improved by 17% in the treatment group and remained the same in the control group. In a repeated-measures analysis of variance, the difference in improvement between the 2 groups was insignificant. Figure 7-8 suggests that the greatest improvement occurred in women in the treatment group, with the worst balance at baseline.

Conclusion.—Single-stance postural sway can be improved with exercise training in older women. Further study is needed to determine whether a combined training program such as that described improves balance more than postural control exercises alone.

▶ After a recent morning of log-splitting, followed by an afternoon of whitewater paddling, I slipped and fell ignominiously in a patch of river ooze that I am sure would not have bothered me if my muscles had not been beginning to protest their workout. In my case, the mud was soft, but if an elderly individual with weakened hip bones slips on a hard surface, this can amount to a slow death sentence. Measures to improve muscle strength and balance are, thus, of great importance when caring for our aging population. This study found therapeutic benefit from such treatment. There was a 17% reduction of postural sway in the subjects receiving both muscle strengthening and postural control exercises, whereas there was no change in the group receiving postural therapy alone. Unfortunately, the sample size was small, and the substantial difference of postural control between the 2 groups was not statistically significant. This highlights the importance of undertaking a minimum sample size calculation before embarking on any experiment.—R.J. Shephard, M.D., Ph.D.

A Controlled Trial of Exercise by Residents of Old People's Homes
McMurdo MET, Rennie L (Univ of Dundee, Scotland)
Age Ageing 22:11–15, 1993   139-94-7–29

Background.—Although young and middle-aged individuals are commonly encouraged to exercise regularly, little attention has been paid to the importance of exercise in elderly persons. Exercise training can at least partially reverse the rate of age-related muscle strength loss. Whether a program of seated exercise produced any significant benefits in an elderly institutionalized population was examined.

Methods.—The subjects were 49 residents of 4 homes for elderly persons (mean age, 81 years). Residents of 2 homes were assigned to receive exercise sessions consisting of twice-weekly, 45-minute sessions of

Changes in Variables (7 Months–Baseline)

	Study group			95% confidence intervals of difference
	Exercise	Reminiscence	p-value	between changes
Mean (SD)				
Body Mass Index	0.24 (1.5)	0.29 (1.4)	NS	−1.0 to 0.9
Sway:				
eyes open	−9.6 (17.7)	−2.9 (16.1)	NS	−18.0 to −4.7
eyes shut	−16.6 (32.3)	−10.9 (34.8)	NS	−28.7 to −17.2
Grip strength (kg)	2.2 (4.2)	−1.0 (3.6)	<0.02	0.6 to 5.8
Spinal flexion (cm)	−12.7 (8.9)	2.2 (8.8)	<0.00001	−20.8 to −9.1
Chair-to-stand time (s)	−0.7 (0.8)	0.3 (0.8)	<0.001	−1.5 to −0.5
Depression scale	−1.8 (1.6)	−0.5 (1.5)	<0.01	−2.3 to −0.3
Life satisfaction index	1.5 (1.6)	0.7 (1.4)	NS	−0.2 to 1.8
Activities of daily living	1.0 (2.8)	−1.0 (2.8)	<0.05	0.1 to 3.8
Mini-mental State Examination	1.4 (1.4)	0.2 (2.4)	NS	−0.2 to 2.6
Median (range)				
Knee flexion:				
right	0 (−5 to 25)	−5 (−15 to 20)	NS	0 to 10
left	0 (−30 to 25)	−5 (−20 to 10)	NS	0 to 10
Knee extension:				
right	0 (0 to 0)	0 (−10 to 10)	NS	0 to 5
left	0 (−10 to 10)	0 (−10 to 10)	<0.05	0 to 10

(Courtesy of McMurdo MET, Rennie L: *Age Ageing* 22:11-15, 1993.)

seated exercise to music. This exercise program was designed to promote full range of motion of the joints of the arms and legs. Residents of the other 2 homes took part in music and reminiscence activities designed to promote social interaction. At baseline and after 7 months, both groups of residents were assessed for postural sway, knee flexion and extension, spinal flexion, activities of daily living, and chair-to-stand time.

Results.—Forty-one subjects completed the study. Neither intervention had any adverse events. The exercise group had a mean improvement in performance on 4 variables—grip strength, spinal flexion, chair-to-stand time, and activities of daily living—whereas the reminiscence group experienced a deterioration (table). Depression decreased in both groups, but more so in the exercise group.

Conclusion.—The exercise program described in this study has proven effective, acceptable, and safe for elderly residents of nursing homes. With seated, low-intensity exercise, even very old individuals can improve their functional capacity.

▶ One challenge in examining the effects of increased physical activity is to devise an appropriate control tactic that mimics the treatment in all respects except the energy expenditure. This study compares favorably with many other studies of the elderly in this respect. It is also useful in confirming that functional improvement is possible even when subjects must remain seated throughout the period of exercise. There was no evidence that the body mass of the experimental group increased relative to the controls, and gains of strength were thus (probably) attributable to better coordination rather than muscle hypertrophy. The largest changes were in flexibility and in body sway, both of which are very important to function in the very old.—R.J. Shephard, M.D., Ph.D.

Risk Due to Inactivity in Physically Capable Older Adults
Simonsick EM, Lafferty ME, Phillips CL, Mendes de Leon CF, Kasl SV, Seeman TE, Fillenbaum G, Hebert P, Lemke JH (Natl Inst on Aging, Bethesda, Md; Yale Univ, New Haven, Conn; Duke Univ, Durham, NC; et al)
Am J Public Health 83:1443–1450, 1993   139-94-7–30

Background.—Research has shown that habitual physical activity improves health, reduces the incidence of coronary heart disease, and increases longevity among middle-aged men and women. Studies of the benefits of habitual activity in elderly persons, however, are limited.

Methods.—The association between recreational physical activity and functional status, incidence of selected chronic conditions, and mortality in capable older adults was investigated over 3 and 6 years. Data were obtained from 3 sites of the Established Populations for Epidemiologic Studies of the Elderly.

Findings.—The likelihood of mortality during 3 and 6 years was reduced by a high level of recreational physical activity. Moderate to high levels of activity decreased the risk of physical impairments over 3 years, but this effect declined after 6 years. There was no consistent association between physical activity and new myocardial infarction or stroke or the incidence of diabetes or angina after 3 or 6 years (table).

Conclusion.—Physical activity appears to be beneficial in physically capable older persons, mainly in reducing the risk of functional decline and mortality.

▶ The authors of this study had the usual difficulty in making an adequate assessment of habitual physical activity on a large sample, and the possibility that some of those who were initially inactive may have been limited by incipient disease could not be entirely excluded. Despite these experimental problems, exercise seemed to offer substantial benefit to patients in the age range studied, a view in keeping with earlier observations by Donahue et al. (1) and supported by a dose/response gradient from moderate to vigorous physical activity.

Those who reported activities such as playing tennis at least once per week were classified as highly active, whereas those who reported walking were classified as only moderately active, even if such individuals in fact en-

Health and Functional Outcomes of Highly and Moderately Active and Inactive Participants After 6 Years

Outcome	n	Activity Level, %			n	Highly Active vs Inactive		Moderately Active vs Inactive	
		High	Moderate	Inactive		Odds Ratio	95% Confidence Interval	Odds Ratio	95% Confidence Interval
East Boston									
Mortality	1874	14.2*	18.1	21.0	1809	0.73	0.48, 1.11	0.85	0.63, 1.15
Myocardial infarction	1728	9.4*	10.9*	15.0	1667	0.69	0.42, 1.16	0.76	0.53, 1.09
Stroke	1728	5.3	6.4	4.7	1667	1.21	0.56, 2.61	1.73	0.98, 3.06
Diabetes	1234[a]	7.6	6.4	8.1	1199	1.11	0.53, 2.30	0.85	0.50, 1.45
Angina	1329[a]	1.7	2.3	2.6	1292	0.79	0.22, 2.89	1.02	0.41, 2.46
Walk a half mile	1387[b]	19.9*	20.6**	28.2	1326	0.82	0.51, 1.32	0.77	0.56, 1.06
Climb stairs	1376[b]	6.4	9.9	10.1	1335	0.65	0.31, 1.37	1.12	0.72, 1.74
Do heavy housework	1373[b]	27.0*	32.4	35.8	1332	0.82	0.53, 1.25	0.94	0.71, 1.26

(continued)

Table *(continued)*

New Haven								
Mortality	1488	19.1**	24.0	26.7	1437	0.66	0.45, 0.95	0.81	0.60, 1.11
Myocardial infarction	1387	9.2	9.7	10.9	1341	0.83	0.47, 1.46	1.23	0.78, 1.95
Stroke	1387	4.9	5.2	4.1	1341	1.05	0.52, 2.12	1.29	0.72, 2.32
Diabetes	906[a]	1.4	5.5	3.3	983	0.59	0.20, 1.77	1.54	0.68, 3.49
Angina	955[a]	0.4*	5.7	3.8	929	0.33	0.08, 1.32	1.71	0.72, 4.03
Walk a half mile	968[b]	24.3**	29.0*	37.9	942	0.63	0.40, 0.98	0.74	0.51, 1.08
Climb stairs	974[b]	11.9*	15.6	18.0	947	0.86	0.50, 1.45	0.97	0.62, 1.51
Do heavy housework	977[b]	27.5	30.0	28.3	950	0.87	0.56, 1.35	0.94	0.65, 1.38
Iowa								
Mortality	1815	9.1**	14.9	15.0	1768	0.59	0.37, 0.92	1.06	0.77, 1.46
Myocardial infarction	1725	8.7	9.9	7.1	1681	1.21	0.72, 2.04	1.41	0.93, 2.14
Stroke	1725	5.0*	7.9	8.6	1681	0.56	0.31, 1.03	0.97	0.64, 1.48
Diabetes	1348[a]	9.2*	4.5	5.5	1310	1.51	0.83, 2.75	0.76	0.42, 1.38
Walk a half mile	1471[b]	17.5*	20.5	23.4	1429	0.70	0.46, 1.05	0.82	0.60, 1.12
Climb stairs	1475[b]	7.3	6.9	6.4	1433	1.23	0.64, 2.35	1.07	0.64, 1.79
Do heavy housework	1477[b]	24.2	25.7	22.3	1435	1.15	0.78, 1.70	1.22	0.89, 1.66

Note: Rates are sex- and age-adjusted. Odds ratios were derived from logistic regression models including age, sex, education, work status, smoking, respiratory symptoms, myocardial infarction, stroke, diabetes, angina, self-rated health, and modified depression score. Sample sizes differ for the rates and adjusted odds ratios because of missing data on variables in the multivariate analyses.

[a] No. of individuals at risk.
[b] Percentage reporting any difficulty among survivors only.
* $P < .05$; ** $P < .01$; *** $P < .001$ (compared with inactive participants).
(Courtesy of Simonsick EM, Lafferty ME, Phillips CL, et al: *Am J Public Health* 83:1443-1450, 1993.)

gaged in 2 miles of brisk walking per day. Benefit was concentrated particularly in those who were classified as highly active.

Despite the advanced age of the sample participants (all were older than 65 years of age and one quarter were older than 75 years of age), highly active individuals had a substantial advantage in terms of their overall mortality rate and risks of myocardial infarction during the 6 years of observation. They also seemed more likely to preserve an ability to walk half a mile and to undertake heavy housework (although the authors admit that the inactive subjects may have exaggerated their initial abilities and, thus, have sustained larger apparent losses of function.—R.J. Shephard, M.D., Ph.D.

Reference

1. Donahue RP, et al: *Am J Public Health* 78:683, 1988.

Effect of Exercise on Cardiovascular Ageing
Kasch FW, Boyer JL, Van Camp SP, Verity LS, Wallace JP (San Diego State Univ, Calif; Indiana Univ)
Age Ageing 22:5–10, 1993   139-94-7–31

Background.—Cardiovascular capacity and other aspects of function diminish with age, reducing the quality of life and the chance of survival in emergencies and increasing the potential for fractures, osteoporosis, and hypokinetic diseases. The decline in peak oxygen intake is the general index of cardiorespiratory aging; reductions of up to 24% per decade have been cited, but there have been few long-term follow-up studies of the same group of subjects. Changes in peak oxygen intake and training regimens were thus documented in a group of men over a 25-year period.

Cardiovascular Function ($\dot{V}o_{2max}$) With 25 Years of Physical Training

Year	Age (years)	n	l/min	$ml \cdot min^{-1} \cdot kg^{-1}$
	44		3.462	45.4
0	(7.0)	12	(444)	(5.1)
	54		3392	46.0
10	(7.3)	12	(575)	(8.3)
	59		3043	41.8
15	(7.7)	12	(763)	(8.8)
	64		2923	40.6
20	(7.3)	12	(611)	(10.3)
	69		2866*	39.5 †
25	(6.7)	12	(645)	(9.3)

Note: Figures in parentheses are standard deviations.
* $P < .02$.
† $P < .10$.
(Courtesy of Kasch FW, Boyer JL, Van Camp SP, et al: *Age Ageing* 22:5–10, 1993.)

Methods.—Twelve men aged 33–57 years at enrollment in the study engaged in individual cardiovascular aerobic training programs or swimming. Exercise mode, frequency, intensity, and duration were recorded daily and reported monthly. At 0, 10, 15, 20, and 25 years, peak oxygen consumption was measured as each subject underwent a maximal exercise test on a motor-driven treadmill or a cycle ergometer.

Results.—At the final assessment, the overall peak oxygen consumption had decreased 13% from baseline, a loss of 5% per decade (table). The sharpest decline occurred between the 10th and 15th years, primarily because of the development of disease in 4 men; the decline was more gradual thereafter. The other 8 men had a minimal loss of 1.6% per decade in cardiovascular function over 25 years. As the subjects aged, the primary decrease in peak oxygen consumption resulted from diminished maximum heart rate and estimated stroke volume.

Conclusion.—The average cardiovascular decline in this aging population was half that reported in the literature. Apparently, sustained physical exercise slows age-associated changes in physical capacity that are common in Western populations.

▶ Kasch and his associates have generated a number of papers from their long-term follow-up of a small population of exercising seniors. They have sometimes argued that a training program can totally halt the aging of cardiorespiratory function, although such claims have ignored the impact of short-term training gains seen at the beginning of their study. The thesis of a minimal rate of aging in those who exercise is maintained in the present paper, in part by a continued use of pretraining data as the starting point for calculations and in part by a post-hoc division of the small group of 12 subjects into 7 healthy individuals and 5 patients with "disease."

The distinction of these 5 people seems rather subjective in that, elsewhere in the paper, it is suggested that 9 of the 12 people had some type of disease by the conclusion of the study. In fact, the current report shows an average loss of aerobic power of 6.5 mL/kg/min from 10 to 25 years of follow-up—a loss of .43 mL/kg/min per year—which is very close to the figure of .43–.45 mL/kg/min that we (1) and others have deduced from personal observations on well-trained subjects and a review of the literature. The figure of .43 mL/kg/min is marginally less than the .5–.6 mL/kg/min per year seen in sedentary individuals (2), but a much stronger argument for persisting with a training regimen into old age is the functional bonus associated with the initial training response.—R.J. Shephard, M.D., Ph.D.

References

1. Kavanagh T, Shephard RJ: *Physician Sportsmed* 18:94, 1990.
2. Shephard RJ: *Physical Activity and Aging.* London: Croom Helm, 1987.

Additive Effects of Age and Silent Myocardial Ischemia on the Left Ventricular Response to Upright Cycle Exercise

Fleg JL, Schulman SP, Gerstenblith G, Becker LC, O'Connor FC, Lakatta EG
(Natl Inst on Aging, Baltimore, Md; Johns Hopkins Univ, Baltimore, Md)
J Appl Physiol 75:499–504, 1993   139-94-7–32

Background.—Age, gender, conditioning status, the presence and severity of cardiac disease, and the nature of the exercise stimulus all affect cardiac response to maximal aerobic exercise. The marked age-associated increase in the prevalence of coronary artery disease may lead to mistaken attributions of an ischemic left ventricular exercise response in asymptomatic subjects to age alone. The hypothesis that age- and exercise-induced silent ischemias have separate but additive effects on the left ventricular exercise response was tested.

Method.—Maximal exercise ergometry was performed in 3 groups of men to separate the independent effects of age and silent myocardial ischemia on the left ventricular response. Eight clinically healthy older men with ischemic responses in prior maximal treadmill exercise made up the old silent ischemia subject group. The old control group was composed of 16 age-matched men with normal ECGs and T1 scan responses. The young control group was composed of 21 healthy young men. The left ventricular ejection fraction, end-diastolic volume index, and end-systolic volume index were similar in the 3 groups at rest.

Findings.—The left ventricular response to upright cycle ergometer exercise was exaggerated in the asymptomatic old silent ischemia group compared to the old and young controls. With increasing work rates, there was a progressive increase in the end-diastolic volume index and a blunted decline in end-systolic volume index in the 2 older groups. At peak effort, both end-diastolic and end-systolic volume indexes were smallest in the young controls, intermediate in the old controls, and largest in the old silent ischemia group. The ejection fraction reversed this pattern, with the lowest value in the old silent ischemia subjects (Fig 7-9). The peak systolic pressure/end-systolic volume index ratio was similar to the pattern for the ejection fraction.

Conclusion.—Asymptomatic older men with prior exercise-induced silent myocardial infarction had diminished aerobic power, cardiac dilatation, and a blunted ejection fraction in response to cycle ergometry. The old silent ischemia group's responses were exaggerated compared to both old and young controls. Advanced age and silent myocardial infarction have qualitatively similar, but additive, effects on left ventricular performance during upright cycle ergometer exercise.

▶ Lakatta and associates long maintained that if patients with silent myocardial ischemia were excluded by exercise ECGs and thallium scans, the remainder of the sample compensated completely for the age-related decrease in their peak heart rate by the Frank-Starling mechanism, an increase of dia-

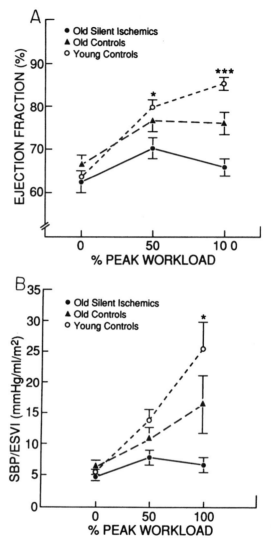

Fig 7–9.—Systolic pump performance as a function of relative work load among 3 groups. **A,** left ventricular ejection fraction. **B,** ratio of systolic blood pressure (*SBP*) to end-systolic volume index (*ESVI*). Values are means ± SE. In both graphs, systolic performance was similar among groups at rest and diverged progressively with increasing effort (significance by repeated-measures analysis of variance). *Young controls significantly different from old men with silent ischemia, P < .05. ***All groups significantly different, P < .05. (Courtesy of Fleg JL, Schulman SP, Gerstenblith G, et al: *J Appl Physiol* 75:499–504, 1993.)

stolic volume leading to a major increase of stroke volume. Their thesis has now been largely abandoned, and the figure taken from their present paper shows much more the difference between young and elderly subjects that we (1) and others have previously illustrated.

One continuing weakness in the Baltimore studies is that what is described as peak work rate is, in fact, substantially less than maximal effort. The average peak heart rate reported for their 65-year-old subjects is only 132 beats per minute, compared with 170 beats per minute in our studies. If a truly maximal effort had been demanded of the elderly individuals, their problems in sustaining stroke volume against a high afterload would have been brought out much more clearly.—R.J. Shephard, M.D., Ph.D.

Reference

1. Niinimaa V, Shephard RJ: *J Gerontol* 33:362, 1978.

Low Bone Mass and High Bone Turnover in Male Long Distance Runners

Hetland ML, Haarbo J, Christiansen C (Ctr for Clinical and Basic Research, Ballerup, Denmark)
J Clin Endocrinol Metab 77:770–775, 1993   139-94-7-33

Objective.—Distance running, although healthy for cardiovascular function and weight control, has been linked to reduced bone mass and the risk of osteoporosis in women. Osteoporosis is also a major cause of morbidity and mortality in men, but there is little information on the potential for bone loss in male runners. The effects of running on bone loss in men were thus studied.

Methods.—The study sample consisted of 120 healthy men with a wide range of running habits. The age range was 19–56 years, and the distance run weekly ranged from 0 to 160 km. Twenty-two subjects were elite runners, whereas 12 had not run regularly for at least 1 year. All subjects underwent measurement of bone mineral content in the lumbar spine, total body, and proximal femurs by dual-energy x-ray absorptiometry and in the forearm by single-photon absorptiometry. Urinary pyridinium cross-links, plasma osteocalcin, and serum alkaline phosphatase were measured to evaluate bone turnover.

Results.—There was a negative correlation between bone mineral content of the lumbar spine and weekly distance run, with a 19% difference between the elite runners and the controls. Results were similar at all sites except the femoral neck. The correlations remained significant for all areas with a high proportion of trabecular bone after adjustment for potential confounding variables. Measurements of bone turnover were 20% to 30% higher in elite runners than in controls. Sex hormone status showed no relationship to running activity.

Conclusion.—There was reduced bone mass and increased bone turnover among male long-distance runners. These athletes appear to have accelerated bone loss, with a possible increased risk of osteoporotic fractures. The pathophysiologic mechanism of this bone loss remains to be determined, but it does not appear to be related to sex hormones.

▶ Because this study is cross-sectional in type, it is unclear how far the self-selecting of running by lightly-boned individuals contributes to the present findings. A low body mass may reduce the stimulus to bone formation during normal daily activities. Nevertheless, the higher rates of bone turnover in the runners point toward some aspect of running as the primary cause of low bone density, and those caring for runners should watch for warning signs of impaired bone health, particularly fatigue fractures. In some runners, low serum testosterone levels have bene reported, mirroring the problems of the female athlete, but this does not seem to explain any osteoporosis observed in the present study. Another variable that can contribute to osteoporosis in the female athlete is an inadequate intake of food energy, and it is unfortunate that this study gives no information regarding the subjects' food intake or reserves of body fat.—R.J. Shephard, M.D., Ph.D.

Bone Mineral Density in Professional Ballet Dancers
Karlsson MK, Johnell O, Obrant KJ (Malmö Gen Hosp, Sweden)
Bone Miner 21:163–169, 1993   139-94-7–34

Introduction.—Postmenopausal women who complete a 40-week exercise program can increase the bone density of the lumbar spine. Whether premenopausal women could also gain bone mineral density (BMD) through heavy training was investigated. Ballet dancers were chosen for study because of their high level of training, especially of the trunk and lower extremities.

Subjects and Methods.—Forty-two professional ballet dancers, 25 women and 17 men, took part in the study. Fourteen had retired from professional dancing and 28 were still actively performing. Controls were 42 healthy age- and sex-matched volunteers. A Lunar DPX apparatus was used to measure BMD in the total body, spine, hip, arms, legs, and the proximal tibia metaphysis. Single-photon absorptiometry (SPA) assessed BMD of the distal forearm.

Results.—Dancers and controls did not differ significantly in BMD, except for lower values in the head of male dancers (Table 1) and and in the arms of female dancers (Table 2), compared to controls. After adjusting for dancers' decreased body mass index, male dancers had higher BMD in the hip (neck) and female dancers had higher BMD in all hip measurements and in the legs. When compared to controls and in relation to age, male dancers had lower BMD in the hips and female dancers had lower BMD in the legs, arms, spine, and total body. There was a significant correlation between SPA measurements in the forearm and all DPX measurements. Twelve of the retired dancers had been measured with SPA in the tibia condyle in 1975, during their active careers. There was no correlation between the 1975 and current SPA measurements.

TABLE 1.—Numeric DPX-Values (BMD in g/cm^2) for Male Dancers and Controls

	Dancers (X_1) $n = 17$		Δ	95% CIΔ	Controls (Y_1) $n = 17$	Δ	95% CIΔ	Active dancers (X_2) $n = 11$		Controls (Y_2) $n = 11$	Δ	95% CIΔ
BMD head	2.08 ± 0.22	*	−0.15	−0.30–0.00	2.23 ± 0.20	−0.14	−0.32–0.04	2.14 ± 0.23	ns	2.28 ± 0.19		
BMD arm	0.93 ± 0.08	ns	−0.04	−0.11–0.03	0.97 ± 0.11	−0.02	−0.10–0.06	0.96 ± 0.08	ns	0.98 ± 0.11		
BMD leg	1.36 ± 0.12	ns	−0.01	−0.09–0.07	1.37 ± 0.12	0.02	−0.07–0.11	1.42 ± 0.09	ns	1.40 ± 0.12		
% fat	13.5 ± 6.0	‡	−7.0	−10.9–(−3.1)	20.5 ± 5.1	−7.8	−11.7–(−3.9)	10.8 ± 4.6	:‡	18.6 ± 4.4		
Lean body mass (kg)	56.9 ± 5.6	†	−6.6	−11.2–(−2.0)	63.5 ± 7.5	−5.5	−10.9–(−0.1)	58.5 ± 5.9	ns	64.0 ± 6.6		
BMI	22.2 ± 1.5	‡	−3.4	−4.7–(−2.1)	25.6 ± 2.2	−3.4	−4.9–(−1.9)	21.6 ± 1.2	†	25.0 ± 2.1		

Abbreviation: ns, not significant.
* $P < .05.$
† $P < .01.$
‡ $P < .001.$
(Courtesy of Karlsson MK, Johnell O, Obrant KJ: *Bone Miner* 21:163–169, 1993.)

TABLE 2.—Numeric DPX-Values (BMD in g/cm^2) for Female Dancers and Controls

	Dancers (X_1) $n = 25$		Controls (Y_1) $n = 25$	Δ	95% CIΔ	Active dancers (X_2) $n = 17$		Controls (Y_2) $n = 17$	Δ	%% CIΔ
BMD head	2.20 ± 0.32	ns	2.36 ± 0.32	-0.16	-0.34–0.02	2.15 ± 0.31	*	2.37 ± 0.24	-0.22	-0.41–(-0.03)
BMD arm	0.77 ± 0.08	*	0.83 ± 0.06	-0.06	-0.10–(-0.02)	0.77 ± 0.06	†	0.83 ± 0.05	-0.06	-0.10–(-0.02)
BMD leg	1.21 ± 0.11	ns	1.17 ± 0.10	0.04	-0.02–0.10	1.22 ± 0.07	ns	1.18 ± 0.09	0.04	-0.02–0.10
% fat	20.9 ± 6.3	‡	31.2 ± 8.2	-10.3	-14.5–(-6.1)	18.3 ± 5.3	‡	30.6 ± 7.9	-12.3	-17.0–(-7.6)
Lean body mass (kg)	41.0 ± 4.8	ns	39.3 ± 3.9	1.7	-0.8–4.2	42.2 ± 5.3	ns	39.8 ± 4.0	2.4	-0.9–5.7
BMI	19.3 ± 1.6	†	21.7 ± 3.2	-2.4	-3.8–(-0.9)	18.9 ± 1.6	†	21.8 ± 3.4	-1.9	-4.8–(-1.0)

Abbreviation: ns, not significant.
* $P < .05$.
† $P < .01$.
‡ $P < .001$.
(Courtesy of Karlsson MK, Johnell O, Obrant KJ: *Bone Miner* 21:163-169, 1993.)

Six dancers had experienced amenorrhea for more than 1 year. Their spine BMD was 7% lower than that of menstruating dancers and they tended to have lower BMD, lower fat content, and higher weight and lean body mass than aged-matched menstruating dancers.

Conclusion.—Weight-bearing activity is widely recommended as a prophylaxis for age-related bone loss. There is little evidence in the literature, however, to suggest that training activity in male weight-lifters has a lasting effect on BMD. The findings of this study indicate that ballet dancers, although more slender, reach the same peak level of BMD as controls. With increasing age and retirement from an active career, ballet dancers appear to lose bone mineral at a faster rate than their peers.

▶ This study provides useful data on BMD in ballet dancers during and after their careers. The low BMD of the cranium (a region that is not extensively involved in ballet performance) is particularly interesting. It is less certain that findings can be extrapolated to the more general issue of weight-bearing exercise and BMD. Ballet dancers are a specialized group, and because of the emphasis on their physical appearance, their nutritional intake is often inadequate relative to their daily energy expenditure. This places them at increased risk of poor bone health relative to others who engage in a similar volume of physical activity. Moreover, it is likely that many ballet dancers try to maintain their thin figures by undereating after they have ceased to be active in their profession, and this could explain why they lose bone mineral rapidly at this stage in their lives.—R.J. Shephard, M.D., Ph.D.

Past and Recent Physical Activity and Risk of Hip Fracture
Jaglal SB, Kreiger N, Darlington G (Univ of Toronto)
Am J Epidemiol 138:107–118, 1993   139-94-7–35

Introduction.—Osteoporosis-related hip fractures result in considerable disability and premature death in elderly persons. Increased physical activity is thought to prevent osteoporosis and reduce the rate of fracture, yet few studies have attempted to document the relationship between exercise and fracture risk. This population-based, case-control study examined the effects of past and recent physical activity on the risk of hip fracture in postmenopausal women.

Methods.—Case subjects were women aged 55–84 years who had a radiologically confirmed diagnosis of hip fracture. Of 934 patients identified from hospital records, 714 were eligible for the study. The time from hip fracture to data collection ranged from 8 to 24 months. Controls comprised a population-based, random sample of women of similar age who lived in the same area (metropolitan Toronto) as case subjects. Of 1,981 controls selected, 1,888 were eligible for the study. Participants responded to questionnaires either by mail or telephone. The survey asked for assessments of physical activity at ages 16, 30, and 50 years and for the year before the study. Participants were also asked

Distribution of Hip Fracture Cases and Controls by Level of Total Past and Recent Physical Activity: Toronto, Canada, 1990–1991

Physical activity	No. of cases*	No. of controls*	Crude OR† estimate	95% CI†	Adjusted‡ OR estimate	95% CI
Total past activity						
Inactive	61	171	1.00		1.00	
Active	154	627	0.69	0.49–0.97	0.66	0.45–0.96
Very active	43	198	0.61	0.39–0.94	0.54	0.33–0.88
Recent activity						
Inactive	56	165	1.00		1.00	
Active	133	628	0.62	0.44–0.89	0.61	0.41–0.90
Very active	69	203	1.00	0.67–1.50	1.15	0.72–1.83

* The numbers of case subjects and controls do not add up to the total number of study subjects because of missing data.
† *Abbreviations:* OR, odds ratio; CI, confidence interval.
‡ Adjusted for the other variable in the table as well as for age, obesity, calcium supplement use, dietary calcium, pack-years of smoking, estrogen use, fluoride use, previous fracture, history of epilepsy, history of osteoporosis, and history of stroke or Parkinson's disease.
(Courtesy of Jaglal SB, Kreiger N, Darlington G: *Am J Epidemiol* 138:107–118, 1993.)

about their dietary calcium intake, use of hormone replacement therapy, smoking history, and other variables. The response rates were 53% for case subjects and 60% for controls.

Results.—Case subjects were slightly older than controls, but the 2 groups were similar in race and education. The level of physical activity was characterized as very active, active, or inactive. After adjusting for recent activity, a protective effect was observed in women who were active (odds ratio [OR], .66) or very active (OR, .54) in the past. After adjustment for past activity, there was a similar protective effect for a recent moderate level of activity (OR, .61). Women who were very active in the past year, however, were not protected from hip fracture (OR, 1.15) (table). Women who had used estrogen therapy for 5 years or more had a lower risk of hip fracture. Factors associated with increased risk were fluoride use and a history of stroke, epilepsy, osteoporosis, or fracture.

Conclusion.—Recent moderate activity and past physical activity both reduced the risk of hip fracture in postmenopausal women. The greatest protection was associated with activity during adolescence. Even though estrogen replacement therapy was more strongly protective, development of bone mass at younger ages appeared to reduce a woman's risk of hip fracture significantly.

▶ There has been an ongoing debate as to whether regular physical activity in younger adult life can build up a bank of bone calcium that protects the older individual against osteoporosis. The substantial advantage of undertaking physical activity as a young adult shown here would seem to point in that direction. Kriska and associates (1) have also noted that physical activity seems to exert its greatest protective effect between 14 and 21 years of age.—R.J. Shephard, M.D., Ph.D.

Reference

1. Kriska AM, et al. *Am J Epidemiol* 127: 1053, 1988.

The Risk of Osteoarthritis With Running and Aging: A 5-Year Longitudinal Study
Lane NE, Michel B, Bjorkengren A, Oehlert J, Shi H, Bloch DA, Fries JF (Univ of California, San Francisco; Univ Hosp, Zurich, Switzerland; Stanford Univ, Calif)
J Rheumatol 20:461–468, 1993   139-94-7-36

Purpose.—Excessive stress on the weight-bearing joints has been associated with joint degeneration and accelerated development of osteoarthritis (OA). The authors here present the 5-year results of a longitudinal study of the effects of aging and running on the development of OA of the knees together with the effects of aging on the hands and lumbar spine.

Methods.—The study sample included 41 members of the 50-Plus Runners Association, aged 50–72 years, and 57 nonrunning community controls matched for age, years of education, and occupation. All study participants underwent rheumatologic and radiographic examination of

| | Lumbar Spine Radiographs (3 Reader Averages) Matched Pairs | | | | | |
| | All Pairs | | Female Pairs | | Male Pairs | |
	50+ Run n=33	Comm. Control n=33	50+ Run n=13	Comm. Control n=13	50+ Run n=20	Comm. Control n=20
Spurs (range 0–60)						
1984	9.3	9.4	9.3	7.5	9.3	10.7
SE	0.6	0.9	1.0	0.7	0.9	1.3
SEM	1.1		1.4		1.5	
1989	10.9	11.0	10.5	8.7	11.1	12.5
SE	0.7	0.9	1.1	0.5	1.0	1.4
SEM	1.2		1.2		1.7	
1989–1984	1.6	1.6	1.2	1.2	1.8	1.8
SE*	0.2	0.2	0.2	0.4	0.3	0.3
SEM	0.3		0.4		0.5	
p Value	$p<0.001$	$p<0.001$	$p<0.001$	$p<0.01$	$p<0.001$	$p<0.001$

Abbreviations: SE, standard error of the mean; *SEM,* standard error of the difference between matched pairs.
* Standard error of the mean of within-subject differences, 1989–1984.
(Courtesy of Lane NE, Michel B, Bjorkengren A, et al: *J Rheumatol* 20:461–468, 1993.)

the hands, lumbar spine, and knee joints and completed comprehensive questionnaires at baseline in 1984 and again in 1989.

Results.—At the end of the 5-year study, 20 male pairs and 13 female pairs were evaluable. Four runners had stopped running, but only 1 of them quit because of knee pain. The hands, knees, and lumbar spine of all study participants showed significant radiographic progression of osteophytes as a result of aging. During the 5-year study, clinical OA of the hand developed in 7 controls and 3 runners and OA of the knee developed in 5 controls and 4 runners. Spurring of the lumbar spine progressed in 16% of the runners and in 17% of the controls (table). None of these differences reached statistical significance. Multivariate analysis revealed that older age and female sex were predictors of OA progression in the hand; older age and higher body mass were predictors of OA progression in the knee; and male sex was predictive of OA progression in the lumbar spine.

Conclusion.—With aging, clinical OA of the hand developed in 13% of all study participants and OA of the knees developed in 12%. Running did not accelerate the development of OA of the knees.

▶ Although moderate amounts of physical stress seem to improve the health of articular cartilage (1), excessive stress has apparently accelerated joint degeneration in both soccer players and ballet dancers (2, 3), particularly if an injury of the joint surface has been sustained. A previous cross-sectional study of distance runners suggested no adverse effect from many years of moderate running (4), but it remained arguable that those in whom symptoms were developing had dropped out of the running clubs. This prospective study is less open to that objection, although, because the age of the subjects at entry averaged 58 years, some selective exclusion of arthritis-prone individuals may have occurred.—R.J. Shephard, M.D., Ph.D.

References

1. Salter RB, Field P: *J Bone Joint Surg (Am)* 42-A:31, 1960.
2. Vincelette P, et al: *Can Med Assoc J* 107:873, 1972.
3. Brodelius A: *Acta Orthop Scand* 30:309, 1961.
4. Lane NE, et al: JAMA 255:1147, 1986.

8 Diet, Obesity, Metabolism, Hormones, and Drug Abuse

Effect of Graded Exercise on Esophageal Motility and Gastroesophageal Reflux in Trained Athletes
Soffer EE, Merchant RK, Duethman G, Launspach J, Gisolfi C, Adrian TE
(Univ of Iowa, Iowa City; Creighton Univ, Omaha, Neb)
Dig Dis Sci 38:220–224, 1993   139-94-8–1

Objective.—The effects of graded exercise on esophageal motor activity and gastroesophageal reflux were examined in trained male cyclists aged 20–32 years. All of the cyclists were healthy, and none of them smoked.

Methods.—Esophageal motility and pH were studied using a catheter with 3 strain-gauge transducers connected to a solid-state datalogger and an ambulatory intraesophageal pH monitor. The subjects exercised on a stationary cycle ergometer for 1 hour at 60% of peak oxygen intake, for 45 minutes at 75% of peak oxygen intake, and for 10 minutes at 90% of peak oxygen intake. They rested for 1 hour before exercising and for 30 minutes between sessions. Only 5% glucose solution was given (intravenously) during the study. Plasma levels of gastrin, motilin, glucagon, pancreatic polypeptide, and vasoactive intestinal peptide were determined before and after each exercise session.

Findings.—Heart rate measurements confirmed that the subjects exercised at different work rates. The amplitude, frequency, and duration of esophageal contractions declined progressively as exercise intensity increased. An esophageal pH less than 4 was present for a significantly longer time during higher intensity exercise (Fig 8–1). The mean number of reflux episodes increased as the subjects exercised more intensively. No significant changes in plasma hormone levels were observed.

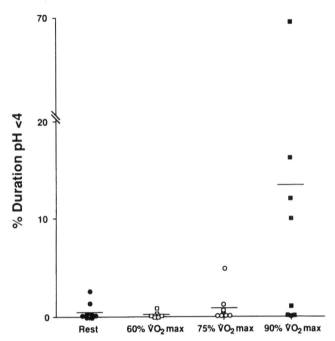

Fig 8–1.—Distribution of percent durations of pH at less than 4 in each subject, in each study period. *Horizontal lines* represent the mean. (Courtesy of Soffer EE, Merchant RK, Duethman G, et al: *Dig Dis Sci* 38:220-224, 1993.)

Conclusion.—Intense exercise depresses esophageal contractility and promotes gastroesophageal reflux through hormone-independent mechanisms.

▶ Very little is known about the behavior of the gastrointestinal tract during exercise. However, there have been reports that endurance activities such as running can induce heartburn, regurgitation, and gastrointestinal reflux (1, 2), giving rise to symptoms that could potentially be confounded with ischemic pain. The dose of exercise used in the present experiments was fairly intense, although the subjects were competitive cyclists; it would be interesting to repeat such observations on older people, in whom gastric reflux is more prevalent.—R.J. Shephard, M.D., Ph.D.

References

1. Moses FM: *Sports Med* 9:159, 1990.
2. Kraus BB, et al: *Ann Intern Med* 112:429, 1990.

Loperamide Abolishes Exercise-Induced Orocecal Liquid Transit Acceleration

Keeling WF, Harris A, Martin BJ (Indiana Univ, Bloomington)
Dig Dis Sci 38:1783–1787, 1993   139-94-8-2

Background.—Loperamide is a popular and effective antidiarrheal agent that possesses both antimotility and antisecretory actions. Recent studies show that acute mild physical activity accelerates the transit of liquids from the mouth to the colon, provoking defecation or even diarrhea in some healthy people. How loperamide might alter this gut response to mild exercise was investigated.

Method.—Twelve healthy individuals with no history of gastrointestinal disease participated in this examination of the effect of loperamide at rest and during exercise. The subjects drank 8 mg of loperamide 1 hour before ingestion of a liquid meal (a dosing schedule that significantly slows orocecal transit). During the exercise experiment, subjects began walking 10 minutes before meal ingestion and continued until the experiment was completed. When studied at rest, the subjects sat in a chair instead of walking.

Results.—With loperamide treatment, exercise failed to hasten increased H_2, a result that contrasted sharply with those in previously studied controls. Loperamide therefore completely halted exercise-induced orocecal transit acceleration. In resting subjects loperamide did not slow transit, although in previous studies it had been shown to do so.

Conclusion.—Loperamide is an effective and safe antidiarrheal medication that abolishes the acceleration of mouth–to–large intestine liquid transit that is sometimes caused by exercise.

▶ The acceleration of orocecal transit is one of the postulated benefits of regular exercise, and it may contribute to the decreased large intestinal cancer rates in regular exercisers. However, sometimes the diarrhea can be sufficiently severe to embarrass a runner; in such patients loperamide may prove to be a useful remedy.—R.J. Shephard, M.D., Ph.D.

Body Weight and Mortality: A 27-Year Follow-Up of Middle-Aged Men

Lee I-M, Manson JE, Hennekens CH, Paffenbarger RS Jr (Harvard School of Public Health, Boston; Harvard Med School, Boston)
JAMA 270:2823–2828, 1993   139-94-8–3

Purpose.—Although it is accepted that gross obesity has negative health effects, there is disagreement regarding the association between body weight and mortality across the weight spectrum. Recent recommendations for desirable weight have been increasing, although it remains unclear whether these increases are justified. A prospective cohort

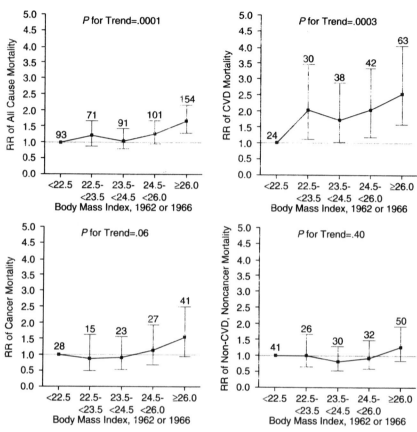

Fig 8–2.—Relative risk (RR) of all-cause mortality, cardiovascular disease (CVD) mortality, cancer mortality, and mortality from causes other than CVD or cancer, 1967/1971 through 1988 (i.e., omitting the first 5 years) among alumni of Harvard University who were never smokers, according to body mass index (weight in kilograms divided by the square of height in meters) in 1962 or 1966. Analyses were adjusted for age (single years) and physical activity (less than 4,200, 4,200–8,399, 8,400–12,599, or 12,600 kJ/wk or greater). *Vertical bars* indicate 95% confidence intervals, and the figures above the bars are the number of mortality events. P values are from tests for linear trend. (Courtesy of Lee I-M, Manson JE, Hennekens CH, et al: *JAMA* 270:2823–2828, 1993.)

study was conducted to assess the nature of the relationship between body weight and all-cause mortality.

Methods.—The subjects were nearly 20,000 male Harvard University alumni who responded to a mailed health questionnaire in either 1962 or 1966. At that time, all respondents were free of self-reported, physician-diagnosed coronary heart disease, stroke, or cancer. The questionnaire included items on weight and height (from which body mass index was calculated) as well as smoking and physical activity. The subjects were followed up through 1988, during which time 4,370 of them had died.

Results.—There was a J-shaped relation between body mass index ι mortality, after multivariate analysis to adjust for age, smoking, and ph, ical activity. Relative risk of death was 1.00 for men with a body ma.., index of less than 22.5, compared with .99 for a body mass index of 22.5 to less than 23.5, .95 for a body mass index of 23.5 to less than 24.5, 1.01 for a body mass index of 24.5 to less than 26.0, and 1.18 for a body mass index of 26.0 or greater. Current smokers had a U-shaped relation, with risk of death being lowest for men with a body mass index of 23.5 to less than 24.5. The curve was also U-shaped for follow-up through 1974, with risk of death being lowest at a body mass index of 24.5 to less than 26.0. A separate analysis for never-smokers only and omitting the first 5 years of follow-up found that the mortality risk of the heaviest individuals was 1.67 times that of the lightest individuals (Fig 8–2).

Conclusion.—This prospective study shows a direct relationship between body weight and mortality. There is no apparent excess mortality among lean men, after adjustment for cigarette smoking and bias caused by illness-related weight loss or inappropriate control for the biological effects of obesity. Men weighing about 20% less than the national average for their age and height appear to have the lowest mortality.

▶ During the past 30 years, recommendations given to American men and women for desirable adult weight have been drifting upward. These recommendations are based on studies of weight and mortality finding U-shaped or J-shaped curves, with higher mortalities in the fattest and the leanest. Many studies, however, are confounded by: failure to account for cigarette smoking; failure to consider bias from illness-related weight loss; and inappropriate control for the biological effects of obesity. In this prospective cohort design of male Harvard alumni, when these variables were properly controlled (adjusting for smoking and illness-related mortality, but not for hypertension or diabetes at baseline), the initial J-shaped curves became almost linear, with no excess mortality among the lean and the fattest one fifth of the men having a 67% higher mortality than the thinnest one fifth. Possible effects from body shape ("apple vs. pear") or weight cycling ("yo-yo dieting") were not studied. The authors conclude that the upward trend in recommended weights is unjustified. Indeed, the lowest mortality was seen in alumni weighing, on average, 20% less than the United States average for men of comparable age and height. In striving for a long life, winners are thinner.—E.R. Eichner, M.D.

Exercise-Induced Bronchospasm in Nonasthmatic Obese Children
Kaplan TA, Montana E (Univ of Miami, Fla)
Clin Pediatr 32:220–225, 1993   139-94-8–4

Background.—Exercise-induced bronchospasm (EIB) is nearly universal in children with asthma, but it is also found in children who are nonasthmatic with other atopic disease and "normal" children. Symptoms

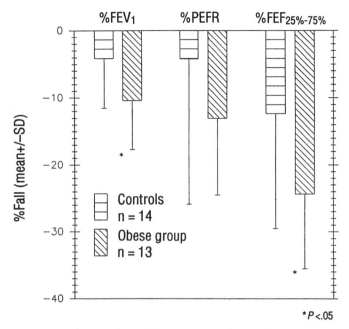

Fig 8–3.—Comparison between obese and control subjects of degree of percentage decrease in pulmonary function after exercise. (Courtesy of Kaplan TA, Montana E: *Clin Pediatr* 32:220–225, 1993.)

include cough, chest tightness, dyspnea, easy fatigue, and wheezing during or after exercise. In an earlier study, a high rate of EIB was observed in obese children and adolescents who were nonasthmatic and nonatopic. Spirometric parameters of obstruction were used to compare bronchial reactivity to exercise in obese and control children.

Method.—Thirteen obese children and 14 control children, aged 6–10 years, performed a 7-minute exercise challenge on a treadmill. Spirometry was performed before and every 3 minutes for 21 minutes after exercise to measure forced expiratory volume in the first second (FEV_1), peak expiratory flow rate (PEFR), and forced expiratory flow between 25% and 75% ($FEV_{25\%-75\%}$) of the forced vital capacity.

Findings.—The obese children had significantly greater mean percentage decreases in FEV_1 in the first second and $FEV_{25\%-75\%}$ compared with the control children. The degree of decrease in the $FEV_{25\%-75\%}$ was significantly correlated with the amount of subcutaneous fat measured by triceps skin-fold thickness (Fig 8–3). The pattern of bronchospasm occurring soon after exercise challenge in the obese children was similar to the pattern for individuals with asthma.

Conclusion.—The findings confirmed earlier observations of bronchial hyperreactivity in obese children. Obese children had a significantly greater frequency and degree of bronchospasm of the smaller airways after exercise challenge than the control children. There was a strong relationship between body fat measured by skin-fold thickness and small-airway reactivity. It is not known whether having EIB predisposes a child to obesity because the child avoids exercise or whether obesity leads to or exacerbates EIB by a biochemical, physiologic, or emotional mechanism.

▶ This article, a study of only a few children, finds that exercise-induced asthma occurs more commonly in nonasthmatic children who are obese, as opposed to lean. This study confirms earlier findings by the same authors of bronchial hyperreactivity in obese children. In regard to exercise-induced asthma, whether obesity is the cart or the horse requires more research. An outstanding review of exercise-induced asthma has just appeared (1).—E.R. Eichner, M.D.

Reference

1. McFadden ER Jr, Gilbert IA: *N Engl J Med* 330:1362, 1994.

The Descriptive Epidemiology of Selected Physical Activities and Body Weight Among Adults Trying to Lose Weight: The Behavioral Risk Factor Surveillance System Survey, 1989
DiPietro L, Williamson DF, Caspersen CJ, Eaker E (Natl Ctr for Chronic Disease Prevention and Health Promotion, Atlanta, Ga)
Int J Obes 17:69–76, 1993   139-94-8-5

Background.—Few researchers have investigated the physical activity patterns of individuals trying to lose weight in population-based studies. Cross-sectional data from an aggregate sample of individuals from 40 states who completed the 1989 Behavioral Risk Factor Surveillance System (BRFSS) survey were analyzed.

Methods.—The self-reported data came from 12,557 women and 6,125 men who stated on the survey that they were trying to lose weight. The BRFSS, a telephone survey of noninstitutionalized adults, used a multistage cluster design based on the Waksberg method of random digit dialing.

Findings.—The most common physical activity was walking, reported by 48% of the study subjects. Eight percent performed aerobic exercises, 5% engaged in gardening, 5% cycled, and 4% ran. Activity choices varied by sociodemographic characteristics. The prevalence of overweight declined significantly with increasing activity level in both men and women. Regression analysis demonstrated that, for both sexes and most age groups, individuals who ran or jogged, performed aerobics, or cycled weighed less than those reporting no activity. This finding was independent of height, race, education, smoking status, and restriction of food intake. Walking was also associated with lower weight in individuals 40 years of age or older (Fig 8–4).

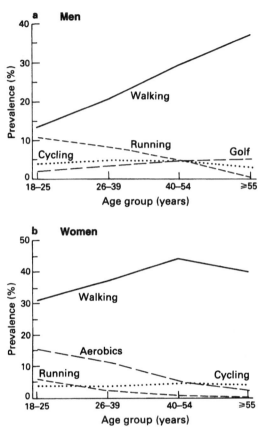

Fig 8–4.—Prevalence of popular activities by age and sex among individuals trying to lose weight. (Courtesy of DiPietro L, Williamson DF, Caspersen CJ, et al: *Int J Obes* 17:69-76, 1993.)

Conclusion.—Because sociodemographic variables are associated with physical activity patterns and choices, these characteristics should be fully considered when developing and implementing physical activity interventions for weight control. Walking is highly prevalent among individuals in most sociodemographic strata, is accessible, and is a low-risk activity. The relative merits of walking should be emphasized when developing interventions.

▶ As in the Canada Fitness Survey and Campbell's Fitness Survey (1, 2), several large United States surveys have shown that walking is by far the most popular form of voluntary physical activity among the general adult population. Many reasons can be postulated for this finding: there is no need to spend a large sum on a club membership or costly equipment; the activity can be performed whenever an individual wishes; it can be performed with family or friends; it is extremely safe; and rather than spending time traveling

---

to a sports facility, a walk can be purposeful, actually saving time over waiting for public transit or a taxi.

As in many epidemiologic studies, DiPietro et al. used the body mass index (body mass/height²) as a surrogate of obesity. If the body mass index is applied to individual patients, someone who is muscular may erroneously be classified as obese; however, in a large sample of the general population, overweight is usually synonymous with fatness. It is often said that walking is as effective or even more effective than jogging as a means of correcting obesity. However, in this study, more vigorous activities such as running, jogging, cycling, and even the use of weights had a closer negative association with body mass.

One probable reason is that many of those who report themselves as walkers during a mass survey are not in fact very serious about their endeavor. If walking is to reduce body mass, it is necessary for an individual to walk briskly for 30–60 minutes per day, not merely to do a little casual walking once or twice per week. A second factor is that those who report engaging in more intense activities are a selected fraction of the overall population sample, people with a strong interest in maintaining good health (including a low body fat content). Despite the somewhat negative findings from their analysis, DiPietro and colleagues conclude by accepting the current wisdom that walking can be an effective public health tactic for containing body weight.—R.J. Shephard, M.D., Ph.D.

References

1. Fitness Canada. *Fitness and Lifestyle in Canada*. Ottawa: Directorate of Fitness and Amateur Sport, 1983.
2. Stephens T, Craig C: *The Well-Being of Canadians: The 1988 Campbell's Survey*. Ottawa: Canadian Fitness and Lifestyle Research Institute, 1990.

Beta-Blockade and Lipolysis During Endurance Exercise
Wijnen JAG, van Baak MA, de Haan C, Struijker Boudier HAJ, Tan FS, Van Bortel LMAB (Univ of Limburg, Maastricht, The Netherlands)
Eur J Clin Pharmacol 45:101–105, 1993   139-94-8–6

Introduction.—Many patients with cardiovascular disorders who are treated with β-adrenoceptor antagonists also engage in dynamic physical exercise. Numerous studies have shown that maximal aerobic power is significantly reduced in normotensive and hypertensive subjects treated by β-blockade. Such impairment of endurance capacity may be related to inhibition of adipose tissue lipolysis. Whether the lower postexercise levels of plasma glycerol and free fatty acid (NEFA) concentrations in such patients are caused by β-adrenoceptor blockade itself or by the shorter time to exhaustion after administration of a β-adrenoceptor blocker was investigated.

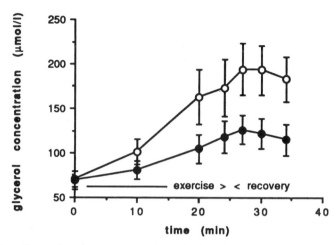

Fig 8-5.—Plasma glycerol concentrations during placebo and propranolol. Means and SEM. *Open circle*, placebo; *filled circle*, propranolol. (Courtesy of Wijnen JAG, van Baak MA, de Haan C, et al: *Eur J Clin Pharmacol* 45:101-105, 1993.)

Subjects and Methods.—The study participants were 11 trained healthy male cyclists. All were normotensive and normally took no medication. Each subject completed an initial progressive maximal cycle ergometer test to determine maximal aerobic power. Two days later, they returned to the laboratory to perform the first endurance test; a second endurance test was conducted 1 week later. One tablet of propranolol (80 mg) was taken before the first test and 1 placebo tablet was taken before the second test in a single-blind study. The second test was stopped at the time of exhaustion found in the previous test.

Results.—The average exercise time was 24 minutes. Plasma glucose was lower during exercise, and plasma lactate and the respiratory exchange ratio were significantly higher when the subjects had received propranolol. Glycerol and NEFA concentrations during exercise showed no significant differences between the 2 conditions. Although exercise times were identical, glycerol (Fig 8-5) and NEFA concentrations during recovery were significantly lower after propranolol treatment.

Conclusion.—This study was designed to examine whether differences resulting from β-blockade would still be seen if the amount of work was fixed. Adipose tissue lipolysis during exercise is inhibited by β-blockade, and thus becomes more apparent during recovery from exercise. Inhibition of lipolysis probably causes a shift from fat to carbohydrate combustion.

▶ One of the interesting findings in this study is that whereas little difference in NEFA could be seen *during* exercise, propranolol treatment reduced NEFA by 75% in the immediate recovery period. It is probable that catecholamine-induced lipolysis continues for some minutes after exercise. At this stage there is little demand for free fatty acids, and blood levels rise. The impact of propranolol thus becomes much more obvious during the recovery period.—R.J. Shephard, M.D., Ph.D.

Theophylline Delays Skeletal Muscle Fatigue During Progressive Exercise

Marsh GD, McFadden RG, Nicholson RL, Leasa DJ, Thompson RT (St Joseph's Health Centre, London, Ont, Canada; Univ of Western Ontario, London, Ont, Canada)
Am Rev Respir Dis 147:876–879, 1993   139-94-8-7

Background.—Researchers have been unable to demonstrate an effect of theophylline on nonrespiratory skeletal muscles. Some reports indicate that overall exercise capacity increases with theophylline, whereas

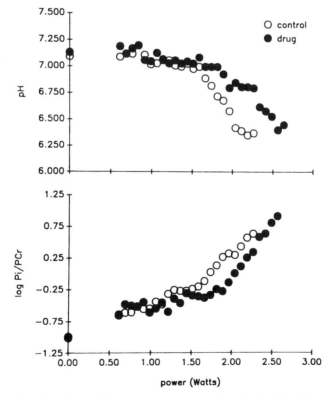

Fig 8–6.—The effect of theophylline on the muscle metabolism of a single individual during progressive exercise. Both the pH response curve (**upper panel**) and the inorganic phosphate/phosphocreatine (*Pi/Pcr*) response curve (**lower panel**) were shifted to the right. In this example, maximal power achieved by the individual increased from 2.25 to 2.55 W, whereas the IT increased from 1.50 to 1.84 W. (Courtesy of Marsh GD, McFadden RG, Nicholson RL, et al: *Am Rev Respir Dis* 147:876–879, 1993.)

others do not. One possible explanation for this discrepancy is that the increase in performance is caused more by CNS stimulation than by any direct action of theophylline on muscle energetics. The effects of theophylline on the metabolism of human wrist flexor muscles during progressive exercise were assessed.

Methods.—The effect of theophylline on human forearm muscle metabolism was determined using ^{31}P nuclear magnetic resonance spectroscopy in 6 healthy men during progressive exercise. The mean age of the subjects was 37 years. The men were assigned in equal numbers to either a control group or a theophylline treatment group. Each man performed 2 dynamic wrist flexion exercise tests to fatigue. The trials were separated by at least 72 hours. The treatment group repeated the protocol after taking 300 mg of sustained-release theophylline every 12 hours.

Findings.—In the control group, power at maximal exercise and at the threshold of intracellular acidosis (IT) was reproducible. In the treatment group, the maximal power attained increased significantly by 19% after theophylline administration. A similar trend was noted at the onset of IT, which was also prolonged by 19%.

Conclusion.—Therapeutic concentrations of theophylline significantly enhanced forearm musculature endurance in these subjects, apparently by delaying the onset of intracellular metabolic acidosis. Theophylline produced a rightward shift of the IT (Fig 8–6) during progressive exercise, suggesting an improvement in oxidative metabolism.

▶ One important statistical exercise at the outset of any investigation is to determine the minimum sample size needed to test the primary hypothesis. In the present instance, some interesting and suggestive findings were obtained, but because only 6 subjects were available, the results did not reach statistical significance.

One trend, which needs to be confirmed on a larger sample, was a rightward shift of both pH and inorganic phosphate/phosphocreatine ratios relative to forearm power output after administration of theophylline. The explanation of the shift in these curves could be either vasodilatation, or (as with the administration of large doses of caffeine) an increased mobilization of fatty acids.

The doses of theophylline used were in the therapeutic range, and it is unlikely that the type of effect described here would be of importance to the performance of an athlete who drinks tea before a competition. However, a theophylline-induced improvement in function of the respiratory muscles may make a helpful contribution to the effort tolerance of patients with chronic obstructive lung disease (1).—R.J. Shephard, M.D., Ph.D.

Reference

1. Murciano D, et al: *J Appl Physiol* 63:51, 1987.

Exercise-Induced Myalgia in Hypothyroidism

Lochmüller H, Reimers CD, Fischer P, Heuβ D, Müller-Höcker J, Pongratz DE
(Ludwig-Maximilians-Universität München, Germany)
Clin Investig 71:999–1001, 1993   139-94-8-8

Background.—Exercise-induced myalgia was an early symptom of hypothyroid myopathy in 1 patient. Muscle biopsy showed recurrent rhabdomyolysis, a finding seen more often in toxic or metabolic myopathies and previously reported in only 3 cases of hypothyroidism.

Case Report.—Woman, 30, experienced myalgia in her lower limbs for several months. Other symptoms included slight periorbital edema, hoarseness, fatigue, and weight gain. The calves were painful if pressed, but no muscle atrophy, hypertrophy, or paresis was present. The thyroid gland was not palpable. Elevated serum creatine kinase (CK) of 2,130 units/L persisted for 3 months. Thyroid-stimulating hormone was also elevated (158 μunits/mL) and triiodothyronine was below normal (15 ng/dL); free thyroxine was not found.

Biopsy specimens from the right medial gastrocnemius muscle revealed disseminated regressive and regenerative fiber changes. Other findings were single-fiber necrosis, macrophages, proliferating satellite cells, and fiber splitting. The histologic diagnosis was a recurrent rhabdomyolysis. Treatment with levothyroxine, starting with 50 μg and increasing to 150 μg daily, brought relief of muscle pain within 1 week. After 6 months, the patient had no muscular complaints, and thyroid hormone and CK values were normal.

Conclusion.—Recurrent rhabdomyolysis was suggested in this patient by clinical symptoms and confirmed by laboratory and myopathologic findings. Rhabdomyolysis is not normally an early sign of hypothyroidism, and exercise-induced myalgias are uncommon signs of hypothyroid myopathy. Because the patient described had only slight classic signs of hypothyroidism, the diagnosis might have been missed. Exercise-induced myalgia should be considered a possible early clinical symptom of hypothyroid myopathy.

▶ An interesting case in which exercise-induced myalgias were an early clue to hypothyroidism is presented. Another interesting thyroid-related report is that of 6 female runners who complained of chronic fatigue and deteriorating running performance; 4 also had high serum cholesterol levels. All had a diagnosis of hypothyroidism secondary to thyroiditis, an easily overlooked cause of chronic fatigue (1). Exercise-related myalgias, apparently from a toxic myopathy, are also being reported in some middle-aged men who begin taking certain cholesterol-lowering drugs, the human menopausal gonadotropin/co-enzyme A reductase inhibitors (2). See the practical review of 6 cases that illustrate the range of diseases besides myositis that can be seen with muscle weakness and laboratory tests reflecting muscle damage (3).—E.R. Eichner, M.D.

References

1. Lathan SR: *Physician Sportsmed* 19:67, 1991.
2. Thompson PD, et al: *JAMA* 264:2992, 1990.
3. Plotz PH: *JAMA* 268:2074, 1992.

Urea Kinetics in Humans at Two Levels of Exercise Intensity
Carraro F, Kimbrough TD, Wolfe RR (Univ of Texas, Galveston)
J Appl Physiol 75:1180–1185, 1993   139-94-8-9

Background.—The role of amino acid oxidation and protein break-down in energy metabolism during exercise is uncertain. Overall protein breakdown and amino acid oxidation do not change at low-intensity exercise. Exercise exceeding the lactate threshold requires high energy substrate metabolism and may elevate amino acid oxidation. Overall protein breakdown and amino acid oxidation are characterized by urea production. The impact of low- and high-intensity exercise on urea production was investigated.

Methods.—After a 2-day liquid diet, 5 normal volunteers performed a treadmill exercise test requiring either 40% maximal oxygen consumption for 3 hours or 70% maximal oxygen consumption for 1 hour. Urea production in response to exercise was quantified using a constant infusion of $[^{15}N_2]$urea. Blood and urine samples were obtained during the rest, exercise, and recovery phases of the protocol. Total rate of urea production from all sources (Ra_t), urea production from recycled N, urea production from nonrecycled N, and urea N recycled back into body protein were calculated.

Results.—Plasma urea concentration remained constant throughout the protocol. Enrichment in the singly and doubly labeled $[^{15}N_2]$urea was at steady state when plasma sampling began during the initial resting phase and did not change during the subsequent exercise and recovery phases for either exercise level. Neither Ra_t nor the amount of $[^{15}N_2]$urea recycled back into urea changed from baseline during exercise or recovery in either exercise protocol. The difference between Ra_t and urea excretion increased significantly during exercise and recovery compared with the rest period in both protocols.

Conclusion.—Total urea production does not change during low-intensity or relatively high–intensity exercise. Thus, exercise does not stimulate urea production, although reincorporation of urea nitrogen into body protein may accelerate.

▶ A number of years ago we noted an increase of plasma urea concentration in postcoronary patients after running a marathon event. The change far exceeded the likely impact of dehydration (1). Even if there had been no excretion of urea while running, the increase would have represented the equivalent of 50 g of protein breakdown in 5 hours, 30 g more than the expected resting rate. The runners were operating at a somewhat greater fraction of their maximal oxygen intake than the subjects studied by Carraro and associates, but the main reason we saw an effect and Carraro et al. did not (despite their sophisticated technology) was that the duration of exercise was too short in the more recent study. Catabolism of protein increases mainly when carbohydrate reserves have been depleted, and this situation does not arise until subjects have been exercising for 90–120 minutes at 70% of maximal oxygen intake. The authors need to undertake a more prolonged experiment before they can conclude that exercise does not increase protein breakdown!—R.J. Shephard, M.D., Ph.D.

Reference

1. Shephard RJ, Kavanagh T: in Howard H, Poortmans JR (eds): *Metabolic Adaptations to Prolonged Exercise*. Basel: Birkhauser Verlag, 1975, pp 245–252.

Increased Reverse Cholesterol Transport in Athletes

Gupta AK, Ross EA, Myers JN, Kashyap ML (Veterans Affairs Med Ctr, Long Beach, Calif; Univ of California, Irvine)
Metabolism 42:684–690, 1993   139-94-8-10

Introduction.—Both long- and short-term exercise will modify lipoprotein metabolism, although the means by which physical activity

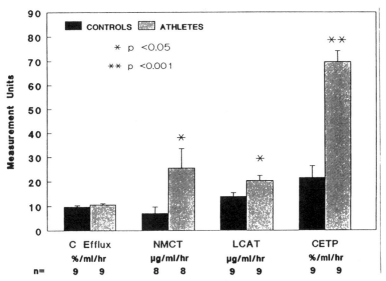

Fig 8–7.—*Abbreviations:* C *Efflux,* cholesterol efflux; NMCT, net mass of free cholesterol transported; LCAT, lecithin:cholesterol acyltransferase; CETP, cholesterol ester transfer proteins. Results of RCT assays for athletes and sedentary control subjects. (Courtesy of Gupta AK, Ross EA, Myers JN, et al: *Metabolism* 42:684–690, 1993.)

achieves cardioprotection are not fully understood. Among the proposed mechanisms for the cardioprotective benefits of exercise are decreased lipid deposition and increased reverse cholesterol transport (RCT). Researchers tested the hypothesis that RCT is enhanced in athletes and that this effect is not necessarily accompanied by large increases in plasma high-density-lipoprotein cholesterol (HDL-C) mass levels.

Subjects and Methods.—Eleven male athletes and 13 sedentary control subjects volunteered for the study. The athletes were exercising at a mean energy expenditure of 21.7 megajoules (5,185 kcal) per week. Controls and athletes were similar in age and body mass index. Venous blood samples were drawn after a 12-hour fast and a 72-hour period of abstaining from alcohol.

Results.—Athletes had similar apolipoprotein (apo) A-1 levels to controls, but their low-density-lipoprotein cholesterol and apo B levels were lower. The athletes had a significantly greater net mass of free cholesterol transported out of cultured human fibroblasts into serum than controls (25.5 vs. 7.1 μg/mL/hr). There was a correlation between the efflux component of this transport and HDL-C and apo A-1 levels, suggesting that antiatherogenic net mass of free cholesterol transported findings in the group of athletes were the result of decreased cholesterol influx into the cells. Compared with controls, athletes had increased plasma lecithin:cholesterol acyltransferase and cholesterol ester transfer protein activities (20.3 vs. 13.9 μg/mL/hr and 69.7 vs. 21.5%/mL/hr, respectively) (Fig 8-7). The net mass of free cholesterol transported inversely correlated with apo B levels and the cardiac risk ratio apo B/A-1 and positively correlated with cholesterol ester transfer protein and plasma lecithin:cholesterol acyltransferase activities. Cholesterol ester transfer protein activities showed an inverse correlation with total cholesterol/HDL-C and low-density-lipoprotein cholesterol/HDL-C ratios.

Conclusion.—Observations that athletes had higher levels of HDL-C raised the possibility of enhanced RCT, the pathway by which cholesterol is removed from peripheral tissues. Exercise is associated with significant increases in the major steps of the RCT pathway. The evidence for increased net flux of free cholesterol out of a peripheral cell model is consistent with the proposed cardioprotective effect of exercise. Measurement of plasma HDL-C and apo A-1 mass does not totally reflect the accelerated transfer of cholesterol.

▶ Individuals must train relatively long and hard to induce quite small increases in blood levels of the scavenging HDL-C. This has led some investigators to question the importance of the HDL-C mechanism in protecting an individual against atherogenesis. Gupta and colleagues have developed techniques to examine 3 components of reversed cholesterol transport: the transfer of free cholesterol from fibroblasts to serum; the esterification of free cholesterol with hepatic excretion (lecithin:cholesterol acyltransferase activity); and the transfer of cholesterol esters from HDL to low-density lipoproteins and very-low-density lipoproteins, again with subsequent hepatic excretion (cholesterol ester transfer protein activity).

Although this study is cross-sectional, it suggests that an active lifestyle speeds all 3 indices of reverse cholesterol transport. Gupta et al. stress that although the athletes and sedentary individuals had similar HDL-cholesterol levels, this is misleading because a static marker is being used to examine a dynamic process.—R.J. Shephard, M.D., Ph.D.

Endurance Exercise Training Reduces Glucose-Stimulated Insulin Levels in 60- to 70-Year-Old Men and Women
Kirwan JP, Kohrt WM, Wojta DM, Bourey RE, Holloszy JO (Washington Univ, St Louis, Mo)
J Gerontol 48:M84–M90, 1993   139-94-8–11

Background.—Older individuals often show a deterioration in glucose tolerance, but it is not known whether this change is related to aging per se or to the decline in physical activity and increase in adiposity that may occur with aging. The effect of a program of endurance exercise on the plasma insulin response in older subjects was determined.

Methods.—Twelve healthy volunteers, 5 men and 7 women aged 60–70 years, participated in the study. For comparative purposes, data were also presented on 12 young subjects. All participants were normally active but had not recently participated in endurance exercise training. All had a normal response to a 75-g oral glucose tolerance test. The older subjects took part in 9 months of endurance exercise training, primarily walking and running on an indoor track or treadmill (approximately 80% of maximal heart rate). Using the hyperglycemic clamp procedure, the effect of this exercise on glucose-stimulated response and glucose disposal rate was evaluated.

Results.—Exercise training brought about modest but significant reductions in body mass and percent body fat. In all subjects, maximal oxygen intake increased 23%. Older subjects achieved a significantly lower insulin, but not glucose, response with training. Their post-training insulin area was not significantly different from that of the younger subjects. In the trained state, fasting insulin levels were similar to those of young sedentary subjects. Individual changes in glucose disposal rate were significantly associated with changes in body mass and waist circumference, but not fat mass (Fig 8–8).

Conclusion.—In the older, healthy subjects who took part in an endurance training program, glucose tolerance was not improved. There were favorable adaptations, however, in a blunted insulin response to glucose and an enhanced insulin action. Such training, performed on a

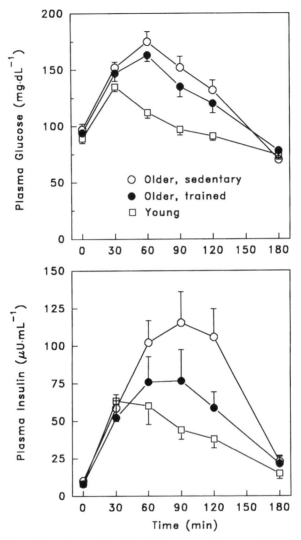

Fig 8–8.—Plasma glucose (**top panel**) and insulin (**bottom panel**) concentrations during an oral glucose tolerance test of older individuals before and after endurance exercise training and of young individuals. (Courtesy of Kirwan JP, Kohrt WM, Wojta DM, et al: *J Gerontol* 48:M84–M90, 1993.)

regular basis, may reduce the risk of certain age-related metabolic disorders developing.

▶ As in other studies of older adults, a period of aerobic training reduced insulin secretion in response to a given glucose challenge, the immediate effect of the exercise program being to bring insulin secretion within the normal range for young adults. The authors make the useful point that the normalization of insulin secretion reflects both short-term responses to the most recent bout of exercise and more long-term consequences of training. For a recent bout of exercise to have a favorable effect on insulin secretion, the activity must have been vigorous, and training is important in helping older subjects to attain this level of activity. The short-term component of the response is reversed very quickly if training is halted. The long-term effects are more persistent and seem to be related to decreased body fat content (1, 2).—R.J. Shephard, M.D., Ph.D.

References

1. Bogardus C, et al: *Diabetes* 33:311, 1984.
2. Gumbiner B, et al: *J Clin Endocrinol Metab* 70:1594, 1990.

Insulin-Dependent Diabetes Mellitus, Physical Activity, and Death
Moy CS, Songer TJ, LaPorte RE, Dorman JS, Kriska AM, Orchard TJ, Becker DJ, Drash AL (Univ of Pittsburgh, Pa)
Am J Epidemiol 137:74–81, 1993   139-94-8-12

Objective.—Regular physical activity is acknowledged as beneficial to the general population, but the long-term effect of increased activity among individuals with insulin-dependent diabetes has received little attention. Accordingly, physical activity was ascertained by a self-administered survey of 548 diabetics followed up in the Pittsburgh Insulin-Dependent Diabetes Mellitus Morbidity and Mortality Study. Physical activity was estimated in 1981 and related to mortality as ascertained through 1987.

Observations.—Compared with the general population, mortality during the 6-year follow-up was more than eightfold higher in male diabetics and thirteenfold higher in female diabetics. A strong inverse relationship was evident between energy expenditure and mortality (Fig 8–9). A lower weekly energy expenditure remained significantly associated with increased mortality in male patients after adjusting for reported complications, age, body mass index, dose of insulin, and drinking and smoking status. In female patients the association was of only borderline significance. A number of lifestyle factors correlated with the level of physical activity. In a case-control analysis, both male and female diabetics were as active as nondiabetic control subjects when patients limited by diabetic complications were excluded. Patients with diabetes were more likely than their sibling controls to be excluded from sports activities.

Implications.—An increased level of physical activity does not appear to place insulin-dependent diabetics at increased risk of dying, and it

A. Males

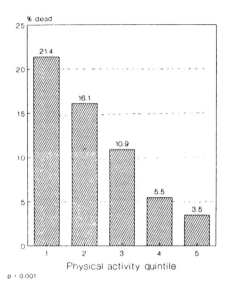

p < 0.001

B. Females

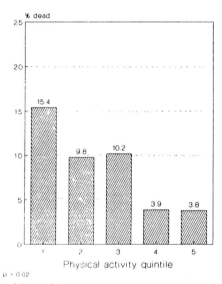

p < 0.02

Fig 8–9.—Proportion of deceased by sex and physical activity quintile. Pittsburgh Insulin-Dependent Diabetes Mellitus Registry prospective mortality cohort, 1981-1987. Quintile cutoffs for male patients were less than 398; 398-1,000; 1,000-2,230; 2,230-4,228; and more than 4,228 kcal/wk. For female patients, the quintiles were less than 168; 168-701; 701-1,330; 1,330-2,360; and more than 2,360 kcal/wk. (Courtesy of Moy CS, Songer TJ, LaPorte RE, et al: *Am J Epidemiol* 137:74-81, 1993.)

may actually extend their longevity. Simple activities such as walking and gardening will suffice.

▶ Given the link between diabetes mellitus and atherosclerotic disease, one might anticipate that physical activity would be at least as beneficial in diabetics as it is in healthy individuals (1). The present report supports this view. The optimal protection, as in normal individuals (2), was seen with a leisure energy expenditure of 8.4 megajoules (2,000 kcal) per week. This need not demand very intensive sport participation, although if walking is to be the main source of the added energy expenditure, it must be persistent and vigorous. For example, walking at 4.8 km/hr (3 mph) is likely to give an energy expenditure of about 20 kJ/min, so that 420 minutes of brisk walking must be undertaken each week to realize an optimal response.—R.J. Shephard, M.D., Ph.D.

References

1. American Diabetic Association Council on Exercise: *Diabetes Care* 13:804, 1990.
2. Paffenbarger RS: *Med Sci Sports Exerc* 20:426, 1988.

Effects of Endurance Training on Hormonal Responses to Prolonged Physical Exercise in Males
Vasankari TJ, Kujala UM, Heinonen OJ, Huhtaniemi IT (Univ of Turku, Finland; Helsinki Research Inst for Sports and Exercise Medicine; Turku Univ, Finland)
Acta Endocrinol 129:109–113, 1993   139-94-8-13

Background.—During acute, prolonged exercise in men, serum testosterone and gonadotropins have been reported to decrease, and serum cortisol and growth hormone have been reported to increase. There are conflicting reports on the effects of endurance training on these hormonal changes. The effect of training background on pituitary, gonadal, and adrenocortical responses to acute, prolonged physical exercise in men was examined in 2 trials.

Study Design.—The first trial consisted of venous blood sampling in 13 athletes before and after a 75-km cross-country ski race and 3 weeks later on a nonrace day. The second trial consisted of venous blood sampling of 10 trained and 8 untrained men before and after a 4-hour bicycle outing on the road at a high performance level.

Results.—In the first trial, serum luteinizing hormone and follicle-stimulating hormone (FSH) concentrations decreased more and cortisol concentrations increased more during the race than on the control day. Serum testosterone decreased during the race, but not on the control day. In the second trial, serum FSH levels were higher in the trained men than in the untrained subjects at all time points (table). Growth hormone

Trial II: Serum Concentrations of Testosterone,
Immunofluorometric Leutinizing Hormone (I-LH), Bioactive LH
(B-LH), FSH, Cortisol, and Growth Hormone (GH) Before
Exercise (A), Immediately After Exercise (B), and 2 Hours After
Exercise (C)

	A	B	C
Testosterone (nmol/l)			
Trained	24.0±1.2	23.8±1.8	21.3±2.1
Untrained	23.4±2.7	16.4±1.0*	16.8±2.6
I-LH (IU/l)			
Trained	4.0±0.6	2.4±0.5	3.0±0.4
Untrained	3.0±0.4	1.5±0.2	2.8±0.4
B-LH (IU/l)			
Trained	12.4±2.6	7.8±1.5	9.4±1.9
Untrained	8.8±1.1	5.3±0.5	8.6±1.2
FSH (IU/l)			
Trained	5.3±0.6	4.6±0.6	4.7±0.5
Untrained	3.5±0.6	2.8±0.5	3.2±0.5
Cortisol (nmol/l)			
Trained	580±39	671±51	407±44
Untrained	393±71	699±80*	428±113
GH (mIU/l)			
Trained	6.1±2.0	38.8±7.5	4.8±1.0
Untrained	1.4±0.2	29.4±8.9	10.7±3.4

Note: Values are means ± SEM; there were 10 trained and 8 untrained subjects. The overall trial effect was significant in testosterone ($P = .0083$), I-LH ($P = .0029$), B-LH ($P = .0147$), FSH ($P = .0001$), and cortisol ($P = .0001$). There was a significant trial-group interaction in GH ($P = .020$) and group difference in FSH ($P = .046$).
* Contrast between groups A and B ($P < .05$).
(Courtesy of Vasankari TJ, Kujala UM, Heinonen OJ, et al: *Acta Endocrinol* 129:109–113, 1993.)

was lower before exercise and higher 2 hours after exercise in the untrained subjects. There were significant differences in preexercise and postexercise levels of testosterone and cortisol between the trained and untrained men.

Conclusion.—Higher FSH levels were detected in trained subjects compared with untrained subjects. This suggests compensated hypogonadism as a result of intensive chronic training or a dysfunction of Sertoli cells. Trained subjects exhibited signs of adaptation to resist the hormonal changes caused by acute physical exercise.

▶ In contrast to some earlier studies, FSH levels seemed to increase in the endurance athletes, helping to maintain serum testosterone levels in the face of prolonged exercise. Probably, as in female competitors, the extent of depression of the sex hormones reflects the adequacy of nutrition among those who engage in frequent and prolonged bouts of exercise. Athletes are sometimes concerned to learn that their testosterone levels may diminish. There are sometimes parallel reductions in sperm count, but these are rarely sufficient to impair fertility (1).—R.J. Shephard, M.D., Ph.D.

Reference

1. Ayers JWT, et al: *Fertil Steril* 43:917, 1985.

Testicular Compression During Exercise: Serum Testosterone Levels
Boustead G, Bornman M, Reif S, Oosthuizen JMC, Luus HG (Med Univ of Southern Africa, Medunsa; Univ of Orange Free State, Bloemfontein, South Africa)
Arch Androl 30:209–211, 1993   139-94-8-14

Introduction.—Levels of serum testosterone (s-T) are known to increase after intensive short-term exercise, and several theories have been proposed to explain this elevation. This study examined whether the mechanical effects of compression on the testes could contribute to the increase in s-T.

Patients and Methods.—The study subjects were 14 men with histologically proved stage D2 carcinoma of the prostate who were scheduled to undergo subcapsular orchiectomy. They volunteered to have pressure applied to the testes via a pneumatic cuff. Baseline levels of s-T were taken when the patients were under general anesthesia. Compression was applied at a pressure of 100 mm Hg for 2 minutes. At the end of this compression and at 1, 1.5, 3, 3.5, 5, and 7 minutes after compression, determinations of s-T were obtained for comparison with baseline values. Samples were also taken directly after and 5 minutes after removal of the testes.

Mean Baseline and $t_{1.5}$ Values of Serum Testosterone in nmol/L

Factor	$n = 6$		$n = 4$	
	Baseline	$t_{1.5}$	Baseline	$t_{1.5}$
Mean s-T	14.22	16.82	13.88	16.20
SD	2.29	3.27	2.37	1.93
% Increase in s-T	18.28		16.71	

(Courtesy of Boustead G, Bornman M, Reif S, et al: *Arch Androl* 30:209–211, 1993.)

Results.—Three patients had to be excluded from the study because they had received diethylstilbestrol before surgery and 5 were excluded because of very low baseline testosterone values. In the remaining 6 patients there was an average increase in s-T of 18.28% at 1.5 minutes after compression (table). The s-T level decreased markedly within 5 minutes after removal of the testes.

Conclusion.—Compression may be a contributing factor, but it does not explain the increase in s-T observed in these patients. Although no specific mechanism has yet been identified, the rise in s-T that occurs with intense short-term exercise is probably multifactorial. Gonadotropin stimulation does not appear to be involved.

▶ Despite major compression of the testes (pressures of 100 mm Hg, values that are unlikely to be encountered except in severe trauma), the observed increase in serum testosterone levels was less than the 37% acute increase seen in endurance exercise (1). Hemoconcentration, altered plasma binding, and decreased hepatic clearance seem to be more probable explanations of the phenomenon than testicular compression (2), particularly during normal running.—R.J. Shephard, M.D., Ph.D.

References

1. Jensen J, et al. *Eur J Appl Physiol* 63:467, 1991.
2. Shephard RJ: *Physiology and Biochemistry of Exercise.* New York: Praeger, 1982.

Overtraining Affects Male Reproductive Status
Roberts AC, McClure RD, Weiner RI, Brooks GA (Univ of California, Berkeley; Univ of California, San Francisco)
Fertil Steril 60:686–692, 1993   139-94-8–15

Background.—Although the effects of strenuous physical exercise on female reproductive function have been extensively documented, there is little information available on the chronic effects of endurance training on reproductive variables in men. Therefore, the effect of strenuous exercise on the hypothalamic-pituitary-gonadal axis was investigated in men by longitudinal evaluation of blood and semen samples.

Study Design.—Five endurance-trained men in their 20s with normal spermatogenic and hormonal profiles recorded their activity, mileage, and duration of exercise. The mileage of their activity was doubled, whereas intensity was held constant for a 2-week period of overtraining. Reproductive variables were examined before, immediately after, and 3 months after overtraining.

Results.—Basal testosterone levels decreased and basal cortisol levels increased immediately after overtraining. That inverse relationship was highly correlated. By 3 months after resumption of normal training, both testosterone and cortisol had returned to baseline levels. Sperm count decreased significantly immediately after overtraining and was further decreased 3 months after overtraining. However, all values remained within the normal range.

Conclusion.—After a period of overtraining, cortisol, testosterone, and sperm concentrations all changed significantly in a group of endurance-trained athletes. Therefore, exercise overtraining has significant effects on both hormonal and semen reproductive variables in men. However, even with these significant changes, all levels were within the normal range and would not be expected to affect fertility.

▶ In this short-term overtraining study, the decrease in basal testosterone level correlated with the increase in basal cortisol level. In fact, the mechanism for the decrease in testosterone may be, at least in part, the increase in cortisol. Sperm count varied greatly from subject to subject, but mean count declined after overtraining and was still down 3 months later (spermatogenesis takes 74 days). This fall in sperm count, however, was only from high to low values, all within the normal range, which would not be apt to affect fertility. The authors claim to be the first to report an effect of physical exertion on sperm count, but a similar trend (declines in testosterone and sperm counts) from a similar study was reported in 1990 (1). A recent cross-sectional study found subclinical decreases in sperm characteristics in endurance runners (2), and a case report documented decreased testosterone and libido in a wrestler with severe weight loss (3). When it comes to exhaustive exercise, then, the question is: Can you keep it up?—E.R. Eichner, M.D.

References

1. Griffith RO: *Physician Sportsmed* 18:54, 1990.
2. Arce JC, et al: *Fertil Steril* 59:398, 1993.
3. Strauss RH, et al: *Physician Sportsmed* 21:64, 1993.

The Effect of Short and Long Duration Exercise on Serum Erythropoietin Concentrations

Klausen T, Breum L, Fogh-Andersen N, Bennett P, Hippe E (Fredriksberg Hosp, Denmark; Univ of Copenhagen)
Eur J Appl Physiol 67:213–217, 1993   139-94-8-16

Background.—The relationship between serum erythropoietin (EPO) concentrations and endurance exercise has attracted attention, especially because endurance athletes have a high total blood volume and red blood cell mass but also lower hemoglobin levels because of high plasma volume. The effects of short- and long-duration exercise on serum EPO levels were investigated.

Methods and Results.—Seven male cross-country skiers and 8 male marathon runners were included. Short-duration exercise was done as 60 minutes of cycling at 80% to 95% of maximal heart rate. Arterial blood oxygen saturations were unchanged throughout exercise. Partial oxygen pressure at which hemoglobin was half-saturated with oxygen and erythrocyte 2,3-diphosphoglycerate did not significantly change during exercise. Blood lactate levels were raised at the end of exercise. Serum EPO levels were also unchanged from before to 30 hours after exercise. These levels were unrelated to earlier parameters. Long-duration exercise consisted of habitual training, a 3-week break, then 2 and 4 weeks of retraining. The serum EPO concentrations, body fat, and serum free testosterone levels were unchanged at the end of each period. Maximal oxygen intakes were reduced after the break and increased during retraining. After the break, body mass was also increased. Serum EPO concentrations were correlated with body fat, body mass, and free testosterone levels.

Conclusion.—Short- and long-duration exercise did not directly affect serum EPO concentrations. However, these concentrations, free testosterone levels, and body composition were associated.

▶ This study adds to the controversy of whether exercise increases the serum EPO concentration. The authors argue that an earlier study showing an increase in EPO 31 hours after a marathon (1) was confounded by the diurnal variation in EPO and that other studies showing exercise-related increases in EPO were done with insensitive assays. In contrast, they argue, no study using the more sensitive radioimmunoassay, as used here, has shown an exercise-related increase in EPO, even after marathons (2). In this study, serum EPO concentrations were not influenced by either brief, intense exercise (meant to simulate hard training or competing) or by longitudinal changes in levels of endurance training. In short, exercise did not directly affect EPO levels.—E.R. Eichner, M.D.

References

1. 1992 YEAR BOOK OF SPORTS MEDICINE, pp 168–170.
2. Weight LM, et al: *Eur J Appl Physiol* 64:444, 1992.

Steroids, Drugs, and Smoking

Sports Nutrition Fraud

Short SH, Marquart LF (Syracuse Univ, NY; Cornell Cooperative Extension, Mexico, NY)
N Y State J Med 93:112–116, 1993   139-94-8–17

Background.—Many athletes use ergogenic aids, including anabolic steroids, blood doping, and nutritional aids to enhance their sports performance. The use of unregulated, worthless sports nutrition products marketed to athletes as part of a multibillion dollar food supplement industry was examined.

Review.—Nutritional supplements for athletes include protein powders and vitamin/mineral products. These supplements are marketed to athletes in general and do not take individual nutritional requirements into account. However, nutritional requirements differ between athletes. Athletes involved in endurance sports have different nutritional requirements than those engaged in short-term events. Furthermore, nutritional guidance should consider body composition, age, amount of time spent in practice and training, and the duration of athletic events. An evaluation of 30 published studies involving athletes and their use of nutritional supplements showed that more than half of those surveyed took dietary supplements. Because of a lack of time and funding, nutritional supplements for athletes are not regulated by the Food and Drug Administration (FDA) and do not have to be proven safe and effective. However, the American public tends to believe that these products have been researched, tested, and inspected by the FDA. Fortunately, most of the dietary supplements are harmless. Sports physicians should question their athletic patients about the use of nutritional supplements and provide them with the correct nutritional information. The amount of money spent on dietary supplements by athletes is substantial and would be better spent on food.

▶ There is no question that many athletes use dietary supplements and other unproven "magical substances" to improve performance. In many instances, the athletes believe they are using substances that have been proven effective through scientific study (1). Although most of these products are harmless, they are not subject to FDA scrutiny and may not be as safe as we think. To improve performance, athletes should follow the sound principles of proper training, good nutrition, and adequate rest. Fads and "magical substances" should be avoided. Sound advice from coaches, athletic trainers, team physicians, and other support personnel is very important to maintain the health of our athletes.—F.J. George, A.T.C., P.T.

Reference

1. 1993 YEAR BOOK OF SPORTS MEDICINE, p 387.

Neuropsychiatric Effects of Anabolic Steroids in Male Normal Volunteers

Su T-P, Pagliaro M, Schmidt PJ, Pickar D, Wolkowitz O, Rubinow DR (Natl Inst of Mental Health, Bethesda, Md; Mental Health Nursing Service, Bethesda, Md)
JAMA 269:2760–2764, 1993   139-94-8–18

Objective.—Several retrospective studies have documented mood changes and psychiatric symptoms associated with anabolic steroid abuse. The acute effects of anabolic steroids on mood and behavior were examined prospectively in a placebo-controlled crossover trial.

Methods.—Twenty healthy men aged 18–42 years volunteered for the study. All had passed rigorous psychiatric screening before admission to the National Institute of Mental Health inpatient research ward. None of the men were involved in athletic training and none had previously used anabolic steroids. Methyltestosterone or placebo was given under 4 drug conditions each lasting 3 days: baseline placebo, low-dose methyltestosterone (40 mg/day), high-dose methyltestosterone (240 mg/day), and withdrawal placebo. Mood and behavioral parameters were measured during each drug condition.

Results.—Anabolic steroids had a significant impact on mood and behavior. High-dose methyltestosterone administration was associated with subtle, although statistically significant, increases in positive mood scores, negative mood scores, and cognitive symptoms when compared with baseline measurements. During high-dose methyltestosterone administration, 1 man who had no personal or family psychiatric history experienced an acute manic episode and another man had major depression. None of the volunteers had psychotic symptoms.

Conclusion.—Anabolic steroids have a significant adverse effect on mood and behavior in normal male volunteers, even when they are given for a short term at relatively low doses.

▶ This is the first placebo-controlled prospective study showing the effects of anabolic steroids (AAS) on mood and behavior. Each participant took the pills in a fixed sequence for only 3 days each: baseline placebo, low-dose AAS, high-dose AAS, and withdrawal placebo. Despite the brief exposure and—compared with what some athletes use—modest doses, significant if subtle changes occurred as a result of the AAS, especially the high-dose segment. Of course, the response to AAS varied greatly between individuals, from negligible to dramatic. During AAS use, 1 subject had major depression develop (he concurrently had a severe post–spinal tap headache) and another had mania develop.

Although self-ratings generally moved in a negative direction on high-dose AAS (e.g., irritability, mood swings, violent feelings, anger, hostility), there was also a significant increase in positive effects (e.g., sexual arousal, energy, euphoria, confidence). This study thus confirms early studies suggesting both activating and adverse moods and behaviors while using AAS.—E.R. Eichner, M.D.

Use of Multiple Drugs Among Adolescents Who Use Anabolic Steroids

DuRant RH, Rickert VI, Ashworth CS, Newman C, Slavens G (Med College of

Georgia, Augusta; Univ of Arkansas, Little Rock; Univ of Alabama, Birmingham)
N Engl J Med 328:922–926, 1993   139-94-8–19

Background.—It has been suggested that adolescents who use anabolic steroids to increase muscle size or enhance athletic performance will not use alcohol, marijuana, or other drugs because they believe these to be harmful to their body. Others are of the opinion that adolescents who use anabolic steroids are likely to also use other substances. A large group of adolescents was surveyed to examine the relationship between anabolic steroid use and the use of other substances.

Methods.—A questionnaire designed to measure risk-taking behavior among adolescents attending public schools was completed by 1,881 high school students (mean age, 14.9 years) attending compulsory health-science classes. The survey contained questions on the use of anabolic steroids and other substances, as well as on the sharing of needles and high-risk behavior for HIV infection.

Results.—The use of anabolic steroids was reported by 6.5% of the boys and 1.9% of the girls. Students in grade 9 reported less use of anabolic steroids than those in grades 10 through 12. Of those who had used anabolic steroids, 24.7% reported having shared needles to inject drugs during the previous 30 days. The frequency of anabolic steroid use was significantly associated with the frequency of use in the previous 30 days of cocaine, injectable drugs, alcohol, marijuana, cigarettes, and smokeless tobacco. Multivariate analysis showed that use of marijuana, shared needles, smokeless tobacco, and cocaine accounted for 33% of the variation in anabolic steroid use.

Conclusion.—Adolescents who use anabolic steroids are likely to use other drugs as well.

▶ The authors bring us more bad news about kids and drugs. In this large survey in Richmond County, Georgia, 5.4% of ninth-grade boys and 1.5% of ninth-grade girls reported using anabolic steroids (AAS). Among the users of AAS, 25% shared needles to inject drugs; those who shared needles were less likely to have received school-based education about HIV and AIDS. In general, the more frequently adolescents used AAS, the more likely they were to use 1 or more other drugs, especially marijuana, tobacco, alcohol, and cocaine. There goes the theory that young AAS users regard the body as a "temple" and so shun other drugs. See also Abstracts 139-94-8–20 through 139-94-8–22. For more on the effects of AAS on mood and behavior, see Abstract 139-94-8–18.—E.R. Eichner, M.D.

▶↓ The following 3 articles illustrate key points about drug use and smoking among young students. Abstract 139-94-8–20, a survey of seventh-grade students in public schools in Modesto, California, found that nearly 5% of boys and over 3% of girls admitted to using anabolic steroids (AAS). Even more alarming, nearly 75% of those who were offered AAS used them at least once. Granted, odds are what they used was not always AAS, but they do tend, alas, to follow the leader. Abstract 139-94-8-21, a survey of tenth graders in 2 suburban Chicago high schools, found that 5% of boys but only 1 girl reported past or present use of human growth hormone (HGH). Those who used AAS were more likely to use HGH; most seemed unaware of the side effects of HGH. Again, they probably were not using genuine HGH, but the point is, they thought they were. Abstract 139-94-8-22 suggests a ray of hope: Students who take part in interscholastic sports are less likely to take up smoking.—E.R. Eichner, M.D.

Rate of Anabolic-Androgenic Steroid Use Among Students in Junior High School

Radakovich J, Broderick P, Pickell G (Hennepin County Med Ctr, Minneapolis; Univ of California, Davis)
J Am Board Fam Pract 6:341–345, 1993   139-94-8-20

Background.—Several studies of the use of anabolic steroids among high school students have reported use rates greater than 4%. Although there is evidence that even junior high school students are using steroids, usage in this age group has not been documented.

Methods.—A 22-item survey of current or previous anabolic-androgenic steroid use, previous abuse of other substances including alcohol, and knowledge about the effects of steroids on the body was administered to 810 seventh-grade students whose parents had given written consent for their children's participation. The survey was confidential and did not contain any identifying information.

Results.—Data from 782 completed surveys were evaluable. Most students were age 12, 13, or 14 years; 11 students were age 15 years. Thirty students (3.8%) admitted to steroid use, 25 of whom were younger than age 15 years. Five steroid users were 12 years of age. Twenty-five users (83%) planned to participate in high school athletics. Steroid users knew significantly less about the effects of steroids on the body than nonusers. African-American race, participation in power sports such as football and wrestling, and past use of alcohol or marijuana were correlated with an increased risk of steroid use in this age group.

Conclusion.—For some, the use of anabolic-androgenic steroids starts in junior high school. Physicians should initiate discussions about steroid use and its potential adverse effects before their patients turn to less qualified individuals for information.

Human Growth Hormone: A New Substance of Abuse Among Adolescents?

Rickert VI, Pawlak-Morello C, Sheppard V, Jay MS (Univ of Arkansas, Little

Rock; Loyola Univ, Chicago)
Clin Pediatr 31:723–726, 1992   139-94-8–21

Introduction.—A recent government study indicates that 5% to 11% of male and 2.5% of female adolescents in high school admit to using anabolic steroids (AS). Prompted by anecdotal reports that athletes may also use human growth hormone (HGH), a study was conducted to examine the prevalence of HGH use in a suburban high school and the relationship between HGH and AS use.

Method.—A 15-item questionnaire was completed by 224 male and 208 female tenth-grade students in 2 suburban midwestern high schools with 83% white, 14% Asian, and 3% black students.

Findings.—Five percent of male students reported past or present use of HGH to increase muscle strength and/or body size and to strengthen their tendons and ligaments. One female student used HGH for medical reasons. Among the male adolescents surveyed, 78% had heard of HGH and 65% had poor knowledge of its effects. Among the 11 HGH users, about half were between 14 and 15 years of age and 70% used HGH more than once per month, but most users were unaware of its side effects. There was a significant association between AS and HGH use, with 7 AS users reporting past or present use of HGH. Users and nonusers of HGH did not differ significantly in sports activity, ethnicity, or age.

Implications.—A small percentage of male adolescents admit to using HGH, and those who admit to AS use appear to be most at risk. Overall, 8.5% of the male adolescents surveyed could be considered abusers of HGH and/or AS. Adolescents may be susceptible at early ages to influences that promise to improve body growth, appearance, and physical strength.

Sports Participation, Age at Smoking Initiation, and the Risk of Smoking Among US High School Students
Escobedo LG, Marcus SE, Holtzman D, Giovino GA (Natl Ctr for Chronic Disease Prevention and Health Promotion, Atlanta, Ga)
JAMA 269:1391–1395, 1993   139-94-8–22

Purpose.—Children and adolescents generally progress from initial favorable attitudes about smoking to initiation, occasional smoking, and regular smoking. Studies have addressed the initiation of smoking and patterns of smoking among youth. However, there are few data on the relationship between sports participation and age at smoking initiation to regular smoking.

Methods.—Using data from the 1990 Youth Risk Behavior Survey, a nationally representative sample of high school students, the incidence and prevalence of smoking initiation and the odds of regular and heavy

in relation to age at initiation and participation in interscholas-
ـs were calculated. The analysis included data on 11,248 stu-
ـents.

Findings.—Seventy-two percent of the students had at least experi-
mented with smoking cigarettes, and 32% had smoked within the past
month. Heavy, regular smoking was more common in older students,
white students, those with low academic performance, and those who
did not participate in interscholastic sports. Adjusted odds ratios of regular, heavy smoking decreased with increasing number of sports played.
Rates of smoking initiation increased rapidly with age, peaking at age
13–14 years and declining after age 16 years. Those who started smoking
at age 12 years or younger were more likely to be regular, heavy smokers
than those who began smoking in later years.

Conclusion.—The risk of heavy, regular smoking in adolescence is increased by starting smoking at a young age. Sports participation appears
to have significant effects on smoking behavior, the nature of which
should be explored in future studies. Efforts to prevent smoking should
begin before age 12 years, and quit-smoking programs should be available for adolescents who smoke.

**Physical Activity, Fitness, and Selected Risk Factors for CHD in Ac-
tive Men and Women**
Bovens AM, Van Baak MA, Vrencken JG, Wijnen JA, Saris WH, Verstappen
FT (State Univ of Limburg, Maastricht, The Netherlands)
Med Sci Sports Exerc 25:572–576, 1993   139-94-8–23

Background.—Past epidemiologic studies demonstrating the inverse
relationship between coronary heart disease (CHD) and physical activity
have involved populations with a high number of inactive individuals,
mostly men. The relationship between physical activity and cardiovascular risk factors in physically active men and women was thus studied.

Methods.—Data on 898 women and 2,009 men older than age 40
years and active in sports were analyzed. Fitness was assessed from peak
cycle ergometer power output. Physical activity included occupational
activity and the use of a bicycle for transport as well as sports participation. The cardiovascular risk factors considered included blood pressure,
body composition, and smoking habits.

Findings.—Correlations between cardiovascular fitness and risk factors indicated that more fit individuals had significantly lower risks than
their peers who were less fit. Except for smoking habits, all risk factors
had stronger associations with fitness in women than in men. The relationship between physical activity indicators and risk factors was weaker
than the fitness–risk factor relationship in both men and women. In addition, joggers of either sex had the best risk profile, compared with individuals who were active in 1 of the other 4 most popular sports (table).

Characteristics of Subpopulations of Men Active in at Least 3 Sports or Active in Only 1 Type of the 5 Most Popular Sports

	Active in at Least Three Sports N = 504 3	Active in Just One Type of Sport				
		Cycling N = 152 A	Jogging N = 133 B	Tennis N = 106 C	Soccer N = 95 D	Volleyball N = 48 E
Age (yr)	47.4 ± 6.7	47.9 ± 7.5	45.1 ± 4.7	47.2 ± 5.5	44.8 ± 4.8	45.7 ± 5.2
Body fat (%)	23.5 ± 5.0	23.1 ± 5.1	21.1 ± 4.9	24.8 ± 4.8	23.4 ± 4.8	23.8 ± 4.9
BMI (kg·m^{-2})	24.7 ± 2.2	25.1 ± 2.3	24.3 ± 2.1	25.2 ± 2.1	25.9 ± 2.0	24.4 ± 2.1
SBP (mm Hg)	136.0 ± 13.0	135.2 ± 12.2	133.8 ± 11.6	135.8 ± 13.9	135.1 ± 13.3	135.1 ± 10.9
DBP (mm Hg)	86.1 ± 7.5	86.6 ± 7.2	85.2 ± 7.2	86.1 ± 7.8	86.5 ± 7.7	86.8 ± 7.4
Smoker (%)	22.0	27.0	19.5	39.6	36.8	29.2
W_{max} (W)	260.8 ± 48.0	269.9 ± 53.1	270.3 ± 35.5	231.3 ± 37.7	244.3 ± 36.5	240.0 ± 39.6
$W_{max} \cdot kg^{-1}$ (W·kg^{-1})	3.4 ± 0.6	3.5 ± 0.7	3.6 ± 0.5	3.0 ± 0.5	3.1 ± 0.5	3.2 ± 0.4
Duration (h·wk^{-1})	6.1 ± 3.4	4.8 ± 3.7	3.6 ± 2.4	3.0 ± 3.0	1.7 ± 1.4	1.7 ± 1.1
Frequency (times·wk^{-1})	4.3 ± 2.2	2.3 ± 1.5	3.2 ± 1.5	1.9 ± 1.0	1.2 ± 0.8	1.1 ± 0.4
Occupational activity (%)	21.6	25.3	22.0	12.5	44.1	19.6
Bicycle for transport (%)	48.4	49.3	47.4	33.0	51.6	56.3

(Courtesy of Bovens AM, Van Baak MA, Vrencken JG, et al: *Med Sci Sports Exerc* 25:572–576, 1993.)

Conclusion.—In an active population, the strength of the relationship between cardiovascular fitness, physical activity, and cardiovascular risk factors is comparable to that in less active populations. Active men and women who are more physically fit have better cardiovascular risk profiles. Joggers have the best risk profiles.

▶ It is a sad commentary on life in Holland that 39.6% of 106 male tennis players are currently smokers! However, this article supports earlier research from North America (1–3) in showing that solitary, aerobic activities are associated with a low prevalence of smoking, and social sports such as tennis are associated with the highest prevalence. It is less clear whether this difference arises because gregarious people are more prone to smoke, or whether activities that are aerobically demanding draw attention to the negative effects of smoking on cardiorespiratory function, thus encouraging smoking withdrawal (3). It is particularly noteworthy that in women, by far the lowest prevalence of smoking is seen in the walkers.—R.J. Shephard, M.D., Ph.D.

References

1. Perrier Great Waters of France: The Perrier Survey. New York: 1979.
2. Shephard RJ: *Br J Sports Med* 23:11, 1989.
3. Shephard RJ, et al: *Br J Sports Med* In press, 1994.

Anabolic-Androgenic Steroid Use in the United States
Yesalis CE, Kennedy NJ, Kopstein AN, Bahrke MS (Pennsylvania State Univ, University Park; Ctr for Substance Abuse Prevention, Rockville, Md; Natl Inst on Drug Abuse, Rockville, Md; et al)
JAMA 270:1217–1221, 1993   139-94-8–24

Introduction.—The use of anabolic-androgenic steroids (AASs) is no longer restricted to elite athletes or adult male subjects, despite the potential adverse impact of these drugs on physical and psychological health. The size of the AAS user population in the United States was estimated, AAS users were characterized, the association between the use of AASs and the use of other illicit drugs was explored, and self-reported aggressive behavior was examined.

Subjects and Methods.—Data were obtained from the 11th United States National Household Survey on Drug Abuse (NHSDA) conducted in 1991, the first year that the survey asked questions about abuse of AASs. The results were based on personal interviews and self-administered questionnaires from 32,594 respondents. The sample design ensured adequate numbers of respondents for 4 age groups: 12–17 years, 18–25 years, 26–34 years, and 35 years or older. Blacks and Hispanics were oversampled to increase the reliability of estimates of drug use by this segment of the population.

Ever and Past-Year Use of Anabolic Steroids

Rate Estimates, %

	Ever Used		**Used Past Year**	
	Observed Estimate	**95% CI**	**Observed Estimate**	**95% CI**
Age, y				
12–17	0.6	0.4–0.9	0.3	0.2–0.6
18–25	1.3	1.0–1.9	0.4	0.2–0.7
26–34	0.6	0.4–0.9	0.1	0.0–0.2
35+	.02	0.1–0.5	0.1	0.0–0.3
Sex				
M	0.9†	0.7–1.2	0.3	0.2–0.4
F	0.1	0.1–0.3	0.1	0.0–0.2
Race				
White	0.6	0.4–0.8	0.2	0.1–0.3
Black	0.4	0.3–0.7	0.1	0.1–0.2
Hispanic	0.4	0.2–0.7	0.2	0.1–0.5
Region				
Northeast	0.4	0.2–0.6	0.1	0.0–0.2
North central	0.3	0.2–0.6	0.1	0.0–0.2
South	0.7	0.5–1.1	0.2	0.1–0.5
West	0.5	0.3–1.0	0.1	0.1–0.3
Total	0.5	0.4–0.7	0.2	0.1–0.3

Abbreviation: CI, confidence interval.
Note: From the National Household Survey on Drug Abuse, 1991.
† Lifetime use, female subjects significantly different than male subjects.
(Courtesy of Yesalis CE, Kennedy NJ, Kopstein AN, et al: JAMA 270:1217-1221, 1993.)

Results.—According to the NHSDA data, the estimated number of current or former AAS abusers in this country is more than 1 million. Slightly more than half of the lifetime abuser population was aged 26 years or older. In the year before the survey more than 300,000 individuals had taken AASs, with 18 years as the median age of initiation. Abuse by age group is shown in the table. Male subjects had higher levels of AAS abuse during their lifetime (.9%) than female subjects (.1%). Male subjects who had ever taken AASs were 2-3 times more likely to report current or recent abuse of other illicit drugs. There were associations between the abuse of AASs and the use of alcohol and cigarettes for some age groups. In the group aged 12-17 years, more than 80% of AAS abusers reported that they had acted in an aggressive way against people or had committed a crime against property in the past year. This association with aggressive behavior was strong for other age groups as well.

Conclusion.—Men, women, and teenagers from various racial groups and in various regions of the United States abuse AASs. It is likely that the survey underreported the actual abuse of such illicit drugs. These findings should enhance the ability to profile the typical AAS abuser.

► Some surveys have reported improbably high levels for the abuse of various substances, and it is easy to see that bravado, illiteracy, and careless completion of questionnaires by 1% to 2% of respondents could translate into an apparent 1% rate of drug abuse. Against such an explanation of the present data are the associations between abuse of anabolic steroids and the abuse of other drugs, and the apparent impact of reported steroid abuse on aggressive behavior. Assuming that the participants responded accurately to the questionnaire, the findings are a sad commentary on the current norms of North American society.—R.J. Shephard, M.D., Ph.D.

Potential Use of Ketoconazole in a Dynamic Endocrine Test to Differentiate Between Biological Outliers and Testosterone Use by Athletes

Kicman AT, Oftebro H, Walker C, Norman N, Cowan DA (King's College London; Norwegian Inst for Sports Medicine Ltd, Oslo; Hormone Lab, Oslo, Norway)

Clin Chem 39:1798–1803, 1993   139-94-8–25

Background.—In athletes, determination of the ratio of testosterone to urinary epitestosterone (T/E) is used to detect testosterone administration. Ratios above 6 are considered as evidence of an offense. The ability of ketoconazole (which inhibits testosterone biosynthesis) to differentiate between those using testosterone and those who naturally produce ratios above 6 was investigated.

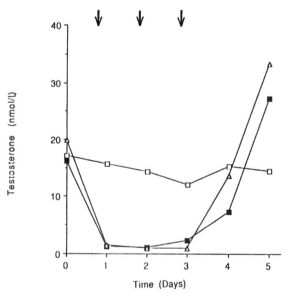

Fig 8–10.—Effect of repeated administration (*arrows*) of ketoconazole (400 mg orally) on serum concentrations of testosterone in the athlete investigated (*open triangle*); the control (*filled square*); and the same control after testosterone heptanoate administration (250 mg intramuscularly) on day −7 (*open square*). (Courtesy of Kicman AT, Oftebro H, Walker C, et al: *Clin Chem* 39:1798–1803, 1993.)

Methods.—Three experiments were performed. In the first, the effects of repeated ketoconazole administration (given orally at 400 mg for 3 days) were evaluated using an athlete with an above normal T/E ratio and a normal adult control. Urine and serum samples were collected daily. The same effects were evaluated 9 months later on the control participant 7 days after the administration of testosterone. The second experiment evaluated the effects of repeated ketoconazole with human chorionic gonadotropin (hCG) administration on the urinary excretion rates of testosterone and epitestosterone in 2 normal men. Ketoconazole was given twice daily at 300 mg for 6 days. On day 2, a single intramuscular dose of 5,000 IU of hCG was administered to both men. Two pooled urine samples were collected from each participant on days 2 through 10. Experiment 3 determined the effect of ketoconazole administration on the urinary ratios in 6 normal participants. A single dose of 400 mg of ketoconazole was given orally. Urine samples were collected before this dose was given and between 0 and 4, 4 and 6, and 8 hours afterward.

Results.—In the first experiment, the serum concentration of total testosterone decreased to very low values in both the athlete and control after administration of ketoconazole (Fig 8–10). In addition, pronounced decreases in the urinary T/E ratios for the athlete and control were noted during ketoconazole administration. Conversely, after testosterone administration, the augmented T/E ratio noted in the control was further increased after ketoconazole was given. In experiment 2, repeated ketoconazole administration resulted in a decrease in the ratio, attributable to a large reduction in the urinary excretion rate of testosterone relative to epitestosterone. Those differences in excretion rates were exacerbated by stimulation with hCG. The third experiment showed that a single administration of ketoconazole to 6 normal participants significantly decreased T/E ratios within 8 hours, this being considered an appropriate time scale for a dynamic test.

Conclusion.—Ketoconazole leads to differential suppression in the urinary excretion rates of testosterone and epitestosterone. The different responses noted suggest that ketoconazole has the ability to distinguish between athletes with naturally large T/E ratios and those who have large ratios caused by testosterone administration. Investigations are now underway to develop the ketoconazole test.

▶ Doping controls are now so efficient that dishonest athletes have switched from synthetic anabolic compounds to naturally occurring testosterone, or substances such as growth hormone that stimulate endogenous testosterone production. Detection of the first (but not the second) type of abuse can be achieved by measuring urinary T/E ratios. Normal males produce 30 times as much testosterone as its inactive epimer, epitestosterone, but excrete 1% of testosterone and 30% of epitestosterone, so that the urinary ratio should be close to 1.0. There is inevitably some dispersion about this mean value, but the International Olympics Committee adopted the generous ceiling ratio of 6.0 in 1983. Some athletes have claimed that they had ratios in the range 6–9 without abuse of steroids (1), and one tactic for further checks has been the calculation of testosterone/luteinizing hormone ratios (2).

Kieman and associates offer another tactic, use of the licensed antifungal agent, ketoconazole, which has the side effect of inhibiting natural testosterone production. If the athlete is innocent, ratios are normalized by ketoconazole administration; if there is exogenous administration of testosterone, the T/E ratio is further increased. The disadvantage of using this test is that the drug has some other side effects, including a transient depression of glucocorticoid and mineralocorticoid synthesis, and (when given with antihistamines) it may induce cardiac arrhythmias. If an athlete has a suspiciously high T/E ratio, other options are to monitor the athlete frequently to see whether this persists or to estimate the testosterone/luteinizing hormone ratio.—R.J. Shephard, M.D., Ph.D.

References

1. Catlin DH, Hatton CK: *Adv Intern Med* 36:399, 1991.
2. Kieman AT, Cowan DA. *Br Med Bull* 48:496, 1992.

Effect of Growth Hormone Treatment on Hormonal Parameters, Body Composition and Strength in Athletes
Deyssig R, Frisch H, Blum WF, Waldhör T (Univ of Vienna; Univ of Tübingen, Germany)
Acta Endocrinol 128:313–318, 1993   139-94-8-26

Purpose.—Growth hormone (GH) is used illegally by bodybuilders and other athletes for its anabolic and lipolytic effects. However, scientific evidence of improved athletic performance after GH administration is not available. The effects of recombinant human GH (r-hGH) administration on physical and endocrine parameters were examined in highly trained male athletes in a double-blind, placebo-controlled study.

Methods.—Twenty-two power athletes, aged 20–28 years, who had engaged in regular weight training for at least 6 months were enrolled in the 6-week study. All athletes were monitored throughout the study for concurrent anabolic steroid abuse. Eleven men were randomly assigned to daily self-administered GH injections and 11 men received vials containing vehicle only. Evaluations were carried out at baseline and at 2-week intervals.

Results.—Three men in the GH-treated group and 1 man in the placebo group did not complete the study. All 18 evaluable athletes had normal baseline serum GH levels, but at 2, 4, and 6 weeks the mean serum GH levels in the GH-treated men were significantly higher than those in placebo-treated controls. Growth hormone therapy did not significantly increase maximal strength during concentric contractions of

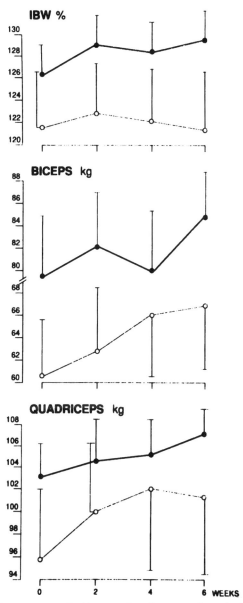

Fig 8–11.—Ideal body weight, strength of biceps and quadriceps muscles in the GH-treated (*shaded circle*) and placebo-treated (*open circle*) athletes before GH therapy and after 2, 4, and 6 weeks (mean ± standard error of the mean). (Courtesy of Deyssig R, Frisch H, Blum WF, et al: *Acta Endocrinol* 128:313–318, 1993.)

the biceps brachii and quadriceps femoris muscles at 2, 4, and 6 weeks (Fig 8–11).

Conclusion.—Growth hormone therapy in highly trained power athletes does not produce significant further increases in lean body mass, muscle size, and muscle strength.

▶ Exercise scientists currently seem to be trying to prevent the abuse of human GH preparations by the same tactic that they adopted with anabolic steroids for many years, claiming that such substances confer no benefit on well-trained athletes. Unfortunately, as in many areas of medicine, the customer knows best! The probable reason that laboratory experiments fail to show an increase of performance when abusers know that such a benefit can be obtained is that much smaller doses are used for much shorter periods in the laboratory than in backstreet administration. Ethical constraints preclude experimental trial of the drug schedules that abusers are prepared to accept in the hope of winning sponsorships in the $10–100 million range.—R.J. Shephard, M.D., Ph.D.

Short-Term Growth Hormone Treatment Does Not Increase Muscle Protein Synthesis in Experienced Weight Lifters
Yarasheski KE, Zachwieja JJ, Angelopoulos TJ, Bier DM (Washington Univ, St Louis, Mo)
J Appl Physiol 74:3073–3076, 1993   139-94-8-27

Objective.—Researchers sought to determine whether short-term administration of growth hormone (GH) to experienced weight lifters would increase the rate of muscle protein synthesis or reduce the rate of whole-body protein breakdown. Such metabolic alterations are necessary to promote muscle protein anabolism.

Methods.—The study participants were 7 healthy young men with a mean age of 23 years. Their typical weight training routines consisted of high-intensity (75% to 90% maximum strength), low-repetition (5–10 lifts) progressive-resistance exercise. All subjects had followed such a program 3-6 days per week for the previous 3 years and maintained this training during the study. The fractional rate of skeletal muscle protein synthesis and the whole-body rate of protein breakdown were determined during a constant IV infusion of $[1\text{-}^{13}C]$leucine or $[1,2\text{-}^{13}C_2]$leucine before and at the end of 14 days of subcutaneous GH administration.

Results.—In these subjects, administration of GH significantly increased fasting serum insulin-like growth factor-I from a mean of 224 ng/mL to 589 ng/mL. The fractional rate of muscle protein synthesis was not increased, however, nor was the rate of whole-body protein breakdown reduced.

Conclusion.—These findings suggest that GH supplementation does not enhance the rate of muscle protein synthesis in experienced weight lifters. Similar findings were reached in a previous study of healthy, sedentary young men who started a 12-week muscle-building exercise program. Thus, 2 weeks of recombinant human GH administration do not enhance conditions that would favor muscle protein accumulation and increase muscle mass.

▶ There are increasingly frequent reports of the abuse of recombinant GH by athletes, and it would be helpful if sports physicians could state categorically that such treatment had no impact on muscle hypertrophy. However, there is an understandable reluctance to make such an incontrovertible statement, given the erroneous early position statement of the American College of Sports Medicine with respect to the use of anabolic steroids (1).

The present study, with its radiocarbon measurements of protein synthesis, goes some way toward providing evidence of the lack of efficacy of recombinant GH preparations. It appears (although is not explicitly stated) that the participants in these experiments were receiving an adequate protein intake (at least 1.5 g/kg per day). However, studies of leucine incorporation were made after an overnight fast, and the subjects were weight lifters who had already reached a plateau of muscle mass. Further, the GH was only administered for 2 weeks, and the dose that was used may have been much less than in some situations in which the product is abused. More data are needed before we can state categorically that GH will not enhance muscle development.—R.J. Shephard, M.D., Ph.D.

Reference

1. American College of Sports Medicine: *Med Sci Sports Exerc* 9:xi, 1977.

9 Cardiorespiratory Fitness, Exercise Testing and Training, and Environmental Medicine

Preferred and Energetically Optimal Gait Transition Speeds in Human Locomotion
Hreljac A (Arizona State Univ, Tempe)
Med Sci Sports Exerc 25:1158–1162, 1993   139-94-9-1

Introduction.—Most previous studies of human locomotion have assumed that gait transition occurs at speeds that minimize metabolic energy consumption. The preferred transition speed (PTS) has been approximated at about 2.5 m/s^{-1}. Whether changing gaits is really an energy-saving mechanism was determined.

Methods.—The subjects were 20 healthy young adults, 10 men and 10 women. All subjects walked on a treadmill at 5 speeds ranging from 70% to 110% of their individually measured PTS and ran at 5 speeds ranging from 70% to 110% of their PTS. Aerobic capacity was monitored throughout this exercise to determine each subject's energetically optimal transition speed (EOTS). The subjects also completed a Rating of Perceived Exertion (RPE) to determine whether their sense of effort was greater for walking or running at the PTS.

Results.—There were no significant differences by sex. The mean PTS was 2.06 m/s^{-1}, which was significantly lower than the mean EOTS of 2.24 m/s^{-1}. Only 1 subject had a slightly greater value for PTS than EOTS. The subjects' RPEs were significantly higher while walking than running at the PTS.

Conclusion.—In contrast to previous assumptions, these data suggest that gait transition during human locomotion does not occur as a means of minimizing metabolic energy consumption. The energetic cost of locomotion does not appear to be a major influence on the speed of the gait transition. In human beings as well as in animals, the energetic cost of running appears to be independent of speed.

▶ It is not intuitively clear to me why the energetic cost–speed curves for walking are so different from the curves for running, but I'll have to trust the research. It is also difficult to understand why the perceived rate of exertion should be higher for walking than for running at the same speed when we know that less energy is actually being used when walking. Hopefully, this laboratory will follow up on its stated intent to consider other factors (e.g., anthropometric, kinematic, and kinetic variables) as possible determinants of gait transition during human locomotion.—Col. J.L. Anderson, PE.D.

A Standard Measure for Exercise Prescription for Aqua Running
Wilder RP, Brennan D, Schotte DE (Baylor College of Medicine, Houston; Houston Internatl Running Ctr)
Am J Sports Med 21:45–48, 1993   139-94-9-2

Background.—Aqua running recently has been advocated as a suitable form of cardiovascular conditioning for the injured athlete and for those who want a low-impact aerobic workout. It consists of simulated running in the deep end of a pool aided by a flotation device that holds the head above water. Until now, no specific measure has been identified for aqua running. To evaluate the usefulness of cadence as a measure for exercise prescription for aqua running, the relationship between cadence and heart rate was investigated.

Method.—Twenty healthy subjects (10 men and 10 women) underwent a graded exercise test of aqua running. The participants were tethered to the pool ladder by an elastic cord, and a T-bar was designed to provide a target to be approached by the flexed knee with each stride. The target discouraged the subjects from shortening their range of motion as cadence increased. Cadence was controlled by use of a metronome. Running began at an initial rate of 48 cycles/min, each cycle consisting of 1 complete cadence cycle with the right knee reaching the target level with each beat of the metronome. Subjects exercised at a rate of 48 cycles/min for a total of 4 minutes; subsequent 2-minute stages followed in succession. Cadence was raised to 66 cycles/min in the second stage, and then to 3–4 cycles/min for each of eleven 2-minute stages up to a maximum of 104 cycles/min. Heart rate during warm-up, exercise, and warm-down was recorded at 15-second intervals.

Results.—The results indicated that cadence and heart rate were highly correlated, both on a group and an individual level.

Conclusion.—Cadence can be used as a quantitative measure for exercise prescription for aqua running. Individuals using aqua running can benefit from periodic graded exercise testing to establish heart rate responses at different levels of cadence. Such information can then be used in exercise prescription.

▶ It is important to point out that conventional methods for exercise prescription, such as heart rate or ratings of perceived exertion, may need to be modified for use in aqua running. As the authors point out, cadence "appears to be an appropriate standard measure for exercise prescription for aqua running."—J.S. Torg, M.D.

Life Style Exercise: A New Strategy to Promote Physical Activity for Adults
Gordon NF, Kohl HW III, Blair SN (Cooper Inst for Aerobics Research, Dallas)
J Cardiopulmon Rehabil 13:161–163, 1993   139-94-9-3

Background.—The exercise stimuli required to improve maximum oxygen intake, the most widely accepted index of cardiorespiratory fitness, have been reasonably well documented. Guidelines for exercise that promotes cardiorespiratory fitness have been based on existing research in this area. However, changes in clinical status do not necessarily parallel increases in maximum oxygen intake. Recent studies have suggested that regular participation in light to moderate exercise, which probably does not have a profound effect on maximum oxygen intake, helps prevent coronary heart disease (CHD) and that more strenuous exercise may not provide markedly greater protection. With this knowledge, many individuals who dislike strenuous exercise may be encouraged to engage in some form of physical activity, with the assurance that they are benefiting from less strenuous exercise.

Promoting Physical Activity in Adults.—In one approach, the focus can be on attaining the desired weekly energy expenditure in patients' exercise programs rather than on the intensity of the exercise. Weekly energy expenditure should be about 2.9–8.4 megajoules (700 to 2,000 calories), according to the American Heart Association. Another approach is to reach a middle ground, encouraging people to attain their weekly energy expenditure while exercising at intensities just above the minimal threshold needed to raise maximum oxygen intake significantly. Patients with documented CHD or other cardiac disorders should be strongly discouraged from exercising at intensities eliciting undesirable cardiovascular responses. Some patients not only dislike strenuous exercise; they dislike any formal exercise at all. In lifestyle approaches to exercising, individuals are taught to integrate multiple short bouts of physical activity into the course of their daily lives. However, the lifestyle approach is not a replacement for more traditional methods of exercise prescription. The approach to prescribing exercise ultimately should be based on medical, logistic, financial, personal preference, and staff availability factors.

Conclusion.—Although various approaches to promoting physical activity for adults have been described, it is clear that exercise scientists and clinicians need to develop further strategies to encourage adults to increase and maintain their physical activity level. Lifestyle exercise is one approach that may be especially useful for sedentary individuals who are not ready for formal exercise training programs.

▶ The recent trend has been away from the advocacy of intensive exercise for the average patient. Cynics have suggested that one reason for this shift of opinion has been a failure of government agencies and sports physicians to achieve the fitness targets that they set for themselves a decade or more ago. However, there are more substantial and scientific reasons for such a change. Modern psychological theory suggests the advantages of slowly shaping behavior rather than attempting a sudden change of personal habits, and the body is also less likely to have an unfavorable reaction to the gradual introduction of a more active lifestyle.

Moreover, a reanalysis of older data plus new findings from several large-scale surveys (1–3), but with one important exception from Britain (4), support the viewpoint that moderate levels of activity, insufficient to change aerobic power, may have appreciable health advantages. Indeed, gains from more intensive effort seem little greater.

One other aspect of the present paper that I liked was its emphasis on everyday activities. Unfortunately, entrepreneurs have made exercise a high-tech process, with an imposed need to purchase vast quantities of clothing and equipment and to drive long distances to exotic fitness centers. However, the same quantity of exercise can be incorporated into such components of daily living as walking, cycling, and a reduced use of power equipment at a much lower cost in time, facilities, and equipment.—R.J. Shephard, M.D., Ph.D.

References

1. Bouchard C, et al: *Physical Activity, Fitness and Health.* Champaign, IL: Human Kinetics, 1994.
2. Leon A, et al: *JAMA* 258:2388, 1987.
3. Magnus K, et al: *Am J Epidemiol* 110:724, 1979.
4. Morris JN, et al: *Br Heart J* 63:325, 1990.

Participation in Community Sports Centres: Motives and Predictors of Enjoyment
Ashford B, Biddle S, Goudas M (Staffordshire Univ, Stoke-on-Trent, England; Univ of Exeter, England)
J Sports Sci 11:249–256, 1993   139-94-9-4

Background.—Promotion of exercise in the community setting requires information on people's motives for taking part in sports and physical recreation activity. Most of the research on this issue has con-

Mean (± 1 SD) Ratings of Participation Motives by Total Sample, Gender, and Age Groups

			Gender		Age		
		Total (n=336)	Males (n=243)	Females (n=93)	16–24 years (n=165)	25–44 years (n=148)	45 years + (n=23)
	n	$\bar{x}\pm$ s.d.	$\bar{x}\pm$ s.d.	$\bar{x}\pm$ s.d.	$\bar{x}\pm$ s.d.	$\bar{x}\pm$ s.d.	$\bar{x}\pm$ s.d.
Health	334	4.41 ± 0.82	4.45 ± 0.78	4.31 ± 1.00	4.30 ± 0.89	4.54 ± 0.72	4.46 ± 0.78
Fitness	329	4.20 ± 0.91	4.28 ± 0.83	3.93 ± 1.16	4.22 ± 0.90	4.19 ± 0.93	4.08 ± 0.95
Relaxation	329	4.15 ± 0.94	4.11 ± 0.93	4.21 ± 0.99	3.95 ± 1.03	4.32 ± 0.79	4.46 ± 0.52
Aesthetic	329	4.05 ± 0.90	4.02 ± 0.90	4.07 ± 0.94	3.93 ± 0.96	4.14 ± 0.84	4.23 ± 0.60
Skills	328	3.92 ± 1.05	3.98 ± 1.07	3.69 ± 0.96	3.94 ± 1.00	3.88 ± 1.08	4.15 ± 1.14
Affiliation	331	3.86 ± 1.20	3.88 ± 1.17	3.72 ± 1.31	3.77 ± 1.26	3.88 ± 1.16	4.38 ± 1.12
Environmental	329	3.49 ± 1.18	3.44 ± 1.19	3.59 ± 1.18	3.48 ± 1.15	3.51 ± 1.20	3.31 ± 1.18
Eustress	327	3.47 ± 1.26	3.58 ± 1.24	3.18 ± 1.23	3.50 ± 1.23	3.42 ± 1.28	3.38 ± 1.56
Excellence	327	3.41 ± 1.23	3.60 ± 1.15	2.81 ± 1.15	3.50 ± 1.17	3.29 ± 1.29	3.31 ± 1.32
Competition	327	3.39 ± 1.47	3.65 ± 1.36	2.49 ± 1.42	3.44 ± 1.43	3.25 ± 1.52	4.00 ± 1.22
Self-learning	328	3.20 ± 1.31	3.28 ± 1.28	2.93 ± 1.35	3.12 ± 1.30	3.30 ± 1.34	3.38 ± 1.12
Achievement	323	3.15 ± 1.32	3.27 ± 1.28	2.76 ± 1.38	3.23 ± 1.30	3.00 ± 1.35	3.31 ± 1.44
Independence	326	3.15 ± 1.30	3.12 ± 1.31	3.09 ± 1.29	3.21 ± 1.27	3.06 ± 1.33	3.15 ± 1.41
Power	327	2.42 ± 1.25	2.44 ± 1.24	2.26 ± 1.26	2.45 ± 1.17	2.33 ± 1.32	2.54 ± 1.45
Aggression	326	2.15 ± 1.26	2.28 ± 1.30	1.74 ± 0.98	2.22 ± 1.26	2.08 ± 1.28	1.61 ± 0.87

Note: Sample sizes vary according to completed data and missing classifications of some subjects. Scores range from 1 to 5.
(Courtesy of Ashford B, Biddle S, Goudas M: *J Sports Sci* 11:249–256, 1993.)

cerned North American children participating in competitive sports programs. The reasons for participation in community sports centers by British adults were thus explored.

Methods and Results.—A total of 336 participants at 6 community sports centers completed a 5-minute questionnaire-interview. Presented with 15 reasons for participating in sports, the subjects were asked to indicate their level of agreement or disagreement with each on a 5-point Likert-type scale. The 3 most highly rated motives were health maintenance, physical fitness, and relaxation. On factor analysis, 4 clear factors emerged: assertive achievement, physical well-being, sociopsychological well-being, and sport mastery and performance. Assertive achievement and sport mastery and performance were more important motivators for men than for women, and sociopsychological well-being was more important for older than for younger subjects. The best predictors of sport enjoyment were sociopsychological well-being, sport mastery and performance, and sport importance, yet even these factors accounted for only 14% of the variance in enjoyment scores.

Conclusion.—Adults participating in sports are more likely to do so for reasons of health, fitness, and general well-being than for achievement or assertive sports behavior. The latter factors are more important for men than for women, although the 2 sexes are equally motivated by the well-being factor. Sports enjoyment appears to vary with sport, location, sociodemographic group, age group, and culture (table).

▶ Although the avowed objective of this study was to see whether motives for participation in community sports were similar in England and North America, the instrument used to assess motives unfortunately has not been used in North America. The subjects were asked to respond to 15 questions, 7 of which had similarities to an instrument previously developed by Kenyon (1) and Alderman and Wood (2). As in North America, maintenance of health and fitness and relaxation were dominant motivators (3).

Given the limited attendance at community exercise facilities on both sides of the Atlantic, future studies could focus on why nonparticipants do not find these particular benefits of community fitness programs rewarding. Another gap in the present research project was the exploration of opportunity cost. This seems to be a major barrier for nonparticipants, but in participants, enjoyment is presumably sufficient to neutralize the cost incurred by travel and exercise class involvement.—R.J. Shephard, M.D., Ph.D.

References

1. Kenyon GS: *Res Q Exerc Sport* 39:566, 1968.
2. Alderman RB, Wood NL: *Can J Appl Sport Sci* 1:169, 1976.
3. Sidney KH, Shephard RJ: *Med Sci Sports* 8:246, 1977.

Minority Patients: Clinical Strategies to Promote Exercise
White J (Assistant Editor, The Physician and Sportsmedicine)
Physician Sportsmed 21:136–144, 1993   139-94-9-5

Introduction.—The health status of minority groups in the United States is known to trail that of the white majority. Many of the conditions that are more prevalent in minority groups (e.g., obesity, hypertension, and diabetes) could be prevented through compliance with certain health measures. Some of the strategies available to physicians for promoting healthy lifestyle choices to minority patients were examined.

Cultural Perspectives.—Physicians need to be aware of their minority patients' attitudes about exercise and physical activity. Not every culture shares the same concept of exercise as a sought-after leisure activity or the value of competitive play and sports. Minority patients with low incomes may view exercise as too expensive. And patients without a clear understanding of physiology may not understand the relationship between exercise and health. Some minority patients do not feel free to ask questions, and some physicians may mistake differences in personal interaction as lack of attention or noncompliance.

Recommendations.—Physicians who recognize the traits of a particular culture can use its existing strengths to increase patient compliance. There are several national organizations that promote improved health status for minority groups, including Native Americans, Hispanics, Asian-Americans, and blacks. The article gives the addresses of these organizations and summarizes their resources.

Conclusion.—Members of minority groups in the United States have a high rate of health problems that might be prevented by exercise and dietary choices. Because of differing communication styles and health care beliefs, physicians need to approach these patients differently than they approach white patients. Exercise should be promoted in a specific, individualized way, with the benefits of such a program clearly presented.

▶ Refugees, both economic and political, are changing the population characteristics and the culture of developed societies such as Canada and the United States. Long-term solutions to the health needs of new immigrants will be found as members of those populations join health care teams and/or become assimilated into the dominant culture. However, in the interim, this article provides some useful tips on how to deal more effectively and sensitively with the needs of minority groups.—R.J. Shephard, M.D., Ph.D.

Relation Between Exercise and Absenteeism Due to Illness and Injury in Manufacturing Companies in Japan
Muto T, Sakurai H (Keio Univ, Tokyo)
J Occup Med 35:995–999, 1993   139-94-9-6

Incidence, Cases of Absence, and Days of Absence (Per 100 Employees and Per Absent
Employee) Resulting From Illness and Injury Per Year by Exercise Group

Diagnostic Group/ Exercise Group	Incidence of Absence (%)	Cases of Absence per 100 Employees	Days of Absence per 100 Employees	Days of Absence per Absent Employee
Cardiovascular				
Nonexercisers	0.6*	0.6	15	23.4
Exercisers I	0.2	0.2	3	13.1
Exercisers II	0.5	0.5	8	16.6
Exercisers III	0.6	0.6	18	26.7
Respiratory				
Nonexercisers	10.7*	13.3	25	2.3
Exercisers I	10.8	13.2	22	2.0
Exercisers II	11.2	13.7	25	2.2
Exercisers III	9.3	11.5	21	2.3
Digestive				
Nonexercisers	2.3†	2.5	41	16.4
Exercisers I	1.7	1.9	21‡	11.2
Exercisers II	1.5	1.6	14‡	9.1‡
Exercisers III	1.6	1.8	21‡	11.9
Musculoskeletal				
Nonexercisers	2.2†	2.5	24	10.6
Exercisers I	1.5	1.7	11‡	7.2
Exercisers II	1.4	1.5	8	5.7
Exercisers III	1.7	1.8	11	6.2
Accidents/poisoning				
Nonexercisers	0.9	0.9	20	20.7
Exercisers I	0.8	0.8	9	11.0
Exercisers II	0.9	0.9	13	14.0
Exercisers III	1.3	1.4	24	17.6
All causes				
Nonexercisers	17.5*	24.2	159	8.9
Exercisers I	16.3	21.9	83‡	5.1‡
Exercisers II	16.4	21.9	90‡	5.4‡
Exercisers III	15.7	20.9	118	7.3

* $P < .05$.
† $P < .01$, χ^2 test.
‡ $P < .05$, compared with nonexercisers by analysis of covariance.
Courtesy of Muto T, Sakurai H: *J Occup Med* 35:995-999, 1993.)

Background.—Studies for North America have reported an encouraging relationship between participation in work-site exercise programs and work attendance. Such relationships were explored in a Japanese industry.

Methods.—Data on exercise and absenteeism resulting from illness and injury were obtained from 21,924 male workers. The study participants who exercised were divided into 3 groups: group 1 consisted of men exercising less than once per week; group 2, once or twice per week; and group 3, more than 3 times per week. These groups were compared with men who did not exercise.

Findings.—All exercisers had a significantly lower incidence of absence than nonexercisers. Absentee rates in groups 1, 2, and 3 were 10%, 10%, and 14% lower, respectively, than that of nonexercisers. The number of days absent in the 3 groups were 48%, 43%, and 26% lower, respectively, than among men who did not exercise. After confounding variables were controlled for in a logistic analysis, the exercisers in all 3 groups still had a significantly decreased relative risk of absence compared with nonexercisers. These risks were .88, .90 and .87, respectively (table).

Conclusion.—In this study, worker exercise was associated with a reduction in absences because of illness and injury. Exercisers had .5–.8 days fewer absences per worker-year than nonexercisers.

▶ North American studies have consistently shown that the introduction of employee fitness programs is associated with a reduction in employee absenteeism (1), although it is less clearly demonstrated that enhanced fitness is the cause of this change. Any beneficial effect is quite small (a one half to one day reduction of absences), but given the cost and inefficiency of replacement workers, even a small change could have a substantial impact on productivity. Conditions of employment are very different in Japan, and it is thus interesting to find a somewhat similar apparent impact of self-determined exercise behavior on work attendance in the Orient. Interpretation must be cautious because the study was limited to reported absences; absences of less than 1 day (which can do much to disrupt production) were excluded from the analysis.—R.J. Shephard, M.D., Ph.D.

Reference

1. Shephard RJ: *Med Sci Sports Exerc* 24:354, 1992.

Work-Site Physical Fitness Programs: Comparing the Impact of Different Program Designs on Cardiovascular Risks
Heirich MA, Foote A, Erfurt JC, Konopka B (Univ of Michigan, Ann Arbor)
J Occup Med 35:510–517, 1993   139-94-9–7

Objective.—More and more employers are considering the establishment of exercise and physical fitness programs for their employees. Although the benefits of exercise and physical fitness are well established, there are few data on how to achieve lasting increases in the level of exercise for the greatest percentage of employees. Three different types of work-site physical fitness programs were compared for their effects on cardiovascular risk reduction.

Three-Year Results for Employees at Risk of Cardiovascular Disease in 4 Auto Plants, 1985–1988

	Site A Control	Results for Employees with Cardiovascular Risks		
		Site B Fitness Facility	Site C Outreach and Counseling	Site D Outreach, Counseling, Plant Organization
Blood pressure results				
Number of hypertensives at screening	102	68	88	71
Percent with their blood pressure under control ‡				
1985	27%	32%	25%	25%
1988*	26%	29%	43%	47%
Weight loss results				
Number overweight at screening §	194	173	150	173
Mean change in weight*	+0.6	+3.1 †	−1.2	−4.7 †
Percent who lost 10 lb or more, 1985–1988	19%	17%	26%	28%
Percent who lost 3 lb or more, 1985–1988*	35%	29%	45%	51%
Smoking cessation results				
Number of smokers and ex-smokers at screening	366	362	362	289
Percent not smoking in 1988*	45.6%	43.9%	52.8%	56.6%

* P < .01 based on analysis of variance.
† P < .01 based on paired Student's t-test.
‡ Blood pressure readings below 140/90.
§ Employees who were 20% overweight or more in 1985.
(Courtesy of Heirich MA, Foote A, Erfurt JC, et al J Occup Med 35:510–517, 1993.)

Methods.—Four plants were randomized to 1 of 4 types of wellness programs. One plant established a staffed physical fitness facility, with a full set of aerobic and muscle-building equipment and certified athletic trainers on staff; another offered direct outreach and one-to-one counseling for employees identified as having cardiovascular risk factors; and another combined one-to-one counseling with work-site organization to encourage peer support and mutual exercise activity, with simple facilities and limited equipment. The fourth plant, with no exercise program, served as a control. Outcomes were assessed from employee health screenings before and 3 years after establishment of the exercise programs and employee reports of participation in the programs.

Results.—Employee participation was lowest at the plant with the extensive exercise equipment, even lower than at the control plant. Those 2 facilities were comparable in terms of cardiovascular risk at follow-up. In contrast, about 45% of employees reported exercising at least 3 times per week at both plants that offered an outreach program. Those programs were also more effective in promoting exercise and reducing risk among employees with cardiovascular risk factors (table).

Conclusion.—Workplace exercise programs with systematic, ongoing outreach to encourage participation appear to be more effective than fitness facilities without outreach. An effective exercise program can be established without the need for expensive fitness facilities. The combination of counseling with peer support and simple exercise activities appears to yield even better results.

▶ I vividly remember being taken to the "best" work-site fitness program in Holland 3 years ago. The company had over 2,000 employees, and a beautiful gymnasium was jam-packed with the latest exercise equipment. When I arrived at around 11 A.M., there were 3 clients. My host explained that the facility became crammed with eager exercisers at lunchtime. I insisted on waiting to see the extent of this cramming, and found attendance rising slowly to the low 20s, including several instructors! This anecdote illustrates the problem of ascertaining program effectiveness—the jobs of those who provide the statistics on attendance at exercise classes are often threatened by the reality of poor recruitment and compliance.

This article by Heirich and associates faces the unfortunate reality of the current situation very honestly—participation is often only 1% to 7% of the labor force, and many of this small minority would exercise somewhere else if the work-site facility were not available. Heirich et al. provide a nice comparison of the health impact between a work site with a well-equipped and staffed gymnasium that waited for clients to appear and a second work site that had an outreach and counseling program that actively recruited employees but had invested little in facilities or gymnasium staff. The latter approach was substantially more effective in reducing body weight, controlling blood pressure, and ensuring smoking cessation among employees.

Further, although the arrangements for exercise were simple at the second work site, many more of the workers chose to adopt an effective amount of physical activity. For those who wish to enhance physical activity, whether in industry or in the community, it seems that a low-tech approach with effective leadership is much more cost-effective than is investment in expensive facilities.—R.J. Shephard, M.D., Ph.D.

Influence of Nasal Airflow and Resistance on Nasal Dilator Muscle Activities During Exercise

Connel DC, Fregosi RF (Univ of Arizona, Tucson)
J Appl Physiol 74:2529–2536, 1993   139-94-9-8

Background.—The alae nasi (AN), or nasal dilator muscles, are accorded a key role in regulating nasal airway resistance, but their neural control is incompletely understood. There are indications that AN muscle activity correlates closely with nasal minute ventilation during exercise, but increasing nasal airflow is accompanied by increased flow turbulence and swings in intranasal pressure, so that the latter may also play a regulatory role.

Objective and Methods.—The effects of nasal airflow and resistance on AN muscle activity at rest and on exercise were separately examined in 10 healthy subjects, 7 men and 3 women aged 23–60 years. Nasal airflow and the AN electromyogram were recorded at rest and during progressive-intensity exercise at levels of 60, 120, and 150–180 W.

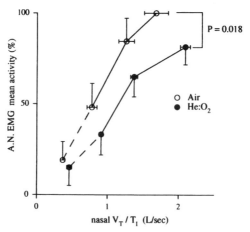

Fig 9–1.—Changes in integrated AN electromyogram (EMG) (mean activity) as function of mean rate of inspiratory nasal airflow (nasal V_T/T_I) in 10 patients breathing air or HE-O_2. Each point represents mean $\pm$ standard error at rest (*point to left of dashed line*) or during exercise at 60, 120, and 150–180 W. Electromyogram data are expressed as percentage of maximal activity that occurred during exercise at highest work rate performed by each subject while breathing air. Nasal V_T/T_I was also maximal at highest work rate, thus, these 2 variables were highly correlated. *Brackets* indicate significant difference between slopes of 2 lines. (Courtesy of Connel DC, Fregosi RF: *J Appl Physiol* 74:2529–2536, 1993.)

Observations.—The AN electromyogram increased significantly as a function of increasing nasal airflow during progressively more intense exercise (Fig 9–1). A similar effect was noted whether subjects breathed air or a mixture of 79% helium and 21% oxygen, although the slope of the relationship was less with the helium/oxygen mixture. Reciprocal changes in nasal airflow and resistance were observed when the helium/oxygen mixture was substituted for air at rest and during exercise. The change to helium breathing decreased airway resistance by about 30% at rest and by 40% to 60% on exercise, as measured by anterior rhinomanometry. Inhaling the helium/oxygen mixture decreased the AN electromyogram by as much as 50% during exercise.

Implications.—Changes in AN muscle activity during exercise are not a simple function of the rate of nasal airflow. It appears that activation of these muscles can lower nasal flow resistance and may prevent collapse of the nasal passages during exercise and other hyperpneic conditions. The findings are in accord with the observation that voluntary "flaring" of the external nares can lower nasal airway resistance by as much as 30%.

▶ Under resting conditions, the nose offers a substantial impedance to respiratory airflow, commonly as much as all of the rest of the respiratory tract. Novelists commonly describe the flaring of the nostrils in animals under the stress of a chase, and it is interesting to see that nasal flaring can allow a substantial reduction of resistance in the nasal air passages in human beings as well. However, exercise-induced catecholamine secretion may also cause a decrease in bronchial resistance, so that the nares remain a high-resistance segment of the airway even during exercise. It is not surprising that when ventilation exceeds about 30–35 L/min (3–3.5 times the resting metabolism) the mouth opens (1), and the normal air-conditioning and filtering mechanisms of the nose are bypassed. This increases exposure of the subject's lungs to air pollutants and cold air, and vigorous city exercisers are well-advised to consider alternative methods of warming and filtering inspired air, especially during the winter months.

In this study, the link between airflow and nasal resistance was explored by surreptitiously switching from air to an oxygen/helium mixture. This tactic increased airflow, but decreased resistance, with a parallel decrease in activity of the alar muscles. It seems that the nasal muscles are sensing either resistance or some expression of nasal turbulence.—R.J. Shephard, M.D., Ph.D.

Reference

1. Niinimaa V, et al: *Respir Physiol* 42:61, 1980.

Tilt Table Testing in the Evaluation and Management of Athletes With Recurrent Exercise-Induced Syncope

Grubb BP, Temesy-Armos PN, Samoil D, Wolfe DA, Hahn H, Elliott L (Med College of Ohio, Toledo)

Med Sci Sports Exerc 25:24–28, 1993   139-94-9-9

Introduction.—Recurrent idiopathic exercise-related syncope in young athletes is a common condition that is often difficult to manage and produces anxiety for patients and coaches. One possible common cause of this condition is vasovagally mediated hypotension and bradycardia, which is difficult to prove. The diagnostic usefulness of head-upright tilt table testing was assessed in young athletes with recurrent idiopathic exercise-related syncope.

Methods.—The study sample comprised 12 male and 12 female trained athletes (mean age, 18 years) with a history of recurrent idiopathic syncope during exertion. In the previous 6 months, all patients had had at least 2 episodes of syncope that were unexplained despite thorough examination. Seven patients had injuries during these episodes. Another 10 conditioned athletes with no such history were also studied. All subjects underwent 30 minutes of upright tilt table testing, with or without infusion of isoproterenol, 1–3 μg/min^{-1} intravenously, to produce bradycardia and/or hypotension.

Results.—Ten of the patients had syncope during baseline tilt testing, and another 9 had syncope during isoproterenol infusion. Therefore, the total positive rate in the patient group was 79%. Of the 19 patients with a positive tilt-test result, 17 had negative results on later testing, after drug therapy, usually with flurohydrocortisone, transdermal scopolamine, or β-blockers (table). They were followed up for a mean of 23 months, during which they had no further syncopal episodes. The other 2 patients refused drug therapy and continued to have syncopal episodes.

Conclusion.—Vasovagally mediated hypotension and bradycardia, or neuroregulatory syncope, appears to be a common cause of exercise-induced syncope among young athletes. Head-upright tilt table testing is a useful method of evaluation for these patients, both in making the initial diagnosis and in assessing the effectiveness of prophylactic drug therapy. Further study of this test will not only clarify its clinical role but will also advance our understanding of this frustrating condition.

▶ This research on tilt table testing to evaluate syncope in athletes supports the view that vasovagally mediated hypotension and bradycardia are common and important in exercise-induced syncope. In the tests here, about 80% of the athletes with past syncope had syncope during the head-up tilt (about half during the baseline tilt and half during isoproterenol infusion) at an average of 18 minutes into the test. None of the 10 control athletes had syncope. Others have studied the head-upright tilt and have pointed out the

Results of Head-Upright Tilt Table Testing

Patient	Age (yr)	Sex	Sport	No. of Syncopal Episodes	Tilt Table Phase Causing Syncope	Tilt Time In Phase Causing Syncope (min)	Therapy
1	16	F	Cross-country	4	Baseline	23	Flurohydrocortisone
2	17	F	Cross-country	6	Isoproterenol 1 $\mu g \cdot min^{-1}$	12	Transdermal scopolamine
3	15	F	Basketball	5	Isoproterenol 3 $\mu g \cdot min^{-1}$	21	Flurohydrocortisone
4	19	F	Volleyball	2	Isoproterenol 2 $\mu g \cdot min^{-1}$	17	Beta blocker
5	16	M	Basketball	2	Baseline	18	Beta blocker + flurohydrocortisone
6	20	M	Track	4			Transdermal scopolamine
7	14	M	Soccer	3	Isoproterenol 2 $\mu g \cdot min^{-1}$	7	Flurohydrocortisone
8	19	M	Cross-country	3	Isoproterenol 3 $\mu g \cdot min^{-1}$	16	Beta blocker
9	16	F	Field hockey	4	Isoproterenol 2 $\mu g \cdot min^{-1}$	5	Beta blocker
10	15	M	Ice hockey	2			Transdermal scopolamine
11	22	M	Cross-country	2	Baseline	23	Flurohydrocortisone
12	14	M	Basketball	3	Isoproterenol 2 $\mu g \cdot min^{-1}$	10	Beta blocker
13	19	M	Football	2			Disopyramide
14	15	F	Track	4	Baseline	25	Beta blocker
15	19	F	Volleyball	2			
16	18	M	Swimming	3	Baseline	19	Flurohydrocortisone
17	15	F	Basketball	4	Baseline	8	
18	17	M	Swimming	3	Isoproterenol 1 $\mu g \cdot min^{-1}$	14	
19	15	F	Volleyball	2	Baseline	24	
20	26	M	Cross-country	2	Baseline	22	
21	14	F	Swimming	3	Baseline	12	Beta blocker + flurohydrocortisone
22	20	M	Wrestling	2			
23	23	F	Cross-country	2	Baseline	28	
24	24	F	Cross-country	2	Isoproterenol 1 $\mu g \cdot min^{-1}$	14	Flurohydrocortisone
Mean	18			3.0		17	
SD	3.4			1.1		6.6	

(Courtesy of Grubb BP, Temesy-Armos PN, Samoil D, et al: *Med Sci Sports Exerc* 25:24–28, 1993.)

profound bradycardia, sinus arrests, and orthostatic syncope that can occur in highly trained endurance athletes (1). See also a practical review on how to diagnose and manage the causes of syncope in athletes (2). Some physicians recommend upper-body resistance training to help mitigate syncope in endurance athletes.—E.R. Eichner, M.D.

References

1. 1990 YEAR BOOK OF SPORTS MEDICINE pp 58–59, 222–224.
2. Cantwell JD, et al: *Physician Sportsmed* 20:81, 1992.

Chronic Endurance Exercise Training: A Condition of Inadequate Blood Pressure Regulation and Reduced Tolerance to LBNP

Raven PB, Pawelczyk JA (Texas College of Osteopathic Medicine, Fort Worth; Univ of Texas, Dallas)
Med Sci Sports Exerc 25:713–721, 1993   139-94-9-10

Introduction.—Reports of dizziness, nausea, and syncopal symptoms in endurance-trained athletes when standing from supine position or a crouch have led to hypotheses that such training affects disposition to

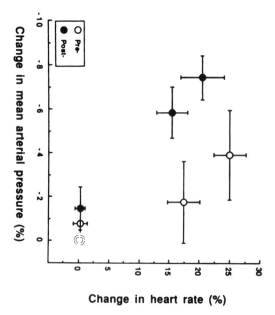

Change in heart rate (%)

Fig 9-2.—The relationship between the relative changes in heart rate and mean arterial pressure during progressive lower-body negative pressure before (*open circles*) and after (*filled circles*) 8 months of endurance exercise training. There is a significantly attenuated heart rate response at −35 and −45 mm Hg lower-body negative pressure, documented by the significantly lower slope of the line relating the 2 variables. (From Raven PB, Pawelczyk JA: *Med Sci Sports Exerc* 25:713–721, 1993. Courtesy of Stegemann J, Meier U, Skipka W, et al: *Aviat Space Environ Med* 46:26–29, 1975.)

orthostatic hypotension. The question now is what is the mechanism of this alteration. The cross-sectional data on this question were reviewed with a focus on whether maximal aerobic power ($\dot{V}O_{2max}$) is a useful predictor of orthostatic tolerance, and the possible role of altered baroreflex responsiveness was explored.

Findings.—The review included cross-sectional studies of unfit subjects and endurance-trained athletes, as well as recent data on changes in orthostatic tolerance and blood pressure regulation occurring after 8 days to 8 months of endurance training. The data suggest that any effect of endurance training on orthostatic tolerance appears only after long periods of intensive training. Maximal aerobic power itself does not appear to be an independent predictor of orthostatic tolerance. However, athletes whose $\dot{V}O_{2max}$ is greater than 65 mL/kg^{-1}/min^{-1} generally have lower orthostatic tolerance than sedentary controls. The explanation for this apparent conflict is probably the selection of highly trained athletes when recruiting subjects with high $\dot{V}O_{2max}$. A fourfold mechanism of orthostatic intolerance in trained athletes is proposed: increased limb vascular compliance; eccentric ventricular hypertrophy; increased total blood volume, possibly attenuating cardiopulmonary baroreflex responsiveness, shifting ventricular function to a steeper part of the ventricular compliance curve, and increasing the inhibitory effect of cardiopulmonary baroreceptors on carotid baroreflex responsiveness; and an independent reduction of carotid and aortic baroreflex responsiveness. The result is not unlike that of pathologic states such as heart failure and hypertension.

Discussion.—The research suggests that orthostatic tolerance in endurance-trained athletes is not directly related to $\dot{V}O_{2max}$. Rather, endurance training may independently affect arterial baroreflex responsiveness, altering both carotid and aortic baroreceptor populations (Fig 9–2). Further studies are needed to determine the endurance training–related changes in aortic baroreflex control of blood pressure or vascular resistance.

▶ The issue reviewed by Raven and Pawelczyk first arose in aerospace laboratories, where it was alleged that (contrary to expectation) fighter pilots who became unusually fit had a poor tolerance of high gravitational accelerations (1). Formal research reduced these fears, showing that tolerance of high G-force was not impaired except in individuals with unusually high levels of fitness.

Endurance athletes also complain sometimes of symptoms of hypotension on moving suddenly from a crouching to an erect position. However, some of the conclusions on the etiology of this phenomenon offered in this review are hard to swallow; indeed, it is difficult to see how Raven and Pawelczyk can justify their views! The threshold for an adverse effect is correctly indicated as a maximal oxygen intake of 65 mL/kg^{-1}/min^{-1}, and from this observation, Raven and Pawelczyk draw the surprising conclusion that training rather than an inherited high maximal oxygen intake is responsible for the orthostatism. Their verdict implies that a sedentary young man would have to train hard enough to increase aerobic power by 50% to be at risk! In fact, there have been at least 9 longitudinal studies of endurance training, all of which have shown either no effect or even a slight improvement of gravity tolerance after training (2, 3). It seems more reasonable to speculate that a tall, thin, and lightly muscled individual who has inherited a high maximal oxygen intake gravitates to a sport such as long-distance running with a constitutionally determined impairment of vasoregulation.—R.J. Shephard, M.D., Ph.D.

References

1. Luft UC, Myhre LG, Loeppky JA, Venters MD. *A study of factors affecting tolerance of gravitational stress stimulated by lower body negative pressure.* Contract NASD 9-14492. Albuquerque, NM, Lovelace Foundation, 1976, pp 1–60.
2. Convertino VA: *Exerc Sports Sci Rev* 15:223, 1987.
3. Greenleaf JE, et al: *Aviat Space Environ Med* 59:152, 1988.

Reduction in Left Ventricular Wall Thickness After Deconditioning in Highly Trained Olympic Athletes
Maron BJ, Pelliccia A, Spataro A, Granata M (Dept of Medicine Italian Natl Olympic Committee, Rome; Natl Heart, Lung, and Blood Inst, Bethesda, Md)
Br Heart J 69:125–128, 1993   139-94-9-11

Background.—The term "athlete's heart" refers to the increase in left ventricular cavity dimension and mass that results from long-term athletic training. Withdrawal from systematic training reportedly reduces left ventricular wall thickening, a clinical phenomenon that might be used to differentiate athlete's heart from hypertrophic cardiomyopathy in conditioned athletes. Echocardiography was used to assess the effects of deconditioning in a group of Olympic athletes.

Subjects and Methods.—The 6 male athletes had a mean age of 24 years. All showed considerable physiologic left ventricular wall thickening ($\geq$ 13 mm). The athletes had competed in rowing or canoeing at the 1988 Olympic Games in Seoul and underwent a substantial period of deconditioning immediately after the event. Echocardiographic studies were performed at peak training and after a period of deconditioning (mean, 13 weeks), followed by a short period of light retraining. An observer, unaware of the identity of the athlete or the state of conditioning, interpreted the echocardiograms.

Results.—During peak training, the mean maximum left ventricular wall thickness in the 6 athletes was 13.8 mm. Deconditioning reduced the maximum wall thickness to a mean of 10.5 mm. Septal thickness decreased by a mean of 3.3 mm, a mean change from trained to deconditioned states of 23%. The mean change in left ventricular mass from peak training to detraining was 22% (Fig 9-3). Overall electrocardiographic voltages also showed a significant decrease. The left ventricular

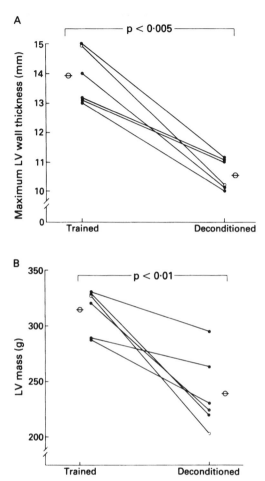

Fig 9–3.—Changes in left ventricular wall thickness (**A**) and mass (**B**) associated with deconditioning in 6 Olympic athletes. *Open symbols* represent the athlete who retired from training and competition after the 1988 Olympic Games and had been deconditioned for 34 weeks at the time of the most recent echocardiographic study. (Courtesy of Maron BJ, Pelliccia A, Spataro A, et al: *Br Heart J* 69:125–128, 1993.)

end-diastolic dimension was not significantly changed during the 2 periods.

Conclusion.—In these elite athletes, deconditioning was associated with a considerable reduction in ventricular septal thickness during a short period. This finding suggests that the athletes had a training-induced physiologic form of left ventricular hypertrophy. Thus, a brief period of forced deconditioning may be clinically useful in differentiating athlete's heart and hypertropic cardiomyopathy.

▶ Some earlier papers (1), using less precise methods such as unblinded examination of the total cardiac shadow, have maintained that the large heart size of the endurance athlete persists for many years after training has ceased. This was always a surprising conclusion, given the rapid deterioration of maximal oxygen intake that occurs during detraining. This paper supports more recent echocardiographic studies (2, 3) and provides convincing evidence of the potential for rapid changes in the amount of ventricular muscle with an alteration of training status.—R.J. Shephard, M.D., Ph.D.

References

1. Grimby G, Saltin B: *Acta Med Scand* 179:513, 1966.
2. Fagard R, et al: *Circulation* 67:896, 1986.
3. Martin WH, et al: *J Am Coll Cardiol* 7:982, 1986.

Re-Examination of the Incidence of Exercise-Induced Hypoxaemia in Highly Trained Subjects
Brown DD, Knowlton RG, Sanjabi PB, Szurgot BT (Illinois State Univ, Normal; Southern Illinois Univ, Carbondale; Herrin Hosp, Ill)
Br J Sports Med 27:167–170, 1993   139-94-9-12

Background.—Previous studies using pulse ear oximetry have reported that approximately 50% of endurance trained athletes will have exercise-induced hypoxemia (EIH) during maximal exercise. However, studies investigating the occurrence of EIH when saturation is determined using arterial blood rather than ear oximetry have not yet been performed.

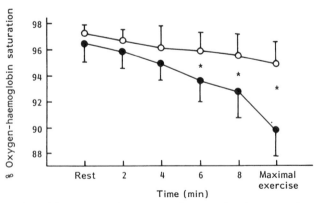

Fig 9–4.—Oxygen-hemoglobin saturation during exercise for arterial blood samples and ear oximetry. *Open circles*, arterial blood; *filled circles*, ear oximetry; *, significantly different. (Courtesy of Brown DD, Knowlton RG, Sanjabi PB, et al: *Br J Sports Med* 27:167–170, 1993.)

Thus, the incidence of arterial oxygen-hemoglobin desaturation during maximal exercise in highly trained athletes was evaluated.

Patients and Methods.—Eleven trained cyclists aged 18–28 years, with a mean maximal aerobic power ($\dot{V}O_{2max}$) of 66.9 $\pm$ 4.8 mL/kg^{-1}/min^{-1} were studied. All participants performed continuous, multistage (270 kpm/min^{-1}) cycle ergometry until exhausted. Arterial oxygen-hemoglobin saturation (%HbO$_2$) measurements were taken simultaneously at rest, every 2 minutes during exercise, and at maximum exercise capacity from arterial blood sampling (%SaO$_2$) and ear oximetry (%SpO$_2$).

Results.—Exercise-induced hypoxemia, defined as %HbO$_2$ of less than or equal to 91%, was noted in 64% of the athletes when pulse oximetry was used, compared with none when %HbO$_2$ was determined using arterial blood samples. The mean resting values were comparable for each method (96.5 $\pm$ 1.6% for %SpO$_2$ and 97.3 $\pm$ 0.6% for %SaO$_2$). However, statistically significant differences in EIH determinations for arterial blood and ear oximetry were noted at 6-minute, 8-minute, and maximal exercise sampling times, which became prevalent at exercise intensities greater than 73% $\dot{V}O_{2max}$ (Fig 9–4).

Conclusion.—When compared with measurements made using arterial blood, ear oximetry overestimates the occurrence of EIH and underestimates the oxyhemoglobin saturation in highly trained athletes during exercise.

▶ Studies using arterial blood specimens have demonstrated fairly conclusively that a small proportion of highly trained athletes can experience some arterial unsaturation (< 5%) during exhausting exercise (1, 2). However, this report is important because it demonstrates that other reports of much greater and more prevalent arterial unsaturation based on ear oximetry may well be fallacious.—R.J. Shephard, M.D., Ph.D.

References

1. Dempsey JA: *Med Sci Sports Exerc* 18:143, 1986.
2. Hopkins SR, McKenzie DC: *J Appl Physiol* 67:1119, 1989.

Coronary Artery Size and Dilating Capacity in Ultradistance Runners
Haskell WL, Sims C, Myll J, Bortz WM, St Goar FG, Alderman EL (Stanford Univ, Calif; Palo Alto Med Research Found, Calif)
Circulation 87:1076–1082, 1993   139-94-9–13

Background.—Some animals have shown evidence of increases in coronary artery size and dilating capacity after endurance training. At autopsy, active men appear to have enlarged epicardial coronary arteries. A cross-sectional study was done to test the hypothesis that, compared with inactive men, highly trained endurance runners have larger epicardial coronary arteries and dilating capacity.

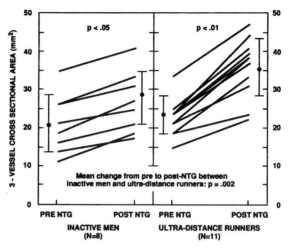

Fig 9–5.—Combined cross-sectional area of the proximal right, left anterior descending, and circumflex coronary arteries before and after nitroglycerin (NTG) for physically inactive men and ultradistance runners. (Courtesy of Haskell WL, Sims C, Myll J, et al: *Circulation* 87:1076–1082, 1993.)

Methods.—Twenty-two men aged 39–66 years volunteered for the study. Eleven had participated in ultradistance running in the preceding 2 years, and 11 were physically inactive men referred for arteriography but with no visible coronary artery disease. Using a computer-based quantitative arteriographic analysis system, the internal diameter of the proximal segments of each major epicardial coronary artery was measured before and after the administration of nitroglycerin.

Findings.—Before nitroglycerin administration, the 2 groups did not differ in the sum of the cross-sectional areas for the proximal right and left anterior descending and circumflex arteries. However, runners had greater increases in the sum of the cross-sectional area for the proximal right and left anterior descending and circumflex arteries after nitroglycerin was given. In addition, the left ventricular mass index was significantly greater for runners, although left ventricular mass was not. In runners, dilating capacity was positively associated with aerobic power and negatively associated with adiposity, resting heart rate, and plasma lipoprotein levels (Fig 9–5).

Conclusion.—These highly trained, middle-aged runners had a significantly greater dilating capacity in the epicardial coronary arteries after nitroglycerin administration than did inactive men. The causes and clinical significance of this greater dilating capacity have yet to be determined.

▶ Postmortem casts have suggested that regular endurance exercise can enlarge the coronary arterial tree both in experimental animals and in human beings. The disadvantage of such postmortem observations is that the normal innervation of the vessels is no longer operative. Haskell and colleagues have adopted a sophisticated system of computerized coronary arteriography to examine the coronary vascular dimensions of healthy adults in vivo. The resting dimensions did not differ between ultradistance runners and sedentary individuals. After nitroglycerin administration, the expansion of the arterial tree was about twice as great in the runners (13.2 mm^2) as it was in the sedentary individuals (6.0 mm^2); accepting the radius^4 hypothesis of coronary vascular resistance, with a total cross-section of 35.9 vs. 27.0 mm^2, the peak coronary flow of the distance runners could have been 70% to 80% greater, supplying hearts with left ventricular mass indices that were 30% greater than those of the sedentary individuals.

The findings are encouraging for those who believe in the preventive value of exercise. However, this study does not indicate whether the coronary vessels of the runners dilated more (as a result of their running) or the vessels of the sedentary group dilated less (because of undetected atherosclerosis). Because the observations were cross-sectional in nature, they cannot prove categorically that either positive or negative activity habits modified coronary vasodilatory capacity. Further, given that the main resistance to blood flow lies in the arterioles, the clinical importance of a more ready chemically induced dilatation of the large vessels has yet to be established.—R.J. Shephard, M.D., Ph.D.

Middle Cerebral Artery Blood Velocity and Cerebral Blood Flow and O$_2$ Uptake During Dynamic Exercise
Madsen PL, Sperling BK, Warming T, Schmidt JF, Secher NH, Wildschiødtz G, Holm S, Lassen NA (Bispebjerg Hosp, Copenhagen; Rigshospitalet, Copenhagen; Univ of Copenhagen)
J Appl Physiol 74:245–250, 1993   139-94-9–14

Background.—The results of external-detector ^{133}Xe clearance tests and studies using Doppler sonography have suggested that dynamic exercise increases the global cerebral blood flow (CBF). Earlier data obtained under less well-defined conditions have contradicted these findings. To investigate the controversy, the Kety-Schmidt technique was used to measure global levels of CBF and the cerebral oxygen consumption (CMRO$_2$) at rest and during a well-defined exercise period.

Methods.—Eleven healthy, nonmedicated volunteers underwent a dynamic exercise test on a Krogh cycle ergometer, performed in a semirecumbent position at a constant pedaling rate of 60 rpm. The global CBF and global CMRO$_2$ were measured during rest and submaximal exercise by using the Kety-Schmidt technique in the desaturation mode with ^{133}Xe infusion as tracer. The middle cerebral artery (MCA) blood flow velocity was measured by transcranial Doppler sonography and was calculated as mean maximal flow velocity.

Results.—When corrected for changes in arterial carbon dioxide tension (PaCO$_2$), the mean CBF of subjects who exercised was unchanged from baseline. The global levels of CMRO$_2$ were identical during exer-

Dynamic Exercises

Subj No.	MCA V_{mean}, cm/s			CBF, ml·100 g^{-1}·min^{-1}			CMRo$_2$, ml·100 g^{-1}·min^{-1}	
	Rest	Exercise	CO$_2$·corr	Rest	Exercise	CO$_2$·corr	Rest	Exercise
1	58.0	65.1	80.3	67.6	51.3	63.3	2.89	3.39
2	34.6	44.0	44.3	43.9	34.1	34.3	3.38	2.62
3	39.6	50.8	54.9	47.4	43.3	46.8	4.04	3.97
4	48.9	62.9	60.4	44.5	50.2	48.2	3.78	3.97
5	30.3	34.3	33.6	52.5	53.3	52.2	4.42	4.28
6	57.7	65.8	64.8	44.0	40.0	39.3	2.91	2.99
7	52.6	54.3	69.1	52.4	43.1	54.7	3.62	3.67
8	58.0	60.8	63.2	46.8	50.6	52.6	3.55	3.91
9	67.3	74.5	73.6	55.8	55.4	54.8	3.79	3.51
10	44.6	45.7	53.7	49.3	44.0	51.7	3.51	3.80
11				55.7	56.5	65.7	3.54	3.50
12	54.6	64.0	70.5	48.1	40.8	45.0	4.18	3.96
Mean ± SD	49.7±11.3 ($P < 0.0003$)	56.6±11.8 ($P < 0.0001$)	60.8±13.5	50.7±6.8 (NS)	46.9±7.0 (NS)	50.7±8.9 (NS)	3.63±0.46	3.63±0.47 (NS)

Subj No.	Oxygen Uptake $\dot{V}O_{2\,max}$, l/min	Oxygen Uptake Exercise %	Pa_{CO_2}, kPa Rest	Pa_{CO_2}, kPa Exercise	Body Temperature, °C Rest	Body Temperature, °C Exercise	Heart Rate, beats/min Rest	Heart Rate, beats/min Exercise	MAP, mmHg Rest	MAP, mmHg Exercise
1	3.5	57	5.45	4.67	37.2	38.5	76	158	79	126
2	3.6	56	4.85	4.83	36.9	37.7	73	138	91	94
3	5.5	45	5.00	4.73	37.0	37.7	62	130	96	110
4	4.4	50	5.12	5.25	36.4	37.6	70	145	97	100
5	4.8	48	4.71	4.78	37.1	38.0	64	131	79	86
6	3.6	36	5.13	5.18	37.1	37.9	67	133	81	90
7	3.6	61	5.55	4.64	37.8	38.6	86	175	90	94
8	3.8	55	4.97	4.84	37.3	37.7	91	150	103	102
9	2.2	41	4.78	4.82	37.2	38.0	71	145	97	102
10	5.2	48	5.06	4.48	36.9	38.6	67	147	94	109
11	2.9	48	4.84	4.30	37.3	38.0	58	153	119	134
12	4.6	52	5.24	4.90	36.8	37.9	56	144	83	90
Mean ± SD	4.0±1.0	50±7	5.06±0.26 ($P < 0.05$)	4.79±0.26	37.1±0.3 ($P < 0.00001$)	38.0±0.4	70±10 ($P < 0.00001$)	146±13	92±12 ($P < 0.02$)	103±15

Abbreviations: MCA V$_{mean}$, middle cerebral artery flow velocity measured by transcranial Doppler sonography; MAP, mean arterial pressure; $\dot{V}O_{2\,max}$, maximal oxygen uptake; *Exercise %*, exercise oxygen uptake in percentage of $\dot{V}O_{2\,max}$; CO_2 -corr, values of global CBF and MCA mean maximal velocity obtained during exercise, corrected for exercise-induced changes in Pa_{CO_2}.
Note: Values are means obtained during rest and dynamic exercise.
(Courtesy of Madsen PL, Sperling BK, Warming T, et al: *J Appl Physiol* 74:245–250, 1993.)

cise and at rest. Exercise significantly increased mean heart rate (109%), mean arterial pressure (12%), hemoglobin (6%), and body core temperature (.9%) (table). The mean maximal flow velocity in the MCA was 14% higher than resting values; correction for alterations in $PaCO_2$ increased the significance of the change.

Conclusion.—In contrast to recent results, these findings suggest that dynamic exercise does not alter the global CBF and levels of $CMRO_2$, but instead it markedly increases the mean maximal flow velocity in the MCA. Thus, any increase in mean maximal flow velocity measured during dynamic exercise does not signify a proportionate increase in overall CBF.

▶ There has been frequent discussion concerning whether exercise can increase CBF, particularly in connection with the postulated impact of regular exercise on mental performance in very old individuals. Certainly, exercise increases systemic blood pressures substantially; other factors being equal, this might be expected to increase cerebral perfusion, at least transiently. However, attempts to measure CBF directly have yielded conflicting results. One difficulty is that a substantial part of the blood flow to the head is directed to the skin, because the head accounts for much of body cooling; here, much vasoconstriction can occur under cold conditions. Further, subjects tend to hyperventilate when laboratory measurements are being made, and the resulting loss of carbon dioxide can cause cerebral vasoconstriction. Finally, there is no simple method of obtaining good measurements of cerebral perfusion.

In this study by Madsen and associates, exercise was relatively mild (about 50% of maximal oxygen intake), and although there was a substantial increase of heart rate, the mean arterial perfusion pressure showed only a small increase. It is therefore not surprising that no increase of overall CBF could be demonstrated. Further studies are needed at intensities of effort that cause a major increase of systemic blood pressure. However, even if more vigorous exercise does augment overall cerebral perfusion, as Madsen et al. point out, the additional flow is not necessarily going to be directed to areas of the brain associated with cognition. Indeed, increased perfusion of the motor and sensory cortex is more probable.—R.J. Shephard, M.D., Ph.D.

Investigation of Circadian Rhythms in Anaerobic Power and Capacity of the Legs
Reilly T, Down A (Liverpool John Moores Univ, England)
J Sports Med Phys Fitness 32:343–347, 1992   139-94-9-15

Background.—Circadian rhythms occur in many biological functions in close association with circadian body temperature fluctuations. Many aspects of exercise performance also vary with the time of day. The effect of the time of day on measures of anaerobic power and capacity was

Circadian Rhythms of Significant Cosine Functions				
	Mesor	Acrophase (time of day)	Amplitude	Amplitude (% of mean)
Rectal temperature	37.25 (°C)	18:11	0.38 (°C)	1.0
Stair run	19.80 (W kg^{-1})	17.26	0.41 (W kg^{-1})	2.1
Broad jump	224.2 (cm)	17:45	7.6 (cm)	3.4

(Courtesy of Reilly T, Down A: *J Sports Med Phys Fitness* 32:343–347, 1992.)

investigated, and any changes in these measures were related to the circadian rhythm in core temperature.

Methods.—Twelve men aged 18–22 years performed 2 series of anaerobic exercise tests at 2, 6, and 10 A.M. 2, 6, and 10 P.M., with at least 24 hours between exercise sessions. The exercise tests included a standing broad jump, a stair run, and the Wingate Anaerobic Test. Diet, preexercise activity, and laboratory temperature were controlled; preexercise rectal temperature was measured on each occasion.

Results.—Rectal temperatures exhibited a circadian rhythm, peaking at 6:11 P.M. (table). The peak to mean variation in the rectal temperature curve was .38°C; the peak to trough variation was .76°C. The first- and second-set data were pooled before applying cosinor analysis. The pooled stair run and standing broad jump results suggested a significant rhythm that was in phase with body temperature. However, no significant rhythm was apparent in Wingate Anaerobic Test peak or mean power scores.

Conclusion.—Circadian rhythms in anaerobic power exist for the stair run and standing broad jump. These rhythms are in phase with rectal temperature. However, a circadian curve in rectal temperature is not reflected in anaerobic power and anaerobic capacity of the legs, as expressed by the Wingate Anaerobic Test after the stair run and jumps.

▶ Reilly and his associates have previously demonstrated cyclic changes in swim bench performance (1), and others (2) have demonstrated a trend toward a circadian rhythm of Wingate scores, with a peak that was 8% higher at 9:00 P.M. than at 3:00 A.M. This data set, likewise, shows peak Wingate readings in the afternoon; the lack of statistical significance of the circadian trend is probably caused by the variability of Wingate performance relative to the sample size (only 12 subjects). The practical lesson is that an athlete can gain an appreciable competitive edge if his or her circadian cycle can be matched with the anticipated time of competition.—R.J. Shephard, M.D., Ph.D.

References

1. Reilly T, Marshall S: *J Swim Res* 7:11, 1991.
2. Hill DW, Smith JC: *Can J Sports Sci* 16:30, 1991.

Physiological Characteristics of Elite and Club Level Female Triathletes During Running

Laurenson NM, Fulcher KY, Korkia P (St Bartholomew's Med College, London)
Int J Sports Med 14:455–459, 1993   139-94-9–16

Objective.—This study was designed to compare the physiologic and training characteristics of elite and club women triathletes who compete at Olympic distances (1.5-km swim, 40-km cycle, 10-km run) and to relate these characteristics to triathlon performance. Ten of the women competed at the national/elite level, and 9 were competitive/club-level triathletes.

Findings.—Personal and anthropometric characteristics were similar in the 2 groups of triathletes, except for a significantly smaller subscapular skinfold thickness in the elite group. In both groups the amount of training varied widely, but the elite athletes swam more often per week than the club athletes. There were no other differences in the training for each event with respect to total time, number of workouts, and distance. Total weekly training times did not differ significantly: 14.8 hours for the elite group and 14.0 hours for the club group. The elite triathletes were faster in each event, but the difference was significant only for running. Peak oxygen uptake was higher in the elite athletes, but there were no significant differences in maximal heart rates or peak ventilation rates (Table 1). Submaximal running tests indicated that the elite athletes ran more economically (Table 2). When running at 15 km/hr^{-1}, the elite athletes had lower blood lactate levels and heart rates and lower values for ventilatory efficiency. Running performance correlated with the percent peak oxygen uptake (% $\dot{V}O_{2max}$) at 15 km/hr^{-1} but not with $\dot{V}O_{2max}$.

TABLE 1.—Results From the Treadmill Ergometer $\dot{V}O_{2max}$ Test

	Elite	Club
$\dot{V}O_2$max (ml.kg^{-1}.min^{-1})	65.6 (6.0)	60.4 (3.1)
Minimum - Maximum	54.3-72.5	55.7-64.6
$\dot{V}$Emax (l.min^{-1})	123.0 (19.7)	123.1 (11.5)
Minimum - Maximum	96.6-154.0	108.2-141.3
HRmax (bpm)	186.6 (4.9)	186.6 (7.4)
Minimum - Maximum	178-196	173-198

Note: Values are means ± 1 SD.
(Courtesy of Laurenson NM, Fulcher KY, Korkia P: *Int J Sports Med* 14:455–459, 1993.)

TABLE 2.—Results of Submaximal Running Test

	Elite	Club
$\dot{V}O_2$ (ml.kg^{-1}.min^{-1}) at 15 kph	51.2 (6.9)	53.8 (3.1)
%$\dot{V}O_2$ max (ml.kg^{-1}.min^{-1}) at 15 kph	78.2 (9.4)	89.2 (6.2)
La (mmol.l^{-1}) at 15 kph	1.8 (0.5)	3.1 (1.5)
$\dot{V}E/\dot{V}O_2$ at 15 kph	29.4 (2.8)	33.1 (2.0)

Note: Values are means ± 1 SD.
(Courtesy of Laurenson NM, Fulcher KY, Korkia P: *Int J Sports Med* 14:455–459, 1993.)

Conclusion.—It has not been possible to predict women's triathlon performance from their anthropometric profiles. The quality of training appears to be a better indicator of success in this activity than its quantity.

▶ This study demonstrates the importance of doing power calculations to determine what sample size is required to identify a significant difference between or within groups in physiologic research. In spite of the large observed differences between elite and club triathletes in distance, duration, and frequency of training for each event, the variability of training regimens within each group plus the small sample size made it impossible for these differences to reach statistical significance. As a result, the authors were forced to infer that it must be the quality rather than quantity of training that explained the difference in performance. Although it is interesting, this study has not been able to provide the definitive answer to the question of whether there are significant differences in the physiologic characteristics and training protocols of elite vs. club triathletes.—B.L. Drinkwater, Ph.D.

The Use of Heart Rates to Monitor Exercise Intensity in Relation to Metabolic Variables

Gilman MB, Wells CL (Arizona State Univ, Tempe)
Int J Sports Med 14:339–344, 1993   139-94-9–17

Background.—Running performance is related to maximal aerobic power $\dot{V}O_{2max}$, to the fractional use of $\dot{V}O_{2max}$ at the onset of blood lactic acid (OBLA), and to running velocity at the onset of blood lactic acid. Exercise intensity can be assessed with the metabolic reference points of ventilatory threshold (VT) and OBLA. Using these metabolic reference points and percentages of maximal heart rate (HR_{max}), individualized training programs can be designed based on heart rates at VT, OBLA,

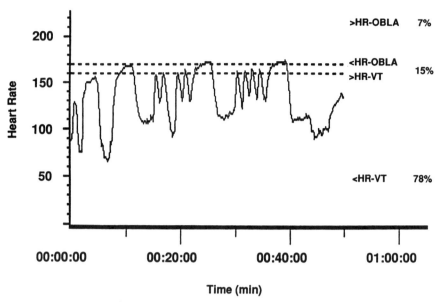

Fig 9–6.—Heart rate during a representative 50-minute training period in reference to heart rate at HR-OBLA and HR-VT for a single patient. (Courtesy of Gilman MB, Wells CL: *Int J Sports Med* 14:339–344, 1993.)

and $\dot{V}O_{2max}$. Heart rates (HR) corresponding to VT and OBLA were used to assess exercise intensity during training and competition in a group of female runners.

Method.—In the first phase, a graded exercise test determined heart rates corresponding to VT and OBLA for each subject. In the second phase, heart rates were recorded during 2 weeks of training. The total weekly training time ranged from 184.3 to 633.2 minutes, with an average total training time of approximately 5 hours. The women were asked to describe each session as easy, moderate, or hard intensity, or as intervals, hills, or long type of training. In the third study phase, heart rate was recorded during an 8-km race.

Findings.—The mean training time above HR-OBLA was 24.3 minutes or 8.5% of the total; the time between HR-OBLA and HR-VT was 140.7 minutes or 45.7% of the total; and the time below HR-VT was 136.2 minutes or 45.8% of the total (Fig 9–6). A comparison of training HRs and monitored HRs revealed that most training was at an easy or moderate intensity. This was significantly different from the subjects' self-reports, which overestimated their hard training time. During the 8-km race, the subjects' heart rate averaged 95.8% of HR_{max}. More than 70% of the race was run at a heart rate exceeding HR-OBLA, and only 3% of the race time was spent at a running intensity requiring less than HR-VT.

Conclusion.—A comparison of training and race intensity revealed that the runners trained at easy to moderate intensity with only 8.5% of their training time at an HR above OBLA. In contrast, nearly three quarters of their race time was at high intensity. The discrepancy between their perceived intensity of training and their actual intensity of training may be attributable to difficulty in objectively selecting an appropriate running intensity. Training intensity can be more accurately judged on the basis of HRs at designated metabolic markers with subsequent HR monitoring.

▶ The discrepancy between an athlete's subjective perception of training intensity and the actual intensity as determined by HR relative to ventilatory and lactate thresholds provides food for thought. It would be interesting to see whether using Borg's Perception of Effort scale and obtaining a finer discrimination of the subjective estimate of effort would have improved the agreement between the subjective and objective measures of intensity. Might a more experienced group of runners have been more successful in estimating the intensity of their workouts? Extension of this research should be useful in assuring that training sessions are being used most effectively to prepare an athlete for competition.—B.L. Drinkwater, Ph.D.

Effects of Stair-Climbing vs Run Training on Treadmill and Track Running Performance
Loy SF, Holland GJ, Mutton DL, Snow J, Vincent WJ, Hoffmann JJ, Shaw S (California State Univ, Northridge)
Med Sci Sports Exerc 25:1275–1278, 1993   139-94-9–18

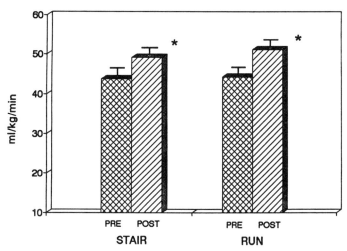

Fig 9–7.—Treadmill maximal oxygen consumption pretraining and post-training for STAIR vs. RUN; *Asterisk* indicates significantly different from pretraining (P < .01). (Courtesy of Loy SF, Holland GJ, Mutton DL, et al: *Med Sci Sports Exerc* 25:1275-1278, 1993.)

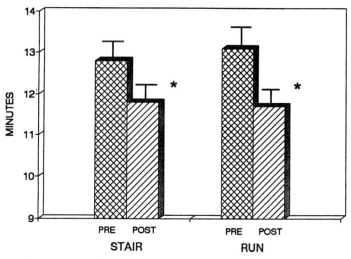

Fig 9–8.—A 2,414-m run performance time pretraining and post-training for STAIR vs. RUN; *Asterisk* indicates significantly different from pretraining ($P < .01$). (Courtesy of Loy SF, Holland GJ, Mutton DL, et al: *Med Sci Sports Exerc* 25:1275–1278, 1993.)

Introduction.—Stair-climbing equipment is popular with the general public. Although this type of exercise training has not been directly compared with running in either laboratory or field studies, those who wish to improve their running performance have been advised to train in a task-specific manner.

Study Plan.—The effects of stair-climbing and run training at equivalent intensities were compared in 23 college-age women who initially were physically active but did not train regularly. They were randomly assigned to train by running or stair-climbing using an automated stair-stepping device. Training of both types began at 70% to 80% of maximal heart rate for 30 minutes, 4 days per week, and progressed to 85% to 90% of peak heart rate for 45 minutes. After 9 weeks of training, subjects completed a maximum oxygen intake ($\dot{V}O_{2max}$) test and submaximal treadmill tests that evaluated performance at similar absolute workloads and relative exercise intensities.

Results.—Peak oxygen uptake on treadmill exercise increased significantly in both training groups (Fig 9–7), and performance times in a 2,414-m run decreased to a comparable degree in the 2 groups (Fig 9–8). The post-test submaximal treadmill run at the same absolute demonstrated significant reductions in $\dot{V}O_{2max}$ and percent maximal heart rate in both training groups. Running at the same relative intensity in the post-test required a significant increase in running speed for both groups. No injuries occurred as a result of stair-climbing training. Two of the runners, however, withdrew from the study because of running-related injuries, and 2 others lost time from training.

Conclusion.—Stair-climbing is a relatively safe form of aerobic training and a viable alternative to running.

▶ An interesting follow-up to this study would be a comparison between a nonautomated stair-climbing device and running. Few women can afford an automated stair-climber for their home, but the self-propelled type is within the financial reach of many more. The difference in injury rates between the 2 modes of exercise should encourage us to focus more attention on the physiologic effects of training on this type of equipment.—B.L. Drinkwater, Ph.D.

Effect of 8 Wk of Bicycle Training on the Immune System of Patients With Rheumatoid Arthritis
Baslund B, Lyngberg K, Andersen V, Kristensen JH, Hansen M, Klokker M, Pedersen BK (Rigshospitalet, Copenhagen; Herlev Amstssygehus, Copenhagen)
J Appl Physiol 75:1691–1695, 1993   139-94-9-19

Background.—Several immune system disturbances have been reported in patients with rheumatoid arthritis (RA). Natural killer (NK) cell activity in such patients reportedly ranges from low to slightly increased. The hypothesis that training in patients with RA would enhance NK cell activity was tested.

Methods.—Eighteen patients with moderate RA participated. Nine patients were randomly assigned to an 8-week program of progressive bicycle training, and 9 were assigned to a control group. Before training and after 4 and 8 weeks of training, the resting levels of various immune parameters were determined.

Findings.—Compared with the control group, maximal oxygen uptake increased significantly in the training group. Heart rate at stage 2 and rate of perceived exertion decreased significantly in the training group. Training had no effect on blood mononuclear cell subpopulations, proliferative response, or NK cell activity. Plasma levels of interleukin-1α, interleukin-1β, and interleukin-6 were also unchanged.

Conclusion.—Conditioning exercise training apparently does not affect immunocompetent cells in the blood of patients with RA. Differences between these and previous findings might be the result of the use of interval training in the current study as well as the fact that the patients were trained for only 8 weeks.

Decreased Salivary Immunoglobulins After Intense Interval Exercise Before and After Training

MacKinnon LT, Jenkins DG (Univ of Queensland, Brisbane, Australia)
Med Sci Sports Exerc 25:678–683, 1993   139-94-9-20

Introduction.—Athletes who participate in intense endurance exercise appear to be at high risk of contracting upper respiratory tract infection. This type of exercise has been shown to decrease the concentration of IgA contained in mucosal secretions. The levels of secretory antibodies such as IgA correlate closely with resistance to respiratory infection caused by certain viruses. The IgA response to brief supramaximal interval exercise was examined before and after an interval training program.

Methods.—Twelve male physical education students at the University of Queensland took part in the experiments. The subjects, aged 17–25 years, were active in recreational athletics but were not in training for any particular sport. The study protocol consisted of five 60-second bouts of supramaximal interval exercise on a cycle ergometer, with each bout separated by a 5-minute rest. Subjects then trained for 8 weeks, performing the same interval exercise protocol 3 times per week. Saliva was collected for measurement of IgA, IgG, and IgM concentrations and calculation of flow rates. The samples of timed, whole unstimulated saliva were obtained before and after the interval exercise protocol both before and after training.

Results.—The subjects exhibited a small but significant increase in anaerobic exercise capacity after the 8-week training period. After each exercise session, IgA and IgM concentrations decreased relative to total protein. There was no exercise-related change in IgG concentration relative to total protein. Flow rates of IgA, IgM, and IgG decreased 50% to 65% after interval exercise. Training had no effect on any immune parameter measured despite an increase in total work performed.

Conclusion.—The output of salivary IgA and IgM decreases after brief supramaximal interval exercise, attributable at least in part to a decrease in saliva flow. Intense exercise does, however, appear to have a specific effect on IgA concentration beyond that attributed to alteration in saliva flow. Thus, decreases in secretory IgA output may contribute to the high incidence of upper respiratory tract infection observed in athletes during intense training and competition. The mechanisms responsible for these changes in saliva flow and secretory IgA output are unclear.

▶ These 2 articles (Abstracts 139-94-9–19 and 139-94-9–20) serve as an update on exercise, natural killer (NK) cells, and salivary immunoglobulins. As covered widely in the 1993 YEAR BOOK OF SPORTS MEDICINE, exercise can change the levels and functions of white blood cells—especially polymorphonuclear leukocytes and lymphocytes—and can affect levels of immunoglobulins and other immune factors (1). Usually, however, exercise-related changes are mild, mixed, and brief, making their clinical import unclear. Exercise-related changes that seem most likely to shape the risk of infection involve NK cells, which defend against some viruses, and salivary immunoglobulins, which defend against microorganisms in the nose and throat. The gist of Abstract 139-94-9–19 is that 8 weeks of aerobic exercise in patients with rheumatoid arthritis improved aerobic capacity but did not change NK cell activity. Nor did it change plasma interleukin levels or lymphocyte numbers, subsets, or function. Thus, this exercise program had no effect on the immune systems studied.

Abstract 139-94-9–20 shows that salivary IgA (and IgM) concentrations decrease after brief, supramaximal interval exercise, as seen earlier in skiers, cyclists, swimmers, and in some studies of runners. Training did not affect salivary IgA levels. The authors suggest that decreases in salivary IgA after exercise are temporally related to upper respiratory tract infections in squash and hockey players. A recent review of exercise and resistance to infection, however, notes that 1 in 500 individuals is born without IgA but may have strong immunity, and that only 1 in 500 lymphocytes is in the blood; therefore, transient increases and decreases in blood levels may mean little (2). Despite much recent research, we still have more questions than answers about athletes, exercise, and immunity.—E.R. Eichner, M.D.

References

1. 1993 YEAR BOOK OF SPORTS MEDICINE, pp 306–317.
2. Cannon JG: *J Appl Physiol* 74:973, 1993.

Urinary Changes in Ultra Long-Distance Marathon Runners
Kallmeyer JC, Miller NM (St Augustine's Hosp, Durban, Natal, South Africa)
Nephron 64:119–121, 1993   139-94-9–21

Purpose.—Exercise-induced hematuria in marathon runners has been well documented. The difference between upper and lower urinary tract hematuria was determined in ultramarathon runners who participated in the Comrades Marathon, a yearly event held in South Africa.

Methods.—The study sample included 39 male and 6 female runners who completed the 90-km race in less than 11 hours. All runners had completed a comprehensive health questionnaire and physical examination before the race. Athletes with a history of renal disease or those taking analgesics were excluded from the study. Urine specimens were collected before the race, immediately after the race, and on days 3 and 7 postmarathon. Urinalysis included a red cell count, red cell morphology, and measurement of the mean corpuscular volume (MCV).

Results.—Eleven runners (24.4%) had red blood cells in the urine immediately after the race. By the third day after the race, only 4 runners still had hematuria, and by the seventh day, all urinary changes had disappeared. Microscopic examination showed that the red cells in the urine were not dysmorphic; the MCV was greater than 72 fL.

Conclusion.—The hematuria seen in runners after an ultramarathon appears to originate from the lower urinary tract. The urinary changes disappear within 1 week after the event. Urologic investigation for post-exercise hematuria should be postponed until at least 4–7 days after the event.

▶ This study on hematuria in ultramarathoners stirs the debate on where the red blood cells originate. As covered before (1), there is agreement that, in distance runners, microscopic hematuria is common and usually transient and benign. However, disagreement reigns on whether the red cells come from the upper or lower urinary tract. Early reports implicated the kidney, but then the focus shifted to the lower tract, especially the bladder, at least in 10-km runners. Studies on "dysmorphic red cells" brought the focus back to the kidney. Then questions were raised on whether dysmorphic red cells always come from the kidney. Red cells probably vary in shape by how long they have been in the bladder, by the milieu of the urine, and by the eye of the beholder. This study finds that microscopic hematuria in ultramarathoners is common, benign, and transient, and suggests that the red cells come from the bladder. So it goes. See also a practical review of causes and management of hematuria in athletes (2), and a case report illustrating that exercise can be a "stress test" to unmask early bladder cancer (3).—E.R. Eichner, M.D.

References

1. 1988 YEAR BOOK OF SPORTS MEDICINE, pp 126–128.
2. 1991 YEAR BOOK OF SPORTS MEDICINE, p 278.
3. 1992 YEAR BOOK OF SPORTS MEDICINE, pp 247–248.

Moderate to High Intensity Conditioning Leisure Time Physical Activity and High Cardiorespiratory Fitness Are Associated With Reduced Plasma Fibrinogen in Eastern Finnish Men
Lakka TA, Salonen JT (Univ of Kuopio, Finland)
J Clin Epidemiol 46:1119–1127, 1993   139-94-9-22

Background.—Reduced plasma fibrinogen may be a mechanism through which physical activity protects against coronary heart disease (CHD). A quantitative study examined the relationship between plasma fibrinogen concentration and conditioning leisure time physical activity (CLTPA) and maximal oxygen uptake ($\dot{V}O_{2max}$).

Patients and Methods.—A total of 1,384 eastern Finnish men aged 42–60 years participated in this study. Each participant completed a CLTPA history, indicating the frequency, duration, and intensity with which they had performed various physical activities during the past 12 months. Each activity was assigned a metabolic value (MET), which represented the intensity of the physical activity. One MET was equal to ap-

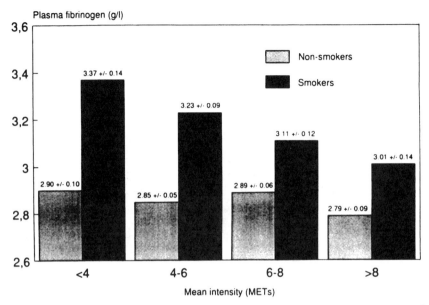

Fig 9–9.—Means and 95% confidence intervals of plasma fibrinogen concentrations in categories of mean intensity of CLTPA among nonsmokers (no. = 935) and smokers (no. = 373). Adjusted for age, examination year, examination day, coffee intake, body mass index, socioeconomic status, regular use of analgesics, and history of rheumatoid arthritis or other rheumatic diseases, diabetes, and stroke. (Courtesy of Lakka TA, Salonen JT: *J Clin Epidemiol* 46:1119-1127, 1993.)

proximately 1 kcal/kg/hr and corresponded to an oxygen uptake of 3.5 mL/kg/min. In addition, a self-administered questionnaire assessing a wide variety of additional variables, such as daily cigarette, cigar, and pipe use; duration of smoking; history of myocardial infarction, angina pectoris, and other CHD; rheumatoid arthritis or other rheumatoid disease, diabetes, and stroke; routine use of analgesics; and socioeconomic status was also completed. Measurements of cardiorespiratory fitness and body mass index were performed, and blood specimens were taken after fasting and abstinence from smoking for 12 hours, abstinence from alcohol for 3 days, and abstinence from analgesic use for 7 days. Plasma fibrinogen concentration was assessed based on clotting of diluted plasma with excess thrombin.

Results.—After adjustment for the strongest covariates, a high mean intensity of CLTPA and a high $\dot{V}O_{2max}$ associated with reduced plasma fibrinogen. The adjusted relative difference in plasma fibrinogen concentration was 6.6% between participants with a mean CLTPA intensity of < 4 and > 8 METs, and 9.1% between the extreme quartiles of $\dot{V}O_{2max}$ (< 2.21 vs. > 2.96L/min). In smokers, the association between the mean intensity of CLTPA and $\dot{V}O_{2max}$ and plasma fibrinogen was stronger than in nonsmokers (Fig 9-9). The correlation between $\dot{V}O_{2max}$ and plasma fibrinogen was also stronger for smokers. Finally, the adjusted

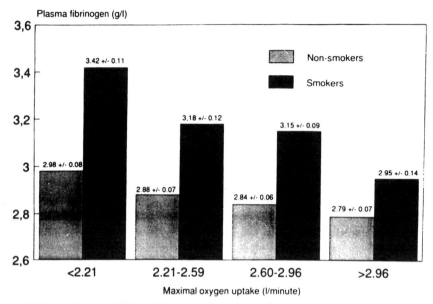

Plasma fibrinogen (g/l)

Maximal oxygen uptake (l/minute)

Fig 9–10.—Means and 95% confidence intervals of plasma fibrinogen concentrations in quartiles of maximal oxygen uptake among nonsmokers (no. = 874) and smokers (no. = 360). Adjusted for age, examination year, examination day, coffee intake, body mass index, socioeconomic status, regular use of analgesics, and history of rheumatoid arthritis or other rheumatic diseases, diabetes, and stroke. (Courtesy of Lakka TA, Salonen JT: *J Clin Epidemiol* 46:1119–1127, 1993.)

relative difference between the extreme quartiles of $\dot{V}O_{2max}$ was 15.9% and 6.8% for smokers and nonsmokers, respectively (Fig 9–10).

Conclusion.—A reduction in plasma fibrinogen may be a mechanism through which moderate to high CLTPA and high cardiorespiratory fitness decrease the risk of CHD.

▶ Lakka and Salonen provide more evidence that exercise is "nature's anti-coagulant." The 6 ways that exercise "thins the blood" were discussed in 1991 (1); the theme was expanded in 1993 (2). A meta-analysis of 6 prospective studies corroborates that fibrinogen is a major cardiovascular risk factor (3). Now, in this first population study of habitual activity, measured fitness, and fibrinogen in middle-aged men, we learn that a lower baseline plasma fibrinogen level (i.e., protection from heart attack and stroke) goes along with increased physical activity and fitness.—E.R. Eichner, M.D.

References

1. 1991 YEAR BOOK OF SPORTS MEDICINE, pp 90–91.
2. 1993 YEAR BOOK OF SPORTS MEDICINE, pp 246–248, 302–306.
3. Ernst E, Resch KL: *Ann Intern Med* 118:956, 1993.

The Effect of Partial Sleep Deprivation on Weight-Lifting Performance

Reilly T, Piercy M (John Moores Univ, Liverpool, England)
Ergonomics 37:107–115, 1994   139-94-9-23

Background.—Even one night of sleep loss can cause a general deterioration in mental performance. Gross motor performance, however, may be reasonably well maintained after partial sleep loss. Thus, it is thought that sleep is needed more for nerve cell restitution than for body tissue restoration. It is unclear whether submaximal efforts and maximal efforts are similarly affected by sleep deprivation. The effects of partial sleep deprivation on submaximal and maximal weight lifting tasks and on subjective states were determined before and after activity.

Subjects and Methods.—The study participants were 8 men, aged 18 to 24 years, who normally slept 8 hours per night and were regularly involved in physical activity. None used weight training on a systematic basis in their fitness program. After baseline measures, the subjects were restricted to 3 hours of sleep on 3 successive nights. A control condition consisted of a 4-day period of normal sleep. Normal and sleep-deprived conditions were separated by 10 days. Weight lifting tasks, performed at submaximal and maximal loads, included the biceps curl, bench press, leg press, and dead lift. Tests conducted each evening determined mood states and subjective sleepiness.

Results.—Sleep loss did not significantly affect the subjects' performance of the maximal biceps curl, but it did significantly alter their ability to perform maximal bench press, leg press, and dead lift. At submaximal load, sleep loss decreased performance for all 4 tasks; the deterioration in performance was significant after the second night of sleep loss. Sleepiness ratings increased linearly with successive days of sleep loss. The sleep-deprivation regimen significantly affected mood states of confusion, vigor, and fatigue, but it did not significantly influence anger, tension, and depression.

Conclusion.—The observed deterioration in mood states after sleep loss probably contributed to the decrease in maximum weights lifted because motivation is crucial to performance in these tasks. Submaximal tasks were affected as well, although a decrease in performance was not always evident after 1 night of deprived sleep. Moods that predispose toward strenuous physical performance exhibited more pronounced changes.

▶ This study on sleep deprivation and weight lifting in men complements recent studies in women and men doing aerobic exercise. In those studies, when 12 young women went 60 hours without sleep, they showed no decrement in endurance performance on cycle ergometry, unlike earlier studies in which men who were deprived of sleep had a decrement on treadmill exercise. In another study involving cycle ergometry, when 15 healthy men went

30 hours without sleep, their maximal exercise capacity was impaired but their exercise endurance was not (1). This study shows that, after only 3 hours of sleep for 3 nights in a row, both mood and strength deteriorated. The changes in mood states (confusion, vigor, fatigue) agree broadly with past research and were not easily reversed by exercise. Both maximal and especially submaximal efforts were attenuated by sleep deprivation, although the effects were not always seen after only 1 night. Tasks involving the larger muscle groups showed greater declines. Maximal lifting decreased most in the last lift performed, suggesting that, in the face of sleep deprivation, negative moods sap the will to perform with maximum effort.—E.R. Eichner, M.D.

Reference

1. 1991 YEAR BOOK OF SPORTS MEDICINE, pp 226–227.

High Prevalence of Asthma in Cross Country Skiers
Larsson K, Ohlsén P, Larsson L, Malmberg P, Rydström P-O, Ulriksen H (Natl Inst of Occupational Health, Solna, Sweden; Swedish Ski Assoc, Stockholm; Hosp of Östersund, Sweden)
BMJ 307:1326–1329, 1993   139-94-9-24

Introduction.—Swedish physicians have observed that asthma symptoms and bronchial responsiveness are more common in cross-country skiers than in nonskiers. In contrast to most other sports, cross-country skiing involves training and competing at low temperatures, with athletes inhaling large amounts of cold air for long periods. The relationship between cross-country skiing and asthma-like symptoms was investigated.

Subjects and Methods.—The study participants were 42 elite skiers from 6 Swedish cross-country teams. The 36 men and 6 women (mean age, 24 years) had competed actively for a mean of 13 years. Twenty-nine healthy controls were age-matched nonskiers who had never smoked. Both groups were examined for bronchial responsiveness, asthma symptoms, and lung function.

Results.—The cross-country skiers had significantly greater vital capacity, total lung capacity, and forced expiratory volume in 1 second than the nonskiing controls. In both winter and summer, skiers had an increased bronchial responsiveness compared with controls. Skiers were significantly more likely than nonskiers to have coughing, abnormal shortness of breath, chest tightness, and wheezing related to exercise, cold, or inhaled stimuli. Fifteen skiers used antiasthmatic drugs regularly, and 13 had physician-diagnosed asthma. Asthma, as defined by the study criteria, was present in 14 of 42 skiers but in only 1 of 29 nonskiers.

Conclusion.—There is a higher prevalence of asthma, asthma-like symptoms, and bronchial responsiveness in cross-country skiers than in the general population and nonskiers. These symptoms occurred even in the summer when the skiers had not been exposed to cold air for several months. Although strenuous training by itself has not been found to increase the risk of asthma, such exercise at low temperatures does appear to be a cause of asthma.

▶ This article brings news about asthma that bears confirmation by others. It finds that asthma is more common in cross-country skiers, both in winter and summer, than in the general population or in nonskiing controls. The authors suggest that breathing large amounts of cold air for several hours per week, several months per year—as skiers do—may cause asthma in healthy people.—E.R. Eichner, M.D.

Cardiovascular Responses to Shoveling in a Thermoneutral, Cold, and Cold With Wind Environment
Emmett JD, Hodgson JL (Pennsylvania State Univ, University Park)
J Cardiopulmon Rehabil 13:43–50, 1993   139-94-9-25

Background.—The cardiovascular effects of shoveling snow in a cold environment result from the combination of high myocardial oxygen consumption accompanied by vasoconstriction of the coronary and peripheral blood vessels caused by exposure to cold. One study of patients with stable cardiac disease in a rehabilitation program determined a safe level of 4.9 times resting metabolism (METs) for shoveling snow. The effect of shoveling at different rates was compared, and the effect of wind as a possible contributor to the level of cardiovascular stress was studied.

Method.—Ten healthy men between the ages of 40 and 61 years shoveled blocks of wood in 3 environmental conditions: thermoneutral with no wind, cold with no wind, and cold with wind. Heart rate and blood pressure were measured during exercise and at rest. Comparisons were made between younger and older men and patients with different percentages of body fat.

Findings.—The mean heart rate at a high shoveling rate and a moderate rate was significantly higher than at a low shoveling rate in all environments. Shoveling in cold conditions with wind significantly lowered the heart rate in comparison with a thermoneutral environment. All cardiovascular responses were higher in men with a higher percentage of body fat in the cold or cold with wind environments. This suggests greater heat storage in subjects with higher body fat percentages, independent of the environment (table). The older men had a lower diastolic blood pressure after shoveling in cold and cold with wind. Systolic blood pressure was significantly higher in the cold environment after shoveling than in the thermoneutral environment. As a result, there was no difference in postshoveling rate–pressure product between environments.

Conclusion.—Shoveling in cold conditions with wind significantly lowered the heart rate compared with shoveling in a thermoneutral envi-

Cardiovascular Responses of Individuals With Low Body Fat and High Body Fat During Shoveling in 3 Environmental Conditions

	Thermoneutral		Cold		Cold with wind	
	Low body fat	High body fat	Low body fat	High body fat	Low body fat	High body fat
Shoveling HR (beats/min)	118.7 ± 4.8	121.7 ± 4.5	104.3 ± 4.5	122.3 ± 4.9*	101.7 ± 5.8	113.1 ± 4.9*
Post-Shoveling SBP (mm Hg)	112.4 ± 2.6	125.8 ± 5.6*	126.7 ± 2.7	139.1 ± 7.5	123.2 ± 3.5	138.1 ± 6.3*
Post-Shoveling RPP (/100)	133.7 ± 6.5	152.5 ± 8.2	131.2 ± 4.8	168.8 ± 10.3	125.4 ± 8.0	155.9 ± 9.8*
Post-Shoveling DBP (mm Hg)	61.5 ± 2.3	74.8 ± 2.5*	67.5 ± 2.9	75.7 ± 1.4*	62.2 ± 2.5	74.5 ± 2.2*

Abbreviations: HR, heart rate; SBP, systolic blood pressure; RPP, rate–pressure product; DBP, diastolic blood pressure; TN, thermoneutral environment (mean temp, 22.2°C); C, cold environment (mean temp, 4.9°C); CW, cold environment with wind (mean temp, 4.8°C with 1.9 m/sec wind).
* P < .05.
(Courtesy of Emmett JD, Hodgson JL: J Cardiopulmon Rehabil 13:43–50, 1993.)

ronment. Age had no significant effect on heart rate. All cardiovascular responses were higher in men with a higher percentage of body fat in the cold or cold with wind environments. Healthy men shoveling at 5 MET or less in a cold environment with or without wind had the protective effect of a lower heart rate. This blunted heart rate response may counter an increase in systolic blood pressure, thus minimizing the increase in rate–pressure product.

▶ Various authors have raised the spectre that shoveling snow precipitates heart attacks in people with silent myocardial ischemia. A search of records in large cities reveals few actual instances in which heart attacks have been linked to shoveling, although epidemiologic studies do suggest some increase in coronary deaths if there has been a major snowfall (1–3). In real life, variables include not only the coldness of the weather but the depth, wetness, and age of the snow; packing by municipal snowplows; and anxiety about clearing a drive against a tight time schedule. In this experiment, a standard 4-kg load of wood was lifted by a 3-kg shovel, and the rate of shoveling was judged to elicit 30% to 47% of maximal oxygen intake; the test thus mimicked leisurely snow clearing rather than a frantic 7 A.M. rush. The cold temperatures would have been better expressed as the corresponding windchill factor; in any event, it is difficult to compare them with normal snow shoveling because the subjects were apparently wearing no more than shoes, socks, and shorts! However, it is interesting that a greater increase of systemic blood pressures during cold exposure can be offset by a slower heart rate, which may be relevant to activities that are performed while wearing more realistic clothing.—R.J. Shephard, M.D., Ph.D.

References

1. Baker-Blocker A: *Am J Public Health* 72:261, 1982.
2. Rogot E, Padgett SJ: *Am J Epidemiol* 103:565, 1976.
3. Glass RI, Zack MM: *Lancet* 1:485, 1979.

Encephalopathy Due to Severe Hyponatremia in an Ultramarathon Runner
Clark JM, Gennari FJ (Univ of Vermont, Burlington)
West J Med 159:188–189, 1993   139-94-9-26

Introduction.—Some athletes who participate in endurance events have acute hyponatremia. In 1 ultramarathon runner, severe hyponatremia with life-threatening encephalopathy occurred about 1 hour after he dropped out of a race because of foot blisters.

Case Report.—Man, 57, previously healthy, became confused and disoriented, then had a seizure after completing 55 miles of a 100-mile ultramarathon. He had decorticate posturing and his neck veins were distended to the angle of the jaw. He had taken ibuprofen for a few days before the race and drank 12 L of a glucose and water solution during the race. Laboratory studies revealed a serum level of sodium of 119 mmol/L and an osmolality of 248 mmol per kg of water. Urinary sodium excretion was 39 mmol/L. Results of noncontrast CT of his head were normal. Anisocoria was noted. He was treated with intravenous furosemide, mannitol, and 3% saline solution. The patient gradually recovered during the next 4 days.

Discussion.—Part of the fluids ingested by the athlete during the race may not have been absorbed, and this sequestered water may have been rapidly absorbed on cessation of the exercise. Reperfusion of the splanchnic bed probably led to the abrupt decrease in serum concentration of sodium and expansion of body fluid volume. Because severe hyponatremia has been reported with the use of nonsteroidal anti-inflammatory drugs (NSAIDs) such as ibuprofen, athletes should be instructed about the effects of NSAIDs on renal function and urinary dilution and warned against overzealous fluid ingestion during endurance exercise.

▶ This is another report of life-threatening hyponatremia during an ultramarathon. Although the mechanism is debated, most experts think the best hypothesis is voluntary overhydration with water (and/or other very hypotonic fluids) in the face of moderate sodium loss in the sweat. I know of 2 severe cases of hyponatremia during or after standard marathons: One is rumored to have played a role in the death of a young woman in California in 1993; the other was reported in 1988 (1). Also, hyponatremia occurred in 4 women who drank only water as they hiked into the Grand Canyon (2). If too little water can kill you, so can too much. To stave off hyponatremia during distance events one must keep the following rules in mind. Don't overhydrate; drink no more water than you lose ("A pint a pound the world around"). Drink not only water (or diluted cola or fruit juice), but also a sports drink with sodium in it, like Gatorade. During an ultramarathon, consume sodium-rich foods (e.g., pretzels, crackers, salted rice balls, or chicken broth). Lightly salt your food daily during hot-weather training.—E.R. Eichner, M.D.

References

1. Nelson PB, et al: *Physician Sportsmed* 16:78, 1988.
2. Backer HD, et al: *Med Sci Sports Exerc* 25:S87, 1993.

Operation Everest II: Spirometric and Radiographic Changes in Acclimatized Humans at Simulated High Altitudes
Welsh CH, Wagner PD, Reeves JT, Lynch D, Cink TM, Armstrong J, Malconian MK, Rock PB, Houston CS (Univ of Colorado, Denver; Univ of California, San Diego; United States Army Research Inst of Environmental Medicine, Natick, Mass; et al)
Am Rev Respir Dis 147:1239–1244, 1993   139-94-9–27

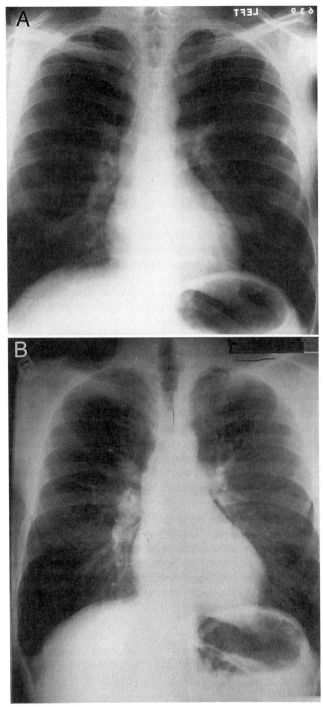

Fig 9–11.—Chest radiographs of patient before descent (**A**) and approximately 1 hour after descent (**B**) from 240 mm Hg. Note hilar prominence and increased vascular markings. (Courtesy of Welsh CH, Wagner PD, Reeves JT, et al: *Am Rev Respir Dis* 147:1239-1244, 1993.)

Objective.—The effects of acute exposure to altitudes of up to 17,000 feet are well recognized. However, there are no data on the effects of higher altitudes, as would occur during a climb of Mount Everest. The restricted lung volumes and flow rates that occur at altitude could be related to a variety of factors, including increased pulmonary or thoracic blood volume, abdominal gas trapping, muscle fatigue, and interstitial edema. As part of Operation Everest II, pulmonary function studies were performed in volunteers subjected to conditions simulating the altitudes experienced during a climb of the Himalayan Mountains.

Methods.—Eight healthy young men were subjected to progressive lowering of barometric pressure during 40 days in an altitude chamber. The conditions were designed to simulate those which would be experienced during a climb of Mount Everest. Subjects were exposed to altitude conditions as high as 8,848 m above sea level. In addition to exercise testing and pulmonary function studies, the subjects underwent chest radiography within 2 hours after descent from maximum altitude to assess the presence of subclinical edema. Airway physiologic and chest radiographic findings were correlated with symptom scores, hemodynamic physiology, and gas exchange.

Findings.—Forced vital capacity declined significantly and progressively by 14% during the 40-day study. This alteration resolved gradually in the 2 days after descent. Midrange forced expiratory flow increased by 82% at altitude, most likely as the result of reduced air density. There was no change in forced expiratory volume in 1 second, however. The postdescent chest radiographs revealed evidence of pulmonary artery enlargement and interstitial edema (Fig 9–11). Mean pulmonary artery pressure measurements were elevated at altitude, both at rest and during exercise; however, pressures were no higher in the subjects with the greatest signs of edema. Ventilation perfusion measurements in 4 subjects showed 1% to 11% of blood flowing through areas of low ventilation-perfusion units.

Conclusion.—A restrictive spirometric change with exposure to high altitudes was demonstrated. This change apparently results from an increase in chest fluid, which is caused by increased pulmonary blood volume and interstitial edema. The 2 causes appear to be about equal in magnitude. Pulmonary edema and increased pulmonary blood volume are thus of potential concern in human beings acutely exposed to high altitude, especially during exercise.

▶ This research was part of the ambitious and productive Operation Everest II (1), in which 8 healthy male volunteers were gradually decompressed during 40 days and 40 nights until they reached the summit of Mt. Everest (6 made it all the way). It shows convincingly, based on clinical data and impressive chest radiographs, that the altitude-related decrease in forced vital capacity is a restrictive change owing mainly to an increase in pulmonary blood volume and interstitial edema. Such a change may play a role in high-altitude pulmonary edema. See also Abstracts 139-94-9–28 and 139-94-9–29. —E.R. Eichner, M.D.

Reference

1. 1993 YEAR BOOK OF SPORTS MEDICINE, pp 409–410.

Treatment of Acute Mountain Sickness by Simulated Descent: A Randomised Controlled Trial
Bärtsch P, Merki B, Hofstetter D, Maggiorini M, Kayser B, Oelz O (Univ Clinic of Medicine, Heidelberg, Germany; Univ Hosp, Zurich, Switzerland; Univ of Geneva)
BMJ 306:1098–1101, 1993   139-94-9–28

Introduction.—High-altitude illness is relatively common in climbers, and acute mountain sickness may progress to the life-threatening conditions of cerebral and pulmonary edema. The treatment of choice, rapid descent, is not always possible. The therapeutic effects of using a portable hyperbaric chamber for treatment of acute mountain sickness were evaluated. Unlike bottled oxygen, the portable chamber is lightweight (4-6 kg) and represents an inexhaustible device for rapid improvement of oxygenation.

Subjects and Methods.—A controlled trial was carried out during 2 mountaineering seasons at a high-altitude (4,559 m) research laboratory in the Alps Valais. The subjects were mountaineers who had ascended by foot and experienced headache and 1 or more additional symptoms of acute mountain sickness. Individuals with clinical signs of high-altitude pulmonary edema and those who had taken acetazolamide or nifedipine during ascent were excluded. The 64 subjects were randomized to 1 hour of treatment in the hyperbaric chamber at pressures of 193 mbar or 20 mbar, or to bed rest. They were evaluated before, immediately after, and 12 hours after treatment. Analgesics and antiemetic drugs were allowed during follow-up.

Results.—The 3 groups did not differ significantly in age or time at altitude before treatment. The median oxygen saturation was 90% during treatment in the 193-mbar group, significantly higher than the 70% overall pretreatment value in the other groups. The decreases in clinical score during treatment and immediately after treatment were significantly greater in the 193-mbar group than in the 20-mbar and rest groups. After 12 hours, however, the 3 groups showed similar improvement in symptom scores.

Conclusion.—One hour of treatment with a portable hyperbaric chamber using a pressure of 193 mbar corresponds to a descent of 2,250 m. This treatment led to a short-term improvement in symptoms of acute mountain sickness, but it was not associated with long-term benefits. The 3 groups had similar intakes of analgesic and antiemetic drugs during follow-up and similar symptom scores after 12 hours.

▶ This controlled trial of the fabric hyperbaric chamber, or Gamow Bag, raises questions about long-term benefit. Experts in altitude medicine feel that the Gamow Bag works acutely for acute mountain sickness and belongs in the "high-altitude therapeutic armament" (1). This article confirms that, immediately after use, the Gamow Bag relieves the symptoms of acute mountain sickness better than control pressurization (only 20 mbar of pressure) or bed rest. However, 12 hours later, all 3 groups had improved to the same extent, suggesting that bed rest alone, along with the feeling of being taken care of, can improve the symptoms of acute mountain sickness despite having no improvement in oxygenation. See also Abstracts 139-94-9–27 and 139-94-9–29.—E.R. Eichner, M.D.

Reference

1. 1993 YEAR BOOK OF SPORTS MEDICINE, pp 412–413.

Acute Mountain Sickness in a General Tourist Population at Moderate Altitudes

Honigman B, Theis MK, Koziol-McLain J, Roach R, Yip R, Houston C, Moore LG (Colorado Altitude Research Inst, Keystone; Univ of Colorado, Denver; Lovelace Med Found, Albuquerque, NM; et al)
Ann Intern Med 118:587–592, 1993   139-94-9–29

Purpose.—Acute mountain sickness (AMS)—the development of headache, fatigue, shortness of breath, sleeplessness, and anorexia after a rapid ascent to high altitude—is common among mountain visitors. Although the population at risk is large (e.g., more than 13 million individuals visited the Colorado mountains in 1990), there are few data on the frequency and severity of AMS in the general population at moderate altitudes. A survey design was used to assess the incidence of AMS in a general population of individuals visiting moderate elevations.

Methods.—The study sample comprised 3,158 adult travelers (mean age, 43.8 years) who were attending conferences at resort locations in the Colorado Rocky Mountains. The resorts were located at elevations of 6,300-9,700 ft. The study questionnaire requested demographic, medical, and other types of information in addition to whether the subjects had any symptoms of AMS. The response rate was 75%.

Results.—Symptoms of AMS were reported by 25% of the respondents (Fig 9-12). In nearly two thirds, the symptoms developed within 12 hours of arrival at the resort. Acute mountain sickness was 3.5 times more common for subjects whose permanent residence was below 3,000 ft. Symptoms were nearly 3 times as common for those who had previously had mountain sickness and twice as common for subjects younger

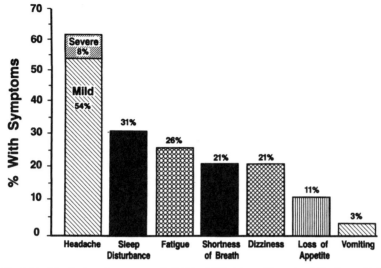

Fig 9–12.—Distribution of symptoms of AMS in 3,072 visitors. (Courtesy of Honigman B, Theis MK, Koziol-McLain J, et al: *Ann Intern Med* 118:587–592, 1993.)

than age 60 years. Symptoms of AMS were also more common in women, obese subjects, individuals who reported themselves to be in average-to-poor physical condition, and individuals with lung diseases (Fig 9–13).

Conclusion.—This study finds a 25% incidence of AMS in a general population of visitors to moderate altitudes. Mountain sickness usually affects an individual's activities. Acute mountain sickness appears to be

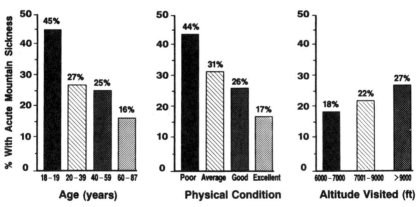

Fig 9–13.—Percentage of AMS in visitors to moderate altitudes according to age, physical condition, and altitude visited. Physical condition was a self-assessed measure. **Left,** no. = 3,143, $P < .001$; **middle,** no. = 3,119, $P < .001$; **right,** no. = 2,812, $P < .001$. (Courtesy of Honigman B, Theis MK, Koziol-McLain J, et al: *Ann Intern Med* 118:587–592, 1993.)

more common in younger individuals and those who are less physically fit, live at sea level, have a history of such symptoms, or have underlying lung problems.

▶ This informative article finds a surprisingly high incidence of AMS in recreational tourists—mainly middle-aged men—who travel to ski resorts in Colorado. Apparently, 25% of such tourists experience symptoms of AMS, most commonly headache and fatigue. In most cases, symptoms begin soon after arrival. Although AMS is usually self-limited, half of those with symptoms reduced their activity or took analgesics. No link to alcohol use was found here, but the authors don't quibble with the conventional wisdom that alcohol can aggravate AMS. Others claim that this study, based only on questionnaires, overestimates the incidence of AMS; but the authors, noting that the incidence of AMS is determined by individual susceptibility, altitude reached, and rate of ascent, successfully defend their findings (1). See also Abstracts 139-94-9–27 and 139-94-9–28.—E.R. Eichner, M.D.

Reference

1. Letters to the editor: *Ann Intern Med* 119:633, 1993.

Pulmonary Function One and Four Years After a Deep Saturation Dive

Thorsen E, Segadal K, Kambestad BK, Gulsvik A (Norwegian Underwater Technology Centre A/S, Ytre Laksevåg, Norway; Univ of Bergen, Norway)
Scand J Work Environ Health 19:115–120, 1993   139-94-9–30

Introduction.—Maintenance of oil and gas production in the North Sea requires diving operations at depths of 50–360 m, which corresponds to pressures of 0.6–3.7 mPa. Adjustment to these pressures is accomplished by saturation diving. Divers are compressed to the working pressure in a hyperbaric chamber complex and then transferred in a diving bell to the work site. The inert atmospheric gas is usually helium, and the partial pressure of oxygen is increased to ensure oxygenation under these conditions. Cross-sectional studies have indicated that airflow limitation develops in divers in relation to their diving exposure. To study these lung function changes, a longitudinal follow-up study of pulmonary function was performed in a group of Norwegian professional saturation divers who had participated in a deep experimental saturation dive to pressures of 3.1–4.6 mPa.

Subjects.—Twenty-four Norwegian professional saturation divers who had participated in deep saturation dives were compared with 28 Norwegian professional saturation divers who performed ordinary saturation diving at pressures of 0.8–1.6 mPa. They were examined 1 and 4 years after the period of the deep dives. There were no significant differences

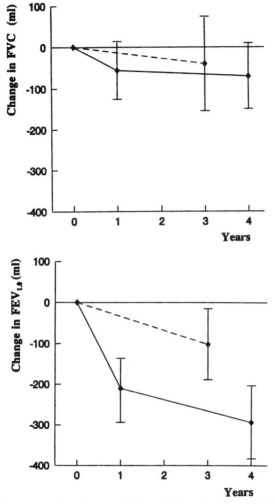

Fig 9–14.—Change in forced vital capacity (FVC) and FEV₁ in deep divers (*solid line*) 1 and 4 years after a deep saturation dive and in reference divers (*dashed line*). The mean reductions in FVC and FEV₁ are shown. (Courtesy of Thorsen E, Segadal K, Kambestad BK, et al: *Scand J Work Environ Health* 19:115-120, 1993.)

between these 2 groups in age, height, weight, smoking history, or initial pulmonary function.

Findings.—Among the deep divers, a significant reduction in forced expiratory volume in 1 second (FEV₁) occurred the first year after the deep dive. After this initial reduction, the annual reduction did not differ from that in the referent saturation divers (Fig 9-14). The forced midexpiratory flow rate and forced expiratory flow rates at low lung volumes were also significantly reduced at 1 year in the deep divers, whereas the closing volume was increased. There were no significant changes in forced vital capacity.

Conclusion.—These findings demonstrate that in the year after the deep dive, there were significant reductions in FEV_1 and forced expiratory flow rates that did not recover in the following 3 years. These results are consistent with the development of airflow limitation in deep saturation divers. The characteristics of their lung function cannot be explained by adaptation or selection. The causes of the changes in lung function have yet to be defined.

▶ An increasing number of divers now spend long periods at great depths. The health consequences of such a lifestyle will only emerge gradually through cumulative experience. The authors' data suggest a substantial (210 mL) loss of FEV_1 in the first year after exposure. The reason for this loss is unknown, but the authors speculate that a toxic reaction to high oxygen pressures (40–60 kPa) may be involved.—R.J. Shephard, M.D., Ph.D.

The Roentgenographic Findings Associated With Air Embolism in Sport Scuba Divers

Harker CP, Neuman TS, Olson LK, Jacoby I, Santos A (Univ of Washington, Seattle; Univ of California, San Diego; Southern Colorado Heart and Lung Group, Pueblo)
J Emerg Med 11:443–449, 1993   139-94-9-31

Introduction.—Arterial gas embolism (AGE) ranks second to drowning as the most common cause of death among scuba divers. The risk for having AGE develop is greatest during panic ascents when pulmonary overinflation may occur. Researchers retrospectively examined the clinical history, physical examinations, and chest roentgenograms (CXR) of 31 scuba divers treated for AGE from 1982 to 1989.

Patients and Methods.—The divers had a mean age of 31.7 years; 26 were male. The range of the maximum depth of the dives was 2.4–61 m (8–200 ft) and 61% of the dives were greater than 18 m (60 ft) in depth. Bottom time, available for 28 divers, was more than 15 minutes in 13 cases. The divers' clinical records were evaluated for signs and symptoms of AGE and a history of aspiration. The approximate time until recompression was also noted. Two of the authors examined the CXRs for each patient, paying attention to conditions possibly predisposing to barotrauma, evidence of pulmonary barotrauma, and signs of pleural effusion or infiltrate.

Results.—Two divers were declared dead and were not recompressed. The average time to recompression was 5.7 hours. Fourteen of 16 divers seen with a history of aspiration had CXRs compatible with this condition. Most (74%) of the patients had significant neurologic deficits ranging from coma and paralysis to decreased coordination and difficulty with constructions. Infiltrates were seen in 16 of 31 CXRs. Eight patients had pneumomediastinum and 1 had a small left pleural effusion. Because radiographic evidence of barotrauma could be subtle, it was overlooked in 4 patients. Extra-alveolar air indicative of barotrauma was often identified along the left cardiac border, descending aorta, aortic arch, and hilar vessels.

Conclusion.—Pulmonary overinflation with AGE can occur even in shallow depths or after apparently normal ascents. Arterial gas embolism is usually diagnosed on the basis of clinical findings and history and is treated by recompression, regardless of radiographic findings. A chest roentgenogram is valuable, however, in excluding pneumothorax, confirming the presence of pulmonary barotrauma, and showing evidence of concomitant near-drowning.

▶ A small tear in the pulmonary vasculature during overdistension of the lungs can allow air emboli to enter the circulation; if such emboli lodge in the cerebral circulation, death can result. Some authors have suggested that such emboli account for as many as 30% of diving deaths (1). Factors that can contribute to such a disaster include breath-holding during ascent, panic, and the sharing of an air supply (2). Much of the research on this topic has concerned submarine escape training rather than the use of scuba equipment; it is important to recognize that in submarine escape training, emergency measures including a high-pressure chamber are much more readily available. Although radiographs can be helpful in showing associated mediastinal emphysema or pneumothorax, the diagnosis often has to be reached on clinical findings of a neurologic deficit.—R.J. Shephard, M.D., Ph.D.

References

1. Kizer KW: *Emerg Med* 16:535, 1987.
2. Dick APK, Massey EW: *Neurology* 35:667, 1985.

Sickle Cell Trait, Heroic Exercise, and Fatal Collapse
Eichner ER (Univ of Oklahoma, Oklahoma City)
Physician Sportsmed 21:51–64, 1993   139-94-9–32

Background.—Although the evidence is incomplete and controversial, it seems likely that the presence of sickle cell trait (SCT) contributes to exercise-related collapse and subsequent death. Of the more than 30 such cases reported since 1970, most were in military recruits or college athletes who collapsed after an unaccustomed level of exertion.

The Sickle Cell Trait.—The trait, which is present in 8% of American blacks, is usually benign. People with SCT have appeared to have a normal exercise capacity. Nevertheless, SCT does pose a small risk of gross hematuria and splenic infarction and may be a serious hazard for people who undertake maximal, unaccustomed exercise. And growing evidence suggests that such exercise can evoke a life-threatening syndrome of sickling, fulminant rhabdomyolysis, lactic acidosis, collapse, acute renal failure, and hyperkalemia.

SCT and Sudden Death.—The first reports of a link between SCT and sudden death came from the military. In 1970, 4 black recruits died during basic combat training at altitude; all had SCT. Four additional trainees, all with SCT, collapsed from 1970 to 1974. All needed dialysis for renal failure and 1 died of hyperkalemia. Three similar cases were reported between 1974 and 1985. The total of such deaths now stands at 20. Similar collapses, and in some cases death, have occurred in black athletes with SCT. In vitro studies suggest that the rate of sickling in SCT is accelerated by the extreme milieu of the exercising limbs: acidosis, hyperthermia, and red cell dehydration. Recent research involving men with SCT who rode cycle ergometers indicates that sickling and symptoms occur during maximal exercise at altitude.

Conclusion.—A review of sudden deaths associated with SCT suggests that brief, "heroic" exercise can take an individual from the peak of health to the brink of death as a result of sickling in the microvasculature of exercising muscles. It is important that physicians and coaches be aware of this syndrome and that athletes train wisely, especially in hot weather or at altitude.

Sickle Cell Trait: A Risk Factor for Life-Threatening Rhabdomyolysis?
Browne RJ, Gillespie CA (Alabama Sports Medicine, Birmingham; Samford Univ, Birmingham, Ala)
Physician Sportsmed 21:80–88, 1993   139-94-9–33

Objective.—Many black athletes are unaware of their sickle cell status and may be at risk for sudden death when exercising in high heat, humidity, and/or altitude. Exertional rhabdomyolysis was diagnosed in an athlete with sickle cell trait.

Case Report.—A black man, 20, had pain in the lower back, thighs, and calves after a run on the first day of football practice at a southeastern college. The patient was known to have sickle cell trait but had not experienced any previous medical problems of note. He was seen in the emergency department in significant discomfort and was admitted for evaluation on the basis of laboratory studies. Treatment consisting of vigorous parenteral hydration and supplemental oxygen was started. The following day, his creatine kinase (CK) peaked at 23,680 units/L with serum glutamic oxaloacetic transaminase (SGOT) at 286 units/L. After about 24 hours, the patient's pain decreased significantly.

At the time of his discharge, 4 days after admission, pain was completely resolved, CK was 6,260 units/L, SGOT was 136 units/L, and serum glutamic pyruvic transaminase was 11 units/L. Exertional rhabdomyolysis and exercise-induced asthma were diagnosed and the patient was started on a program of monitored exercise and allowed to return to full practices and games within 2 weeks. He was advised to remain well hydrated and not to resume distance running. During games, he received oxygen on the sidelines.

Discussion.—Many black athletes have sickle cell trait, some of whom are unaware of their status. Although the trait is normally considered a harmless carrier state or condition, some individuals may be at risk for rhabdomyolysis, acute renal tubular necrosis, disseminated intravascular coagulopathy, or even sudden death. When deprived of fluids, individuals with sickle cell trait become dehydrated, which predisposes them to impaired blood flow and hypoxemia. The resultant lactic acidosis initiates the sickling process.

Conclusion.—Team physicians should test athletes whose sport requires prolonged exertion—especially in extremes of heat, humidity, or altitude—for sickle cell trait. An athlete in whom the trait is identified needs to take special precautions, possibly choosing a college in a northern climate.

▶ These 2 articles (Abstracts 139-94-9–32 and 139-94-9–33) emphasize a rare yet grave hazard of "heroic exercise" among athletes with sickle cell trait (SCT). Fortunately, SCT is generally benign and consistent with top athletic performance. There are the expected number of athletes with SCT in the NFL, in high school football, and among elite athletes and runners in Africa. In rare individuals with SCT, however, as shown in this review and case report, all-out exercise, especially in hot weather or when new at altitude, can evoke a life-threatening syndrome of sickling in working limbs, fulminant rhabdomyolysis, lactic acidosis, shock, collapse, acute renal failure, and hyperkalemia.

Physicians and coaches must know that this unique syndrome can mimic other causes of collapse, and that prompt diagnosis and therapy can save lives. The review outlines the scope of the problem; the case report shows that not all cases are life-threatening, that early diagnosis can prevent problems, and that special care can enable the athlete to compete. Coaches (especially in the South or at altitude) should enforce preseason conditioning of athletes and stop trying to "separate the men from the boys" on the first day of practice. All athletes should train wisely, stay hydrated, heed environmental stress and early warning signs (e.g., severe cramping), and never bolt into heroic exercise. Why die to make the team? Schools and colleges should consider informed, voluntary screening of all athletes for SCT.—E.R. Eichner, M.D.

Toxic Effects From Nitrogen Dioxide in Ice-Skating Arenas
Soparkar G, Mayers I, Edouard L, Hoeppner VH (Univ of Saskatchewan, Saskatoon, Canada)
Can Med Assoc J 148:1181–1182, 1993   139-94-9–34

Introduction.—Malfunctioning ice-resurfacing machines can cause nitrogen dioxide to accumulate in poorly ventilated indoor ice-skating arenas. One hockey player had nitrogen dioxide poisoning, a potentially lethal condition.

Case Report.—Man, 43, was seen with a cough with blood-stained sputum, severe orthopnea, and cyanosis. His symptoms had started 3 days earlier after he had played in an ice hockey tournament. The man was afebrile and tachypneic, and crackles were heard in all lung fields. A chest radiograph showed bilateral centrifugal airspace disease, and lung function tests revealed a diffusing capacity of 82% of the predicted norm. The patient received oxygen and diuretics when left ventricular failure was erroneously diagnosed. Two days later, a chest radiograph showed resolution of the airspace disease.

Findings.—After a similar cough occurred in all the other hockey players and several officials, it was determined that the ventilation fans in the arena had not been working the day of the tournament and that the ice-resurfacing machine was not functioning properly. A gas-detector tube system tested the air in the arena 30 days after the tournament. When the fans were operating normally, the nitrogen dioxide levels were below the safe maximum. The exhaust fumes of the resurfacing machine, however, had levels twice that of the recommended maximum of 1 ppm.

Conclusion.—Nitrogen dioxide poisoning, unlike carbon monoxide poisoning, may not produce immediate symptoms. Irritation of the upper respiratory tract is often not apparent until the day after exposure. Patients with nitrogen dioxide poisoning have symptoms of acute pulmonary edema and frequently receive a misdiagnosis. Proper precautions need to be taken in facilities used for ice skating and hockey. Nitrogen dioxide poisoning is potentially lethal and may even affect the spectators in a poorly ventilated arena.

▶ Acute exposure to nitrogen dioxide concentrations above 5–10 ppm may produce severe cough, hemoptysis, chest pain, and pulmonary edema. Asthmatics are especially vulnerable. Because the gas is heavier than air, it settles above the ice. This patient had the most severe symptoms because he had played at the end of the day and had skated longer and harder than the other players, thereby having the highest minute ventilation.

The few reports in the literature of nitrogen dioxide poisoning in arenas probably underrepresent the problem because the condition is poorly recognized. In a 1994 survey, the 1-week average nitrogen dioxide concentration was above 1 ppm in 10% of 70 northeastern American ice-skating rinks. Considering that short-term peak concentrations were likely to have reached 2–5 times the measured 1-week average, this suggests that nitrogen dioxide levels in such rinks may be a public health hazard (1). Others have studied the acute pulmonary effects of nitrogen dioxide exposure during treadmill running (2).—E.R. Eichner, M.D.

References

1. Brauer M, Spengler JD: *Am J Publ Health* 84:429, 1994.
2. 1992 YEAR BOOK OF SPORTS MEDICINE, pp 163–164.

10 Cardiorespiratory and Miscellaneous Diseases

Increased Life Expectancy of World Class Male Athletes
Sarna S, Sahi T, Koskenvuo M, Kaprio J (Univ of Helsinki)
Med Sci Sports Exerc 25:237–244, 1993   139-94-10-1

Introduction.—Moderate physical activity is known to decrease the risk of cardiovascular disease and increase life expectancy (LE). Little is known, however, about the long-term effects of training at maximal level on chronic diseases and LE. Therefore, Finnish male world-class athletes in a number of sports were studied to compare their estimated LE with that of healthy young Finnish men.

Subjects and Methods.—The athletes had represented Finland at least once in the Olympic Games, World or European championships, or intercountry competitions between 1920 and 1965. Sports selected for the study were track and field, cross-country skiing, soccer, ice hockey, basketball, boxing, wrestling, weight lifting, and shooting. The 2,613 athletes were compared with 1,712 twenty-year-old Finnish men who were classified as completely healthy at the time of induction to compulsory military service. Vital status of the athletes and conscripts was recorded as of May 1989. A questionnaire was sent in 1985 to the 2,851 survivors of the original cohort.

Results.—Athletes were more likely than referents to belong to the executive or clerical class in 1985 (70% vs. 30%) and to be married (94.1% vs. 85.8%). After adjustment for occupational group, there was a statistically significant difference between the survival curves of referents and cross-country skiers and long-distance runners. The mean LE adjusted for occupational group, marital status, and age at entry to the cohort ranged from 71.5 years for power-sports participants to 75.6 years for athletes in endurance sports; the adjusted LE for referents was 69.9 years. A decrease in cardiovascular mortality accounted for most of the difference between athletes and referents.

Conclusion.—Surviving athletes had a healthier and physically more active lifestyle than the referents. Life expectancies were increased significantly for both endurance athletes and team athletes, mainly because of lower rate of cardiovascular and cancer mortality in former world-class athletes. It is also likely that the athletes had a higher social status and a wider social support network than average members of their socioeconomic class.

▶ Perhaps the true explanation for this observed phenomenon lies less in the athletes' healthier and physically more active lifestyle and more in accord with the basic tenets of the Darwinian theory of evolution and the survival of the fittest.—J.S. Torg, M.D.

Preventing Sudden Death: The Role of Automated Defibrillators
Simons SM, Berry J (Univ of Notre Dame, Ind)
Physician Sportsmed 21:53–54,57–59, 1993   139-94-10-2

Value of Early Defibrillation.—A King County, Washington study reported that, when physician attention followed a paramedic response using a standard defibrillator, the rate of survival from cardiac arrest was 17%. The response time for the paramedic team averaged nearly 9 minutes, whereas firefighters equipped with the automated external defibrillator (AED) responded in an average of $3^1/_2$ minutes. Once at the scene, the AED saves further valuable time compared with the standard defibrillator. Clinical outcome reports provide compelling evidence for the value of AEDs in the field.

Safe Operation.—The AED possesses sophisticated circuitry and complex computer algorithms that are able to identify potentially lethal arrhythmias, rendering the presence of a skilled observer unnecessary. Most models are designed to recognize and shock for ventricular fibrillation and rapid ventricular tachycardia, either automatically or with a machine prompt. Using the AED, members of the sports medicine team who are likely to be on the scene first can provide early defibrillation. The device is reportedly totally specific when used in patients in full cardiac arrest who lack a pulse and are not breathing. Hands-on practice, critical feedback, and verbal reinforcement all are vital aspects of initial training. From 2 to 4 hours of training are required.

Planning for Success.—Early defibrillation requires close medical supervision and the authorization of a local medical director for Emergency Medical Services. Local and state regulations must be thoroughly understood before instituting the use of AEDs. Athletic trainers, especially those responsible for many athletes in practice or competition, should be trained in using the AED and should have immediate access to it.

▶ Automatic and semiautomatic external defibrillators are usually operated by Emergency Medical Services personnel authorized by a sponsoring hospital's emergency physician. Presumably, on the sideline setting the team physician would need to assume this role. As the article points out, "it may be necessary to ascertain whether legal immunity exists for trained operators working under a physician's supervision." In view of the safety of the device and its lifesaving potential, eliminating legislative restrictions based on old technology is warranted.—J.S. Torg, M.D.

▶ Simons and Berry present a clear, cogent, and eloquent plea for the wider use of the AED in the sports medicine setting. A supervising physician—in this case, the team physician—must buy the AED (prices begin at about $4,000), establish standing orders and protocols, certify skill levels, and provide periodic retraining and assessment of the program. The authors are convinced that the lives of athletes will be saved if team physicians become actively involved in the trainers' education, practice, and emergency use of the AED. See Abstract 139-94-10–3 for one athletic setting in which the AED may save lives.—E.R. Eichner, M.D.

Commotio Cordis in Two Amateur Ice Hockey Players Despite the Use of Commercial Chest Protectors: Case Reports
Kaplan JA, Karofsky PS, Volturo GA (Office of the Chief Med Examiner, Concord, NH; Univ of Wisconsin, Madison; Univ of Massachusetts, Amherst)
J Trauma 34:151–153, 1993   139-94-10–3

Background.—Ice hockey is becoming increasingly popular among teenagers. This relatively violent sport can result in serious injury and death. Two boys, aged 15 years, who died of commotio cordis after being struck in the chest with the puck, despite the use of commercially designed and manufactured chest protectors, were studied.

Case Report.—In 1 case, the boy had a generalized tonic seizure of about 30 seconds immediately after being struck. The boy had been in excellent health with no underlying cardiac, metabolic, or neurologic disorders. After this convulsion, he rose to his feet briefly, then fell again and had a seizure lasting 2–3 minutes. He became cyanotic during the second convulsion. A pediatrician and a surgeon were present during this seizure and noted an absence of carotid and femoral pulses. Cardiopulmonary resuscitation was begun immediately. Paramedics, arriving 15 minutes after CPR was started, intubated the boy. An ECG revealed ventricular fibrillation, which remained unchanged during 20 minutes of various treatment.

After 25 minutes of resuscitation on the ice, the boy was taken to the hospital, where further resuscitation efforts were attempted unsuccessfully. At autopsy, an oval bruise was found over the left part of the precordium. Gross and microscopic examinations of the heart, lungs, and brain were normal. The boy's chest protector covered both shoulders with dense preformed plastic matrix, but the mid and lower precordium and lateral chest regions were protected by thinner, more conformable closed-cell plastic foam, .7 cm thick, sandwiched between woven synthetic cloth. The puck had struck this thinner part of the chest protector.

Conclusion.—Commotio cordis, a manifestation of concussive injury to the heart, results in ventricular dysrhythmia and ultimately cardiac standstill. Younger age groups are apparently predisposed to commotio cordis. The sports medicine community is alerted to the materials and designs used in the manufacture of commercial ice hockey chest protection, especially for younger players.

▶ In the second case presented in this article, the boy experienced cardiac arrest after being struck in the left chest by a puck. A pediatrician began CPR within 1 minute, to no avail. Autopsy showed a bruise that fit the shape of the puck on the left chest (under the thinner part of the chest protector), associated fracture of the fifth rib, contusion of the lingula and left anterolateral pericardial sac, and no significant injury to the heart, which was normal. Similar cases in baseball were covered in the 1993 Year Book of Sports Medicine (1). *Sports Illustrated* covered a case in which a seemingly harmless stick-slash to the chest killed an Italian hockey player and led to a manslaughter trial (2). Also relevant is the 41-year-old man with underlying coronary artery disease who had traumatic coronary artery thrombosis and myocardial infarction after being hit in the chest by a spiked volleyball (3).—E.R. Eichner, M.D.

References

1. 1993 Year Book of Sports Medicine, pp 14–16.
2. Swift EM: *Sports Illustrated* 79:66, 1993.
3. Grossfield PD, et al: *Med Sci Sports Exerc* 25:901, 1993.

Effects of Different Training Intensities on 24-Hour Blood Pressure in Hypertensive Subjects
Marceau M, Kouamé N, Lacourcière Y, Cléroux J (Laval Univ, Quebec)
Circulation 88:2803–2811, 1993   139-94-10-4

Background.—After a number of studies found that physical training exerted a significant antihypertensive effect, the World Hypertensive League recommended exercise as part of the management of essential hypertension. Some later studies, however, did not report any difference in ambulatory blood pressure after training. The effects of endurance training at different intensities on ambulatory blood pressure and on blood pressure load were compared.

Methods.—The participants were 11 sedentary patients, 10 men and 1 woman, with uncomplicated mild to moderate primary hypertension. They were evaluated in a crossover fashion after a sedentary control period and after 2 training periods. Training sessions were held 3 days per week for 10-week periods, 1 at 50% of maximal oxygen intake and the other at 70% of maximal oxygen intake. The patients exercised on cycle ergometers under supervision of trained personnel.

Results.—Nine patients, 8 men and 1 woman, completed all 3 periods; 2 patients withdrew for reasons unrelated to the study. Three patients were included in each of 3 sequences: train 70%—sedentary—train 50%; sedentary—train 50%—train 70%; and train 50%—train 70%—sedentary. Training at moderate (70%) intensity, but not at low (50%) intensity, resulted in a higher maximal oxygen intake compared with sedentary values. Both low and moderate training intensities exerted a similar antihypertensive effect of about 5 mm Hg for systolic and diastolic 24-hour blood pressures. Training at low intensity reduced blood pressure only during the waking hours, whereas training at moderate intensity reduced blood pressure only during evening and sleeping hours. Waking blood pressure load decreased significantly (from 66% to 49%) after training at low intensity. Training at moderate intensity resulted in a significant decrease in sleeping blood pressure load (from 61% to 34%).

Conclusion.—The findings of this study may explain some of the discrepancies in previous reports on the antihypertensive effects of training. Each training intensity may interfere with different pathogenic effects associated with different blood pressure profiles; thus, both may be beneficial in preventing cardiovascular events linked to hypertension.

▶ This intriguing study tries to clarify mixed results from prior studies on exercise for hypertension by showing that 10 weeks of exercise training at low intensity (50% of maximal oxygen intake, equivalent to brisk walking) or moderate intensity (70% of maximal oxygen intake, equivalent to jogging) exert similar antihypertensive effects (about 5 mm Hg for 24-hour systolic and diastolic blood pressures). However, the effect of low-intensity exercise is seen mainly during the morning, whereas that from moderate-intensity exercise is apparent mainly during the evening and sleeping periods. See an elegant, comprehensive review by an expert on exercise, training, and hypertension (1).—E.R. Eichner, M.D.

Reference

1. Tipton CM: *Exerc Sports Sci Rev* 19:447, 1991.

Determination of the Readability of Educational Materials for Patients With Cardiac Disease
Owen PM, Porter KA, Frost CD, O'Hare E, Johnson E (Roger Williams Med Ctr, Providence, RI)
J Cardiopulmon Rehabil 13:20–24, 1993   139-94-10–5

Background.—Patient education is more important than ever as patients struggle to manage their own health care needs. Professionals are also relying more on printed materials to supplement their efforts to educate patients. However, many questions about patient education remain

Mean Readability Scores After Elimination of Medical Terminology

	Before	After
A Patient's Guide to Anticoagulation (DuPont Pharmaceuticals)	17.2	9.6
Living with your Pacemaker (American Heart Association)	11.6	9.3
Heart Attack. What Now? (Prichett-Hull Company)	9.2	8.6

(Courtesy of Owen PM, Porter KA, Frost CD, et al: *J Cardiopulmon Rehabil* 13:20–24, 1993.)

unanswered. The readability of educational materials for patients with cardiac disease was assessed.

Methods.—Readability was determined by dividing the average sentence length by the number of polysyllabic words and multiplying the result by the constant .04. Samples of educational materials currently given to cardiac patients were obtained from 14 inpatient and outpatient cardiac programs in Rhode Island. Twenty-four commercially prepared samples and 13 materials written by nurses were analyzed.

Findings.—The entire sample had a mean readability score equivalent to an educational grade of 12.2. Grade levels ranged from 8 to 17.2. The mean readability scores for commercial vs. nurse-prepared materials were 12.3 vs. 12.1, respectively. No significant differences were found in readability among content areas. Eliminating polysyllabic technical terms lowered the readability scores to between 8.6 and 9.6 (table).

Conclusion.—Most printed patient education materials are beyond the reading ability of most patients. Substituting commonly understood words for medical terminology improves readability as determined by the formula used. Medical terms that patients need to learn can be taught as a separate vocabulary or incorporated gradually into the material.

▶ If medicine is to realize its full potential in the prevention of disease, it will need to make much greater use of the media—print, audiotapes and videotapes—available for patient education. When we attempt to prepare such educational materials, it is easy to fall into the trap of assuming that everyone who enters a physician's office has both postdoctoral training and perfect fluency in English. We have recently reviewed one Canadian screening tool, the Physical Activity Readiness Questionnaire (PAR-Q), in this context. We found that a number of the sentences in the text were unduly long, and polysyllabic words often were used where simpler expressions could be substituted. This paper by Owen and associates provides another example of how educational materials must be reviewed for readability and suggests modifications that can be adopted so they will be comprehensible for someone having a tenth-grade education.—R.J. Shephard, M.D., Ph.D.

Suggested Guidelines for Rating Cardiac Disability in Workers' Compensation
Clark WL, Alpern HL, Breall WS, Hyman RM, Markovitz A, O'Brien JB, Starke RD (State of California, San Francisco; Cedars-Sinai Med Ctr, Los Angeles; Univ of California, San Francisco; et al)
West J Med 158:263–267, 1993   139-94-10-6

Background.—Currently, cardiac disability ratings in workers' compensation cases lack a consistent scientific basis. Medical evidence used by different examiners may vary in the same case. Opinions on the extent of disability may vary, delaying resolution of the case and the delivery of benefits to the patient. Guidelines for determining cardiac impairment were presented.

Guidelines for Rating Cardiac Disability.—Eight guidelines for assessing disabilities at various anatomical sites have been presented by an advisory committee to the California Division of Industrial Accidents (table). Exercise stress testing provides the best reproducible data on cardiac ability. Alternative or supplemental testing is needed when exercise stress testing is not possible or adequate. Ejection fraction may be used to estimate cardiac impairment when exercise testing is not done. The most accurate way to determine ejection fraction is cardiac catheterization, with the direct measurement of cardiac output and cardiac index. Ejection fraction may also be determined using the findings of an echocardiogram or a multigated angiogram. Exercise testing may be supplemented with information from the patient's history. Conditions such as hypertension, arrhythmias, coronary artery spasm, and a history of coronary artery surgery or myocardial infarction may also affect cardiac ability without being reflected in exercise testing.

Conclusion.—Cardiac disability may be rated accurately when it is based on a summary of the medical evidence. Currently, exercise testing is the most productive way to quantitate a worker's impairment. In some cases, however, such testing is not possible or sufficient. Alternative or supplemental testing is needed in such instances.

▶ Given the present drive to "get people off welfare," there may be a substantial increase in formal assessments of cardiac disability during the next decade. The starting point in such an assessment is determining the fraction of maximal oxygen intake that a worker can reasonably be expected to sustain during an 8-hour day. Clark and associates assume the fairly heavy loading of 45% of maximal oxygen intake (self-paced workers typically adopt 40% of maximal oxygen intake) (1). The next step is to see what fraction of the current labor market demands more energy expenditure than the pa-

Guidelines for Evaluating Disabilities of the Heart

Paragraph	Standard Disability Rating, %†	Description
a	10	*Disability precluding very heavy lifting* contemplates that an employee has lost about a fourth of preinjury lifting capacity; a statement such as "unable to lift 50 lbs" is not meaningful; the total lifting effort, including weight, distance, endurance, frequency, body position, and similar factors, should be considered
b	15	*Disability precluding very heavy work* contemplates that an employee has lost about a fourth of preinjury capacity for performing activities such as bending, stooping, lifting, pulling, and climbing or other activities involving comparable physical effort
c	20	*Disability precluding heavy lifting* contemplates that an employee has lost about half of preinjury lifting capacity
d	25	*Disability precluding heavy lifting, repeated bending, and stooping* contemplates that an employee has lost about half of preinjury capacity for lifting, bending, and stooping
e	30	*Disability precluding heavy work* contemplates that an employee has lost about half of preinjury capacity for performing activities such as bending, stooping, lifting, pushing, pulling, and climbing or other activities involving comparable physical effort
f.	50	*Disability resulting in limitation to light work* contemplates that an employee can do work in a standing or walking position, with a minimum of demands for physical effort
g	60	*Disability resulting in limitation to semisedentary work* contemplates that an employee can do work about half the time in a sitting position and about half the time in a standing or walking position with a minimum of physical effort, whether standing, walking, or sitting
h	70	*Disability resulting in limitation to sedentary work* contemplates that an employee can do work predominantly in a sitting position at a bench, desk, or table with a minimum of physical effort and with some degree of walking and standing permitted

Note: Guidelines are from the State of California Department of Industrial Relations.
† Ratings are modified administratively to take into account age and occupation.
(Courtesy of Clark WL, Alpern HL, Breall WS, et al: *West J Med* 158:263–267, 1993.)

tient's 45% performance ceiling. The assessor then subtracts from this the job exclusions that would result from normal age and gender effects.

If maximal oxygen intake can be measured directly, the calculation is fairly straightforward. However, malingering may cause some people to stop exercise prematurely, in which case the true maximal performance must be judged from such indices as peak heart rate and subjective impressions of how far short of maximum effort the individual has stopped. Ejection fraction is suggested as another measure that does not require patient cooperation, although in view of the poor correlation between resting ejection fraction and exercise performance (Abstract 139-94-10–22), the use of this variable seems open to legal challenge.—R.J. Shephard, M.D., Ph.D.

Reference

1. Hughes AL, Goldman RF: *J Appl Physiol* 29:570, 1970.

Associations Between Changes in Physical Activity and Risk Factors for Coronary Heart Disease in a Community-Based Sample of Men and Women: The Stanford Five-City Project
Young DR, Haskell WL, Jatulis DE, Fortmann SP (Stanford Univ, Calif)
Am J Epidemiol 138:205–216, 1993   139-94-10–7

Introduction.—Higher levels of physical activity are associated with a number of health benefits, including lower body mass index and improved lipid profiles. Most physical activity training studies, however, are of limited application because of their rigorous inclusion criteria, relatively short-term protocols, and small sample sizes. The effects of a change in physical activity were studied in a large community sample during a 5-year period.

Subjects and Methods.—The study sample consisted of 380 men and 427 women between the ages of 18 and 74 years. All were participants in the Stanford Five-City Project, a trial of the effects of community-based cardiovascular health education. The subjects were evaluated for changes in self-reported physical activity and in total cholesterol, high-density-lipoprotein (HDL) cholesterol, systolic blood pressure, resting pulse rate, and body mass index from baseline to 60-month follow-up.

Results.—At baseline, premenopausal women (the majority of the female sample) generally had a favorable cardiovascular risk status compared with similarly aged men. Change in physical activity among men had a significant positive correlation with change in HDL cholesterol and a significant negative correlation with change in body mass index. Among women, change in the physical activity score at follow-up was associated with a significant positive change in HDL cholesterol and a negative correlation with change in the resting pulse rate. Men and women were grouped according to whether their physical activity score decreased, was maintained, or increased. In general, decreases in activity level were related to increases in estimated 10-year coronary heart disease risk scores and increases in activity were related to lowered coronary heart disease risk scores (table).

Conclusion.—Physical activity can change cardiovascular risk factors in a community-based sample as well as among subjects in controlled, structured trials. Body mass index and HDL cholesterol levels changed

Changes in Cardiovascular Risk Factors for the Cohort Sample Aged 18–74 Years Who Decreased, Did Not Change, or Increased Their Composite Physical Activity Score

	Total cholesterol change (mg/dl)		HDL cholesterol* change (mg/dl)		Systolic blood pressure change (mmHg)		Resting pulse rate change (beats/minute)		Body mass index change (kg/m²)		Smokers who quit (%)		Estimated CHD* risk change (events/ 1,000 persons)	
	Men	Women	Men	Women	Men	Women	Men	Women	Men	Women	Men	Women	Men	Women
Decreased activity†	8.2 ± 27.0‡	9.0 ± 24.6	-4.1 ± 9.6	-3.4 ± 10.5	-5.4 ± 16.5	-4.2 ± 14.7	3.4 ± 11.4	1.5 ± 9.6	1.01 ± 1.7	0.96 ± 2.1	26.5	31.0	8.4 ± 33.3	-0.1 ± 17.2
No activity change§	-1.1 ± 27.9	4.9 ± 31.1	-2.5 ± 10.9	-0.7 ± 12.2	-7.1 ± 13.6	-1.3 ± 16.4	-0.1 ± 10.7	0.7 ± 10.1	0.42 ± 1.6	0.61 ± 1.7	29.5	21.2	-0.5 ± 37.2	1.2 ± 22.9
Increased activity‖	4.3 ± 29.6	4.1 ± 25.2	-0.4 ± 10.7	-0.4 ± 12.1	-6.0 ± 15.3	-5.5 ± 13.2	1.8 ± 12.0	-2.1 ± 10.4	0.32 ± 1.8	0.50 ± 1.7	32.3	33.3	-1.2 ± 26.6	-2.0 ± 12.3

Note: Source is Stanford Five-City Project (California), 1979–1985.
* HDL, high-density lipoprotein; CHD, coronary heart disease.
† For men, no. = 108; for women, no. = 119.
‡ Mean ± standard deviation.
§ For men, no. = 178; for women, no. = 193.
‖ For men, no. = 94; for women, no. = 115.
(Courtesy of Young DR, Haskell WL, Jatulis DE, et al: Am J Epidemiol 138:205–216, 1993.)

favorably for both men and women who increased their physical activity. Community-wide promotions of physical activity have the potential to influence cardiovascular risk factors and cardiovascular risk positively.

▶ A growing number of large-scale community exercise projects are now looking not only at cross-sectional associations between physical activity and health status, but also at the consequences of a change in reported activity patterns during a period of 5–10 years. This is one such study. It demonstrates the health benefit of an increase of physical activity in terms of HDL cholesterol, resting pulse rate, body mass index, and smoking withdrawal. In the case of smoking, the differential benefit from increased exercise was greater in men than in women. In part because of a greater impact on smoking prevalence, the estimated risk of future cardiac events decreased more in male than in female exercise adopters. In subjects older than 50 years of age, the changes in risk factor prevalence were in the same general direction as for younger adults. However, either because of a smaller sample size or because activity is more difficult to assess in the elderly, the effects were not statistically significant.—R.J. Shephard, M.D., Ph.D.

Exercise, Fibrinogen, and Other Risk Factors for Ischaemic Heart Disease: Caerphilly Prospective Heart Disease Study
Elwood PC, Yarnell JWG, Pickering J, Fehily AM, O'Brien JR (Llandough Hosp, Penarth, Wales; St Mary's Hosp, Portsmouth, England)
Br Heart J 69:183–187, 1993   139-94-10–8

Background.—Although recent studies have suggested a relative risk of ischemic heart disease with a sedentary lifestyle compared with an active lifestyle, the association between physical activity and risk factors is not well understood. The debate continues about the nature of physical activity, the amount of such activity, and the mechanism by which it affects the risk of ischemic heart disease. The relationship between physical activity and risk factors for ischemic heart disease, including fibrinogen concentration and plasma viscosity and triglyceride, was examined.

Methods.—Data were drawn from 2,398 men, aged 50–64 years, who were examined as part of the follow-up of the Caerphilly Prospective Heart Disease Study. Validated questionnaires were used to quantify energy expenditure on leisure activities and to grade occupational activities. Blood pressure, lipids, fibrinogen, and plasma viscosity—all risk factors for heart disease—were examined. Data were standardized for 3 possible confounding variables: smoking, employment vs. lack of employment, and prevalent ischemic heart disease.

Findings.—Fibrinogen concentration and viscosity were lower in the men who were most active in their leisure activities. Triglyceride concentrations also appeared to be substantially lower in the active men, but the findings were not consistent. There was a weak positive relation with high-density-lipoprotein cholesterol. The results for total cholesterol, fasting glucose concentrations, and blood pressure showed no relation to activity level. Work-related activity level was related to lipid concentrations but not to the hemostatic test findings.

Conclusion.—A beneficial relationship between leisure activities of all levels and hemostatic and lipid factors was found. Exercise was associated with lower triglyceride concentrations, a risk factor strongly predictive of heart disease for men in this cohort. For the men enrolled in this study, exercise seemed to reduce the risk of an ischemic heart disease event by about 3% to 4% with respect to triglyceride concentrations and 7% to 8% for either fibrinogen or viscosity.

▶ Now that the American Heart Association has recognized hypertension, smoking, a high level of serum cholesterol, and a lack of physical activity as the primary risk factors for ischemic heart disease, this study is more properly described as an examination of physical activity and blood coagulability. Given the review done by Tipton (1), the authors' comment dismissing the effect of exercise training on blood pressure is also surprising. Fibrinogen levels and plasma viscosity were only related to leisure activity in individuals who were not employed, after data had been controlled for age, smoking habits, and prevalent ischemia. The authors attribute this somewhat unexpected paradox to the fact that there was a broader range of activity levels in the unemployed individuals.—R.J. Shephard, M.D., Ph.D.

Reference

1. Tipton CM: *Exerc Sport Sci Rev* 19:447, 1991.

Increased Response of Diastolic Blood Pressure to Exercise in Patients With Coronary Artery Disease: An Index of Latent Ventricular Dysfunction?
Paraskevaidis IA, Kremastinos DT, Kassimatis AS, Karavolias GK, Kordosis GD, Kyriakides ZS, Toutouzas PK (Athens Univ, Greece)
Br Heart J 69:507–511, 1993   139-94-10-9

Background.—The behavior of systolic blood pressure during exercise has been extensively studied and has been shown to correlate with both myocardial oxygen consumption and the number of obstructed blood vessels. Changes in diastolic blood pressure during exercise stress testing in patients with coronary artery disease were investigated and attempts were made to correlate changes with numbers of obstructed arteries and left ventricular systolic function at rest.

Method.—A total of 50 patients with coronary artery disease (38 men and 12 women with a mean age of 57 years) entered the study. Inclusion criteria comprised an intact atrioventricular and intraventricular conduction system, shown by ECG; left ventricular wall thickness within normal limits shown by echocardiography; absence of unstable angina, acute or myocardial infarction in the previous 3 months, and arterial hypertension. Diastolic blood pressure was measured invasively during exercise stress testing, and coronary angiograms and left ventriculograms were taken at rest. The abnormal diastolic blood pressure response was compared with the number of obstructed coronary arteries and with left ventricular systolic function.

Results.—The patients were split into 2 groups depending on their intra-arterial diastolic blood pressure response. Group 1 consisted of 10 patients (3 with 1-, 4-, with 2-, and 3 with 3-vessel coronary artery disease) with abnormal increase in diastolic pressure during the stress test. Nine of those had symptomatic and 1 had asymptomatic ST segment depression. The increased diastolic pressure preceded the ST depression by 1.2 minutes and returned to normal .9 minutes after the ST segment returned to normal. Group 2 consisted of 40 patients (12 with 1-, 16 with 2-, and 12 with 3-vessel coronary artery disease) with no abnormal increase in diastolic blood pressure. Nine experienced symptomatic ST segment depression, 18 had asymptomatic ST segment depression, and 13 had a normal stress test. The ejection fraction and cardiac index in group 1 were less than in group 2. The end systolic volume was greater in group 1 than in group 2.

Conclusion.—In patients with coronary artery disease, an abnormal increase in diastolic blood pressure during exercise stress testing correlated well with left ventricular systolic function at rest. However, it did not correlate with the number of obstructed arteries. It is likely that the abnormal response of diastolic blood pressure reflects deterioration of myocardial function.

▶ An increase of systolic pressure that is less than expected is correlated quite closely with severe (2- or 3-vessel) coronary artery vascular disease (1). The extent of abnormalities in diastolic pressure reported here is greater than others have observed (2, 3), perhaps because direct intra-arterial pressures were recorded. The findings also differed from earlier reports in showing that the increase in diastolic pressure was associated with deterioration of left ventricular function rather than with the number of obstructed arteries.—R.J. Shephard, M.D., Ph.D.

References

1. Willerson JT, et al: *Ischemic Heart Disease.* New York, Raven Press, 1983.
2. Akhras F, et al: *Br Heart J* 53:598, 1985.
3. Sheps SD, et al: *Am J Cardiol* 43:708, 1979.

Effect of a Standardized Meal on the Threshold of Exercise-Induced Myocardial Ischemia in Patients With Stable Angina

Colles P, Juneau M, Grégoire J, Larivée L, Desideri A, Waters D (Montreal Heart Inst; Univ of Montreal)
J Am Coll Cardiol 21:1052–1057, 1993   139-94-10-10

Background.—Exercise tolerance in patients with angina is thought to be decreased after a meal. However, the findings of studies addressing this phenomenon have been contradictory and inconclusive. The effect of a standardized meal on the ischemic threshold and exercise capacity was determined in patients with stable angina, exercise-induced ischemia, and reversible exercise-induced perfusion defects.

Methods.—Twenty subjects performed 2 exercise tests using the Bruce protocol with ^{99m}Tc-sestamibi on consecutive days in a random order.

Fasting and Postprandial Measurements During Exercise

	Fasting	Postprandial	Change (%)	p Value
At onset of 1-mm ST depression				
Duration of exercise (s)	248 ± 93	197 ± 87	−20	0.0007
Heart rate (beats/min)	122 ± 16	120 ± 12		0.41
Blood pressure (mm Hg)				
Systolic	172 ± 17	166 ± 13		0.13
Diastolic	87 ± 6	83 ± 5	−4	0.02
Rate-pressure product ($\times 10^{-3}$)	21.0 ± 3.6	20.0 ± 2.6		0.14
At onset of angina				
Duration of exercise (s)	340 ± 82	287 ± 94	−15	0.002
Heart rate (beats/min)	136 ± 14	135 ± 16		0.46
Blood pressure (mm Hg)				
Systolic	181 ± 19	182 ± 22		0.61
Diastolic	88 ± 8	86 ± 6		0.42
Rate-pressure product ($\times 10^{-3}$)	24.7 ± 4.0	24.9 ± 4.7		0.72
At peak exercise				
Duration of exercise (s)	376 ± 65	344 ± 86	−9	0.002
Heart rate (beats/min)	142 ± 12	140 ± 13		0.53
Blood pressure (mm Hg)				
Systolic	184 ± 18	184 ± 20		0.87
Diastolic	89 ± 9	86 ± 6		0.23
Rate-pressure product ($\times 10^{-3}$)	26.1 ± 3.6	25.9 ± 4.2		0.89
Work load (METs)	7.2 ± 1.1	6.6 ± 1.4	−8	0.008
Maximal ST depression (mm)	2.6 ± 1.0	2.6 ± 0.9		0.69
Defect score at rest*	3.2 ± 4.1	3.2 ± 4.1		0.33
Defect score on exercise	7.4 ± 5.5	6.7 ± 5.3		0.37
Ischemia score (exercise − rest)	4.2 ± 3.2	3.5 ± 2.6		0.33

Note: Data are expressed as mean value ± SD.
Abbreviation: METS, metabolic equivalents.
* On ^{99m}Tc-sestamibi single-photon emission CT.
(Courtesy of Colles P, Juneau M, Grégoire J, et al: *J Am Coll Cardiol* 21:1052–1057, 1993.)

One test was performed while fasting, and one was performed 30 minutes after a 4-megajoule (1,000-calorie) meal.

Findings.—Exercise time to ischemia was decreased by 20% in the postprandial state. Time to angina was reduced by 15%, and exercise tolerance was reduced by 9%. Rate-pressure products at these end points did not differ significantly between the fasting and postprandial tests. The quantitative ^{99m}Tc-sestamibi ischemia score was also unaffected (table).

Conclusion.—A 4-megajoule meal significantly reduced time to ischemia, time to angina, and exercise tolerance in these patients with stable angina. These effects resulted from a more rapid increase in myocardial oxygen demand with exercise. There were no effects on extent or severity of exercise-induced ischemia.

▶ The impact of meals on exercise tolerance has practical importance both in advising patients about when they should exercise, and in interpreting the results of laboratory tests when it is not possible to arrange for observations to be made in the fasting state.

Colles and associates have shown that the problem of a lowering of the ischemic threshold is not caused by a postprandial decrease in coronary perfusion. Rather, an increased fraction of the cardiac output is diverted to the gastrointestinal tract after a meal. Thus, there is a more rapid increase of heart rate and cardiac work rate during exercise, which in turn shortens the time needed to reach a critical rate-pressure product (1, 2).

The effect of a meal is not negligible. Whereas exposure to cold reduces exercise tolerance in only about one third of patients with myocardial ischemia, eating adversely affected exercise tolerance in 18 of 20 patients, commonly by 20% or more.—R.J. Shepard, M.D., Ph.D.

References

1. Kelbaek H, *Br Heart J* 61:506, 1989.
2. Yi JJ, et al: *Br Heart J* 63:22, 1990.

Seven-Year Prognostic Value of the Electrocardiogram at Rest and an Exercise Test in Patients Admitted for, but Without, Confirmed Myocardial Infarction

Fruergaard P, Launbjerg J, Jacobsen HL, Madsen JK (Frederiksborg County Central Hosp, Hillerød, Denmark; Univ of Copenhagen)
Eur Heart J 14:499–504, 1993   139-94-10-11

Background.—Patients in whom acute myocardial infarction (AMI) is suspected but not confirmed and who have no other apparent cause of pain have a high incidence of death from cardiac causes or AMI after hospital discharge. These patients may be at increased risk beyond the first year. A study was done to determine the long-term prognostic value

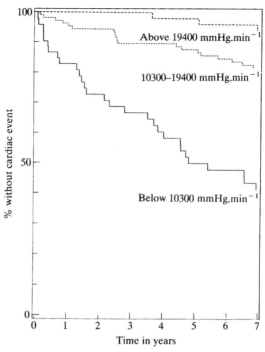

Fig 10–1.—Kaplan-Meier estimate of percentage of patients without cardiac events in relation to the increase in rate-pressure product during exercise. (Courtesy of Fruergaard P, Launbjerg J, Jacobsen HL, et al: *Eur Heart J* 14:499–504, 1993.)

of ECG at rest and of an exercise test in patients admitted for myocardial infarction without a confirmed diagnosis.

Methods.—A total of 217 patients admitted for chest pain without confirmed AMI made up the study group. The median follow-up was 88 months. The patients' 7-year prognosis for cardiac events after discharge was related to an ECG at rest and a symptom-limited exercise test.

Findings.—The study patients had a better 7-year prognosis than a comparable group of patients with confirmed AMI. However, the overall frequency of cardiac events for the former group was still very high. At high risk were patients with negative T waves, ST depression or elevation, intraventricular block or Q waves at rest, ST abnormalities during exercise, or a combination of these. Patients without these ECG abnormalities had a significantly better prognosis. Fifty-three percent and 92% of these 2 groups, respectively, had had no cardiac events in the 7 years of follow-up. The 7-year prognosis was significantly impaired in patients with a low exercise-induced increase in the rate-pressure product (indicating reduced function of the left ventricle) and in patients in whom angina pectoris developed during exercise (Fig 10–1).

Conclusion.—Although non-AMI patients had a better prognosis after hospital discharge than patients with confirmed AMI, one fourth of the former group had a cardiac event within 7 years. The noninvasive approach to risk stratification described in this study identified a subgroup of patients at high risk for cardiac events as well as a group comprising more than half the patients who were at very low risk.

▶ It is common for a patient to be admitted to hospital with a suspected myocardial infarction, but firm confirmation of the diagnosis can prove elusive. This paper by Fruergaard and associates provides interesting prognostic data on the long-term fate of such individuals. Although it is better to have a suspected rather than a confirmed diagnosis of myocardial infarction, the long-term prognosis of a patient with a suspected infarction is on average still quite grave; there is a 27% chance of a definitive infarction within 7 years. Before passing this disturbing news on to the patient, it is a good idea to apply some of the tactics listed by Fruergaard and associates, using the resting ECG and exercise stress test responses to distinguish those patients in whom future cardiac events are very likely (47% risk) from those whose long-term prospects are much better (8% risk).—R.J. Shephard, M.D., Ph.D.

Impedance Cardiography During Exercise in Patients With Coronary Heart Disease
Thomas SHL, Crowther A (United Med and Dental School, London; St Thomas' Hosp, London)
Eur Heart J 14:150–159, 1993   139-94-10–12

Background.—Patients with coronary heart disease commonly have abnormalities in left ventricular response to exercise. Impedance cardiography may offer a simple, inexpensive method of measuring these responses. Impedance responses to exercise were compared with later cardiac catheterization findings in patients with suspected coronary heart disease.

Methods.—The study sample comprised 102 consecutive men referred for cardiac catheterization. Too few women were referred for analysis. All underwent impedance cardiography at rest and during cycle ergometry to exhaustion. They underwent cardiac catheterization for clinical indications of coronary vascular disease 2–7 weeks later. The findings of cardiac catheterization were used to divide the patients into 4 groups: group A, normal; group B, 1- or 2-vessel disease; group C, 3-vessel disease; and group D, 3-vessel disease with a left ventricular ejection fraction (LVEF) less than 55%. In groups A, B, and C, LVEF was greater than 55%.

Results.—Significant correlations were noted between a number of impedance measures taken immediately after exercise and resting LVEF, particularly peak range of change in transthoracic impedance (dZ/dt_{max}) and Heather index. The latter was the best parameter for differentiation

Sensitivity, Specificity, Predictive Value, and Risk Ratio of Abnormal Measurements Immediately After Maximal Exercise for Detection of (A) Any Coronary Heart Disease (> 70% Narrowing in One or More Vessels) or (B) Triple-Vessel Disease

Measurement	Limit*	Sensitivity (%)	Specificity (%)	Predictive value (%)	Risk ratio
(A) Any coronary disease					
ST depression	$>0{\cdot}15\,mV$	36	92	97	1·17
Systolic BP	$<138\,mmHg$	12	100	100	1·16
dZ/dt_{max}	$<1{\cdot}88\,\Omega\,s^{-1}$	10	100	100	1·16
PEP	$>85\,ms$	32	83	93	1·10
PEP/VET	$>0{\cdot}564$	1	100	100	1·15
Heather index	$<15\,\Omega\,s^{-2}$	16	100	100	1·17
Stroke index	$<36\,ml\,.\,m^{-2}$	7	100	100	1·16
Cardiac index	$<6{\cdot}21\,.\,min\,.\,m^{-2}$	41	92	97	1·19
TPR	$<1282\,dyn\,.\,s\,.\,cm^{-5}\,.\,m^{-2}$	55	75	94	1·17
ST depression or reduced Heather index		45	92	97	1·12
(B) Triple vessel disease					
ST depression	$>0{\cdot}15\,mV$	41	71	35	1·42
Systolic BP	$<138\,mmHg$	26	96	70	2·97
dZ/dt_{max}	$<1{\cdot}88\,\Omega\,s^{-1}$	19	96	62	2·47
PEP	$>85\,ms$	63	82	59	3·87
PEP/VET	$>0{\cdot}564$	4	100	100	3·62
Heather index	$<15\,\Omega\,s^{-2}$	33	94	69	3·15
Stroke index	$<36\,ml\,.\,m^{-2}$	15	97	67	2·58
Cardiac index	$<6{\cdot}21\,.\,min\,.\,m^{-2}$	52	71	43	2·14
TPR	$<1282\,dyn\,.\,s\,.\,cm^{-5}\,.\,m^{-2}$	63	53	35	1·42
ST depression or reduced Heather index		63	81	45	2·57

Abbreviations: PEP, pre-ejection period; *VET*, ventricular ejection time; *TPR*, total peripheral resistance.
* Limits of normality defined as mean ± 2 SD of measurements taken from a separate group of 34 healthy male volunteers.
(Courtesy of Thomas SHL, Crowther A: *Eur Heart J* 14:150–159, 1993.)

of disease groups, with mean values of 26 Ωs^{-2} for group A, 22 Ωs^{-2} for group B, 18 Ωs^{-2} for group C, and 15 Ωs^{-2} for group D. However, the groups overlapped considerably, with a risk ratio of 1.17 for any coronary disease and 3.15 for triple-vessel disease.

Conclusion.—In patients with suspected coronary heart disease, impedance cardiography is of little value in identifying patients with abnormal left ventricular responses to exercise. In most patients with abnormal responses, diagnosis is more simply made on the basis of poor exercise tolerance or abnormal blood pressure responses. Although it appears to be specific, impedance cardiography is not a sensitive indicator of coronary heart disease; a positive test suggests triple-vessel disease, with or without abnormalities of resting ventricular function (table).

▶ Impedance cardiography began almost 40 years ago, with Nyboer's studies on the specific conductivity of various body tissues (1). The idea is relatively simple—a high-frequency electrical current passes readily through blood or fluid-filled tissues, but not through fat or air. In theory, the method can thus be used to examine the blood content of the heart and limbs, the air content of the chest, and body fatness. However, in practice, there are many problems in obtaining useful data. In particular, the electrical currents are easily deflected by tissue membranes, and it is necessary to make rather specific assumptions about the geometry of the body parts that are being examined.

There have been some claims that impedance technology can measure cardiac stroke volume, and the method could conceivably demonstrate an impairment of cardiac performance in patients with severe myocardial ischemia. However, as Thomas and Crowther demonstrate, exercise tolerance and the blood pressure response to a standard exercise test protocol provide simpler and more useful indications of failing cardiac function.—R.J. Shephard, M.D., Ph.D.

Reference

1. Nyboer J: *Electrical Impedance Plethysmography.* Springfield, IL: C.C. Thomas, 1959.

Diagnostic Accuracy of Seismocardiography Compared With Electrocardiography for the Anatomic and Physiologic Diagnosis of Coronary Artery Disease During Exercise Testing

Wilson RA, Bamrah VS, Lindsay J Jr, Schwaiger M, Morganroth J (Oregon Health Sciences Univ, Portland; Med College of Wisconsin, Milwaukee; George Washington Univ, Washington, DC; et al)
Am J Cardiol 71:536–545, 1993   139-94-10–13

Background.—Seismocardiography, a noninvasive technique, measures seismic waves on the anterior chest surface emanating from the motion of the heart. It is safe, inexpensive, and easy to use, but its sensitivity in detecting patients with coronary artery disease (CAD) has not been validated. In this multicenter study, the diagnostic accuracy of seismocardiography was compared with that of ECG for physiologically and anatomically significant ischemic CAD during exercise stress testing.

Methods.—A total of 129 patients were enrolled by 5 centers. The patients underwent simultaneous seismocardiography and 12-lead ECG at the time of their exercise treadmill stress tests. Coronary artery disease was defined as both anatomically and physiologically significant disease.

Findings.—Seismocardiography was significantly more sensitive than ECG in detecting anatomical CAD. The sensitivities of the 2 modalities were 73% and 48%, respectively. The specificities of the 2 were comparable at 78% and 80%, respectively. Exercise seismocardiography provided significant incremental diagnostic data beyond what exercise ECG provided. Seismocardiography was more sensitive in women and in patients not achieving maximal predicted heart rate. It was also significantly more sensitive than, and just as specific as, ECG in patients with physiologically significant CAD.

Conclusion.—Seismocardiography is significantly more sensitive than ECG for detecting anatomical and physiologic CAD. Seismocardiography may be a useful adjunct in exercise stress testing.

▶ The force of ventricular contraction sets up substantial shock waves around the body. Indeed, there was a time when many of us attempted to use ballistocardiograms both for cardiovascular diagnosis and for the estimation of cardiac stroke volume. The present seismographic technique derives from the ballistocardiographic lineage. A small piezoelectric transducer is mounted over the lower part of the sternum to record vibrations induced by cardiac contractions, and one presumes that changes of body posture or slipping of the recorder could make a substantial difference to the tracings obtained. Myocardial ischemia apparently induces a substantial change of the immediate postexercise waveform (1). The method is interesting and merits further study. However, the claim that the new method has a better sensitivity and specificity than the exercise ECG must be accepted with some reserve, because this conclusion rests largely on the authors' figures for exercise ECG, which are poor relative to what many other investigators have suggested.—R.J. Shephard, M.D., Ph.D.

Reference

1. Salerno DM, Zanetti J: *J Cardiovasc Technol* 9:111, 1990.

Variables Associated With a Poor Prognosis in Patients With an Ischemic Thallium-201 Exercise Test
Travin MI, Boucher CA, Newell JB, LaRaia PJ, Flores AR, Eagle KA (Massachusetts Gen Hosp, Boston; Spaulding Rehabilitation Hosp, Boston)
Am Heart J 125:335–344, 1993   139-94-10-14

Introduction.—Data obtained from thallium-201 exercise tests are useful in predicting subsequent cardiac events in patients with known or suspected coronary artery disease. Multivariate analysis was used to determine the exercise work rate, ECG, and thallium-201 image parameters most closely associated with a poor prognosis in patients who had evidence of ischemic heart disease.

Methods.—From a review of the records of 4,900 patients, 752 patients with exercise-induced myocardial ischemia were identified. Of these, 268 patients were selected for analysis, all with unequivocal exercise-induced thallium-201 ischemia. Their thallium-201 images were reviewed without knowledge of the patients' clinical, exercise, and follow-

Multivariate Analysis: Variables Predictive of Poor Outcomes

Parameter	Chi square	p Value
Elective CABG/PTCA ≤6 months after test (n = 54)		
LV dilatation	9.72	0.0020
CP during exercise	8.54	0.0038
Pattern of MVD	8.16	0.0046
CABG/PTCA > 6 months after test (n = 27)		
Stage I ischemia	7.01	0.0081
CP during exercise	3.00	0.0834
Nonfatal myocardial infarction (n = 12)		
Ischemic index >1.25	6.91	0.0086
LV dilatation	3.49	0.0616
<9.6 METS	3.36	0.0667
Cardiac death (n = 12)		
Lung uptake	6.98	0.0082
Absence of ECG ischemia	6.11	0.0134
<9.6 METS	5.99	0.0144

Abbreviations: CABG, coronary artery bypass grafting; CP, chest pain; LV, left ventricular; MVD, multivessel disease; PTCA, percutaneous transluminal coronary angioplasty.
(Courtesy of Travin MI, Boucher CA, Newell JB, et al: *Am Heart J* 125:335–344, 1993.)

up data. Outcomes defined as adverse cardiac events were cardiac death, nonfatal myocardial infarction, and a revascularization procedure performed more than 6 months after the exercise test or at any time when required by clinical deterioration (table).

Results.—Follow-up data were obtained up to a mean of 25 months after the exercise test. In 156 of the 261 patients, no adverse cardiac events occurred during follow-up. Fifty-four patients underwent a revascularization procedure within 6 months, generally because of thallium exercise test results. Twenty-seven patients had a revascularization because of clinical deterioration or on an elective basis more than 6 months after the test. There were 12 cardiac deaths and 12 patients who had a nonfatal myocardial infarction. Patients who had the most abnormal thallium images frequently underwent early revascularization. In the remaining patients, the outcome of nonfatal myocardial infarction was most closely associated with the amount of thallium ischemia. Parameters reflecting left ventricular dysfunction, including abnormal lung uptake of thallium and an inability to exercise to 9.6 times resting metabolism (METs) were associated with cardiac death.

Conclusion.—Patients with cardiac death were no more likely to have extensive ischemia than patients with no cardiac event. As with the findings of many previous investigations, mortality correlated most strongly with parameters that reflected ventricular function.

▶ The question that must be asked when any laboratory test is performed is how much information does the procedure contribute to patient management? This is particularly important in the case of a relatively costly procedure such as thallium scintigraphy. However, it is surprisingly difficult to acquire such information. In this paper by Travin and associates, a sample of 4,900 patients underwent a thallium test, but only 752 of these showed "unequivocal" myocardial ischemia; this in itself suggests the procedure is being grossly overused. Of the 752 patients in whom the result was said to be "unequivocal," the results of a further 100 of the patients became doubtful when the test was repeated! The sample actually analyzed was further decreased to 268 cases, and of these, 54 had to be excluded because the initial testing led to the individual being placed on a waiting list for coronary revascularization. A further 5 patients seem to have disappeared.

During the next 25 months, only 51 of the residual 207 patients sustained measurable clinical events, 27 of which were coronary surgery. Although some of this group may have deteriorated during the period of observation, it also seems likely that further review of the original documents influenced the decision to operate in many of the 27. Thus, the only unequivocal new events from 4,900 scintigrams were 12 myocardial infarctions and 12 coronary deaths. The thallium test did help to identify those with a risk of subsequent infarction, 9 of 12 showing an ischemic index of > 1.25, and 11 of 12 having left ventricular dilatation. However, 8 of these 12 patients also showed a poor exercise tolerance, which could have been observed without the thallium scan and might well have been detected by careful clinical questioning. The poor exercise tolerance was also a feature of those who sustained a coronary death (10 of 12 patients). Clearly, there remains a lot of scope for more careful audit of expensive laboratory tests.—R.J. Shephard, M.D., Ph.D.

Diagnostic Value of Postexercise Systolic Blood Pressure Response for Detecting Coronary Artery Disease in Patients With or Without Hypertension

Tsuda M, Hatano K, Hayashi H, Yokota M, Hirai M, Saito H (Univ of Nagoya, Japan)

Am Heart J 125:718–725, 1993   139-94-10–15

Background.—Exercise-induced ST-segment depression is used for noninvasive detection of coronary artery disease (CAD), but it has low sensitivity and specificity. The diagnostic value of 1 alternative, postexercise systolic blood pressure (SBP), has not been resolved. Postexercise

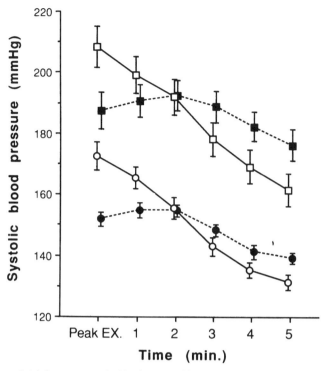

Fig 10–2.—Serial changes in systolic blood pressure (during recovery periods. In normotensive control subjects (no. = 48, *open circle*) and hypertensive control subjects (no. = 27, *open square*), SBP decreased steadily. In normotensive patients wtih CAD (no. = 82, *filled circle*) and hypertensive patients with CAD (no. = 24, *filled square*), SBP increased or did not change between 1 and 3 minutes after exercise. Data are expressed as mean ± SEM. (Courtesy of Tsuda M, Hatano K, Hayashi H, et al: *Am Heart J* 125:718-725, 1993.)

SBP was examined in patients with and without CAD to evaluate its diagnostic potential.

Subjects.—Treadmill testing was conducted in 181 predominantly male and middle-aged subjects who also underwent coronary angiography. Of these, 130 had normal blood pressure and 51 had hypertension. Among those with normal blood pressure, 82 had CAD; among those with hypertension, 24 had CAD.

Findings.—After treadmill exercise, SBP decreased immediately in the subjects without CAD. However, in those with CAD, SBP either increased or remained stable between 1 and 3 minutes after exercise (Fig 10-2). The postexercise SBP response was defined as SBP at 3 minutes of recovery divided by SBP at peak exercise. An SBP ratio greater than .9 was considered abnormal. In those with normal blood pressure, the abnormal SBP response identified CAD as accurately as did ST-segment depression. In patients with hypertension, diagnostic accuracy was significantly increased by combining the abnormal SBP response and ST-segment depression. The SBP ratio increased with the number of diseased coronary arteries.

Conclusion.—An abnormal postexercise SBP response was useful in the diagnosis of CAD, with a diagnostic value similar to that of ST-segment depression. In patients with hypertension, a combination of the abnormal SBP response and ST-segment depression was the most accurate in diagnosing CAD. The SBP response also appears to provide information about the severity of CAD.

▶ Although ST-segment depression can identify a group of patients with an increased risk of clinically manifest coronary vascular disease, it is less successful in predicting the prognosis of individual patients. The search continues for ways of improving the sensitivity and specificity of this test. This paper by Tsuda and colleagues suggests that persistent hypertension after exercise may be useful information, either when combined with ST-segment depression or when used as an independent sign of myocardial ischemia in conditions in which interpretation of the exercise ECG is difficult.

However, the reason for the persistent hypertension needs to be clarified before the authors' proposal can be accepted with enthusiasm. Acanfora et al. (1) suggested that persisting postexercise hypertension might reflect a poor exercise tolerance. Poor cardiac function is certainly a common accompaniment of myocardial ischemia, but a low cardiac output could also arise from other causes. If this is indeed the physiologic basis for the hypertensive phenomenon, it seems unlikely that it will provide a specific index of myocardial ischemia.—R.J. Shephard, M.D., Ph.D.

Reference

1. Acanfora D, et al: *Circulation* 77:1306, 1988.

Relative Importance of Psychologic Traits and Severity of Ischemia in Causing Angina During Treadmill Exercise
Davies RF, Linden W, Habibi H, Klinke WP, Nadeau C, Phaneuf DC, Lepage S, Dessain P, Buttars, JA; and the Canadian Amlodipine/Atenolol in Silent Ischemia Study (CASIS) Investigators (Univ of Ottawa, Ont, Canada)
J Am Coll Cardiol 21:331–336, 1993   139-94-10–16

Introduction.—Some patients with heart disease are more likely than others to have angina for reasons that remain uncertain. Why this is the case is clinically relevant, because patients without angina are less likely to seek medical help. Asymptomatic ischemia has been associated with altered sensory thresholds, decreased sensitivity to physical symptoms in general, and certain personality and behavioral traits.

Study Plan.—The influence of psychological traits on the ischemic threshold and exercise tolerance during treadmill exercise was examined by stepwise logistic regression analysis of 122 patients known to have

Univariate Comparison of Patients With and Without Angina

	Angina (n = 66)	No Angina (n = 56)	p Value
Results of psychologic testing			
Sensitivity to physical symptoms	112.7	90.5	0.001
Type A behavior	5.6	4.6	0.021
Depression	8.84	6.84	0.032
Hostility	121.9	117.7	0.063
Daily stress	28.0	20.1	0.140
Deception of others	10.0	10.9	0.205
Self deception	8.94	9.59	0.276
Marital adjustment	109.2	113.0	0.341
Suppressed anger	17.4	16.6	0.311
Anger control	24.2	24.7	0.584
Expressed anger	14.1	14.4	0.739
Measures of ischemic threshold			
Rate-pressure product at 1 mm ST $\downarrow$ (beats/min × mm Hg)	18,947	21,008	0.009
Time to 1-mm ST $\downarrow$ (s)	226	280	0.024
HR at 1-mm ST $\downarrow$ (beats/min)	118.2	125.8	0.020
SBP at 1-mm ST $\downarrow$ (mm Hg)	159.9	166.0	0.153
Peak ST $\downarrow$ (mm)	2.18	2.25	0.647
Ischemia on AECG (Y/N, n = 106)	43/14	38/11	0.823
DBP at 1 mm ST $\downarrow$ (mm Hg)	87.2	87.2	0.97
Measures of exercise performance			
Exercise time (s)	357.0	467.3	<0.001
Peak HR (beats/min)	132.2	145.2	<0.001
Peak rate-pressure product (HR × SBP)	22,818	25,569	0.005
Peak SBP (mm Hg)	172.7	176.1	0.45
Peak DBP (mm Hg)	89.0	87.6	0.60

Abbreviations: AECG, ambulatory electrocardiogram; *HR*, heart rate; *ST ↓*, ST-segment depression; *DBP*, diastolic blood pressure; *SBP*, systolic blood pressure.
(Courtesy of Davies RF, Linden W, Habibi H, et al: *J Am Coll Cardiol* 21:331–336, 1993.)

coronary artery disease. Psychological tests measured sensitivity to physical symptoms, denial and deception, type A behavior, anger and hostility, depression, marital adjustment, and the amount of external stress.

Findings.—On univariate analysis, patients who had angina during exercise were more sensitive to physical symptoms, had more type A behavior, and experienced more depression than those without angina (table). In addition, their threshold work rates for ischemia were lower and their exercise tolerance was poorer. On multivariate analysis, angina was independently related to greater sensitivity to physical symptoms, a lower work rate threshold for ischemia, and poor exercise performance.

Implications.—Individual differences in sensory and perceptual mechanisms probably have an important effect on whether myocardial ischemia will produce symptoms. The findings emphasize the need to assess ischemia objectively in patients with coronary artery disease who are relatively asymptomatic.

▶ Many psychological measures are rather imprecise, and this analysis would have been strengthened by using a larger sample size than 122 patients. The main conclusion that there are differing personality structures and/or sensory thresholds between patients who have silent ischemia and those whose diagnosis is manifest at first inspection seems logical. However, it is dangerous to assume causality. If a patient has symptomatic exercise-induced angina, depression and a variety of related symptoms are likely to develop, and exercise performance is also likely to be poorer than in those who are symptom-free.

Even the association of angina with type A behavior is not immune from this criticism—type A individuals are more likely to push themselves when exercising, and thus to have symptoms develop. The authors point out that when their trial becomes "unblinded," they may have better answers to some of their questions, in that they can then determine whether anti-ischemic treatment modifies the symptom reporting of their subjects or whether symptoms are independent of the extent of ischemia, as would be predicted from their hypothesis.—R.J. Shephard, M.D., Ph.D.

Physical Exertion as a Trigger of Acute Myocardial Infarction
Willich SN, for the Triggers and Mechanisms of Myocardial Infarction Study Group (Free Univ of Berlin)
N Engl J Med 329:1684–1690, 1993   139-94-10–17

Study Plan.—Continuing controversy over whether identifiable events such as physical exertion actually precipitate acute myocardial infarction prompted a study of 1,194 patients (74% of whom were men) who were interviewed a mean of 13 days after infarction. The findings were compared with those in the general population of Augsburg, Germany, a city of 330,000 residents. Control subjects and cases were matched for age, gender, marital status, type of work, educational level, and the usual frequency of physical exertion.

Observations.—The patients were nearly twice as likely as the control subjects to have engaged in physical exertion (defined as 6 or more metabolic equivalents) at the onset of infarction of the control event. The frequency of exertion was 7.1% in case patients and 3.9% in controls. A case-crossover comparison yielded a relative risk of 2.1 for having engaged in strenuous activity within 1 hour before the onset of infarction. Patients who regularly exercised less than 4 times per week had a relative risk of 6.9, compared with 1.3 for those who exercised more frequently. Infarction was most frequent in the hours after awakening in the morning (Fig 10–3). Unusual emotionally upsetting events were more often described by the case patients.

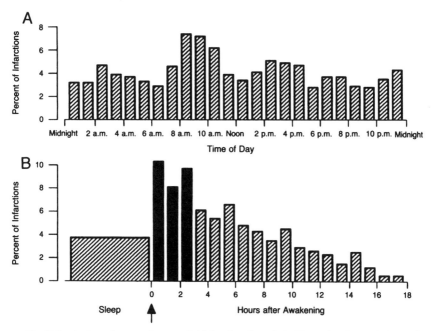

Fig 10–3.—A, time of onset of myocardial infarction showed significant circadian variation, with peak incidence from 8 to 11 AM (**A**). Relative risk of myocardial infarction during this period, as compared with other times of day, was 1.8. **B,** after adjustment for individual patients' times of awakening, morning peak was more pronounced. The relative risk of myocardial infarction during the initial 3-hour period after awakening was 2.7. (Courtesy of Willich SN, for the Triggers and Mechanisms of Myocardial Infarction Study Group: *N Engl J Med* 329:1684–1690, 1993.)

Implications.—Both strenuous physical activity and routine morning activities appear to relate to an increased risk of myocardial infarction in some individuals. It is possible that taking long-acting cardiac medication at night or dosing before arising in the morning would be more protective than scheduling medication for some time after arising.

▶ Willich and his associates are particularly well known for their discovery of the increased risk of heart attacks during the morning hours. Multivariate analyses show that this effect is independent of the exertion that begins on waking. Nevertheless, the combined effects of morning changes in blood coagulability and the inherent acute risk of exercise may be enough to precipitate an infarction, and in coronary-prone individuals there may be some advantage in exercising later during the day.—R.J. Shephard, M.D., Ph.D.

Triggering of Acute Myocardial Infarction by Heavy Physical Exertion: Protection Against Triggering by Regular Exertion

Mittleman MA, for the Determinants of Myocardial Infarction Onset Study Investigators (Deaconess Hosp, Boston)
N Engl J Med 329:1677–1683, 1993   139-94-10–18

Background.—There is considerable anecdotal evidence suggesting that heavy physical exertion sometimes precedes, and may actually trigger, the onset of acute myocardial infarction. There have been, however, no controlled studies of the risk involved in heavy exertion, the interval before symptoms appear, or whether the risk may be reduced by regular exercise.

Study Plan.—To quantify the relative risk of myocardial infarction after heavy exertion, as compared with periods of lighter exertion or no exertion, a case-crossover study was designed. Interviews were conducted with 1,228 patients an average of 4 days after acute infarction. Heavy exertion was defined as 6 or more metabolic equivalents, and its

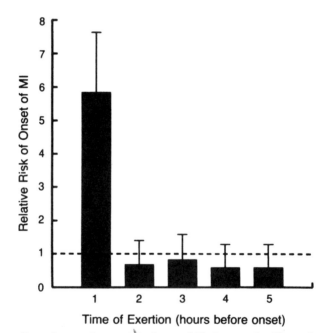

Fig 10–4.—Time of onset of myocardial infarction (MI) after episode of heavy physical exertion (induction time). Each of the 5 hours before onset of MI was assessed as an independent hazard period, and exertion during each hour was compared with that during the control period. Only exertion during the hour immediately before the onset of MI was associated with an increase in the relative risk, suggesting that the induction time for MI is less than 1 hour. Ninety-five percent confidence limits are represented by the T *bars. Dotted line* indicates the baseline risk. (Courtesy of Mittleman MA, for the Determinants of Myocardial Infarction Onset Study Investigators: N *Engl J Med* 329:1677–1683, 1993.)

frequency was validated by comparing data from a population-based control group of 218 individuals.

Findings.—Fifty-four patients, 4.4% of the total, had engaged in heavy exertion within 1 hour before the onset of infarction. Mixed isometric and aerobic activities, such as gardening and splitting wood, were most frequent. In more than 80% of patients the symptoms began during the activity (Fig 10–4). The relative risk of infarction for individuals engaging in heavy exertion during the 1-hour hazard period was 5.6. Those who exerted themselves less than once per week were at a much higher risk of infarction within 1 hour of heavy exertion than those who exercised vigorously at least 5 times per week.

Conclusion.—Heavy physical exertion is able to trigger acute myocardial infarction, particularly in habitually sedentary individuals.

▶ The authors of this report have omitted several significant papers in their review of the literature. Analysis of data from the Toronto Rehabilitation Centre (1) demonstrated that prior exercise was a significant immediate precipitant of nonfatal infarction many years ago, and Vuori et al. (2) showed a dose/response relationship between the intensity of such exercise and sudden cardiovascular death. The results of the Ontario Multicentre Trial (3) further showed that exercise continued to be an immediate risk factor for infarction after recovery from a first infarction. Our analyses emphasized that although all types of physical activity could be triggers, the most common history was of undertaking an activity for which the subject was ill-prepared, e.g., a 1-km canoe portage on closing up the cottage for the winter. Despite the acute risk of an attack while exercising, the prospects of the exerciser are improved for the remainder of the day. The acute dangers are a reminder to exercise with discretion, but they are not a reason for remaining sedentary.—R.J. Shephard, M.D., Ph.D.

References

1. Shephard RJ: *Br J Sports Med* 8:101, 1974.
2. Vuori I, et al: *Med Sci Sports Exerc* 14:114, 1982.
3. Shephard RJ: *Br Heart J* 42:133, 1979.

Long-Term Reduction of Cardiac Mortality After Myocardial Infarction: 10-Year Results of a Comprehensive Rehabilitation Programme
Hedbäck B, Perk J, Wodlin P (Oskarshamn District Hosp, Sweden)
Eur Heart J 14:831–835, 1993   139-94-10-19

Objective.—Comprehensive rehabilitation programs aim to help patients who have had myocardial infarction (MI) resume as normal a lifestyle as possible. One important goal is to help patients develop cardioprotective habits in the areas of smoking, diet, and exercise. The 10-year

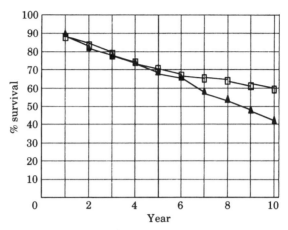

Fig 10–5.—Ten-year survival in intervention group (*open square*) vs. reference group (*closed triangle*). (Courtesy of Hedbäck B, Perk J, Wodlin P: *Eur Heart J* 14:831–835, 1993.)

results were compared for 2 different types of post-MI care: a comprehensive program vs. standard post-MI care.

Methods.—A total of 147 patients, all below age 65 years, participated in a comprehensive rehabilitation program, which included patient and family education; standardized follow-up, including smoking and dietary counseling; and regular physical training, both in groups and at home. They were compared with 158 patients of the same age group from another hospital in a neighboring district who received standard post-MI care. The 305 patients were followed for 10 years.

Findings.—The 2 groups were comparable in their pre-MI, socioeconomic, and acute MI characteristics. As reported previously, the comprehensive rehabilitation program significantly reduced the incidence of smoking and poorly controlled hypertension at 5-year follow-up. Also at 5 years, the recurrence rate of nonfatal MI was 17% in the intervention group vs. 33% in the control group. The total incidence of cardiac events was also lower in the intervention group, 40% vs. 53%. Fifty-two percent of the intervention group were still at work, compared with 27% of the control group. At 10 years, total mortality was 42% in the intervention group vs. 58% in the control group (Fig 10–5). Cardiac mortality was 37% vs. 48%, respectively. The ten-year incidence of nonfatal reinfarction was 29% in the intervention group vs. 40% in the control group. Fifty-nine percent of patients younger than retirement age who took part in the comprehensive rehabilitation program were still at work, compared with 22% of those receiving standard post-MI care.

Conclusion.—The comprehensive rehabilitation program described appears to reduce total and cardiac mortality significantly among patients with myocardial infarction. The mortality benefits of the program were not observed in patients who continued to smoke. Although the study was not randomized, its design essentially eliminated the risk of the intervention influencing the behavior of the control group.

▶ Studies at the Toronto Rehabilitation Centre have shown little change of smoking habits during several years of follow-up. Typically, the prevalence of smoking decreases from around 80% preinfarction to around 35% postinfarction. This study shows that the usual treatment of MI in Sweden has a similar result; however, with a comprehensive program of lifestyle education, the prevalence of smoking can be approximately halved relative to currently accepted practice. It further demonstrates very clearly that the vigorous promotion of smoking withdrawal can have a major effect on subsequent prognosis.—R.J. Shephard, M.D., Ph.D.

Various Intensities of Leisure Time Physical Activity in Patients With Coronary Artery Disease: Effects on Cardiorespiratory Fitness and Progression of Coronary Atherosclerotic Lesions
Hambrecht R, Niebauer J, Marburger C, Grunze M, Kälberer B, Hauer K, Schlierf G, Kübler W, Schuler G (Medizinische Universitätsklinik, Heidelberg, Germany)
J An. Coll Cardiol 22:468–477, 1993   139-94-10–20

Introduction.—For patients with coronary artery disease, regular physical exercise has important protective effects, including reduced coronary risk factors, increased efficacy of oxygen extraction in the peripheral skeletal muscles, and decreased stress-induced myocardial ischemia. However, there are no established guidelines about what training intensity is needed to achieve these benefits. The effect of different levels of leisure physical activity on cardiorespiratory fitness and progression of coronary atherosclerotic lesions in 62 unselected patients with coronary artery disease was defined in a randomized, prospective study.

Methods.—The patients were assigned in roughly equal numbers either to an intervention group, which participated in regular physical exercise, or to a control group, which received care as usual. The standardized questionnaires and data collected during group exercise sessions were used to estimate energy expenditure in leisure activities. Coronary angiography with quantitative digital image processing was performed before and after 1 year of participation.

Results.—Oxygen uptake increased in the intervention group, by 7% at ventilatory threshold and 14% in peak exercise, compared with a significant decrease in the control group. Patients had to expend about 5.9 megajoules (1,400 kcal)/wk in leisure activities to obtain significant improvement in their state of cardiorespiratory fitness; the intervention group expended a mean of 7.85 megajoules (1,876 kcal)/wk, compared with 4.97 megajoules (1,187 kcal)/wk in the control group. Coronary artery disease regressed in 28% of the exercise group compared with just 6% in the controls; the rate of disease progression was 10% in the exercise group vs. 45% in the controls. No change was noted in 62% and 49% of subjects, respectively. Overall, patients with disease progression had the lowest level of leisure activity at 4.28 megajoules (1,022 kcal)/wk, compared with 6.42 megajoules (1,533 kcal)/wk for patients with no change and 9.23 megajoules (2,204 kcal)/wk for patients with disease regression.

Conclusion.—For patients with coronary artery disease, about 5.9 megajoules (1,400 kcal)/wk of leisure physical activity is needed to achieve measurable improvement in cardiorespiratory fitness. About 6.3 megajoules (1,500 kcal)/wk is needed to halt progression of coronary atherosclerotic lesions, whereas 9.2 megajoules (2,200 kcal)/wk—about 5 or 6 hours of physical exercise is needed for disease regression. Patients with high activity levels and good compliance may still show disease progression.

▶ Most formal studies of postcoronary programs have used a fixed amount of exercise. In this study, patients were allowed to select their exercise involvement and the resulting differences of outcome were measured. Although the findings are interesting, when the patients are allowed to determine their own weekly energy expenditure, the question of cause and effect arises. Are the less active individuals limited by more severe disease, or does disease become more severe because such patients are less active?—R.J. Shephard, M.D., Ph.D.

Economic Evaluation of Cardiac Rehabilitation Soon After Acute Myocardial Infarction
Oldridge N, Furlong W, Feeny D, Torrance G, Guyatt G, Crowe J, Jones N (McMaster Univ, Hamilton, Ont, Canada)
Am J Cardiol 72:154–161, 1993   139-94-10–21

Background.—Decisions about the allocation of increasingly scarce health care resources to interventions such as cardiac rehabilitation requires both clinical and economic evaluation. Although there have been many clinical evaluations of cardiac rehabilitation after acute myocardial infarction (AMI), a complete economic evaluation has not been published. Therefore, a randomized trial of cardiac rehabilitation was carried out with economic evaluation as the primary outcome.

Study Design.—Patients with AMI who have mild to moderate anxiety or depression were randomized in the hospital, with 99 receiving an 8-week rehabilitation intervention and 102 receiving standard care. During a 1-year trial, comprehensive costs and health-related quality of life, measured with the time trade-off preference score, were used wth survival data derived from meta-analysis to estimate cost-utility and cost-effectiveness of the rehabilitation. The time trade-off preference score is an interval-scale measure based on determining the maximal number of years of life one would be willing to trade-off to live in full health rather

Cost-Utility/Quality-Adjusted Life-Year (QALY) and Cost-Effectiveness/Life-Year
Gained (LYG) of Selected Cardiovascular Health Care Interventions in 1991
U.S. Dollars

	1991 U.S. $
Cost-utility ($/QALY) for selected interventions and therapies	
Coronary artery bypass surgery[23]	
Left main disease	7,900
1-vessel disease in patients with mild angina	68,200
Treatment of diastolic hypertension in 40-year-old men[23]	
Severe (> 104 mm Hg)	17,700
Mild (95–104 mm Hg)	35,900
Rehabilitation/QALY (from Table III; 1 year)	9,200
Rehabilitation/QALY gained (from Table IV; 3 years)	6,800
Cost-effectiveness ($/LYG) for selected interventions and therapies	
Brief smoking cessation advice during office visit (55-year-old men)[24]	
2.7% cessation (10% relapse)	1,200
1% cessation (50% relapse)	9,500
Aspirin for all AMI[25]	3,100
β-adrenergic antagonist therapy (55-year-old, high-risk men)[26]	5,300
Monotherapies for hypertension (> 94 mm Hg)[27]	
Propanolol hydrochloride	16,000
Captopril	106,900
Hypercholesterolemia (> 272 mg/dl)[28]	
Lovastatin (40 mg/day)	17,000
Lovastatin (80 mg/day)	73,000
Hypercholesterolemia (> 265 mg/dl)[29]	
Colestipol (bulk price)	104,500
Rehabilitation/LYG (from Table IV; 3 years)	21,800

Note: United States/Canadian currency exchange rate for 1987 = .81; and United States medical care
consumer price index changes determined from the Economic Report of the President, February 1992.
(Courtesy of Oldridge N, Furlong W, Feeny D, et al: *Am J Cardiol* 72:154–161, 1993.)

than in one's present state. Quality-adjusted life-years are calculated by
multiplying time trade-off scores by duration of suboptimal health in
years.

Results. —The best estimate of the incremental 1-year costs for patient
rehabilitation was $480 per patient. During a 1-year follow-up, those pa-
tients who had received rehabilitation had significantly fewer follow-up

rehabilitation visits and gained .052 quality-adjusted life-years more than the patients who received standard care. The cost-utility ratio was $9,200 per quality-adjusted life-year gained with cardiac rehabilitation during the 1-year follow-up (table).

Conclusion.—Brief cardiac rehabilitation initiated promptly after AMI for patients with mild to moderate anxiety or depression may be an efficient use of health care resources and may be economically justified.

▶ Early economic analyses of exercise programs examined cost/benefit ratios, e.g., the dollar return in terms of lower medical costs and greater productivity for each dollar that was invested in exercise programs. Such an approach had the major disadvantage that greater worth was ascribed to the rehabilitation of those patients with a high earning potential. Further, many items on the benefit side of the equation were of uncertain dollar magnitude (1).

More recently, the move has been toward cost-effectiveness analyses. These provide answers to questions such as how many years of life are gained by a given investment in exercise programming, relative to the years that would be gained by a similar investment in some alternative tactic such as a smoking cessation program or even the provision of coronary bypass surgery after myocardial ischemia has developed. Such analyses still do not address the important issue that a mere prolongation of life may be undesirable—the ideal objective is to maximize the patient's quality-adjusted life span. Given the extent of terminal disability, an improvement of quality-adjusted life expectancy is often a more important justification for exercise than is a mere extension of life span.

A cost-utility analysis is a variant of cost-effectiveness analysis that seeks to answer the question of the quality of survival. It measures the cost of achieving a given quality-adjusted extension of life span by various tactics. The big stumbling block remains how to estimate quality-adjusted life span. Oldridge and associates have adopted the simple tactic of "time trade-off," asking patients how many years of survival they would be willing to forego to achieve a good quality of life. During the first year of a cardiac rehabilitation program, the cost/utility ratio that they estimate ($9,200 per quality-adjusted life-year) is of the same order as that for the provision of bypass surgery. Surgery, of course, has a short-term economic advantage because it is focused on patients who are in particular and immediate need, whereas exercise rehabilitation is a "blunderbus" type of therapy, offered to all regardless of their current risk status.

Other types of treatment (e.g., physican counseling on smoking, or the use of aspirin) also have a better immediate cost/utility ratio than exercise-centered rehabilitation. However, it is doubtful whether a categorical verdict on the cost-utility of exercise programs can be provided through a 1-year study. The key issue is a likely change in quality-adjusted life span when life is followed through to the terminal years of disability; at this stage of a patient's life, I believe that exercise will show large dividends relative to alternative types of treatment.—R.J. Shephard, M.D., Ph.D.

Reference

1. Shephard RJ: *The Economic Benefits of Enhanced Fitness.* Champaign, IL: Human Kinetic Publishers, 1986.

Pulmonary and Peripheral Vascular Factors Are Important Determinants of Peak Exercise Oxygen Uptake in Patients With Heart Failure

Kraemer MD, Kubo SH, Rector TS, Brunsvold N, Bank AJ (Univ of Minnesota, Minneapolis)
J Am Coll Cardiol 21:641–648, 1993   139-94-10-22

Background.—The mechanisms underlying exercise intolerance in patients with heart failure are not well understood. Previous research has shown that peripheral factors, such as regional blood flow, may be more closely related to exercise capacity than to cardiac function. The role of pulmonary function has received less attention.

Methods.—Fifty patients with stable heart failure were comprehensively examined to determine the relationships among exercise capacity and pulmonary, peripheral vascular, cardiac, and neurohormonal factors in patients with chronic heart failure. Evaluation included a symptom-limited maximal cardiopulmonary exercise test, right heart catheteriza-

	Stepwise Linear Regression for All Variables vs. Peak Oxygen Uptake		
	Sequential R Value	p Value	R^2
Minimal forearm resistance	0.57		
FEV_1	0.71	< 0.001	0.50
FEV_1	0.56		
Plasma norepinephrine	0.67	< 0.001	0.45
FEV_1	0.55		
DLCO	0.65	< 0.001	0.42
Minimal forearm resistance	0.57		
FVC	0.67	< 0.001	0.44
FVC	0.50		
Plasma norepinephrine	0.61	< 0.01	0.37
DLCO	0.47		
FVC	0.58	< 0.001	0.33

Abbreviations: FEV_1 signifies expiratory volume in 1 second; DLCO, diffusing capacity for carbon monoxide; FVC, forced vital capacity.
(Courtesy of Kraemer MD, Kubo SH, Rector TS, et al: *J Am Coll Cardiol* 21:641–648, 1993.)

tion, pulmonary function tests, determination of neurohormonal levels, radionuclide ventriculography, and forearm blood flow at rest and after 5 minutes of brachial artery occlusion.

Findings.—Mean ejection fraction was 19%, and peak oxygen uptake was 16.5 mL/min per kg. Univariate analysis indicated no significant associations between peak oxygen uptake and rest cardiac output, pulmonary wedge pressure, ejection fraction, and pulmonary or systemic vascular resistance. By contrast, the forced expiratory volume in 1 second, forced vital capacity, and diffusing capacity for carbon monoxide were all significantly associated with peak oxygen uptake, even in the absence of arterial desaturation during exercise. Also significantly related to peak oxygen uptake were peak postocclusion forearm blood flow, the corresponding minimal forearm vascular resistance, and plasma norepinephrine level at rest. Multivariate analysis showed that minimal forearm vascular resistance and forced expiratory volume in 1 second were independently associated with peak oxygen uptake. Other bivariate models showed correlations between forced expiratory volume and plasma norepinephrine and diffusing capacity (table).

Conclusion.—Compared with rest indexes of cardiac performance, measures of pulmonary function and peripheral vasodilator capacity were more closely related to peak exercise oxygen uptake in patients with heart failure. The relationships were independent of each other, together accounting for half the variance in peak oxygen uptake. Pulmonary and peripheral vascular adaptations may be important determinants of exercise intolerance in patients with heart failure.

▶ It is widely recognized that resting cardiac performance provides little indication of how the heart will respond to all-out exercise (1). In young and healthy individuals, the ejection fraction may increase, but in those with chronic cardiac failure, it is likely to decrease as afterloading is increased by exercise. We and others have previously drawn attention to the relationship between peak postexercise peripheral blood flow and maximal oxygen intake (2, 3). The other determinant of maximal oxygen intake noted by Kraemer and associates (1-second forced expiratory volume) presumably reflects the influence of pulmonary edema on the compliance of the lungs and the work of breathing, possibly with some influence of poor perfusion of the respiratory muscles (4).—R.J. Shephard, M.D., Ph.D.

References

1. Franciosa JA, et al: *Am J Cardiol* 47:33, 1981.
2. Reading JL, et al: *J Appl Physiol* 74:567, 1993.
3. Sullivan MJ, et al: *Circulation* 80:769, 1989.
4. Minotti JR, et al: *J Clin Invest* 88:2077, 1991.

Physical Training Improves Skeletal Muscle Metabolism in Patients With Chronic Heart Failure

Adamopoulos S, Coats AJS, Brunotte F, Arnolda L, Meyer T, Thompson CH, Dunn JF, Stratton J, Kemp GJ, Radda GK, Rajagopalan B (John Radcliffe Hosp, Oxford, England)

J Am Coll Cardiol 21:1101–1106, 1993   139-94-10–23

Introduction.—Exercise intolerance is a major limiting symptom in heart failure. When peripheral blood flow is increased, exercise capacity and skeletal muscle oxygen use do not immediately respond, indicating that intrinsic abnormalities of skeletal muscle are involved in exertional fatigue in chronic heart failure. However, this abnormality can be reversed with long-term vasodilator therapy. There are many similarities between the skeletal muscle abnormalities associated with chronic heart failure and those of physical deconditioning. Therefore, the effects of physical training on skeletal muscle metabolism were investigated in patients with chronic heart failure.

Methods.—Phosphorus-31 nuclear MR spectroscopy was used to study muscle metabolism during exercise in 12 patients with stable ischemic chronic heart failure who underwent 8 weeks of home cycle ergometer exercise training in a randomized crossover controlled trial. Changes in muscle pH and concentrations of phosphocreatine and adenosine diphosphate (ADP) were measured in calf muscle at rest, throughout incremental work load plantar flexion until exhaustion, and during recovery from exercise. The results were compared with those of 15 age-matched subjects who performed 1 study only.

Results.—Before training, phosphocreatine depletion, muscle acidification, and ADP increase during the first 4 minutes of exercise were all significantly increased compared with control values. Training produced a highly significant increase in exercise tolerance, accompanied by changes in phosphocreatine depletion and ADP increase. After training, changes in ADP were not significantly different from those in controls. The phosphocreatine recovery half-time was significantly shorter after training. The initial rate of phosphocreatine resynthesis after exercise was significantly increased by training, so that it was not significantly different from control values.

Conclusion.—The reduction in phosphocreatine depletion and increase in ADP during exercise and the increase in the rate of phosphocreatine resynthesis during recovery from exercise all indicate that exercise training can correct the impaired oxidative capacity of skeletal muscle in patients with chronic heart failure.

▶ The more successful immediate treatment of myocardial infarction and an aging population are together creating a growing burden of patients with chronic heart failure. Accordingly, research interest has increasingly turned to this category of patients, with a particular focus on the ability of cardiologists to improve the exercise tolerance of such individuals by progressive aerobic training programs.

It would be surprising if a few weeks or months of aerobic training could reverse the adverse hemodynamic consequences of major myocardial scarring, and most authors have concluded that even where benefit is observed, a change in the skeletal rather than cardiac muscle is responsible. A strengthening of the skeletal muscles may allow a given rhythmic activity to proceed at a smaller fraction of peak muscle force, thereby reducing afterloading of the left ventricle. Compensatory peripheral vasoconstriction may also be reversed by training. Finally, if the patient has been sedentary, the activity of aerobic enzymes is initially very low, and (as Adamopoulos and associates suggest) even aerobic training may help to restore this aspect of peripheral function.

The nuclear MR technique used in this study only allowed patients to perform a simple plantar flexion exercise to exhaustion. Such activity is heavily dependent on phosphocreatine depletion, and the findings cannot be applied directly to the performance of aerobic exercise. In parallel aerobic tests, Adamopoulos et al. found that the peak oxygen intake of their patients increased by the sort of margin that we and others have previously described, from 12.2 to 14.1 mL/kg^{-1}/min^{-1}. There was also an increase of cardiac output during submaximal exercise, suggesting that improved perfusion of the skeletal muscles, rather than local enzyme alterations, explained any benefits observed during aerobic activity. Nevertheless, changes in the rate of creatine phosphate depletion during the nuclear MR test were also induced by cycle ergometer training, with beneficial consequences as a result of the performance of such exhausting activities.—R.J. Shephard, M.D., Ph.D.

Exercise Performance After Lung Transplantation
Levy RD, Ernst P, Levine SM, Shennib H, Anzueto A, Bryan CL, Calhoon JH, Trinkle JK, Jenkinson SG, Gibbons WJ (McGill Univ, Montreal; Univ of Texas Health Sciences Ctr, San Antonio)
J Heart Lung Transplant 12:27–33, 1993   139-94-10–24

Background.—Combined heart/lung, isolated double lung, or single lung transplantation may provide benefits for patients with advanced cardiopulmonary disorders. Indications for these procedures overlap and depend on recipient cardiac function, pulmonary infectious status, surgical technique, and potential operative difficulties. The need for cardiopulmonary bypass, the potential for accelerated coronary artery atherosclerosis in the cardiac allograft, donor organ availability, and local surgical experience must also be considered. Exercise capacity anticipated after transplantation may be a useful factor in selecting the best procedure. Exercise performance was compared in patients who had undergone different lung transplantation procedures.

Exercise Performance

	Group 1-Heart-lung	Group 2-Double lung	Group 3-Single lung (obstructive)	Group 4-Single lung (restrictive)	Group 5-Control	Statistical significance*
Subjects (n)	11	6	10	6	28	
Maximum workload (watts)	85.9 ± 22.7	85.0 ± 40.0	66.0 ± 16.5	68.3 ± 33.1	192.6 ± 43.6	5≠1,2,3,4
Peak $\dot{V}O_2$ (ml/min)	988.0 ± 243.0	1265.0 ± 528.0	827.0 ± 271.0	992.0 ± 404.0	2140.0 ± 519.0	5≠1,2,3,4
Peak $\dot{V}O_2$ (ml/kg/min)	15.6 ± 3.2	23.5 ± 9.1	12.2 ± 2.8	13.8 ± 2.9	33.7 ± 7.5	5≠1,2,3,4
Peak $\dot{V}O_2$ (% predicted)	52.1 ± 17.3	59.4 ± 19.7	44.2 ± 16.6	41.0 ± 12.2	85.5 ± 16.2	5≠1,2,3,4
Peak $\dot{V}CO_2$ (ml/min)	1288.0 ± 331.0	1296.0 ± 565.0	922.0 ± 284.0	1209.0 ± 579.0	2733.0 ± 635.0	5≠1,2,3,4
Ventilatory responses						
Peak ventilation (L/min)	43.5 ± 8.6	52.8 ± 9.6	34.2 ± 11.3	59.5 ± 24.3	81.3 ± 26.0	5≠1,2,3,4
Peak ventilation (% predicted)	38.7 ± 10.2	53.7 ± 13.9	47.9 ± 13.0	70.1 ± 6.8	57.6 ± 22.2	1≠4
Peak respiratory rate (/min)	31.5 ± 5.9	32.4 ± 8.4	28.0 ± 5.9	40.4 ± 6.3	38.0 ± 8.7	3≠4,5
Peak tidal volume (ml)	1522.0 ± 219.0	1785.0 ± 777.0	1216.0 ± 237.0	1518.0 ± 655.0	2185.0 ± 486.0	5≠1,2,3,4
Peak tidal volume (% vital capacity)	47.9 ± 7.7	56.6 ± 9.7	50.8 ± 5.8	56.9 ± 5.9	49.4 ± 10.6	NS
$\dot{V}_E/\dot{V}O_2$ at anaerobic threshold	45.5 ± 8.3	42.5 ± 9.2	38.7 ± 7.9	50.6 ± 13.8	31.0 ± 5.4	5≠1,2,4; 4≠3,5

(continued)

Method.—Eleven heart/lung, 6 double lung, and 16 single lung recipients and 28 control subjects were included in the study. All underwent maximal symptom-limited incremental exercise testing on a cycle ergometer.

Table *(continued)*

$\dot{V}_E/\dot{V}CO_2$ at anaerobic threshold	35.0 ± 4.4	43.2 ± 11.3	36.8 ± 5.9	53.6 ± 23.2	27.0 ± 3.6	4≠1,2,3,5;2≠5
Oxygen saturation (%) at peak exercise	97.1 ± 1.5	96.7 ± 1.5	94.4 ± 3.2	90.2 ± 6.8	97.4 ± 1.4	4≠1,2,3,5
Cardiovascular responses						
Resting heart rate (/min)	106.9 ± 14.8	102.7 ± 9.4	96.4 ± 14.5	93.3 ± 15.8	76.0 ± 11.9	5≠1,2,3,4; 1≠3,4
Peak heart rate (/min)	141.6 ± 20.1	163.2 ± 15.6	133.9 ± 14.6	142.3 ± 10.8	170.8 ± 14.6	2,5≠1,3,4
Peak heart rate (% predicted)	81.4 ± 12.3	89.9 ± 9.8	79.9 ± 8.0	85.2 ± 10.1	95.5 ± 7.7	5≠1,3
Peak oxygen pulse (ml/min/beat)	7.1 ± 1.8	7.6 ± 2.7	6.2 ± 2.1	6.9 ± 2.6	12.7 ± 3.9	5≠1,2,3,4
Anaerobic threshold (% predicted $\dot{V}O_{2max}$)	33.8 ± 9.3	42.9 ± 13.8	32.0 ± 11.4	30.8 ± 8.4	57.0 ± 12.8	5≠1,2,3,4

Abbreviations: $\dot{V}O_2$, oxygen uptake; $\dot{V}CO_2$, carbon dioxide production; NS, not significantly different; $\dot{V}_E$, minute ventilation.
° Numbers refer to subject groups.
Significantly different from.
(Courtesy of Levy RD, Ernst P, Levine SM, et al: *J Heart Lung Transplant* 12:27–33, 1993.)

Results.—There were no substantial differences in performance related to the specific lung transplantation procedure used. Transplant recipients in the different groups reached maximal oxygen intakes at peak exercise in the range of 40% to 60% of predicted values. After peak exercise, all the study groups had similar ventilatory patterns and there was no indication that ventilatory factors limited exercise. Overall, patients who underwent transplants demonstrated a reduced aerobic power and diminished oxygen pulse, indicating abnormal cardiovascular performance (table). These limitations may result from chronic deconditioning or peripheral muscle dysfunction related to steroid therapy.

Conclusion.—The heart/lung, double lung, and single lung transplant recipients all demonstrated a reduced aerobic power and diminished oxygen pulse, indicating abnormal cardiovascular performance. However, their aerobic and peak exercise capacities were adequate to permit a comfortable lifestyle and moderate levels of work and exercise. The absence of substantial differences in exercise capacity among the transplant groups suggests that selection of the optimal lung replacement procedure for an individual should be based on other considerations.

▶ The authors of this report claim no difference of maximal oxygen intake between single lung, double lung and heart/lung transplant patients. However, the comparison is clouded by substantial differences of age between the 3 patient groups: patients receiving double lung transplants had an average age of 28 years; patients undergoing heart/lung transplants were an average age of 38 years; and single lung transplants were done on patients whose average age was 47–48 years. It is encouraging that 6 months after a heart/lung transplant, the peak oxygen intake was 52% of population norms, even if specific exercise rehabilitation was limited to the period of hospital stay. However, the corresponding peak oxygen intake (about 4.5 times the resting metabolism) remains insufficient to give any great quality of life to a 38-year-old patient, and there is plainly scope to improve on this figure through a more aggressive program of exercise training.—R.J. Shephard, M.D., Ph.D.

Hemodynamic Responses to Exercise After Lung Transplantation
Ross DJ, Waters PF, Mohsenifar Z, Belman MJ, Kass RM, Koerner SK (Cedars-Sinai Med Ctr, Los Angeles; Univ of California, Los Angeles)
Chest 103:46–53, 1993   139-94-10-25

Background.—Patients who have undergone unilateral or bilateral lung transplantation have been reported to have a reduced maximal oxygen intake ($\dot{V}O_{2max}$) and moderate restrictive ventilatory defects associated with a variable degree of airflow obstruction. The mechanisms of the reduced exercise tolerance in these patients are not clear. Putative mechanisms include deconditioning, chronic anemia, submaximal cardiac rate response, muscle atrophy, and limitation in pulmonary vascular capacity. This study investigated hemodynamic responses to exercise after lung transplantation, examining the possible mechanisms of reduced exercise tolerance.

Hemodynamic Data at Rest and Maximum Exercise Before and After Lung Transplantation

Data	Case 1	Case 2	Case 3	Case 4	Case 5	Case 6	Case 7	Case 8	Mean ± SEM
HR, beats per min									
Rest									
Before	124	106	114	130	81	120	112	...	112±6
After	109	106	79	120	77	91	80	91	94±6*
Exercise									
Before	131	118	140	...	90	133	142	...	126±8
After	133	141	102	180	136	114	118	138	133±8
Cardiac index, L/min/m²									
Rest									
Before	2.88	3.17	2.56	3.08	2.40	2.53	2.42	...	2.72±0.12
After	2.64	2.83	3.47	2.91	2.53	3.12	2.17	2.52	2.77±0.14
Exercise									
Before	3.55	4.55	4.78	4.55	3.80	3.68	6.59	...	4.50±0.39
After	7.66	7.27	7.67	5.68	7.13	5.38	5.93	5.85	6.57±0.34*
MPAP, mm Hg									
Rest									
Before	19	...	12	24	26	19	21	...	20±5
After	11	25	10	19	23	14	18	28	18±2*
Exercise									
Before	36	...	28	31	42	32	31	...	33±2
After	19	37	16	52	48	34	33	50	36±5
PCW, mm Hg									
Rest									
Before	5	14	12	4	9	10	10	...	9±1
After	...	8	4	3	9	7	10	10	7±1
Exercise									
Before	18	...	22	6	21	15	12	...	16±2
After	...	15	8	25	13	25	14	24	18±3

	1	2	3	4	5	6	7	8	Mean ± SD
PVR, Wood units									
Rest									
Before	3.0	...	0.7	5.0	3.5	2.0	2.9	...	2.9 ± 0.6
After	...	3.2	1.0	4.0	2.8	1.4	2.2	3.4	2.6 ± 0.4
Exercise									
Before	4.0	...	0.7	4.2	2.8	2.7	1.8	...	2.7 ± 0.5
After	...	1.6	0.6	3.5	2.5	1.0	1.9	2.5	1.9 ± 0.4
SVI, ml/beat/m²									
Rest									
Before	23	30	22	24	30	21	22	...	25 ± 1
After	24	27	44	24	33	34	27	28	30 ± 2
Exercise									
Before	31	39	34	38	42	28	46	...	37 ± 2
After	58	52	75	32	52	47	50	42	51 ± 4*
Systemic O$_2$ delivery, ml/min/kg									
Rest									
Before	...	12.5	14.0	17.6	12.2	14.2	12.2	...	13.8 ± 0.8
After	12.5	11.8	14.3	15.7	11.1	15.8	9.8	10.1	12.6 ± 0.8
Exercise									
Before	...	17.6	27.8	22.9	13.2	19.7	27.6	...	21.5 ± 2.4
After	39.5	...	34.1	31.0	30.7	28.0	25.9	22.4	30.2 ± 2.1*
ER, %									
Rest									
Before	...	47	48	29	40	37	36	...	40 ± 3
After	35	40	19	30	40	34	38	...	34 ± 3
Exercise									
Before	...	57	55	39	42	53	63	...	52 ± 4
After	59	...	54	48	63	48	60	57	56 ± 2

Abbreviations: HR, heart rate; MPAP, mean pulmonary artery pressure; PCW, pulmonary capillary wedge pressure; PVR, pulmonary vascular resistance; SVI, stroke volume index; ER, oxygen extraction ratio.

* P < .05 for before vs. after.

(Courtesy of Ross DJ, Waters PF, Mohsenifar Z, et al: *Chest* 103:46–53, 1993.)

Method.—The hemodynamic responses to incremental cycle ergometry were assessed before and after lung transplantation in 8 patients (table). After transplantation, the patients had a formal 6-week exercise training program and were encouraged to continue a similar level of physical activity.

Findings.—The $\dot{V}O_{2max}$ and peak work rate improved significantly after lung transplantation. The transition thresholds for arterial standard bicarbonate were abnormally low and there was an early rise in arterial lactate. The maximum stroke volume index increased in 6 of 7 patients. The mean arterial pulmonary pressure during exercise was elevated in 6 patients. Pulmonary vascular resistance was mildly elevated after transplantation, but it decreased appropriately during exercise and was associated with normal cardiac output responses.

Conclusion.—The 8 recipients of lung transplantation had significant improvement in $\dot{V}O_{2max}$ and peak work rate with transplantation, but the mean values were only 42% of the predicted $\dot{V}O_{2max}$ for age-matched peers. In 5 transplant recipients pulmonary vascular abnormalities during hemodynamic exercise testing were attributed to cardiovascular limitation or to deconditioning. In the remaining 3 patients the exercise study was considered to be submaximal because of low peak heart rates. The limitation to maximum exercise was associated with a persistent state of cardiovascular deconditioning. Therefore, exercise training after lung transplantation may have considerable value.

▶ In the patient undergoing cardiac transplant, exercise performance is initially limited by muscle weakness and poor cardiovascular condition, which can be corrected largely by participation in a sustained training program (1). Training has previously extended for periods as long as 16 months, and the large gains of maximal oxygen intake (45%) observed with only 6 weeks of training are quite surprising. The 6-week period of exercise began immediately after discharge from the hospital, and because the study did not include controls, it is quite likely that much of the apparent training response is really caused by spontaneous recovery. The main value of the study is it shows that in lung transplantation, as in cardiac transplantation, the biggest functional limitation arises from a postsurgical loss of cardiac function and/or muscle weakness rather than from pulmonary vascular problems.—R.J. Shephard, M.D., Ph.D.

Reference

1. Shephard RJ: *Exerc Sports Sci Rev* 20:297, 1992.

Lifelong Exercise and Stroke

Shinton R, Sagar G (Univ of Birmingham, England; Dudley Road Hosp, Birmingham, England)

BMJ 307:231–234, 1993   139-94-10-26

Introduction.—Exercise is acknowledged to reduce the risks of coronary heart disease and hypertension, but the protection afforded against stroke has received less attention. The potential of lifelong patterns of increased physical activity to prevent stroke was investigated.

Subjects and Methods.—During a 24-month period, 125 men and women aged 35–74 years who had just had their first stroke entered the case-control study. The controls were 198 randomly selected subjects from the general practice population in the same area (west Birmingham, England), matched for age and sex with the stroke patients. Excluded were subjects with a history of any of the following: stroke, mitral valvular heart disease combined with atrial fibrillation, primary or metastatic cerebral neoplasm, coagulation disorder, or myeloproliferative disease. Both stroke patients and controls completed questionnaires related to exercise, diet, smoking, alcohol consumption, and health status.

Results.—Most stroke patients were assessed within 14 days of the start of the stroke. The median ages of the patients with stroke and the controls were 66 years and 63 years, respectively. The odds ratio for stroke was most reduced among subjects reporting vigorous exercise in youth. (The table shows the protective effect of vigorous exercise in youth examined separately by age, sex, and smoking. A similar benefit was seen in all groups.) This reduction was not appreciably affected by adjustment for a number of variables: race, social class, peak body mass index, subscapular skinfold thickness, dietary intake of saturated fat, family history of stroke, and histories of hypertension, diabetes mellitus, and cardiac ischemia. There were minimal effects on the odds ratios

Relative Risk of Stroke After Regular Vigorous Exercise Undertaken at Age 15–25 Years, Stratified by Sex, Age, and Cigarette Smoking

| | Exercise not undertaken | | Exercise undertaken | |
	Odds ratio	No of cases: no of controls	Odds ratio (95% confidence interval)	No of cases: no of controls
Sex*:				
Male	1·0	30:16	0·30 (0·1 to 0·6)	43:82
Female	1·0	40:52	0·37 (0·2 to 0·8)	12:48
Age group (years)†:				
35-54	1·0	9:11	0·20 (0·1 to 0·8)	5:26
55-64	1·0	17:22	0·34 (0·1 to 1·0)	19:47
65-74	1·0	44:35	0·36 (0·2 to 0·8)	31:57
Cigarette smoking‡:				
Never	1·0	14:36	0·65 (0·2 to 2·0)	8:33
Former	1·0	28:14	0·19 (0·1 to 0·5)	26:55
Current	1·0	28:18	0·30 (0·1 to 0·8)	21:42

Note: Odds ratio adjusted for *age; †sex; ‡age and sex.
(Courtesy of Shinton R, Sagar G: *BMJ* 307:231–234, 1993.)

with adjustment for recent vigorous exercise and recent walking. Increasing years of participation in vigorous exercise between the ages of 15 and 55 years resulted in an increasing protection from stroke.

Conclusion.—Vigorous exercise in early adulthood (ages 15–25 years) encourages lifelong habits of physical activity and results in a reduced age- and sex-adjusted odds ratio for stroke (.33 in this group of subjects). Continuing this level of activity throughout life can offer increased protection against stroke.

▶ This paper supports another recent study from the United Kingdom that suggested that habitual physical activity could protect against stroke (1), although it is at variance with an earlier American study of nonfatal strokes (2). The emphasis on benefits from sports participation between the ages of 15 and 25 years is a little puzzling. Because the findings were adjusted only for age and sex, it is possible that some of the apparent benefit from teenage activity may reflect differences of social class and related smoking habits. Many working-class youths leave school at an age of 15 or 16 years in England, whereas those in higher socioeconomic strata attend universities and thus have ready access to sports programs throughout their early twenties.—R.J. Shephard, M.D., Ph.D.

References

1. Wannamethee G, Shaper AG: *BMJ* 304:597, 1992.
2. Paffenbarger RS, Wing AL: *Am J Epidemiol* 94:524, 1971.

Effort Thrombosis in a Young Wrestler: A Case Report
Medler RG, McQueen DA (St Francis Regional Med Ctr, Wichita, Kan)
J Bone Joint Surg (Am) 75-A:1071–1073, 1993   139-94-10–27

Introduction.—Effort thrombosis, or Paget-Schroetter syndrome, is the term applied to the occurrence of venous thrombosis in an otherwise healthy subject after some strenuous activity that is usually athletic in nature. Effort thrombosis usually occurs in the upper extremities but has also been reported in the lower extremities. Effort thrombosis of the upper extremity was studied in a high school wrestler.

Case Report.—Boy, 15 years, was referred to an orthopedist 3 days after competing in a wrestling match. Although he had no apparent injury during the match, he had since experienced diffuse swelling of his right arm, from the fingers to the shoulder. Biceps diameter was 3 cm greater on the right than the left. The patient had prominent superficial veins, with pain on palpation of the deltopectoral groove and on all extremes of motion. Venography and digital venous imaging demonstrated total occlusion of the axillary and subclavian veins (Fig 10–6).

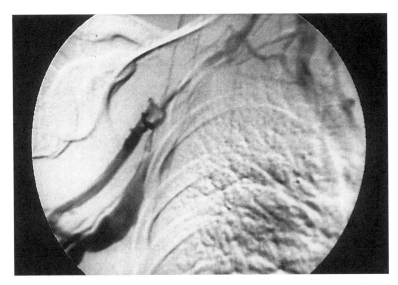

Fig 10–6.—Digital vascular imaging study of the right arm, showing total occlusion of the axillary and subclavian veins and marked collateral venous return. (Courtesy of Medler RG, McQueen DA: *J Bone Joint Surg (Am)* 75-A:1071–1073, 1993.)

In the intensive care unit, the patient received tissue-plasminogen activator, 5 mg by intravenous bolus, followed by 55 mg during the first hour and 20 mg/hr during the next 2 hours. Heparin and warfarin were added later and titrated to achieve a partial thromboplastin time and prothrombin time of 1.5–2 times the control value. Symptoms resolved during the next 5 days, and the patient was discharged on warfarin therapy. The swelling resolved by 1 month after discharge; and after 6 months, warfarin treatment was stopped and he was allowed to return to wrestling gradually.

Discussion.—Effort thrombosis syndrome can occur in athletes who use their arms in an overhead position, including swimmers, baseball players, and tennis players. The diagnosis may be difficult to make; symptoms include pain and swelling after strenuous activity. Venography confirms the diagnosis.

Coagulopathy Presenting as Calf Pain in a Racquetball Player

Wong C, Bracker M (Univ of California, San Diego, La Jolla)
J Fam Pract 37:390–393, 1993   139-94-10-28

Introduction.—Leg pain is a common complaint among athletes that usually results from musculoskeletal injury. In a young athletic patient, leg pain with an unusual cause—protein S deficiency—was seen.

Case Report.—Man, 27, who was a fourth-year medical student experienced a progressively worsening, poorly localized pain in the calf of his left leg. He attributed the pain to muscle strain because he had been playing racquetball 2 days before the onset of symptoms. The pain resolved with aspirin and a period of inactivity, then returned after the patient was on his feet most of the day or performed stretching exercises. At the time of evaluation, circumferential leg measurements revealed the left leg to be 2.5 cm greater than the right. Duplex ultrasound showed evidence of a deep venous thrombosis in the left leg extending to the level of the adductor canal. The patient was hospitalized, received 4 days of heparin treatment, and was discharged receiving warfarin therapy. After 3 months of treatment, a repeat Doppler ultrasound showed only a small area of noncompressibility of the left popliteal vein. Tests for hypercoagulable states yielded total protein S at the lower limit of normal range; free protein S was less than 12% by rocket immunoelectrophoresis.

Conclusion.—Protein S deficiency, the most frequent cause of idiopathic venous thrombosis, is inherited as an autosomal dominant trait with incomplete penetrance. The incidence of this condition is currently unknown. Among those with protein S deficiency there is a 68% probability of a thrombotic event by age 35 years. Treatment is identical to that of acute venous thrombosis resulting from any cause. Asymptomatic patients need not receive long-term warfarin prophylaxis. Patients should be counseled about the risks associated with protein S deficiency, and their family members should be evaluated for risk of thrombosis. Aspirin (81 mg daily) or placement of a Greenfield filter are possible alternatives to lifelong low-dose warfarin.

▶ These companion articles (Abstracts 139-94-10–27 and 139-94-10–28) illustrate problems in diagnosing and managing venous thrombosis in athletes. The case report of effort thrombosis in a wrestler presented by Medler and McQueen (Abstract 139-94-10–27) complements another report of a lower limb vein in a football player with tight pants (1) as well as a report of axillary and subclavian veins in a football player who, just before his arm became mottled and swollen, had bench-pressed weights (2). In 2 of 3 patients, thrombolysis was used. Guidelines have been offered for return to sports after deep venous thrombosis (DVT) of the calf (3), but not after effort thrombosis per se.

Abstract 139-94-10–28 shows that DVT can mimic calf strain, and that an inherited hypercoagulable state can underlie or spur DVT. A good review of inherited and acquired hypercoagulable states appeared in 1993 (4). A recent editorial estimates that, in otherwise healthy patients younger than 45 years of age who are referred for DVT, inherited deficiency of antithrombin III, protein C, and protein S each account for about 5% of cases (5). New inherited deficiencies, however, such as resistance to activated protein C (which seems to be much more common than the above deficiencies), continue to be discovered (6). Some experts now say that inherited defects in "natural anticoagulants" may account for up to half of patients younger than 45 years of age with DVT (5).—E.R. Eichner, M.D.

References

1. 1991 YEAR BOOK OF SPORTS MEDICINE, pp 276–277.
2. 1993 YEAR BOOK OF SPORTS MEDICINE, pp 300–302.
3. Roberts WO, Christie DM Jr: *Med Sci Sports Exerc* 24:2, 1992.
4. Nachman RL, Silverstein R: *Ann Intern Med* 119:819, 1993.
5. Bauer KA: *N Engl J Med* 330:566, 1994.
6. Svensson PJ, Dahlback B: *N Engl J Med* 330:517, 1994.

Pleurodynia Among Football Players at a High School: An Outbreak Associated With Coxsackievirus B1
Ikeda RM, Kondracki SF, Drabkin PD, Birkhead GS, Morse DL (New York State Dept of Health, Albany)
JAMA 270:2205–2206, 1993   139-94-10–29

Introduction.—Epidemic pleurodynia (epidemic myalgia, Bornholm disease) is characterized by sudden pain in the chest or abdomen and is usually associated with fever. It is generally a result of coxsackievirus B infection, but other enteroviruses have been identified in those affected. An outbreak of pleurodynia occurred among football players at a public high school in upstate New York in the fall of 1991.

Epidemiology.—Of 84 players on 3 school teams, 17 (20%) described an illness that met the case definition. All were members of the junior varsity and varsity teams. Eating ice cubes from the team ice chest carried a relative risk of 9.2, and drinking from the team water cooler carried a risk of 6.3. Those who made oral contact with the cooler spout were at increased risk of becoming ill (table). Stool specimens from 4 of 8 players who had had symptoms in the previous week yielded coxsackievirus B1. Throat swab specimens were negative on viral culture. Analysis of water samples yielded normal coliform counts.

Risk of Acquiring Pleurodynia Among Football Players, New York, September 1991

Behavior	No. (%) Ill With Behavior	No. (%) Ill Without Behavior	RR*	95% CI†
Eating ice cubes from the team ice chest‡	13/34 (38)	1/24 (4)	9.2	1.3-65.5
Drinking water from the team cooler§	15/43 (35)	2/36 (6)	6.3	1.5-25.7
Direct oral contact with spout on team cooler‖	5/9 (56)	9/33 (27)	2.0	0.9-4.6

* Relative risk determined in univariate analysis.
† 95% confidence interval.
‡ Information missing for 26 respondents.
§ Information missing for 5 respondents.
‖ Information missing for 1 respondent.
(Courtesy of Ikeda RM, Kondracki SF, Drabkin PD, et al: JAMA 270:2205-2206, 1993.)

Conclusion.—It appears that common water containers were contaminated by coxsackievirus B1 from an infected player. Some of the illness may have resulted from repeated contamination of water sources or person-to-person spread. In addition to discouraging direct oral contact with common drinking containers, disposable cups should be used. Ice packs should be used rather than ice cubes for treating injuries. Information on enteroviral illness should be provided to students and coaching staff.

▶ This recent report of enteroviral transmission among football players reminds us that, as in prior outbreaks of hepatitis and aseptic meningitis in football players (1), because of common-source contamination of water or breaches in hygiene, the risk of infection comes not from the exercise, but from the team. Will athletes ever learn to avoid grabbing ice from common containers, sharing drinking cups, and mouthing the spout of water coolers? A practical review of infectious disease in sports has just appeared (2).—E.R. Eichner, M.D.

References

1. Eichner ER: *Physician Sportsmed* 21:15, 1993.
2. Goodman RA, et al: *JAMA* 271:862, 1994.

The Relationship Between Comfortable and Most Metabolically Efficient Walking Speed in Persons With Unilateral Above-Knee Amputation
Jaegers SMHJ, Vos LDW, Rispens P, Hof AL (Univ of Groningen, The Netherlands; Rehabilitation Centre Beatrixoord, Haren, The Netherlands)
Arch Phys Med Rehabil 74:521–525, 1993   139-94-10-30

Purpose.—For healthy individuals, the most comfortable walking speed is similar to the most metabolically efficient speed—that at which energy expenditure is lowest per distance covered. It is unknown whether the walking speed selected by above-knee amputees is also close to their most efficient speed. The association between the most comfortable and the most efficient walking speed was assessed in 11 healthy men with unilateral above-knee amputation.

Methods.—Six normal men were also studied as controls. The subjects were studied both at rest and at 6 incremental walking speeds, based on their self-selected comfortable walking speed. Subjects walked at each speed for 6 minutes as their oxygen uptake, heart rate, and step rate were monitored. At each speed, energy expenditure was measured per second and per meter.

Results.—In controls, comfortable walking speed was the same as most efficient speed. For most of the amputees, however, comfortable walking speed was lower than the most efficient walking speed. The am-

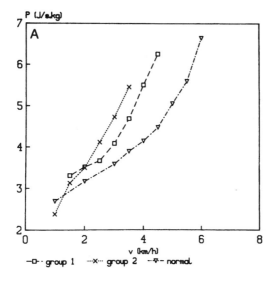

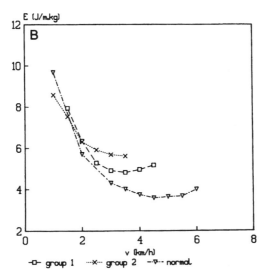

Fig 10–7.—Mean energy expenditure and standard deviation per second, per kilogram of body weight (**A**) and per meter, per kilogram of body weight (**B**) of normal subjects (*triangles*), group 1 (*squares*), and group 2 (X) of the above-knee amputees. (Courtesy of Jaegers SMHJ, Vos LDW, Rispens P, et al: *Arch Phys Med Rehabil* 74:521–525, 1993.)

putees had higher energy expenditure at comfortable walking speed than controls. At most efficient speed, the energy expenditure per second was the same for both amputee and normal subjects (Fig 10-7). Step rate at comfortable walking speed was also the same for both groups, but the amputee group showed a smaller increment in step rate at increased walking speeds.

Conclusion.—Energy expenditure at comfortable walking speed is higher for unilateral above-knee amputees than for normal subjects. For amputees, comfortable walking speed is lower than the most efficient walking speed. Some of the higher energy expenditure of above-knee amputees, both above and below comfortable walking speed, appears to be attributable to their deviating step rate.

▶ There have been quite a number of papers on the oxygen cost of walking in amputees. Most of these reports make the point underlined by Jaegers and associates that such individuals are not able to walk fast enough to attain an economical speed of walking. However, almost all of these papers have fallen into the trap of expressing oxygen cost in units of mL/[kg·m] of body mass, based on the *gross* oxygen cost of covering a fixed distance. The slower the pace, the larger the contribution of resting oxygen consumption to the apparent cost of the task, so that gross efficiency almost inevitably improves with the speed of ambulation!

If data are expressed (more correctly) as *net* oxygen costs, then we do not see a sharp minimum of energy expenditures with increasing speeds; values are consistent over a wide range of speeds, although costs do rise at the extremes of very slow and very rapid movement. Further, we then find that the majority of amputees are able to reach or approach their optimum cost of movement (1).—R.J. Shephard, M.D., Ph.D.

Reference

1. Shephard RJ, et al: *Can J Rehabil:* In press.

Exercise and Multiple Sclerosis
Ponichtera-Mulcare JA (Wright State Univ, Dayton, Ohio)
Med Sci Sports Exerc 25:451–465, 1993   139-94-10–31

Background.—Multiple sclerosis (MS), a neurologic disease, produces a variety of potentially debilitating symptoms. Many patients have a normal life expectancy and remain ambulatory all their lives. Little is known about how MS affects basic physiologic responses during exercise.

Exercise and MS.—Some patients with MS have abnormalities in cardiovascular reflexes during quiescent testing. However, heart rate and blood pressure responses during exercise are not consistent with these findings. Cardiorespiratory deficits seem to be present in moderately impaired patients but not always in the minimally impaired (Table 1). Skeletal muscle function abnormalities have also been reported in some patients with MS but not in others. Both cardiorespiratory fitness and skeletal muscle function appear to be enhanced through training. The level of study subjects' physical impairment appears to influence findings

TABLE 1.—Summary of Investigations Examining Cardiorespiratory Response to Exercise Among Individuals With MS

Investigators (Sample Size)	Control Group	Mode of Ergometry	Direct Metabolic Data	Power Output Maximum (W)	$\dot{V}O_{2max}$ (ml · kg⁻¹ · min⁻¹)
Senaratne et al. (52) (N = 21)	Yes	ARM	No	70	NM
Schapiro et al. (48) (N = 25)	Yes *	ARM/LEG	No	121	NM
Ponichtera (36) (N = 9)	Yes	RLEG	Yes	126	28.7
Ponichtera et al. (37) (N = 10)	Yes	RLEG	Yes	112	38.2
	Yes	ARM	Yes	58	23.8
	Yes	ARM/LEG	Yes	118	40.1

Note: All data are reported as group means.
Abbreviations: NM signifies data not measured; ARM, arm cycling ergometry; RLEG, recumbent leg ergometry; ARM/LEG, combined arm and leg ergometry.
* Control subjects were also individuals with MS; all other control groups were healthy subjects without MS.
(Courtesy of Ponichtera-Mulcare JA: *Med Sci Sports Exerc* 25:451–465, 1993.)

TABLE 2.—Summary of Clinical Thermal Perturbations and Related Symptom Instability in MS

Investigator(s)	Type of Perturbation	General Results with Thermal Stress
Guthrie (17) (N = 10)	Total body hot water immersion; arm immersion; leg immersion	Reduction in grip strength and leg strength; reduced visual acuity (VA); increased central scotoma; dysarthria
Watson (59) (N = 8)	Cold water immersion; cold air exposure; and ice	Reduction in core temperature corresponded with an improvement of MS symptoms
Nelson and McDowell (31) (N = 14)	Infrared body heating; hot water immersion	Increase in core temperature elicited the appearance of at least 1 MS symptom
Noronha et al. (34) (N = 60)	Heat cradle; pilocarpine; and bladder distention	Abnormal sweating response to heat cradle and pilocarpine, no response to bladder distention
Cartlidge (5) (N = 50)	Hot water arm immersion	Various abnormal sweating responses
Namerow (28) (N = 1)	Circadian variation; refrigerated blanket; hydrocortisone sodium succinate; nicotinic acid; bicycle exercise nicotinic acid	VA improved with a concomitant reduction in core temperature and worsened with an increase in core temperature; no changes in VA with hydrocortisone or no change with exercise when there was no core temperature change
Hopper et al. (19) (N = 1)	Acute ambient temperature increase; ice emulsion ingestion hot water ingestion; epinephrine; hand immersion in ice	VA worsened with increased ambient temperature; no change in VA with hot water ingestion; improved VA with epinephrine and with ice immersion of hand
Ponichtera (39) (N = 11)	Acute and prolonged recumbent leg cycling in air and water	No significant change in core temperature during acute or prolonged test in either environment

(Courtesy of Ponichtera-Mulcare JA: *Med Sci Sports Exerc* 25:451–465, 1993.)

indirectly. Several researchers have elicited symptoms in response to thermal stressors, but unreliable methods were used to measure core temperature. When more valid methods were used during rest and exercise, no relationship between symptoms and core temperature changes was found. Thermal sensitivity, which is reported by most patients with MS, may be a symptom unique to each patient, and sample selection may have indirectly contaminated past findings (Table 2).

Conclusion.—The effects of MS on basic physiologic responses during exercise are not well understood. Four topics related to this issue were addressed: autonomic control of heart rate and arterial blood pressure, cardiorespiratory fitness, skeletal muscle function, and symptom instability under thermal stress.

▶ Multiple sclerosis has substantial implications for population health, both in terms of the numbers of people affected (probably a quarter of a million in the United States alone) and the length of the disease process (three quarters living at least 25 years after the diagnosis of MS). However, there has been surprisingly little research on the potential benefits of exercise in this condition. Demyelination is a local phenomenon, and there is little evidence that exercise accelerates progression of the disease. It thus makes sense to institute programs to maximize residual function in both heart and muscle.—R.J. Shephard, M.D., Ph.D.

Low-Back Pain in Sports: Managing Spondylolysis in Young Patients
Johnson RJ (Hennepin County Med Ctr, Minneapolis)
Physician Sportsmed 21:53–59, 1993   139-94-10-32

Pars Injury.—Injuries of the pars interarticularis—the narrow part of bone lying between the superior and inferior articular facets of the vertebral arch—range from a stress reaction with negative radiographs to fracture, which on radiographs is seen as a collar in the "Scottie dog." Typically, radiographs are not abnormal for 2–3 weeks after injury. Symptomatic injury is most prevalent in athletes aged 10–15 years. Most often there is a history of overuse caused by repetitive motion. Weight-loading activities, rotation-associated sports including baseball, and back-arching movements like those in football and tennis are the riskiest pursuits.

Clinical Assessment.—Unilateral low back pain present for longer than 2–3 weeks should raise a suspicion of pars injury in an adolescent athlete. Pain is felt in the paraspinal region near the midline and can usually be localized with "one finger" tensors. A positive radiograph with a negative bone scan may suggest a poor outlook for bone healing, whereas a positive bone scan, regardless of the radiographic findings, suggests a more acute fracture that is relatively likely to unite.

Management.—It is important to reduce or cease the offending activity, to stretch the hamstrings and gluteal muscles, and to strengthen the abdominal and back extensors. The role of antilordotic bracing is uncertain. The recommended duration of treatment ranges from 6 weeks to 6 months. Most recommend that active rehabilitation not be started until symptoms have been absent for 4 weeks. Conservative measures usually prove effective, and recurrence is infrequent after fibrous or bony healing.

Complications.—If a pars injury heals with elongation of the pars, the entire segment may be overloaded, thus increasing the risk of rapid degenerative changes. A unilateral pars defect may heighten stress on the other pars, resulting in bilateral spondylolysis. It is not clear whether fibrous union promotes degenerative changes.

▶ Johnson presents a thoughtful, informative, practical approach to diagnosing and managing spondylolysis in young patients. Spondylolysis, a stress fracture of the pars interarticularis, differs from other stress fractures in that it develops at a younger age, usually heals with less periosteal callus or a fibrous union, and has a strong family history. The typical patient with spondylolysis has unilateral, "finger-point" localized, near-midline back pain, usually at the L5 level, and a positive one-legged lumbar hyperextension test. The most sensitive diagnostic test is the bone scan enhanced by single photon emission CT, as covered in the 1992 YEAR BOOK OF SPORTS MEDICINE (1). Early diagnosis and conservative therapy help the patient return to sports quickly. See also a comprehensive, practical review on low back pain in young athletes (2) and Abstract 139-94-7–19 in this issue.—E.R. Eichner, M.D.

References

1. 1992 YEAR BOOK OF SPORTS MEDICINE, pp 40–42.
2. Harvey J, Tanner S: *Sports Med* 12:394, 1991.

Heart Rate, Physical Activity, and Mortality From Cancer and Other Noncardiovascular Diseases
Wannamethee G, Shaper AG, Macfarlane PW (Royal Free Hosp, London; Royal Infirmary, Glasgow, Scotland)
Am J Epidemiol 137:735–748, 1993   139-94-10–33

Introduction.—Elevated resting heart rate has been associated with an increased risk of ischemic heart disease and may also be positively related to noncardiovascular mortality. Several studies suggest that physical activity may be protective against cancer. This study examined the relation between heart rate, physical activity, and 9.5-year mortality from noncardiovascular diseases.

Subjects and Methods.—The study participants were 7,735 British men, aged 40–59 years, drawn from general practices in 24 towns. The subjects were examined and were administered questionnaires during 1978–1980, and then were followed until December 1989. Information was obtained on their cigarette smoking status, alcohol consumption, usual pattern of physical activity, and occupation. Resting heart rate was determined from the three-orthogonal-lead ECG.

Results.—There were 691 deaths from all causes during follow-up. Cardiovascular disease was the cause of 356 deaths and cancer was the cause of 255 deaths. The mean heart rate for the entire study population was 70.7 beats per minute. Mortality rates for all causes increased significantly with increasing heart rate. There was a significant positive association between heart rate and both cancer and other noncardiovascular causes of death. For cancer mortality, the highest risk was seen in men with a heart rate of 80–89 beats per minute. Mean heart rate decreased significantly and progressively with increasing physical activity.

Conclusion.—Resting heart rate and high levels of physical activity are independent prognostic factors for cancer mortality in middle-aged men. The positive associations observed here persisted even after adjustment for age, lung function, blood cholesterol, body mass index, heavy alcohol consumption, smoking, preexisting ischemic heart disease, social class, and systolic blood pressure.

▶ In principle, the resting heart rate is a good indicator of physical condition, and a few epidemiologists have sought correlations between resting heart rate and cancer in occupational studies (1). One immediate difficulty is that, in a large study like this one by Wannamethee and associates, it is not possible to ensure that subjects have abstained from smoking before heart rate determination, and smoking increases the resting heart rate by 5–10 beats per minute. Given the substantial impact of smoking on many disease processes, including a variety of cancers, it is not surprising that a high heart rate becomes associated with a high noncardiovascular mortality.

Despite a 10-year follow-up, a survey based on 7,735 men also yielded only 255 associated cases of cancer, another major difficulty in conducting this type of research. As expected, the impact of physical activity was greatest on cancers of the digestive system, although even here the relative risk of .46 was statistically no different from 1.0. The impact of exercise on cancer of the lungs (relative risk, .53; 95% confidence interval, .78–1.28) merits further exploration on a larger sample.—R.J. Shephard, M.D., Ph.D.

Reference

1.   Persky V, et al: *Am J Epidemiol* 114:477, 1981.

Occupational Physical Activity and the Incidence of Cancer of the Breast, Corpus Uteri, and Ovary in Shanghai

Zheng W, Shu XO, McLaughlin JK, Chow W-H, Gao YT, Blot WJ (Shanghai Cancer Inst, China; Natl Cancer Inst, Bethesda, Md)

Cancer 71:3620–3624, 1993   139-94-10-34

Background.—A sedentary lifestyle has been consistently associated with an increased risk of colon cancer. Recently, it has also been associated with breast and other gynecologic cancers. This new evidence is limited. The role of occupational physical activity in the risk of cancer of the breast, corpus uteri, and ovary was studied in Shanghai, where the rates of these cancers are relatively low.

Methods and Findings.—Occupational data on 3,783 incident patients with cancer diagnosed from 1980 to 1984 were obtained and compared with 1982 census data in Shanghai urban areas. Professionals, government officials, and clerical workers were found to have a significantly increased incidence of breast cancer. The incidence was reduced among service workers and craftswomen. Occupational physical activity was inversely associated with breast cancer incidence. The standardized incidence ratios were 127–131 for inactive jobs and 79–93 for active jobs. Similar relationships were seen among patients with cancer of the corpus uteri and ovary but to a lesser extent (table).

Conclusion.—Women in occupations involving minimal physical activity had an increased incidence of breast, corpus uteri, and ovarian cancer. This incidence was reduced among women with high-activity jobs. These data are consistent with previous reports and provide further evidence that physical activity may decrease the risk of these female hormone–dependent cancers.

▶ There is increasing evidence that a sedentary lifestyle exposes women to risks of reproductive tract cancers (1, 2). This report supports this view, although unfortunately the authors lacked the data to control for other risk factors that may have been greater in women of higher socioeconomic status (e.g., dietary fat intake, obesity, age at first live-birth, and number of pregnancies.).—R.J. Shephard, M.D., Ph.D.

References

1. Frisch RE, et al: *Am J Clin Nutr* 45:328, 1987.
2. Vena JE, et al: *Am J Clin Nutr* 45:318, 1987.

Number of Observed Cases and Standardized Incidence Ratios According to Cancer Sites and Occupational Physical Activity Indexes (Urban Shanghai, 1982–1984)

Occupational physical activity index	Cancer site					
	Breast		Corpus uteri		Ovary	
	No.	SIR	No.	SIR	No.	SIR
Sitting time						
Long	516	127*	74	110	97	112
Moderate	1070	110*	162	103	220	110
Short	1150	93†	216	97	278	102
Energy expenditure						
Low	1105	131*	144	110	205	118
Moderate	1377	95	260	101	318	100
High	254	79*	48	80	72	102

Abbreviation: SIR, standardized incidence ratio.
* $P \leq .01$.
† $P \leq .05$.
(Courtesy of Zheng W, Shu XO, McLaughlin JK, et al: *Cancer* 71:3620–3624, 1993.)

Past and Present Physical Activity and Endometrial Cancer Risk

Sturgeon SR, Brinton LA, Berman ML, Mortel R, Twiggs LB, Barrett RJ, Wilbanks GD (Natl Cancer Inst, Bethesda, Md; Univ of California, Irvine, Orange; Milton S Hershey Med Ctr, Hershey, Pa; et al)
Br J Cancer 68:584–589, 1993   139-94-10–35

Background.—The risk for endometrial cancer is markedly higher in overweight women. Excess body weight is related to physical inactivity and may increase risk of endometrial cancer through obesity-mediated hormonal mechanisms. The relationship between recent and lifetime physical activity and the risk for endometrial cancer was evaluated in a case-control study.

Methods.—Four hundred five women who had had epithelial endometrial cancer and 297 controls were interviewed to obtain information regarding possible risk factors for endometrial cancer. The risk factors included demographics; pregnancy, menstrual history, contraceptive and exogenous hormone use, family cancer, and medical events; body weight changes; diet and alcohol intake; and recreational and nonrecreational physical activity.

Results.—After adjustment for age, study area, level of education, parity, cigarette smoking, oral contraceptive and menopausal estrogen use, women who rarely or never engaged in housecleaning, stair-climbing, walks or hikes, active sports, or in walking or standing on the job had increased risk for endometrial cancer. Adjustment for body mass diminished the association between risk and walks or hikes and active sports. Adjusted risk was twofold higher in recreationally and nonrecreationally inactive women than in their active counterparts (table). However, when

Relation Between Recent Physical Activity and Risk of Endometrial Cancer

Measure	Cases	Controls	Adjusted * RR	Adjusted * † RR (95% CL)
Recreational activity				
Active	83	73	1.0	1.0 ‡
Average	148	122	1.2	1.0 (0.6–1.5)
Inactive	167	102	1.9	1.2 (0.7–2.0)
Unknown	7	0		
Nonrecreational activity				
Active	83	98	1.0	1.0 §
Average	126	110	1.3	1.2 (0.8–2.0)
Inactive	190	89	2.2	2.0 (1.2–3.1)
Unknown	6	0		

* Adjusted for age, study area, education, parity, years of use of oral contraceptives, years of use of menopausal estrogens, and cigarette smoking.
† Adjusted for current body mass.
‡ Adjusted for nonrecreational activity.
§ Adjusted for recreational activity.
(Courtesy of Sturgeon SR, Brinton LA, Berman ML, et al: *Br J Cancer* 68:584–589, 1993.)

adjusted for body mass index and nonrecreational activity, the association in the recreationally inactive women decreased to 1.2. The 2.2 relative risk for nonrecreational inactive women did not change appreciably when adjusted for body mass and recreational activity. Lifelong recreationally inactive women with a body mass of 25 kg/m^{-2} or more were at risk for endometrial cancer, whereas lifelong nonrecreationally inactive women in every body mass category were at risk.

Conclusion.—Risk for endometrial cancer may be higher in inactive women because they tend to be overweight or obese. Physical inactivity per se may increase endometrial cancer risk, but additional studies with more data relative to the type, intensity, and duration of activity are required to establish this relationship.

▶ Although it is intriguing to speculate that physical activity per se may be responsible for decreasing a woman's risk for endometrial cancer, the data from this study can only support previous studies that show a relationship between obesity and endometrial cancer risk. In every category of recreational and nonrecreational activity, women with a body mass index greater than 28 are at a higher risk than those with a body mass index less than 25, regardless of lifetime activity. On the other hand, nonrecreational activity appears to have an effect independent of body mass (table).

As the authors point out, confounding factors that were not accounted for in the analysis might have altered the results. It would be premature to suggest that physical activity, either recreational or nonrecreational, plays a role in reducing a woman's risk for endometrial cancer independent of the obesity factor.—B.L. Drinkwater, Ph.D.

Gender Difference in Aerobic Capacity in Adolescents After Cure From Malignant Disease in Childhood
Matthys D, Verhaaren H, Benoit Y, Laureys G, De Naeyer A, Craen M (Univ Hosp, Gent, Belgium)
Acta Paediatr 82:459–462, 1993   139-94-10–36

Background.—The late effects of anthracycline treatment for malignant disorders in childhood include cardiac toxicity, growth retardation, cognitive impairment, early puberty, and excessive weight gain. Female patients appear to be affected more than male patients. This study examined gender differences in aerobic power after cure from malignant disease in childhood.

Method.—Eighteen male patients aged 11–19 years and 17 female patients aged 10–18 years were studied a minimum of 2 years after cessation of therapy. Twelve male and 11 female patients had received comparable doses of anthracyclines during treatment. None of the patients had received mediastinal radiation therapy. Maximal exercise tests were performed on a cycle ergometer.

Findings.—The female patients who had been treated for malignant disease in childhood had a lower aerobic power than their controls, but

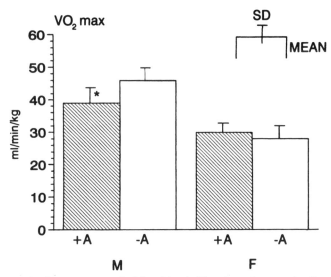

Fig 10–8.—Aerobic capacity in male (M) and female (F) patients after cure of malignant disease in childhood: anthracycline (+A)-treated group vs. nonanthracycline (−A)-treated group. *Abbreviations:* $\dot{V}o_{2max}$, maximal oxygen consumption; *SD*, standard deviation. *$^*P$ < .001. (unpaired *t*-test). (Courtesy of Matthys D, Verhaaren H, Benoit Y, et al: *Acta Paediatr* 82:459–462, 1993.)

the male patients who had been treated did not (Fig 10-8). The gender difference could not be attributed to radiation therapy because none of the subjects had received mediastinal irradiation. Two causes were postulated: female patients were relatively smaller than their controls, possibly because of a higher vulnerability to cranial irradiation than is seen in boys. The smaller height of the female patients with an equal body mass meant a relative obesity that resulted in a lower aerobic power. Secondly, the female patients were less involved in sports than the male patients when compared with their controls.

Conclusion.—After cure of childhood malignant disease, female patients had a lower level of aerobic fitness than male patients when compared with their controls. The smaller height of the female patients and the more sedentary lifestyle may explain the gender difference apparent at maximal exercise. In planning therapy for malignant disease this gender difference should be considered. Both male and female patients should be encouraged to participate in regular physical activity after treatment.

▶ There have been relatively few studies of exercise rehabilitation after the successful treatment of neoplasms. Immediate therapy with agents such as anthracyclines often causes a long-lasting and severe debility. Signs of impaired cardiac performance may persist for 5–10 years (1, 2), and there is considerable scope for an appropriately designed training program. The prescribed exercise must take due account of the patient's initial condition, and it is important to avoid overtraining, which can depress natural killer cell function and thus predispose to a recurrence of the tumor. There is often a need to overcome parental fears and encourage greater activity in both boys and girls (3). The gender difference in loss of function seen in this study is probably more cultural than biological in origin. Parents are more willing to accept that a girl is no longer able to participate in sports and games than would be the case for a boy.—R.J. Shephard, M.D., Ph.D.

References

1. Steinherz LJ, Steinherz P: *Am J Cardiol* 62:205, 1988.
2. Goorin AM, et al: *J Pediatr* 116:144, 1990.
3. Calzaolari A, et al: Longitudinal physical evaluation of off-therapy leukemic children, in: *Children and Exercise.* Pediatric Work Physiology XV. Budapest, Hungary: National Institute for Health Promotion, 1991, pp 49–51.

Supervised Exercise Training Improves Cardiopulmonary Fitness in HIV-Infected Persons
MacArthur RD, Levine SD, Birk TJ (Med College of Ohio, Toledo)
Med Sci Sports Exerc 25:684–688, 1993   139-94-10-37

Introduction.—Many HIV-infected individuals have significant muscle wasting and fatigue in the later stage of illness. In a recent report, progressive resistance exercise was found to improve muscle function in a group of patients with AIDS. The potential benefits of supervised exercise training were assessed in individuals who were moderately to severely immunocompromised by HIV infection.

Subjects and Methods.—The participants, 24 men and 1 woman, were invited to participate in a 24-week exercise study and assigned to either a low-intensity or high-intensity training group. To keep energy expenditures approximately equal and avoid possible orthopedic problems, interval training was used for both groups. The low-intensity group started at four 10-minute work intervals at 50% to 60% of maximal oxygen consumption, and the high-intensity group started at six 4-minute work intervals at 75% to 85% of maximal oxygen consumption. A submaximal evaluation was scheduled for all participants at 12 and 24 weeks.

Results.—Only 6 participants attended more than 80% of the planned sessions. These patients had evidence of a significant training effect, with a 24% improvement in maximal oxygen intake. Minute ventilation increased 13% in these patients and oxygen pulse increased 24%. The mean baseline score on the General Health Questionnaire for all 25 subjects was 5.7. High scores correlated with low CD4 counts but did not predict the degree of compliance with the exercise program. Seventeen participants—including the 6 who were compliant, 5 who were somewhat compliant, and 6 who were noncompliant—had blood drawn for lymphocyte subset analysis at 12 weeks. There were no significant changes in mean CD4 count or mean CD4% between baseline and 12 weeks. Values also remained unchanged from 12 to 24 weeks in the 8 subjects (6 compliant, 2 noncompliant) who were available for subset analysis at 24 weeks. Because so few participants completed the program, low- and high-intensity regimens could not be compared.

Conclusion.—Although the dropout rate was disappointingly high, HIV-infected patients who completed the exercise program did show improvements in cardiopulmonary fitness. Exercise training can benefit some individuals who are moderately to severely immunocompromised by HIV infection. There were no adverse hematologic or immunologic effects, and CD4 counts remained stable or were nonsignificantly improved.

▶ In some large North American cities, HIV infections now affect as much as 1% of the population, including both homosexual and heterosexual individuals. Physiologic measures to improve the quality of life have major attractions relative to very costly and rather ineffective medication. Muscle wasting normally leads to severe fatigue in later stages of the disease, and there have been suggestions that muscle function can be sustained or even improved by progressive resistance exercise (1). The danger of such training is that it may impair the function of an already weakened immune system, and therefore the dose of exercise must be titrated with care. However, as this paper demonstrates, it is possible to improve function (and associated psychological responses) without evidence of any adverse change in T-helper (CD4+) counts.—R.J. Shephard, M.D., Ph.D.

Reference

1. Spence DW, et al: *Arch Phys Med Rehab* 71:644, 1990.

Physical Fitness Training in Patients With Fibromyalgia
Mengshoel AM, Førre Ø (Oslo Sanitetsforening Rheumatism Hosp, Norway)
J Musculoskel Pain 1:267–272, 1993   139-94-10-38

Purpose.—Whether patients with fibromyalgia, a chronic pain syndrome, can perform low-intensity dynamic endurance training without increased pain and fatigue was determined.

Study Design.—Women with fibromyalgia were randomly assigned to participate in the training group (11 subjects) or the control group (14 subjects) (table). The training consisted of low-impact aerobic dance twice per week. Pain was monitored at 0, 10, and 20 weeks by using the McGill Pain Questionnaire.

Results.—There were no significant changes in either pain or fatigue ratings during the 20-week period for the training group. There were no significant differences between the 2 groups at any point.

Patient Characteristics

	Training group (N = 11)		Control group (N = 14)	
	Median (range)	Percent	Median (range)	Percent
Age (yrs)	30 (21-42)		34.5 (25-37)	
Duration of symptoms (yrs)	9 (4-20)		9 (3-21)	
Number of tenderpoints	16 (11-18)		16 (11-18)	
Pain during last week (mm VAS)*	51 (4-78)		59 (33-85)	
Fatigue during last week (mm VAS)*	67 (32-93)		69.5 (33-93)	
Sleep during last week (mm VAS)*	60 (2-90)		51.5 (0-100)	
Full or partly employment (%)		54.5		36.4
Weekly exercising >30min causing sweating (%)		27.3		35.7

* Measured on a 100-mm visual analogue scale (VAS).
(Courtesy of Mengshoel AM, Førre Ø: *J Musculoskel Pain* 1:267–272, 1993.)

Conclusion.—The results of this small study suggest that patients with fibromyalgia can participate in low-intensity endurance training without an exacerbation of symptoms.

▶ A common reaction to rheumatic pain in an older patient is a decrease of physical activity, leading to a vicious cycle of immobilization and functional loss. This small study suggests that fibromyalgia is not worsened by exercise. The observations merit repetition on a larger sample.—R.J. Shephard, M.D., Ph.D.

Exercise Performance and Fatiguability in Patients With Chronic Fatigue Syndrome

Gibson H, Carroll N, Clague JE, Edwards RHT (Univ of Liverpool, England)
J Neurol Neurosurg Psychiatry 56:993–998, 1993   139-94-10–39

Objectives.—Twelve patients given a diagnosis of chronic fatigue syndrome (CFS) were evaluated to learn whether delayed recovery of peripheral muscle function after exercise contributes to the fatigue experi-

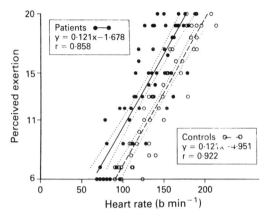

Fig 10–9.—Relationship between perceived exertion and heart rate during incremental exercise. A parallel shift in slope to the left is seen for the patient group demonstrating a change in threshold for greater perception of effort compared with the control subjects. Data pooled, regression lines, and 95% confidence intervals shown for in each group (no. = 12). (Courtesy of Gibson H, Carroll N, Clague JE, et al: *J Neurol Neurosurg Psychiatry* 56:993–998, 1993.)

enced by these patients. Another goal was to determine whether perceptions of effort limit exercise performance in patients with CFS.

Study Plan.—The patients with CFS, 6 men and 6 women aged 17–47 years, were compared with 12 sex- and age-matched sedentary control subjects. Incremental, symptom-limited exercise was carried out on a cycle ergometer. The contractile function of the quadriceps muscle was examined by percutaneous electrical stimulation and maximum isometric voluntary contraction for up to 48 hours after exercise. The 20:50 Hz tetanic force ratio and maximum relaxation rate also were determined.

Results.—At baseline, all the patients with CFS were able to achieve maximum force production when verbally encouraged. All exercised to their subjective maximum exercise capacity. Exercise times varied widely in both the patient and control groups, with no significant difference between groups. There also was a significant difference in blood lactate levels 5 minutes after exercise. The increase in perceived effort with heart rate during exercise was similar in patients with CFS and control subjects, but the threshold for perceiving effort was reduced in the patient group once exercise had commenced. (Fig 10–9). Parameters of muscle physiology were normal in the patients with CFS both before and after exercise.

Conclusion.—Muscle contractility and recovery from exercise appear to be normal in patients with CFS. They do not exercise to full functional capacity, however, and tend to perceive greater effort. Patients with CFS should know that they can participate in a graduated exercise program without risk of damaging their muscles.

▶ Argument continues over the etiology of CFS. I can recall one graduate student who developed such a syndrome apparently as a reaction to the news that her thesis was unacceptable! Her symptoms continued for several years. Some people, including her physician, have attributed the syndrome to the Epstein-Barr virus. However, even if the prevalence of the virus is increased in patients affected by chronic fatigue (and this assertion is hotly debated), viral proliferation could be a secondary manifestation of stress and impaired immune function. This article deals with CFS as it affects ordinary patients rather than high-level athletes who have been overtrained or have failed to achieve their competitive goals. It shows that in affected patients, the rating of perceived exertion on the Borg scale is 3–4 units higher than normal for a given heart rate. However, there is no essential difference in muscle physiology or the rate of muscle recovery after sustained exertion. The primary basis of CFS in general practice is thus a lack of central neural drive rather than peripheral muscular weakness, although a lack of exercise can undoubtedly have secondary consequences for peripheral muscle function. There seems to be good evidence allowing doctors to assure their patients that it is safe for them to exercise and that they will not strain their muscles doing so.—R.J. Shephard, M.D., Ph.D.

Subject Index*

A

A-angle
  in patellar alignment measurement, efficacy, 93: 106
Abdomen
  acute, after trauma, 93: 240
  injuries, 94: 27
  muscle training in sport, 94: 252
  trauma, occult injury may be life threatening, 94: 47
Absenteeism
  due to illness and injury in manufacturing companies, and exercise, 94: 367
Abuse
  androgenic anabolic steroids, and platelet aggregation in weight lifters, 93: 386
  of drugs, 94: 319
  of growth hormone during adolescence, 94: 348
Accelerometer
  measurements of shoe during walking, cushioning properties, 93: 28
Accidents
  ski, severity of, alcohol and benzodiazepines in, 93: 385
Acetazolamide
  for mountain sickness, acute, 93: 414
  in ventilatory response to high altitude hypoxia, 93: 413
Achilles tendon
  allograft reconstruction of anterior cruciate ligament deficient knee, 94: 134
  pain
    peritendinitis causing, 93: 92
    steroids and outcome, 93: 91
  repair, functional postoperative treatment, 93: 92
  rupture
    early controlled motion after surgical repair, 93: 93
    operative repair, early mobilization after, 94: 168
    operative vs. nonoperative treatment, 94: 167
Achillis, tendo (see Achilles tendon)
ACOG guidelines
  for exercise during pregnancy, and pregnancy outcome, 94: 280
Acromioclavicular
  dislocation, third-degree, strength testing after, 93: 38
  joint, arthroscopic resection of, 93: 42

Adolescence
  anabolic steroid use in, 93: 389
  anterior cruciate ligament tears during, 93: 135
  athletes, bronchospasm of, unrecognized exercise-induced, 93: 271
  ballet dancers as model of female athlete, menstrual cycle and exercise, 93: 322
  body image and attitudes toward anabolic steroid use during, 93: 390
  bone mineral density during, diet, hormonal and metabolic factors in, in amenorrhea and eumenorrhea in female runners, 93: 320
  gender difference in aerobic capacity after cancer cure in childhood, 94: 479
  girls during, calcium supplement and bone mineral density in, 94: 268
  growth hormone abuse during, 94: 348
  hypertension during, exercising non-pharmacologic control, 93: 252
  multiple drugs with anabolic steroid use during, 94: 346
  strength training during, weighing the risks, 94: 290
Adrenaline
  levels in serial squash matches, 93: 249
βAdrenergic
  receptor properties, myocardial, influence of exercise and age on, 93: 366
$β_2$-Adrenoceptor agonist
  salbutamol increasing skeletal muscle strength in young men, 93: 292
Aerobic
  capacity
    failure to attain peak, during bicycle exercise in congestive heart failure, 93: 264
    gender difference during adolescence after cancer cure in childhood, 94: 479
    in peripheral vascular disease, 93: 445
    in rheumatoid arthritis, 93: 436
  exercise
    cerebral performance indices during, in older adults, 93: 235
    and thermoregulation during pregnancy, 94: 285
    fitness, maternal, in cardiorespiratory responses to exercise, 94: 282

---

* All entries refer to the year and page number(s) for data appearing in this and the previous edition of the YEAR BOOK.

487

M

improving slowly after anterior
cruciate ligament reconstruction,
93: 164
of rotator muscles in professional
baseball pitchers, 93: 196
shoe for lower leg strength and
flexibility development, 94: 178
of shoulder external rotation and
abduction, isokinetic and isometric
measurement of, 93: 195
suture anchor failure strength, 94: 63
testing after acromioclavicular
dislocation, third-degree, 93: 38
training
of immature athlete, overview,
94: 251
muscle soreness during, prevention,
93: 206
weighing the risks during childhood
and adolescence, 94: 290
trunk muscle, and leisure time physical
activity in 15 year old school
children, 94: 289
Strengthening
of scapular muscles, four exercises for,
93: 41
Streptokinase
for acute myocardial infarction, 93: 252
Stress
fracture
femoral neck, negative bone scan in,
93: 430
femoral neck in long distance runner,
biomechanics, 94: 97
malleolar, medial, clinical and imaging
features, 93: 97
navicular, management outcome in
athletes, CT in, 93: 98
olecranon, in throwing, 93: 71
(See also Fracture, stress)
glenohumeral joint, fluoroscopic
evaluation in anterior shoulder
instability, 93: 54
thermoregulatory, during exercise in
heat in spinal cord injury, 93: 438
Stretch
low-load prolonged, thermal agents in
effectiveness of, 93: 205
shortening drills for upper extremities,
theory and clinical application,
94: 78
to stretch or not to stretch, warm-up
procedure, 94: 254
Stretching
method, effect on hamstring muscle
flexibility, 93: 83
Stroke
lifelong exercise and, 94: 462

modification relieving tennis elbow,
93: 70
Student
high school, sports participation, age at
smoking initiation and risk of
smoking of, 94: 349
junior high school, anabolic androgenic
steroid use, 94: 348
Stumble
recovery from, kinematics of, 94: 293
Subacromial
arthroscopic decompression
clinical review, 93: 49
technique, 93: 47
Subdural
hematoma, acute, and second impact
syndrome, 93: 32
Subscapularis
electromyography of, intramuscular
wire, 93: 183
Sudden death
prevention
by automated defibrillators, 94: 420
by cardiovascular screening in young
athletes, 93: 241
during snow shoveling, 93: 244
Suprascapular
nerve
entrapment, MRI of, 93: 51
syndrome, MRI of, 94: 47
Supraspinatus
tendon deep surface impingement on
posterosuperior glenoid rim,
arthroscopy of, 93: 61
Surfing
body surfing accidents resulting in
cervical spine injuries, 93: 34
Surveys of physical activity (see Physical
activity, surveys)
Suture
anchor
failure strength, 94: 63
pull-out strength of, 94: 65
pull-out strength of, in rotator cuff
and Bankart lesion repairs, 94: 65
Bankart suture repair, arthroscopic,
94: 62
methods for flexor tendon repair,
biomechanical analysis, 94: 93
technique in arthroscopic Bankart
procedure, indications, technique
and results, 93: 56
Swelling
arm, painless, in high school football
player, 93: 300
Swimmers
bathers in polluted seawater, morbidity
in, 93: 448

X

Y

Author Index

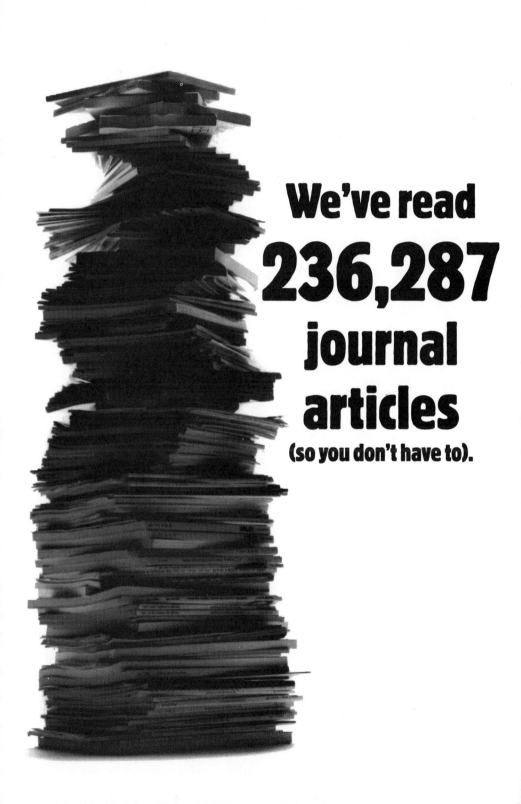

We've read
236,287
journal
articles
(so you don't have to).

The Year Books–
The best from 236,287 journal articles.

At Mosby, we subscribe to more than 950 medical and allied health journals from every corner of the globe. We read them all, tirelessly scanning for anything that relates to your field.

We send everything we find related to a given specialty to the distinguished editors of the **Year Book** in that area, and they pick out *the best*, the articles they feel *every practitioner in that specialty should be aware of.*

For the **1994 Year Books** we surveyed a total of 236,287 articles and found hundreds of articles related to your field. Our expert editors reviewed these and chose the developments you don't want to miss.

The best articles–condensed, organized, and with personal commentary.

Not only do you get the past year's most important articles in your field, you get them in a format that makes them easy to use.

Every article that the editors pick is condensed into a concise, outlined abstract, a summary of the article's most important points highlighted with bold paragraph headings. So you can quickly scan for exactly what you need.

In addition to identifying the year's best articles, the editors write concise commentaries following each article, telling whether or not the study in question is a reliable one, whether a new technique is effective, or whether a particular trend you've head about merits your immediate attention.

No other abstracting service offers this expert advice to help you decide how the year's advances will affect the way you practice.

With a special added benefit for Year Book subscribers.

In 1994, your **Year Book** subscription includes a new added benefit. Access to **MOSBY Document Express**, a rapid-response information retrieval service that puts copies of original source documents in your hands, in a little as a few hours.

With **MOSBY Document Express**, you have convenient, *around-the-clock-access to literally every article* upon which **Year Book** summaries are based. What's more, you can also order journal articles cited in references—or for that matter, virtually any medical or scientific article that can be located. Plus, at your direction, we will deliver the article(s) by FAX, overnight delivery service, or regular mail.

This new added benefit is just one of the enhanced services that makes your **Year Book** subscription an even better value—it's your key to the full breadth of health sciences information. For more details, see **MOSBY Document Express** instructions at the beginning of this book.